CHAPMAN & NAKIELNY'S

AIDS TO RADIOLOGICAL DIFFERENTIAL DIAGNOSIS

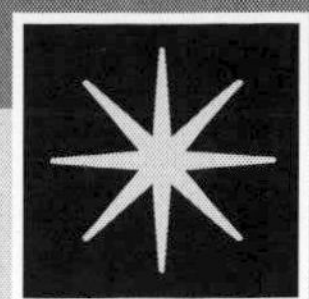

CHAPMAN & NAKIELNY'S

AIDS TO RADIOLOGICAL DIFFERENTIAL DIAGNOSIS

Edited by

Hameed Rafiee, MBBS FRCR
Consultant Radiologist and Training Programme Director,
Norfolk and Norwich University Hospitals,
Norwich, UK

SEVENTH EDITION

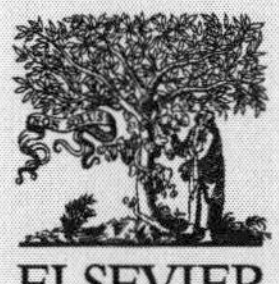

Edinburgh London New York Oxford Philadelphia St Louis Sydney 2020

First edition 1984
Second edition 1990
Third edition 1995
Fourth edition 2003
Fifth edition 2009
Sixth edition 2014
Seventh edition 2020

Notices

Practitioners and researchers must always rely on their own experience and knowledge in evaluating and using any information, methods, compounds or experiments described herein. Because of rapid advances in the medical sciences, in particular, independent verification of diagnoses and drug dosages should be made. To the fullest extent of the law, no responsibility is assumed by Elsevier, authors, editors or contributors for any injury and/or damage to persons or property as a matter of products liability, negligence or otherwise, or from any use or operation of any methods, products, instructions, or ideas contained in the material herein.

ISBN: 978-0-7020-7539-1

Content Strategist: Laurence Hunter
Content Development Specialist: Helen Leng
Project Manager: Louisa Talbott
Design: Brian Salisbury
Illustration Manager: Muthukumaran Thangaraj
Illustrator: MPS North America LLC
Marketing Manager: Deborah Watkins

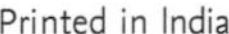

Printed in India

Last digit is the print number: 9 8

Contents

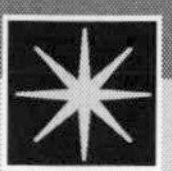

Preface and explanatory notes

I am very fortunate to find myself in the position of editing this well-loved core radiology text, and at the same time very anxious to do the book justice to maintain its reputation. Radiology has expanded rapidly in recent years, and as such this 7th edition is the biggest revision this book has had in its long history. Nearly every section in every chapter has undergone major changes, with the addition of a new Nuclear Medicine chapter to reflect its importance in modern medical imaging. Part 2 has been restructured to focus on multisystem disorders which cannot be fully covered in individual chapters—many of these are a favourite of the long cases in the FRCR Part 2B exam. Where these multisystem disorders are listed as differentials in the various chapters of Part 1, they are denoted by an asterisk (*) to enable the reader to check Part 2 for the imaging features of the disease in other organ systems.

Important discriminating features have been added to nearly every differential to aid the reader in developing a strategy for reaching a diagnosis. Diagnoses are still listed in the approximate order of commonness, but note that this order is less clear-cut for rarer diagnoses due to less reliable epidemiological data. Also, the presence or absence of discriminating features has significant impact on the relative likelihood of the differentials. In view of this, and the large variability of data in the literature, I have reduced the amount of 'percentages' in this book. These are far less important than learning the discriminating features. Finally, the top differentials in each list which are considered most important for radiology trainees to learn are underlined. The number of diagnoses underlined varies from list to list—some of the more important lists have all of their differentials underlined, whereas other lists which are aimed at specialists may have no underlined differentials at all.

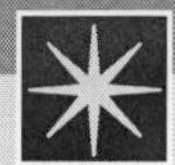

List of Contributors

In addition to those listed, the editors would like to acknowledge and offer grateful thanks for the input of all previous editions' contributors, without whom this new edition would not have been possible.

Syed Babar Ajaz MBBS MCPS FCPS DMRD FRCR
Consultant Radiologist and Honorary Senior Lecturer, Imperial College Healthcare NHS Trust, London, UK

Hifz-ur-Rahman Aniq MBBS FRCR
Consultant Radiologist, Royal Liverpool University Hospital; Honorary Lecturer, University of Liverpool, UK

Clare Beadsmoore MBBS MRCP FRCR
Consultant Radiologist and Radionuclide Radiologist, Norfolk & Norwich University Hospital, Norwich, UK

Nishat Bharwani BSc(Hons) MBBS(Hons) MRCP FRCR
Clinical Radiologist and Training Programme Director, Imperial College Healthcare NHS Trust, London, UK; Honorary Clinical Senior Lecturer, Imperial College London, London, UK

Elena Boyd MBBS FRCR
Consultant Radiologist, Wexham Park Hospital, Frimley NHS Trust, Wexham, UK

Sajid Butt MBBS FCPS FRCR
Consultant Radiologist, Royal National Orthopaedic Hospital NHS Trust, London, UK

Erika Denton MBBS FRCP FRCR DSc
Medical Director and Honorary Professor of Radiology, Norfolk & Norwich University Hospitals, Norwich, UK; National Advisor for Imaging, NHS Improvement

Luke Dixon BSc(Hons) MBBS MRCS FRCR
Neuroradiology Fellow, Charing Cross Hospital, Imperial College NHS Trust, London, UK

Swamy Gedela FRCR MBBS
Consultant Cardiothoracic Radiologist; Cardiac MRI Unit Director; Cardiothoracic Imaging Lead, Essex Cardiothoracic Centre, Basildon University Hospital, Basildon, UK

Chris J Harvey BSc(Hons) MBBS MRCP FRCR
Consultant Radiologist and Honorary Senior Lecturer, Imperial College Healthcare NHS Trust, Hammersmith Hospital, London, UK

Chandrashekar Hoskote MBBS DMRD MD DM(Neuro) FRCR
Specialty Doctor, The National Hospital for Neurology and Neurosurgery, London, UK

Nabil Hujairi MD FRCR
Consultant Radiologist and Nuclear Medicine Physician, Royal Marsden Hospital, London, UK

Arne Juette FRCR
Consultant Radiologist and Director of Breast Screening, Norfolk & Norwich University Hospital, Norwich, UK

Musa Kaleem MBBS MRCPCH FRCR
Consultant Paediatric Radiologist, Alder Hey Children's Hospital NHS Foundation Trust, Liverpool, UK

Sami Khan MBBS MCPS FCPS FRCR
Consultant Radiologist, Basildon and Thurrock University Hospitals NHS Foundation Trust; Associate Lecturer, Anglia Ruskin University, Chelmsford, UK; Honorary Clinical Senior Lecturer, University College London, UK

Joseph Lansley BSc MBBS FRCR EDiNR
Consultant Neuroradiologist, Barts Health NHS Trust, London, UK

James MacKay MA MB BChir MRCP FRCR
Radiology Registrar, Norfolk & Norwich University Hospital, Norwich, UK

Qaiser Malik BSc(Hons) MBBS MRCP FRCR
Clinical Director Radiology, Basildon and Thurrock University Hospital NHS Trust; Honorary Senior Clinical Lecturer, University College London, London, UK

Simon Morley MA BM BCh MRCP FRCR
Consultant Radiologist, University College Hospital, London, UK

Andrew Plumb BA BMBCh MRCP FRCR PhD
Associate Professor of Medical Imaging, University College London; Consultant Radiologist, University College London Hospitals, London, UK

Jeremy Rabouhans BSc(Hons) MBBS(Hons) MRCS FRCR
Consultant Interventional Radiologist, Basildon and Thurrock University Hospitals NHS Foundation Trust, Basildon, UK

Hameed Rafiee BSc(Hons) MBBS FRCR
Consultant Radiologist and Training Programme Director, Norfolk & Norwich University Hospital, Norwich, UK

Alessandro Ruggiero MD PhD
Consultant Cardiothoracic Radiologist, Royal Papworth Hospital, Cambridge, UK

Janak Saada MBBS BSc MRCP FRCR
Consultant Radiologist, Norfolk & Norwich University Hospital, Norwich, UK

Thomas Semple BSC(Hons) MBBS FRCR
Consultant Paediatric and Adult Cardiothoracic Radiologist, The Royal Brompton Hospital, London, UK

Susan Shelmerdine BSc(Hons) MBBS PGCertHBE FHEA MRCS FRCR
Paediatric Radiology Research Fellow, Great Ormond Street Hospital for Children NHS Foundation Trust, London, UK

Victoria Stewart BMed Sci BMBS MRCP FRCR
Consultant Radiologist, Imperial College Healthcare NHS Trust, London, UK

Imran Syed MBBS BSc(Hons) FRCP FRCPEd FRCR
Consultant Interventional Radiologist, Basildon and Thurrock University Hospitals NHS Foundation Trust, Basildon, UK

Stuart Taylor BSc MBBS MD MRCP FRCR
Consultant Radiologist and Professor of Medical Imaging, University College Hospital, London, UK

Andoni Toms PhD FRCR
Consultant Radiologist and Honorary Professor, Norfolk & Norwich University Hospital, Norwich, UK

Bhavin Upadhyay BSc(Hons) MBBS MRCS FRCR
Consultant Musculoskeletal Radiologist, Royal National Orthopaedic Hospital NHS Trust, London, UK

Neil Upadhyay BSc(Hons) MBBS MRes MEd FRCR
Consultant Radiologist and Honorary Senior Lecturer, Imperial College Healthcare NHS Trust, London, UK

Patrick Wong MBBS FRANZCR
Radiology Fellow, Royal Brompton Hospital, London, UK

Acknowledgements

This project has been a monumental task, and would not have been possible without the expertise of the 32 contributors who have worked on this with me. Special thanks go to Sami Khan for his additional invaluable assistance in the planning stage of the project and for helping me find contributors for various chapters, as well as Stuart Taylor and the publishing team at Elsevier for giving me the opportunity to take on this project in the first place. A huge thank you also goes to my fantastic colleagues at Norfolk & Norwich University Hospital, many of whom have contributed to this edition. The culture of excellent radiology education and support in our department makes it a wonderful place to train and work, and has quite literally made me the radiologist I am today. For this reason I am donating 50% of my royalties to the Norwich Radiology Academy Charitable Fund, to help train and support current and future radiology trainees at the Academy.

Lastly, and most importantly of all, I cannot thank my family enough for all of the support they've shown me throughout this project – my delightful daughters Elika and Suri, for being my raison d'être and for tolerating a part-time father; my wonderful wife Hoda, for being my rock and for tolerating a part-time husband whilst raising a newborn and a toddler; Hoda's amazing family, for supporting her whilst I was preoccupied; my parents Abdi & Sima, for being the best parents I could wish for and inspiring me to become a teacher and author; and my incredible brother Siam, for whom I am donating the other 50% of my royalties to the charity PSC Support.

Abbreviations

99mTc-DMSA	Technetium-99m-2,3-dimercaptosuccinic acid
αFP	Alpha-fetoprotein
AAA	Abdominal aortic aneurysm
ABC	Aneurysmal bone cyst
ABPA	Allergic bronchopulmonary aspergillosis
ACE	Angiotensin-converting enzyme
ACTH	Adrenocorticotropic hormone
AD	Autosomal dominant
ADC	Apparent diffusion coefficient
ADPKD	Autosomal dominant polycystic kidney disease
AIDS	Acquired immune deficiency syndrome
AKI	Acute kidney injury
AML	Angiomyolipoma
ANCA	Anti-neutrophil cytoplasmic antibody
AP	Anteroposterior
AR	Autosomal recessive
ARDS	Acute respiratory distress syndrome
ARPKD	Autosomal recessive polycystic kidney disease
ARVC	Arrhythmogenic right ventricular cardiomyopathy
ARVD	Arrhythmogenic right ventricular dysplasia
ASD	Atrial septal defect
AV	Atrioventricular
AVM	Arteriovenous malformation
AVN	Avascular necrosis
AVSD	Atrioventricular septal defect
AXR	Abdominal X-ray
BCC	Basal cell carcinoma
BFH	Benign fibrous histiocytoma
BPH	Benign prostatic hyperplasia
CADASIL	Cerebral autosomal dominant arteriopathy with subcortical infarcts and leukoencephalopathy
CBD	Common bile duct
CEA	Carcinoembryonic antigen
CF	Cystic fibrosis

CHD	Common hepatic duct
CJD	Creutzfeldt–Jakob disease
CMC	Carpometacarpal
CMV	Cytomegalovirus
CNS	Central nervous system
COPD	Chronic obstructive pulmonary disease
CPPD	Calcium pyrophosphate deposition disease
CRMO	Chronic recurrent multifocal osteomyelitis
CSF	Cerebrospinal fluid
CT	Computed tomography
CTA	CT angiography
CTPA	Computed tomography pulmonary angiogram
CXR	Chest X-ray
DAI	Diffuse axonal injury
DCIS	Ductal carcinoma in situ
DCM	Dilated cardiomyopathy
DIP	Distal interphalangeal
DISH	Diffuse idiopathic skeletal hyperostosis
DMSA	Dimercaptosuccinic acid
DNET	Dysembryoplastic neuroepithelial tumour
DPM	Ductal plate malformation
DVT	Deep vein thrombosis
DWI	Diffusion-weighted imaging
EBV	Epstein–Barr virus
ELISA	Enzyme-linked immunosorbent assay
EPI	Echo-planar imaging
ESR	Erythrocyte sedimentation rate
FAP	Familial adenomatous polyposis
FDG	Fluorodeoxyglucose
FIGO	International Federation of Gynecology and Obstetrics
FLAIR	Fluid-attenuated inversion recovery
FMD	Fibromuscular dysplasia
FNA	Fine needle aspiration
FNH	Focal nodular hyperplasia
GB	Gall bladder
GCSF	Granulocyte-colony stimulating factor
GCT	Giant cell tumour
GGO	Ground-glass opacification
GI	Gastrointestinal
GIST	Gastrointestinal stromal tumour

HAART	Highly active antiretroviral therapy
HCC	Hepatocellular carcinoma
hCG	Human chorionic gonadotropin
HCM	Hypertrophic cardiomyopathy
HHT	Hereditary haemorrhagic telangiectasia
HIDA	Hepatobiliary iminodiacetic acid
HIV	Human immunodeficiency virus
HOA	Hypertrophic osteoarthropathy
HPB	Hepatic pancreatic biliary
HPV	Human papillomavirus
HRCT	High-resolution computed tomography
HSP	Henoch-Schönlein purpura
HSV	Herpes simplex virus
HU	Hounsfield units
HUS	Haemolytic uremic syndrome
IBD	Inflammatory bowel disease
IHD	Ischaemic heart disease
IPF	Idiopathic pulmonary fibrosis
IPMN	Intraductal papillary mucinous neoplasm
IUD	Intrauterine device
IV	Intravenous
IVC	Inferior vena cava
IVF	In vitro fertilization
IVU	Intravenous urogram
LAM	Lymphangioleiomyomatosis
LBO	Large bowel obstruction
LCH	Langerhans cell histiocytosis
LGE	Late gadolinium enhancement
LIP	Lymphoid interstitial pneumonia
LV	Left ventricle
LVF	Left ventricular failure
MAC	*Mycobacterium avium* complex
MALT	Mucosa-associated lymphoid tissue
MCA	Middle cerebral artery
MCP	Metacarpophalangeal joint
MEN	Multiple endocrine neoplasia
MI	Myocardial infarction
MIBG	Meta-iodo-benzyl-guanidine
MPA	Main pulmonary artery
MPNST	Malignant peripheral nerve sheath tumour

MR	Magnetic resonance
MRA	MR angiography
MRCP	Magnetic resonance cholangiopancreatography
MRI	Magnetic resonance imaging
MS	Multiple sclerosis
MTPJ	Metatarsophalangeal joint
NAI	Nonaccidental injury
NEC	Necrotizing enterocolitis
NET	Neuroendocrine tumour
NF	Neurofibromatosis
NHL	Non-Hodgkin lymphoma
NICE	National Institute for Health and Clinical Excellence
NM	Nuclear medicine
NMO	Neuromyelitis optica
NOF	Nonossifying fibroma
NRH	Nodular regenerative hyperplasia
NSAID	Nonsteroidal antiinflammatory drug
NSIP	Nonspecific interstitial pneumonia
OCP	Oral contraceptive pill
OPG	Orthopantomogram
PA	Posteroanterior
PAN	Polyarteritis nodosa
PAS	Periodic acid–Schiff (stain)
PBC	Primary biliary cholangitis
PCP	*Pneumocystis carinii* pneumonia
PD	Pancreatic duct
PDA	Patent ductus arteriosus
PE	Pulmonary embolism
PEEP	Positive end-expiratory pressure
PET	Positron emission tomography
PID	Pelvic inflammatory disease
PIP	Proximal interphalangeal
PKD	Polycystic kidney disease
PMF	Progressive massive fibrosis
PNET	Primitive neuroectodermal tumour
POEMS	Polyneuropathy, organomegaly, endocrinopathy, monoclonal gammopathy, skin changes
PRES	Posterior reversible encephalopathy syndrome
PSC	Primary sclerosing cholangitis
PSV	Peak systolic velocity

PTLD	Posttransplant lymphoproliferative disorder
PUJ	Pelviureteric junction
PV	Portal vein
PVNS	Pigmented villonodular synovitis
RCC	Renal cell carcinoma
RFA	Radiofrequency ablation
RPF	Retroperitoneal fibrosis
RTA	Road traffic accident
RV	Right ventricle
SAH	Subarachnoid haemorrhage
SAM	Segmental arterial mediolysis
SAPHO	Synovitis, acne, pustulosis, hyperostosis, osteitis
SBC	Simple bone cyst
SBO	Small bowel obstruction
SCC	Squamous cell carcinomas
SCD	Sickle cell disease
SDH	Subdural haemorrhage
SIJ	Sacroiliac joint
SLE	Systemic lupus erythematosus
SMA	Superior mesenteric artery
SMV	Superior mesenteric vein
SPECT	Single-photon emission computed tomography
STI	Sexually transmitted infection
STIR	Short tau inversion recovery
SUFE	Slipped upper femoral epiphysis
SVC	Superior vena cava
SWI	Susceptibility weighted imaging
TACE	Transarterial chemoembolization
TAPVD	Total anomalous pulmonary venous drainage
TB	Tuberculosis
TCC	Transitional cell carcinoma
TE	Echo time or time to echo
TFCC	Triangular fibrocartilage complex
TGA	Transposition of the great arteries
TI	Terminal ileum
TORCH	Toxoplasmosis, other infections, rubella, cytomegalovirus, herpes simplex
TURP	Transurethral resection of prostate
UC	Ulcerative colitis
UIP	Usual interstitial pneumonia

URTI	Upper respiratory tract infection
US	Ultrasound
UTI	Urinary tract infection
vHL	von Hippel Lindau
VSD	Ventricular septal defect
VUJ	Vesicoureteric junction
VUR	Vesicoureteric reflux
VZV	Varicella-Zoster virus
XD	X-linked dominant
XGP	Xanthogranulomatous pyelonephritis
XR	X-linked recessive

Part 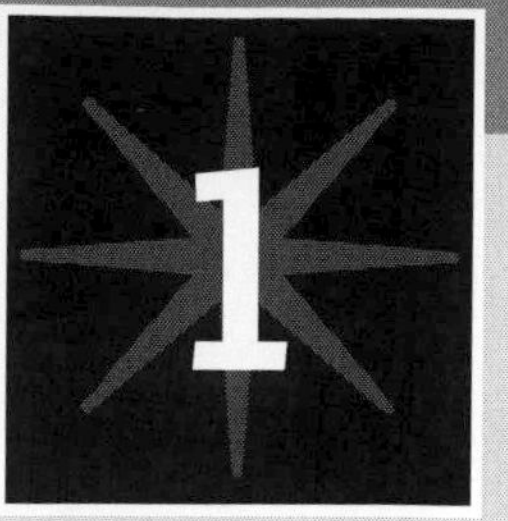

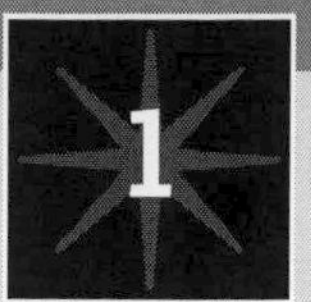

Bones

Bhavin Upadhyay, Sajid Butt, Syed Babar Ajaz, Andoni Toms, James MacKay

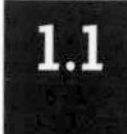

1.1 GENERALIZED INCREASED BONE DENSITY IN AN ADULT

Most common

1. Metastases—prostate and breast most common. Heterogeneous; generally not diffuse.
2. Sickle cell disease—medullary sclerosis and bone infarcts. Growth arrest of long bones. H-shaped vertebrae.
3. Myelofibrosis—older patients. Diffuse medullary sclerosis, loss of corticomedullary differentiation. No heterogeneity.

Less common

4. Renal osteodystrophy—axial > appendicular. Rugger jersey spine.
5. Osteopetrosis—thickened cortices with reduced marrow space. Pathological transverse fractures.
6. Paget's disease—coarse trabeculae and bone expansion. Multiple bones rather than generalized.
7. Systemic mastocytosis—lytic, sclerotic or mixed. Usually diffuse affecting spine and epiphyses of long bones.

Rare

8. Fluorosis—diffuse osteosclerosis, particularly ribs and spine, with entheseal ossification.
9. Pyknodysostosis—narrow medullary cavities with multiple long bone fractures.
10. **Hypoparathyroidism**—diffuse sclerosis in 10%. Dense metaphyseal bands and skull vault thickening.
11. **Progressive diaphyseal dysplasia (Camurati-Engelmann disease)**—young patients. Fusiform enlargement and sclerosis of long bones sparing the epiphyses.
12. **Myeloma**—rare osteosclerosing form. Associated with POEMS syndrome.

1.2 SOLITARY SCLEROTIC BONE LESION

Most common

1. **Bone island (enostosis)**—ovoid with long axis parallel to long axis of bone and a feathered border.
2. **Enchondroma**—confluent punctate or nodular calcification, denser centrally than peripherally. Enchondromas in the large long bones are often more calcified than those in the fingers.
3. **Metastasis**—prostate, breast, mucinous adenocarcinoma of GI tract, carcinoid, lymphoma, TCC in adults. Medulloblastoma and neuroblastoma in children.
4. **Callus**—usually associated with a fusiform swelling in long bones.
5. **Bone infarct**—usually a central metadiaphyseal lucency with thin serpentine calcified margins.

Less common

6. **Paget's disease**—blastic phase causes sclerosis accompanied by bone expansion, and cortical and trabecular thickening.
7. **Osteoma**—arises from membranous bone: skull and paranasal sinuses. Ivory osteomas contain no trabeculae. Mature osteomas have visible marrow. If multiple consider Gardner syndrome.
8. **Osteoid osteoma/osteoblastoma**—sclerosis caused by eccentric periosteal thickening. Osteoid osteoma: radiolucent nidus <2 cm. Osteoblastoma: more common in the posterior elements of spine, larger nidus with thin shell.
9. **Healed or healing bone lesion**—treated metastasis, NOF, simple bone cyst, brown tumour, eosinophilic granuloma.
10. **Primary bone sarcoma**—aggressive features: poorly defined margins, aggressive periosteal reaction, Codman's triangles, bone destruction, soft tissue mass.
11. **Fibrous dysplasia**—usually lytic with ground glass areas but can calcify in later life.
12. **Chronic osteomyelitis**—usually associated with an area of lysis, chronic periosteal reaction and occasionally a sequestrum.
13. **Chronic recurrent multifocal osteomyelitis (CRMO)**—idiopathic inflammatory disorder. Most commonly affects clavicles and tibias in children. Often multifocal.
14. **Lymphoma**—primary bone lymphoma rare. More common as secondary involvement. Large extraosseous soft tissue mass with relative preservation of bone.
15. **Cement and bone graft substitutes**—history of surgery.

1.3 MULTIPLE SCLEROTIC BONE LESIONS

Most common

1. Metastases—prostate, breast, mucinous adenocarcinoma of GI tract, carcinoid, lymphoma, TCC in adults. Medulloblastoma and neuroblastoma in children.
2. Multiple healed bone lesions—lytic metastases following radiotherapy or chemotherapy. Eosinophilic granulomas and brown tumours following treatment.
3. Paget's disease—often polyostotic.

Less common

4. Multiple bone infarcts—consider an underlying disorder, e.g. sickle cell or Gaucher disease.
5. Multiple stress fractures—callus formation around fractures.
6. Lymphoma.
7. Osteopoikilosis—multiple symmetrically distributed bone islands in the metaphyses and epiphyses of long bones and the pelvis. Some ovoid, some round.
8. Multifocal osteosarcoma.
9. Multiple osteomas—Gardner syndrome.
10. Fibrous dysplasia—long lesions in long bones, often hemimelic (McCune-Albright syndrome). Usually lytic but can calcify.
11. CRMO and SAPHO.

Rare

12. Osteopathia striata (Voorhoeve disease)—linear striations along long axis of long bone.
13. Erdheim-Chester disease—bilateral symmetrical metadiaphyseal sclerosis in long bones, most commonly femora and tibias.
14. **Multiple myeloma**—sclerotic in 3%.
15. **Tuberous sclerosis.**
16. **Intramedullary osteosclerosis**—diaphyseal endosteal sclerosis typically involving the tibia or femur, usually bilateral and in women.

1.4 BONE SCLEROSIS WITH A PERIOSTEAL REACTION

Most common

1. **Healing fracture**.
2. **Metastasis**—osteoblastic metastases from prostate.
3. **Osteoid osteoma/osteoblastoma**—solid or lamellated periosteal reaction.
4. **Chronic osteomyelitis**—look for sequestrum.
5. **Osteosarcoma**—classically sunray spiculation.

Less common

6. **Ewing sarcoma**—often onion-skin or lamellated periosteal reaction.
7. **Chondrosarcoma**—chondroid matrix with regions of enchondral ossification.
8. **Lymphoma**.
9. **CRMO**—clavicles and tibias in children and adolescents.
10. **SAPHO syndrome**—similar to CRMO but in adults. Although similar long bone changes may be seen, anterior chest wall and pelvic involvement predominate.
11. **Infantile cortical hyperostosis (Caffey's disease)**—infants <6 months of age. Multiple bones, especially mandible, ribs and clavicles.

Rare

12. **Melorheostosis**—sclerotomal distribution. Cortical and medullary sclerosis likened to dripping candle wax.
13. **Tertiary syphilis**—usually bilateral periostitis involving skull, clavicles, ribs and tibias. Mixed sclerotic and lytic 'gummatous' lesions can also be seen.

1.5 SOLITARY SCLEROTIC BONE LESION WITH A LUCENT CENTRE

Most common

1. Osteoid osteoma/osteoblastoma—lucent nidus.
2. Brodie's abscess.
3. Medullary bone infarct—irregular serpentine outline.
4. Stress fracture—lucent fracture line may be visible.

Less common

5. Looser's zone of osteomalacia.
6. Liposclerosing myxofibrous tumour—characteristic location in the intertrochanteric region of the femur.
7. Tuberculosis.

Rare

8. Syphilis.
9. Yaws.

1.6 COARSE TRABECULAR PATTERN

1. Paget's disease.
2. Osteoporosis.
3. Osteomalacia.
4. Haemoglobinopathies.
5. Haemangioma.
6. Gaucher disease.

1.7 SKELETAL METASTASES

Nearly all malignant tumours can metastasize to bone, but 80% are from prostate, breast, lung or kidney. Mainly involves the axial and proximal appendicular skeleton (red marrow)—distal appendicular bone metastases are rare and usually from lung or, less commonly, breast. Most bone metastases are lytic; sclerotic or mixed metastases have a more limited differential, though treated lytic metastases can become sclerotic. The lists below cover the more common sources.

Lytic

1. Lung.
2. Breast—usually lytic but can be sclerotic or mixed.
3. Myeloma.
4. Nonmucinous adenocarcinomas of the GI tract.
5. Most other primary sources.

Lytic and expansile

1. Renal cell carcinoma.
2. Thyroid.
3. **Hepatocellular carcinoma.**
4. **Melanoma.**
5. **Phaeochromocytoma.**

Sclerotic

1. Prostate.
2. Breast—particularly post treatment.
3. **Carcinoid.**
4. **Mucinous adenocarcinomas of the GI tract.**
5. **Transitional cell carcinoma.**
6. **Small cell lung cancer.**
7. **Lymphoma**—particularly Hodgkin lymphoma; rare.

Mixed

1. Breast.
2. Lung.
3. Lymphoma.
4. **Cervix.**
5. **Testis.**
6. **Transitional cell carcinoma.**
7. **Melanoma.**
8. **Neuroblastoma**—in children.

1.8 SITES OF ORIGIN OF COMMON PRIMARY BONE LESIONS

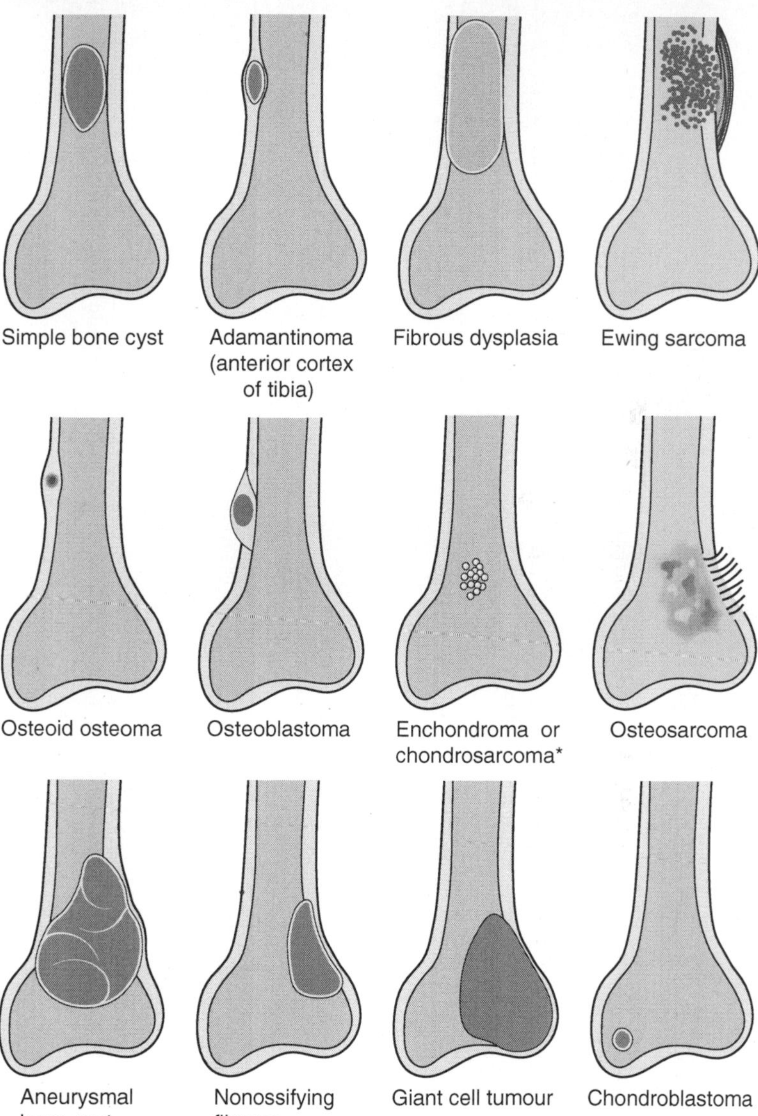

* These two lesions have overlapping imaging features. A larger size and presence of endosteal scalloping would favour chondrosarcoma.

1.9 COMMON FEATURES OF SOLITARY INTRAOSSEOUS LESIONS

	Peak age (years)	Location	Centrality[a]	Density	Margin	Expansile[a]	Periosteal Reaction[b]	Notes
Generally well-defined predominantly lytic lesions								
Simple bone cyst	5–20	Met±Dia	**Central**	**Lucent**	**Well+Scl**	–/+	–	Unilocular. **'Fallen fragment'** if fractured
Aneurysmal bone cyst	5–30	**Met**	Eccentric	**Lucent**	**Well+Scl**	++	–	**Expansile, bubbly**. May occur 2° to another lesion
Giant cell tumour	**20–50**	**Met+Epi**	Eccentric	**Lucent**	Well/ Poor	+	–	**Nonsclerotic margin, often abuts articular surface**
NOF/FCD*	5–25	**Met**	**Cortical**	**Lucent**	**Well+Scl**	–/+	–	NOF >3 cm; FCD <3 cm. Sclerose after healing
Benign fibrous histiocytoma	**25–40**	Met/Dia	Eccentric	Lucent	Well±Scl	–/+	–	Rare; **similar to NOF but in older patients** + any location
Chondromyxoid fibroma	10–30	Met	Eccentric	Lucent	Well±Scl	+	–	Rare; can mimic NOF, ABC and BFH
Osteoid osteoma	10–30	**Dia**/Met	**Cortical**	Lucent± Ost	**Scl**	-	**Solid**	**Lucent nidus <2 cm + surrounding sclerosis**

Osteoblastoma	10–30	Dia/Met	Eccentric	Lucent± Ost	Well±Scl	+	Solid	**Lucent nidus >2 cm; spine>** flat bones>long bones>talus
Chondroblastoma	5–20	**Epi**	Eccentric	**Lucent± Chon**	**Well+Scl**	–	–/Solid	Classically **epiphyseal**; also in apophyses, patella, tarsals
Intraosseous lipoma	>20	Met	Any	Lucent± Scl	Well±Scl	–/+	–	Lucent ± **central sclerosis. Calcaneus**>prox femur>other
Fibrous dysplasia*	>3	**Dia**	**Central**	**Ground glass**	Well±Scl	+	–	Variable density. Commonest in long bones, ribs, skull
LSMFT	>20	Met	Central	**Lucent±** Scl	**Well+Scl**	–/+	–	**Intertrochanteric region of femur**
Adamantinoma	10–35	**Dia**	**Cortical**	**Lucent±** Scl	**Well+Scl**	+	–	**Anterior cortex of tibial diaphysis**
Osteofibrous dysplasia	**<10**	Dia	Cortical	Lucent± Scl	Well±Scl	+	–	**Similar to adamantinoma but in younger age group**
Desmoplastic fibroma	10–50	Met/Dia	Central	Lucent	Well	+	–	Rare. Lytic + **pseudotrabeculations**
Haemophilic pseudotumour	>10	Any	Any	Lucent	Well±Scl	++	–	Male ± **signs of haemophilia** ± pseudotrabeculations
Brown tumour	>40	Any	Any	Lucent	Well	+	–	**Look for other features of hyperparathyroidism**

Continued

	Peak age (years)	Location	Centrality[a]	Density	Margin	Expansile[a]	Periosteal Reaction[b]	Notes
Generally well-defined sclerotic/mixed lesions								
Bone island	>20	Any	Any	**Scl**	**Well**	–	–	**Round/oval ± spicules, uniformly dense, <2 cm**
Bone infarct[c]	Any	Any	**Central**	**Scl+** Lucent	**Well+Scl**	-	–	**Serpiginous sclerosis**, can mimic enchondroma
Enchondroma*	>10	Met/Dia	**Central**	**Lucent/ Chon**	**Well**	–/+	–	Lytic in phalanges, **chondroid calc** in larger bones
Chondrosarcoma[d]	**>30**	Met	Central	**Lucent/ Chon**	Poor/ Well	–/+	–	Can mimic enchondroma, chondroblastoma or GCT
Haemangioma*[,e]	>10	Met	Any	Lucent± Scl	Well	–/+	–/Spic	**Spine** > skull > other. Appearance depends on site
Paget's disease	>40	All	All	Lucent/ Scl	Well	–	–	Appearance depends on stage and location; see Part 2

Aggressive lesions in children and adolescents								
Osteomyelitis	Any	**Met/Epi**	Any	**Lucent**	**Poor**	–	Lam	If chronic: sclerosis ± sequestrum ± cloaca
Brodie's abscess	0–20	**Met/Epi**	Any	**Lucent**	**Scl**	–	Solid	**Discrete lucency + surrounding sclerosis**
Eosinophilic granuloma	0–30	Any	Any	Lucent	Poor/ Well	–	Lam	Variable site/appearance, **usually aggressive**
Ewing sarcoma	5–20	**Dia**	Central	**Mixed**	**Poor**	–	**Lam**	Often subtle, ± noncalcified soft tissue mass
Osteosarcoma[f]	10–25	**Met**	Any	**Ost**	**Poor**	–	**Spic**	± Characteristic **osteoid matrix in soft tissue mass**
Aggressive lesions in adults								
Metastasis	**>40**	Any	Any	Lucent/ Scl	Poor/ Well	–/+	–/Spic if sclerotic	Usually multiple, variable appearance; see Section 1.7
Plasmacytoma	**>40**	Any	Central	**Lucent**	**Well**	**++**	–	**Axial and proximal appendicular skeleton**
Bone lymphoma	>30	Any	Central	**Mixed**	**Poor**	–	Lam	**Large soft tissue mass + only subtle bone changes.** 2°>1°

Continued

1

	Peak age (years)	Location	Centrality[a]	Density	Margin	Expansile[a]	Periosteal Reaction[b]	Notes
Chordoma	>30	N/A	Central	**Lucent+** Scl	Well±Scl	++	–	Lytic + foci of calcification. **Sacrum** > **clivus** > vertebrae
Fibrosarcoma and UPS	>20	Met/Dia	Any	Lucent	Poor	–	Any	Nonspecific. Can arise from Paget's, infarct and others
HP/HE/ angiosarcoma	>20	Any	Any	Lucent	Poor	+	–	Rare. A **regional cluster of lytic lesions** is suggestive

Key**: Dia=diaphysis, Met=metaphysis, Epi=epiphysis, Chon=chondroid matrix, Ost=osteoid matrix, Scl=sclerotic, Well=well-defined, Poor=poorly defined; Lam=lamellated, Spic=spiculated, NOF=nonossifying fibroma, FCD=fibrous cortical defect, LSMFT=liposclerosing myxofibrous tumour, HP=haemangiopericytoma, HE=haemangioendothelioma, UPS=undifferentiated pleomorphic sarcoma.* ***Bold text *represents key features. Note that items in the table have been loosely grouped together based on their features, but there is some overlap between the categories.*

**These lesions, when in their polyostotic form, often occur in atypical locations and have atypical appearances; e.g. Jaffe-Campanacci syndrome (NOFs), McCune-Albright syndrome (fibrous dysplasias), Ollier disease and Maffucci syndrome (enchondromas), cystic angiomatosis (haemangiomas).*

[a]*Note that eccentric and nonexpansile lesions may appear central and expansile if large or within a small/thin bone.*

[b]*Note that any lesion may show a periosteal reaction if fractured.*

[c]*Note that acute bone infarcts are usually occult on plain film. If seen in children, suspect underlying sickle cell or Gaucher disease. Termed avascular necrosis when located in the epiphysis. Bone infarcts can transform into various sarcomas.*

[d]*Low-grade chondrosarcomas can occur in young adults and can look nonaggressive or mimic enchondroma—features favouring chondrosarcoma include size >5 cm, deep endosteal scalloping or cortical breach, atypical location (e.g. pelvis, axial skeleton, epiphysis) and history of pain. The clear cell variant of chondrosarcoma arises in epiphyses and can mimic chondroblastoma (though usually in an older age group). Chondrosarcomas can also arise from an existing enchondroma or osteochondroma.*

[e]*Vertebral haemangiomas are common and show coarse vertical trabeculae. In flat bones haemangiomas are often expansile with a sunburst periosteal reaction. In long bones the trabecular coarsening often creates a honeycomb appearance.*

[f]*Osteosarcoma has a second peak in old age due to malignant degeneration of other lesions, e.g. Paget's disease, bone infarct, fibrous dysplasia. Also beware the telangiectatic variant (mimics ABC).*

1.10 LUCENT BONE LESIONS

Well-defined, sclerotic margin

1. Nonossifying fibroma—young patients, eccentric metaphyseal location. Consider benign fibrous histiocytoma if patient >25 years or atypical location.
2. Bone cysts—both SBCs and ABCs usually have a thin sclerotic margin. ABCs are more eccentric and expansile.
3. Fibrous dysplasia—variable appearance, typically diaphyseal.
4. Chondroblastoma—epiphyseal location, young patients. If patient >20 years, consider clear cell chondrosarcoma.
5. Brodie's abscess—typically young patients, most common in metaphysis. Discrete lucency with surrounding ill-defined sclerosis.
6. Healing metastases or primary malignant bone lesions—sclerotic rim indicates a good response to treatment.
7. Osteoblastoma—large lucent nidus with a sclerotic margin. Most common in spine.
8. Intraosseous lipoma—typically in calcaneus or intertrochanteric region of femur. Thin sclerotic margin. Focus of central calcification is pathognomonic but not always present.
9. Liposclerosing myxofibrous tumour—characteristic location: intertrochanteric region of femur. Usually a thick sclerotic margin.
10. Adamantinoma/osteofibrous dysplasia (OFD)—characteristic location: anterior cortex of tibial diaphysis. Both can look identical but OFD occurs in a younger age group (<10 years).
11. **Chondromyxoid fibroma**—rare; can mimic NOF, BFH and ABC.
12. **Haemophilic pseudotumour**—usually very expansile + other signs of haemophilia.

Well-defined, nonsclerotic margin

1. Metastasis—usually older patients, in axial or proximal appendicular skeleton.
2. Myeloma/plasmacytoma—older patients, usually in axial or proximal appendicular skeleton. Typically 'punched-out' appearance, may be expansile.
3. Low-grade chondral lesions—e.g. enchondroma, low-grade chondrosarcoma. Both can be lytic without chondroid matrix.
4. Giant cell tumour—typically has a well-defined nonsclerotic margin. Adults 20–50 years.
5. Simple/aneurysmal bone cyst—both may have no perceptible sclerotic margin.
6. Eosinophilic granuloma—may appear well-defined.

7. Brown tumour—often expansile. Look for other signs of hyperparathyroidism.
8. Lytic phase of Paget's disease—well-defined flame-shaped advancing edge without sclerosis.
9. **Desmoplastic fibroma**—rare. Often contains pseudotrabeculations.

Poorly defined margin

1. Metastasis—usually ill-defined.
2. Myeloma—usually discrete but may appear ill-defined.
3. Osteomyelitis—ill-defined and lytic in the acute phase.
4. Bone lymphoma—typically ill-defined subtle bone destruction with a large soft tissue mass. Can occur at any age but more common in older patients.
5. Primary bone sarcomas—e.g. Ewing sarcoma, osteosarcoma, chondrosarcoma, fibrosarcoma, undifferentiated pleomorphic sarcoma, angiosarcoma. Internal matrix may be absent.
6. Eosinophilic granuloma—patients <30 years. Can occur anywhere, often has an aggressive appearance indistinguishable from infection or malignancy.
7. Giant cell tumour—can appear ill-defined. Adults 20–50 years.

1.11 GROSSLY EXPANSILE LUCENT BONE LESION

Most common

1. Plasmacytoma—older patients, usually in axial or proximal appendicular skeleton.
2. Metastases—RCC, thyroid, HCC, phaeochromocytoma, melanoma. Usually in axial or proximal appendicular skeleton.
3. Aneurysmal bone cyst—in children and young adults. Usually has a thin sclerotic margin.
4. Giant cell tumour—usually older patients than ABC. Often abuts articular surface, no sclerotic margin.

Less common

5. Telangiectatic osteosarcoma—mimics ABC.
6. Fibrous dysplasia—usually fusiform expansion rather than a discrete expansile mass.
7. Brown tumour—look for other signs of hyperparathyroidism.
8. Haemangioma—often expansile when in flat bones, e.g. skull or pelvis, with a sunburst periosteal reaction.
9. Chordoma—in sacrum, clivus or vertebral bodies.

Rare

10. **Haemophilic pseudotumour**—look for other signs of haemophilia.
11. **Slow growing central bone sarcoma.**
12. **Hydatid cyst.**

1.12 LUCENT EPIPHYSEAL BONE LESION

This includes carpal and tarsal bones since they are epiphyseal equivalents.

1. **Lesions related to joint pathology**—e.g. geode, intraosseous ganglion, erosion, osteochondral defect, PVNS.
2. **Giant cell tumour**—nonsclerotic margin, extends from metaphysis to epiphysis. Mainly in adults.
3. **Chondroblastoma**—perilesional sclerosis ± chondroid calcification. Typically 10–20 years.
4. **Infection**—including Brodie's abscess.
5. **Location-specific lesions**—e.g. intraosseous lipoma (calcaneus, central calcification), simple bone cyst (calcaneus, no central calcification), osteoblastoma (talus).
6. **Clear cell chondrosarcoma**—mimics chondroblastoma but usually occurs >20 years.
7. **Bone lesions which can occur anywhere**—e.g. metastasis, brown tumour, lymphoma, myeloma, haemophilic pseudotumour.

1.13 LUCENT BONE LESION CONTAINING CALCIUM OR BONE

Most common

1. **Enchondroma**—chondroid matrix.
2. **Osteoid osteoma and osteoblastoma**—lucent nidus can contain calcification.
3. **Avascular necrosis and bone infarction**.
4. **Metastases**—some are mixed lytic and sclerotic.

Less common

5. **Chondroblastoma**—chondroid matrix. Epiphyseal location.
6. **Chondrosarcoma**—chondroid matrix. Usually metaphyseal.
7. **Osteosarcoma**—osteoid matrix. Usually metaphyseal.
8. **Fibrous dysplasia**—usually ground-glass density but can be sclerotic.
9. **Osteomyelitis with sequestrum**.
10. **Eosinophilic granuloma**—'button sequestrum'.
11. **Intraosseous lipoma**—characteristic central focus of calcification, especially in calcaneus.
12. **Haemangioma**—contains coarsened trabeculae. Most common in spine.

13. <u>Liposclerosing myxofibrous tumour</u>—classically intertrochanteric region of femur.
14. **Fibrosarcoma/undifferentiated pleomorphic sarcoma.**

1.14 EXOPHYTIC AND JUXTACORTICAL BONE LESIONS

1. <u>Callus</u>—can be profuse, e.g. after an avulsion fracture, if bones misaligned or in malunion.
2. <u>Osteochondroma</u>—well-defined exophytic bony mass (sessile or pedunculated), usually arising from metaphysis and pointing away from the joint. The cortex and trabeculae within the lesion should be continuous with those in the metaphysis. Can transform to chondrosarcoma: worrying features include continued growth or change in morphology after physeal closure, bone destruction, soft tissue mass and cartilage cap >1 cm thick (on ultrasound/MRI).
3. <u>Heterotopic ossification and myositis ossificans</u>—well-defined with dense ossification in the periphery and less density centrally. May mimic surface osteosarcoma in the early stage; follow up can help differentiate by showing maturation of ossification.
4. <u>Surface osteosarcoma</u>—three types:
   (a) **Parosteal**—low grade, arises from outer periosteum, usually metaphyseal. Pedunculated 'cauliflower' appearance with a narrow stalk + partial cleft between the mass and underlying bone. Mature osteoid matrix within the mass which is more dense centrally (in contrast to myositis ossificans).
   (b) **Periosteal**—intermediate grade, arises from inner periosteum, usually diaphyseal. Broad-based with cortical erosion and spiculated periosteal reaction. Less organized osteoid matrix.
   (c) **High grade**—amorphous osteoid matrix + larger soft tissue mass ± underlying cortical destruction. Usually diaphyseal.
5. <u>Periosteal chondroma/chondrosarcoma</u>—both typically arise on the metaphyseal surface as a soft tissue mass ± chondroid matrix. The underlying cortex is mildly scalloped. Difficult to differentiate the two on imaging; size >3 cm is more suggestive of chondrosarcoma.
6. <u>Cortical desmoid</u>—characteristic location: distal posteromedial femoral metaphyseal cortex (at muscle insertion site). Well-defined scalloping of cortical surface, typically small.
7. **Parosteal lipoma**—juxtacortical radiolucent mass with an associated irregular bony excrescence arising perpendicularly from the periosteum.
8. **Bizarre parosteal osteochondromatous proliferation (BPOP)**—typically arises from the periosteum of bones in the hands and

feet. Mimics an osteochondroma but does not show medullary continuity with the underlying bone.

9. **Trevor's disease**—developmental disorder, presents in children with an osteochondroma-like mass arising from an epiphysis, usually at the ankle. May involve >1 joint in the same limb, e.g. knee + ankle. Overgrowth of nearby bones is usually also seen.
10. **Melorheostosis**—lobulated cortical hyperostosis (both periosteal and endosteal) with a 'flowing candle wax' appearance in a sclerotomal distribution, often crossing joints.
11. **Osteoma**—usually located within the paranasal sinuses but can arise from the surface of the skull, mandible or long bones in Gardner syndrome. Small, well-defined, uniformly dense osseous nodule on the cortical surface; typically sessile in the long bones with no periosteal reaction. Can be multiple and lobulated, mimicking melorheostosis, but no endosteal involvement or sclerotomal distribution.
12. **Subperiosteal abscess**—usually in children; lamellated periosteal reaction ± erosion of cortex. Can progress to osteomyelitis.
13. **Subperiosteal haemorrhage**—e.g. due to scurvy or haemophilic pseudotumour.
14. **Periarticular lesions**—e.g. ganglion cysts, PVNS. These can scallop the cortex.
15. **Other rare lesions not specific to this site**—e.g. metastasis, subperiosteal osteoid osteoma, ABC.

1.15 'MOTH-EATEN BONE' IN AN ADULT

Multiple scattered lucencies of variable size with no major central lesion. Coalescence may occur later. Cancellous and/or cortical bone is involved.

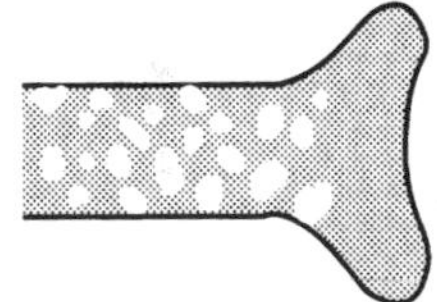

1. Metastases.
2. Multiple myeloma—numerous punched-out lytic lesions.
3. Bone sarcomas—e.g. Ewing sarcoma, osteosarcoma, chondrosarcoma.
4. Bone lymphoma—subtle ill-defined bone destruction, usually with a large soft tissue mass.
5. Langerhans cell histiocytosis—young adults only.
6. Osteomyelitis.
7. Osteoporosis—extensive cortical tunnelling can mimic an aggressive process.
8. Hyperparathyroidism—extensive subperiosteal bone resorption + brown tumours can mimic malignancy.

1.16 REGIONAL OSTEOPENIA

Definition: Decreased bone density confined to a region or segment of the appendicular skeleton.

Most common

1. **Disuse**—typically distal foot and ankle, hand and wrist.
2. **Complex regional pain syndrome**—typically unilateral upper limb. Triple phase uptake on bone scintigraphy.
3. **Inflammatory arthropathy**.
4. **Septic arthritis**.

Less common

5. **Transient osteoporosis of the hip**.
6. **Regional migratory osteoporosis**.
7. **Haemophilic arthropathy**.
8. **Soft tissue arteriovenous malformation.**

1.17 GENERALIZED OSTEOPENIA

Definition: Generic description for nonquantitative radiographic finding of reduced bone density.

1. **Osteoporosis**.
2. **Diffuse infiltrative bone disease**—multiple myeloma in adults, leukaemia in children.
3. **Osteomalacia/rickets**.
4. **Hyperparathyroidism**.

1.18 OSTEOPOROSIS

Definition: Systemic skeletal disease characterized by reduced bone mass, increased bone fragility and fracture susceptibility. Also defined by the WHO as 2.5 standard deviations below peak bone mass for postmenopausal women and men >50 years.

Radiographic findings

1. **Increased radiolucency of bone**—can be affected by radiographic factors.
2. **Cortical thinning**—most commonly endosteal resorption in the elderly. Pencil-line cortex, vertebral picture framing.
3. **Prominent secondary trabeculae**—caused by preferential resorption of primary trabeculae.
4. **Vertebral fractures**—anterior wedge or biconcave vertebral compression.
5. **Insufficiency fractures**—sacrum, pubis, femoral neck, tibial plateau, ankle and foot.

Causes

Primary

1. Postmenopausal.
2. Age-related.
3. **Juvenile**—rare self-limiting condition occurring in children of 8–12 years. Spontaneous improvement is seen.

Secondary

1. Endocrine—e.g. hypogonadism, Cushing's, diabetes, acromegaly, hyperprolactinaemia, Addison's disease, hyperthyroidism, hyperparathyroidism (subperiosteal resorption), mastocytosis (mast cells produce heparin; may also produce diffuse sclerosis).
2. Disuse.
3. Iatrogenic—e.g. steroids, heparin, aromatase inhibitors, androgen deprivation, antiepileptics, proton pump inhibitors.
4. Deficiency states—e.g. vitamin C (scurvy), protein, chronic renal/liver disease, anorexia, malabsorption, alcohol excess.
5. Chronic and systemic disease—e.g. rheumatoid arthritis, amyloidosis, COPD.
6. Congenital—e.g. osteogenesis imperfecta, Turner syndrome, homocystinuria, neuromuscular diseases, mucopolysaccharidoses, trisomy 13 and 18, pseudo and pseudopseudohypoparathyroidism, glycogen storage diseases, progeria.

1.19 OSTEOMALACIA AND RICKETS

Most common causes

1. **Vitamin D deficiency**—either low dietary intake, poor sunlight exposure or malabsorption.

Other causes

2. **Renal disease**.
   (a) **Glomerular disease**—results in renal osteodystrophy.
   (b) **Tubular disease**—e.g. renal tubular acidosis, Fanconi syndrome or hypophosphataemic rickets.
3. **Hepatic disease**—parenchymal failure or chronic cholestasis.
4. **Anticonvulsants**—phenytoin and phenobarbital.
5. **Tumour-associated**—paraneoplastic phenomenon, usually due to a benign phosphaturic mesenchymal tumour which may be small and hard to find; PET-CT can aid localization.

Conditions which mimic rickets/osteomalacia

1. **Hypophosphatasia.**
2. **Metaphyseal chondrodysplasia (Schmid type)**—metaphyseal cupping and irregularity, bowed long bones, short-limbed dwarfism.

In infants <6 months of age

1. **Biliary atresia.**
2. **Metabolic bone disease of prematurity**—combined dietary deficiency and hepatic hydroxylation of vitamin D.
3. **Hypophosphatasia.**
4. **Vitamin D-dependent rickets**—rachitic changes are associated with a severe myopathy in spite of adequate dietary intake of vitamin D.

1.20 PERIOSTEAL REACTIONS—TYPES

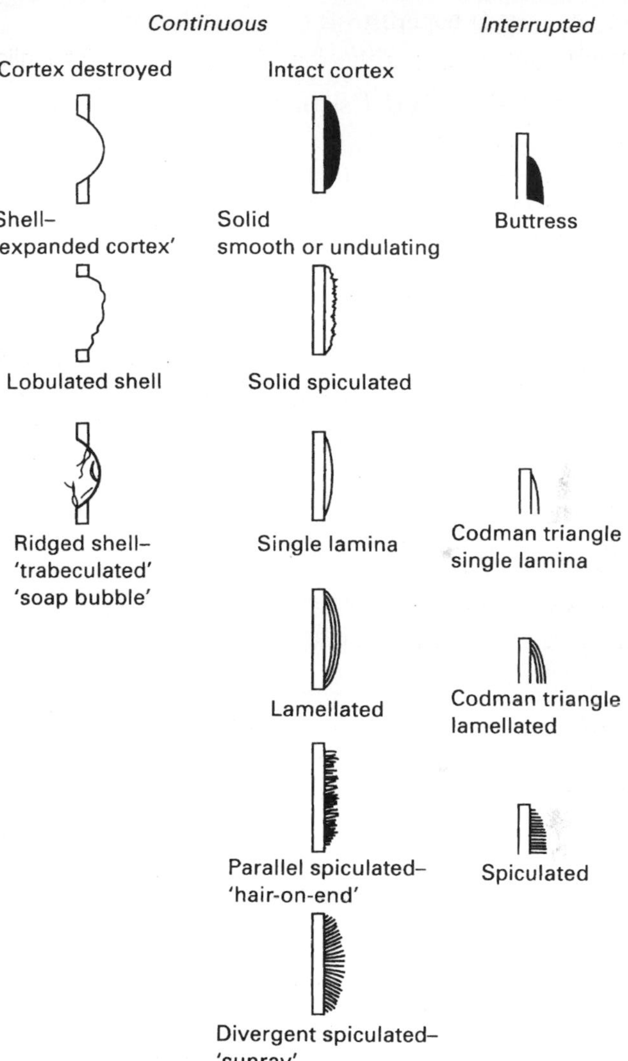

(Modified from Ragsdale, B.D., Madewell, J.E., Sweet, D.E., 1981. Radiologic and pathologic analysis of solitary bone lesions. Part II: Periosteal reactions. Radiol Clin North Am 19, 749–783.)

The different types are, in general, nonspecific, having multiple aetiologies. However, the following comments can be made.

Continuous with destroyed cortex

This is the result of an expansile lesion; see Section 1.11.

Parallel spiculated ('hair-on-end')

1. Ewing sarcoma.
2. Infantile cortical hyperostosis (Caffey's disease).
3. Syphilis.

Divergent spiculated ('sunray')

1. Osteosarcoma.
2. Metastases—especially from sigmoid colon and rectum.
3. Ewing sarcoma.
4. Haemangioma—when in flat bones, e.g. skull, pelvis.
5. Meningioma—skull only.
6. Tuberculosis.
7. Tropical ulcer—typically involves the foot or lower leg.

Codman triangle (single lamina or lamellated)

1. Aggressive malignant bone tumour.
2. Osteomyelitis.

1.21 PERIOSTEAL REACTIONS—SOLITARY AND LOCALIZED

1. Trauma—fracture, periosteal haematoma.
2. Insufficiency and stress fractures.
3. Inflammatory.
4. Neoplastic—e.g. malignant primary bone tumour, metastasis, or benign bone lesion + pathological fracture.

1.22 PERIOSTEAL REACTION—BILATERALLY SYMMETRICAL IN ADULTS

1. Hypertrophic osteoarthropathy (HOA)—aka HPOA or secondary HOA. See Section 1.24.
2. Vascular insufficiency—most common in lower limbs due to venous stasis/varicose veins. Often associated with phleboliths.
3. Thyroid acropachy—predominantly radial sided in the thumbs and index fingers.
4. Pachydermoperiostosis—aka primary HOA. Solid periosteal reaction + skin thickening.
5. Fluorosis—solid undulating periosteal new bone along long bones with calcification/ossification of tendon and ligament insertions.
6. Hypervitaminosis A.

1.23 PERIOSTEAL REACTIONS—BILATERALLY ASYMMETRICAL

1. **Metastases**.
2. **Osteomyelitis**.
3. **Reactive and psoriatic arthritis**.
4. **Nonaccidental injury**—in infants and children.
5. **Osteoporosis**—increased liability to fracture.
6. **Osteomalacia**—associated with Looser's zones.
7. **Bleeding diathesis.**
8. **Sickle cell dactylitis**—in young children due to infarction of persistent red marrow in long bones of hands and feet. Hard to differentiate from osteomyelitis.

1.24 HYPERTROPHIC OSTEOARTHROPATHY

Primary

Pachydermoperiostosis—rare, autosomal dominant inheritance. Presents in children and young adults, mainly males. Skin thickening is also seen.

Secondary

Most common

1. **Lung cancer**—>60% of cases.
2. **Bronchiectasis**—frequently due to cystic fibrosis.
3. **Lung metastases**.

Less common

4. **Other pleuropulmonary causes**—e.g. pleural fibroma (rare, but has the highest incidence of accompanying HOA), mesothelioma, COPD, pulmonary fibrosis, sarcoidosis, chronic infection (e.g. abscess, empyema, TB), pulmonary AVM.
5. **GI disorders**—irritable bowel disease, coeliac disease, Whipple's disease, polyposis, malignancy.
6. **Cyanotic congenital heart disease**—produces clubbing but only rarely a periosteal reaction.
7. **Cirrhosis and hepatobiliary malignancies**.
8. **Other malignancies**—lymphoma, nasopharyngeal carcinoma, RCC, breast phyllodes tumour, thymic carcinoma, melanoma.

1.25 EXCESSIVE CALLUS FORMATION

Most common

1. Hypertrophic fracture nonunion.
2. Neuropathic arthropathy—including congenital insensitivity to pain. Accompanied by joint destruction, fragmentation, sclerosis and osteophyte formation.
3. Steroid therapy and Cushing's syndrome.

Less common

4. **Osteogenesis imperfecta.**
5. **Paralysis**—more common in lower extremities.
6. **Renal osteodystrophy.**
7. **Multiple myeloma.**

Children

8. Nonaccidental injury.

1.26 OSTEONECROSIS/AVASCULAR NECROSIS

Common

1. Corticosteroids—both exogenous and endogenous (Cushing's syndrome).
2. Alcohol.
3. Idiopathic—e.g. Perthes' disease in children.
4. Fractures—especially femoral neck, talus and scaphoid.
5. Chemotherapy.

Less common

6. Haemoglobinopathies—especially sickle cell anaemia.
7. Radiotherapy—localized to the treatment field, e.g. pelvis/sacrum.
8. Metabolic and endocrine—e.g. pregnancy, diabetes, hyperlipidaemia, gout, Gaucher disease.
9. **Connective tissue diseases**—e.g. SLE, rheumatoid arthritis, scleroderma.
10. **Toxic**—e.g. immunosuppressives, anti-inflammatories (NSAIDs).
11. **Haemopoietic disorders**—e.g. polycythaemia vera, haemophilia.
12. **Thrombotic and embolic**—including vasculitis, fat embolism and dysbaric osteonecrosis.
13. **Others**—e.g. pancreatitis, severe burns, amyloidosis.

1.27 EROSIONS OF THE MEDIAL METAPHYSIS OF THE PROXIMAL HUMERUS

1. **Normal variant**.
2. **Chronic rotator cuff tear**—results in elevation of humeral head and impingement of medial metaphysis on glenoid, causing mechanical erosion.
3. **Hyperparathyroidism**—subperiosteal resorption.
4. **Rheumatoid arthritis**.
5. **Malignancy**—e.g. leukaemia, metastases (including neuroblastoma in children).
6. **Lysosomal storage disorders**—e.g. Gaucher disease, Hurler syndrome, Niemann-Pick disease.

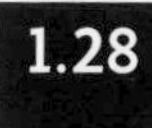

1.28 EROSION OR ABSENCE OF THE OUTER END OF THE CLAVICLE

Common

1. **Posttraumatic osteolysis**.
2. **Postoperative**—e.g. following subacromial decompression.
3. **Rheumatoid arthritis**—typically bilateral and symmetrical.

Less common

4. **Malignancy**—metastasis, myeloma.
5. **Septic arthritis**—erosion involves both sides of joint.
6. **Hyperparathyroidism**—typically bilateral and symmetrical, ± resorption at other sites, e.g. coracoclavicular ligament insertion, sternoclavicular joint, greater and lesser tuberosities of humerus.
7. **Cleidocranial dysplasia**.
8. **Pyknodysostosis**—hypoplastic clavicles also associated with hypoplastic mandibles, acroosteolysis and osteosclerosis.
9. **Scleroderma**—juxtaarticular soft tissue calcification highly suggestive.
10. **Gout**.

1.29 MADELUNG DEFORMITY

Primary

The isolated congenital form is often associated with Vicker's ligament connecting the distal radius to the lunate and TFCC. The radiographic findings include:

- Short bowed distal radius with increased radiocarpal angle.
- Long dorsally subluxed ulna.
- V-shaped proximal carpal row.

Secondary

The term secondary Madelung is often applied to similar bowing deformities of the distal radius that do not always include a long ulna. Causes include:

1. **Growth arrest following radial growth plate injury or infection**.
2. **Multiple hereditary exostoses**.
3. **Turner syndrome**.
4. **Achondroplasia.**
5. **Leri-Weill dyschondrosteosis.**

1.30 CARPAL FUSION

Congenital

Isolated

Tends to involve bones in the same carpal row (proximal or distal). More common in Afro-Caribbeans.

1. **Lunate-triquetral**—most common site. 1% of the population.
2. **Capitate-hamate**.
3. **Trapezium-trapezoid**.

Syndrome-related

Tend to exhibit massive carpal fusion affecting bones in different rows (proximal and distal).

1. **Acrocephalosyndactyly (Apert syndrome)**—craniosynostosis, syndactyly.
2. **Arthrogryposis multiplex congenita**—multiple congenital contractures.
3. **Diastrophic dwarfism**—short-limbed dwarfism.
4. **Ellis-van Creveld syndrome**—short-limbed dwarfism, polydactyly.
5. **Dyschondrosteosis**—mesomelic dwarfism + bilateral Madelung deformities.

6. **Hand-foot-genital syndrome**—scaphoid-trapezium coalition.
7. **Nievergelt syndrome**—mesomelic dwarfism, club foot, metatarsal synostoses.
8. **Oto-palato-digital syndrome**—deformed carpals, ear and palatal anomalies.
9. **Holt-Oram syndrome**—radial ray anomalies and cardiac malformations.
10. **Turner syndrome**—Madelung deformity and lunate-triquetral coalition may be seen.
11. **Symphalangism**—interphalangeal joint fusions and carpal coalitions.
12. **Fetal alcohol syndrome**—capitate-hamate coalition + radioulnar synostoses.

Acquired

1. **Inflammatory arthritides**—especially juvenile idiopathic arthritis and rheumatoid arthritis.
2. **Pyogenic arthritis.**
3. **Chronic tuberculous arthritis.**
4. **Posttraumatic.**
5. **Postsurgical.**

1.31 SHORT METACARPAL(S) OR METATARSAL(S)

1. **Idiopathic**.
2. **Posttraumatic**—iatrogenic, fracture, growth plate injury, thermal or electrical.
3. **Postinfarction**—e.g. sickle cell anaemia.
4. **Turner syndrome**—4th ± 3rd and 5th metacarpals.
5. **Pseudo and pseudopseudohypoparathyroidism**—4th and 5th metacarpals.

1.32 ARACHNODACTYLY

Elongated and slender tubular bones of the hands and feet ('spider fingers'). The metacarpal index aids diagnosis and is estimated by measuring the lengths of the 2nd to 5th metacarpals and dividing by their breadths at the exact midpoints. These four figures are then added together and divided by 4. NB: this is a poor discriminator between Marfan syndrome and constitutional tall stature.

Normal range 5.4–7.9.
Arachnodactyly range 8.4–10.4.

Most common

1. Marfan syndrome—although arachnodactyly is not necessary for the diagnosis.
2. Normal variant—constitutional tall stature.

Less common

There are several disorders that have a marfanoid phenotype that can include arachnodactyly. These include:

3. Homocystinuria.
4. Ehlers-Danlos syndrome.
5. Klinefelter syndrome.
6. **Loeys-Dietz syndrome.**
7. **Congenital contractural arachnodactyly (Beals syndrome).**
8. MEN 2B.
9. **Myotonic dystrophy.**
10. **Stickler syndrome.**

1.33 DISTAL PHALANGEAL DESTRUCTION

Resorption of the tuft (acroosteolysis)

Most common

1. Scleroderma—look for soft tissue thinning and calcification.
2. Raynaud disease—and other vasculopathies, e.g. SLE.
3. Psoriatic arthropathy—look for joint erosions.
4. Hyperparathyroidism—look for subperiosteal bone resorption.
5. Trauma—including burns and frostbite.

Less common

6. Peripheral neuropathy—e.g. due to diabetes, leprosy, congenital insensitivity to pain. Results in recurrent trauma.
7. **Other arthritides**—e.g. juvenile idiopathic arthritis, reactive arthritis, multicentric reticulohistiocytosis.
8. **Other skin disorders**—dermatomyositis, epidermolysis bullosa, congenital erythropoietic porphyria.
9. **Phenytoin toxicity**—in infants of treated epileptic mothers.
10. **Snake and scorpion venom.**
11. **Pyknodysostosis (mimic)**—look for diffuse bony sclerosis.

Resorption of the midportion

1. Hyperparathyroidism.
2. Polyvinyl chloride tank cleaners.
3. **Acroosteolysis of Hajdu and Cheney**—very rare.

1.34 LYTIC LESIONS OF THE PHALANGES

Poorly defined

1. <u>**Osteomyelitis**</u>—particularly in diabetic feet. Also consider tuberculous dactylitis, sickle cell dactylitis and syphilitic dactylitis.
2. <u>**Metastasis**</u>—lung is the most common primary site.

Well-defined

1. <u>**Enchondroma**</u>—often purely lytic without chondroid matrix.
2. <u>**Joint-based lesions**</u>—e.g. subchondral cysts, erosions.
3. <u>**Implantation epidermoid**</u>—palmar scalloping, distal phalanx only.
4. <u>**Glomus tumour**</u>—dorsal scalloping, distal phalanx only.
5. <u>**Sarcoidosis**</u>—multiple well-defined lace-like lytic lesions.
6. **Other rare lesions not specific to the phalanges**—e.g. fibrous dysplasia, ABC, GCT, SBC, brown tumour, LCH, fibrous cortical defect.

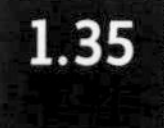

1.35 FLUID–FLUID LEVELS IN BONE LESIONS ON CT AND MRI

Benign

1. <u>**Aneurysmal bone cyst**</u>.
2. **Chondroblastoma.**
3. **Giant cell tumour.**
4. **Simple bone cyst.**
5. **Fibrous dysplasia.**

Malignant

1. <u>**Telangiectatic osteosarcoma**</u>.
2. **Any necrotic bone tumour.**

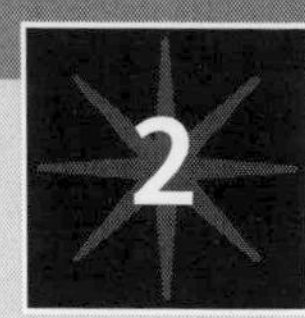

Spine

Sajid Butt, Bhavin Upadhyay, Sami Khan, Andoni Toms, James MacKay

2.1 SCOLIOSIS

Scoliosis is a lateral spinal curve on a PA radiograph with a Cobb angle >10 degrees. If <10 degrees then it should be described as spinal asymmetry.

Idiopathic (80%)

1. **Congenital**—0–3 years, M>F. Left side convex. Usually regresses.
2. **Juvenile**—4–9 years, females. Right side convex. Usually progresses.
3. **Adolescent**—females. Right-sided thoracic convexity. Progressive if the Cobb angle at skeletal maturity is >30 degrees. If <30 degrees, the chance of progression is only 5%.

Congenital anomalies (10%)

Progressive in 75% of patients.

1. **Vertebral**—either failure of formation (wedge-shaped vertebrae, hemivertebrae, butterfly vertebrae), failure of segmentation (unilateral bar) or mixed anomalies.
2. **Neurological**—Chiari malformation, syringomyelia, tethered cord, diastematomyelia.

Others

1. **Developmental dysplasias**—diffusely involve multiple bones, e.g. achondroplasia, neurofibromatosis, osteogenesis imperfecta.
2. **Neuromuscular**—cerebral palsy, spinocerebellar degeneration, poliomyelitis, muscular dystrophies (e.g. Duchenne).
3. **Tumour-related**—osteoid osteoma, osteoblastoma, aggressive haemangioma, intraspinal tumours. Usually painful.
4. **Degenerative**—acquired secondary to degenerative spondylosis. Most common in lumbar spine.
5. **Posttraumatic.**
6. **Infection.**

Most cases are idiopathic and do not require further imaging; indications for cross-sectional imaging (usually MRI) include:

1. **Clinical findings**—age of onset <10 years, spinal pain (suggests an underlying osteoid osteoma, osteoblastoma, intraspinal tumour or infection), headaches, neurological deterioration, foot deformities or prior to surgical correction.
2. **Radiological findings**—left thoracic curve, double or triple curves that do not straighten on bending views, long thoracic curve (associated with neuromuscular disorders), progression beyond skeletal maturity, or signs of intraspinal pathology, e.g. thinned pedicles, widened spinal canal, features of dysraphism, widened neural foramina.
3. **Nonidiopathic causes**—MRI and/or CT imaging is almost always needed for assessment and follow-up.

2.2 SOLITARY COLLAPSED VERTEBRA

NB: vertebra plana = almost complete loss of anterior and posterior vertebral body height.

1. **Osteoporosis**—generalized osteopenia. Coarsened trabecular pattern in adjacent vertebrae due to resorption of secondary trabeculae.
2. **Neoplastic disease**.
   (a) **Metastasis**—breast, lung, prostate, kidney and thyroid account for most patients with a solitary spinal metastasis. The disc spaces are preserved until late. The bone may be lytic, sclerotic or mixed ± pedicle destruction.
   (b) **Multiple myeloma/plasmacytoma**—a common site, especially for plasmacytoma. May mimic an osteolytic metastasis or be expansile and resemble an aneurysmal bone cyst.
   (c) **Lymphoma**—secondary > primary bone involvement.
3. **Trauma**.
4. **Infection**—with destruction of vertebral endplates and adjacent disc spaces. TB, in particular, can cause vertebra plana with relative preservation of the discs.
5. **Eosinophilic granuloma**—commonest cause of solitary vertebra plana in childhood. The posterior elements are usually spared.
6. **Benign tumours**—haemangioma, GCT and ABC.
7. **Paget's disease**—diagnosis is difficult when a solitary vertebra is involved. Neural arch is involved in most cases. Hallmarks are trabecular coarsening and bone expansion. If other noncollapsed vertebrae are affected, then diagnosis becomes much easier.

2.3 MULTIPLE COLLAPSED VERTEBRAE

1. **Osteoporosis**.
2. **Neoplastic disease**—most commonly multiple myeloma, leukaemia and lymphoma. Disc spaces are usually preserved until late. Paravertebral soft-tissue mass is more common in myeloma than metastases.
3. **Trauma**—unusual to involve >2–3 levels. Visible cortical discontinuity and angular deformity.
4. **Scheuermann's disease**—children and young adults; wedging of ≥3 adjacent vertebrae in the lower thoracic spine with irregular endplates, disc space narrowing and kyphosis.
5. **Infection**—destruction of endplates adjacent to a destroyed disc.
6. **Langerhans cell histiocytosis**—children and adolescents. Disc spaces often enlarged.
7. **Sickle cell anaemia**—characteristic step-like depression centrally in the endplates, resulting in H-shaped vertebrae. Small calcified spleen may be visible on plain film.
8. **Gaucher disease**—also causes H-shaped vertebrae, but the spleen is typically enlarged. Also associated with other pathological fractures, AVN and Erlenmeyer flask deformity.
9. **Osteogenesis imperfecta**—osteopenia with multilevel compression fractures.
10. **Osteomalacia**—coarse trabeculae with "fuzzy" demineralization.
11. **Hyperparathyroidism**—subperiosteal bone resorption and brown tumours.

2.4 EROSION, DESTRUCTION OR ABSENCE OF A PEDICLE

1. **Metastasis**—lumbar > thoracic > cervical, but neural compression is most common at thoracic level due to a smaller spinal canal.
2. **Multiple myeloma**.
3. **Intraspinal tumours**—e.g. ependymoma, nerve sheath tumours. Usually cause erosion or flattening of pedicles + widening of the interpedicular distance.
4. **TB* and other infections.**
5. **Radiotherapy.**

2.5 SOLITARY DENSE PEDICLE

1. **Osteoblastic metastasis**—no change in size.
2. **Osteoid osteoma**—some enlargement of the pedicle ± radiolucent nidus ± scoliosis.

3. Bone island.
4. Secondary to unilateral spondylolysis—stress-induced sclerosis of the contralateral pedicle.
5. **Congenitally absent/hypoplastic contralateral posterior elements.**
6. **Osteoblastoma**—lucent nidus is larger than osteoid osteoma (>2 cm), therefore usually presents as a lucency with a sclerotic margin rather than a purely sclerotic pedicle.
7. **Other sclerotic bone lesions**—e.g. Paget's disease, fibrous dysplasia, sarcoidosis, tuberous sclerosis.

2.6 ENLARGED VERTEBRAL BODY

Generalized

1. Gigantism—occurs prior to growth plate fusion.
2. Acromegaly—particularly in AP dimension, with widened disc spaces, osteopenia and posterior vertebral body scalloping.

Local (single or multiple)

1. Paget's disease—trabecular coarsening and cortical thickening. Can involve body or entire vertebra. 'Picture frame' appearance in mixed phase, ivory vertebra in diffuse sclerotic phase.
2. Benign bone tumour.
   (a) Aneurysmal bone cyst—typically purely lytic and expansile. Involves both anterior and posterior elements more commonly than one part alone. Rapid growth; fluid–fluid levels on MRI.
   (b) **Haemangioma**—with a prominent vertical trabecular pattern.
   (c) **Giant cell tumour**—involvement of the body alone is most common. Expansion is minimal.
3. Fibrous dysplasia—commonly ground-glass matrix. Spine lesions are more common in polyostotic disease. The neural arch is more commonly involved than the vertebral body.
4. **Hydatid**—over 40% of cases of osseous hydatid disease occur in vertebrae. Osteolytic expansile lesions, typically associated with paraspinal cystic lesions extending into adjacent ribs.

2.7 SQUARING OF ONE OR MORE VERTEBRAL BODIES

1. Seronegative spondyloarthropathies—most commonly ankylosing spondylitis.
2. Paget's disease.
3. **Rheumatoid arthritis.**

2.8 BLOCK VERTEBRAE

1. **Klippel-Feil syndrome**—C2/3 and C5/6 are most commonly affected. Narrowing of the vertebrae at the site of a fused/ rudimentary disc space ('wasp-waist' sign). Fusion of posterior elements is also common. Often associated with other anomalies, e.g. other segmentation anomalies, scoliosis, dysraphism, spinal cord anomalies, Sprengel's deformity of the scapula (± omovertebral bar), cervical ribs, genitourinary anomalies (e.g. unilateral renal agenesis), cardiac/aortic anomalies and deafness.
2. **Isolated congenital**—failure of segmentation, frequently associated with hemivertebra and absent vertebra adjacent to block vertebra, ± posterior element fusion.
3. **Juvenile idiopathic arthritis**—can mimic Klippel-Feil syndrome, but there may also be angulation at the fusion site (not a feature of congenital fusion), and typically the spinous processes do not fuse in juvenile idiopathic arthritis.
4. **Ankylosing spondylitis**—squaring of anterior vertebral margins, syndesmophytes, calcification of intervertebral discs and adjacent ligaments. No wasp-waist sign.
5. **Infectious spondylodiscitis**—fusion across the disc space occurs late in the course of the disease. Features suggesting TB include a calcified or thin-walled paravertebral abscess, gibbus deformity, subligamentous spread ≥3 vertebral levels and involvement of an entire vertebral body or multiple noncontiguous levels.
6. **Surgical fusion**—no wasp-waist sign.
7. **Posttraumatic**—no wasp-waist sign.

2.9 IVORY VERTEBRAL BODY

Single or multiple very dense vertebrae. The list excludes those causes where increased density is due to compaction of bone following collapse.

1. **Metastasis**—prostate and breast are the most common sources.
2. **Paget's disease**—vertebra is also mildly enlarged.
3. **Haemangioma**.
4. **Low-grade infection**—including TB.
5. **SAPHO syndrome**.
6. **Lymphoma**—more common in Hodgkin disease.
7. **Sarcoidosis.**

2.10 ATLANTOAXIAL SUBLUXATION

Atlantodental interval = gap between the anterior arch of C1 and the odontoid peg in the sagittal plane. Abnormal if >3 mm in adults and older children, or >5 mm in younger children or if the gap changes considerably between flexion and extension.

Trauma

1. Osseous injury—C1/C2 fracture.
2. Ligamentous injury—disruption of transverse ligaments.

Arthritides

1. Rheumatoid arthritis—in 20–25% of patients with severe disease. Associated erosion of the odontoid ± pannus.
2. Psoriatic arthropathy—in 45% of patients with spondylitis.
3. Juvenile idiopathic arthritis—most commonly in seropositive juvenile onset rheumatoid arthritis.
4. CPPD—calcified inflammatory tissue may surround the dens, and can cause crowned dens syndrome in the acute setting.
5. Hydroxyapatite deposition disease (HADD)—can also cause crowned dens syndrome with bone erosions, similar to CPPD.
6. **Systemic lupus erythematosus**—in 10%; reported association with length of disease, Jaccoud's arthropathy and hypermobility.
7. **Ankylosing spondylitis**—in 2% of cases. Usually a late feature.

Congenital hypoplasia/absence of the dens

NB: in children <9 years it is normal for the tip of the odontoid to fall well below the top of the anterior arch of the atlas. Congenital hypoplasia can be isolated or occur as part of various syndromes including Down's (20%), Morquio, spondyloepiphyseal dysplasia and achondroplasia.

Infection

1. **C1/C2 infection**—associated epidural phlegmon or abscess.
2. **Grisel syndrome**—laxity of transverse/alar ligaments usually occurring in young children, caused by hyperaemia following a nearby infectious process, e.g. retropharyngeal abscess, otitis media, pharyngitis or upper respiratory tract infection.

2.11 INTERVERTEBRAL DISC CALCIFICATION

Most common

1. Degenerative spondylosis—common, can involve any part of the disc.
2. Following spinal fusion.
3. Ankylosing spondylitis—peripheral annulus calcification + other characteristic features.

Less common

4. DISH—anterior annulus calcification + flowing osteophytes.
5. CPPD—calcification of annulus ± pulposus, ligaments and facet joints, but usually no ankylosis. Can cause acute calcific disc inflammation ± endplate erosion, which can mimic infection (disc calcification aids differentiation).
6. HADD—can cause calcific disc inflammation similar to CPPD.

Rare

7. **Alkaptonuria/ochronosis**—multilevel central disc calcification, disc space narrowing and severe osteopenia.
8. **Haemochromatosis**—similar to CPPD.
9. **Gout**—together with erosions and tophi.
10. **Poliomyelitis.**
11. **Acromegaly.**
12. **Hyperparathyroidism.**
13. **Amyloidosis.**
14. **Idiopathic**—a transient painful phenomenon in the cervical spine of children.
15. **Juvenile chronic arthritides.**

2.12 BONY OUTGROWTHS OF THE SPINE

Osteophytes

Arise from endplate margins from Sharpey fibres, usually horizontal or claw-like. Represents degenerative disc disease. Very common.

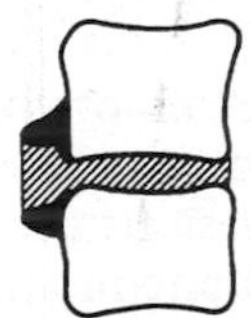

Lateral

Syndesmophytes

Ossification of the annulus fibrosus. Thin, vertical and symmetrical. When severe, results in 'bamboo spine'.

AP

1. Ankylosing spondylitis—classic cause of syndesmophytes, usually as a later feature of the disease (after corner erosions, 'shiny corners' and squaring of the vertebral bodies). Other classic features include ossification of interspinous ligaments, ankylosis of facet joints and erosion/ankylosis of costovertebral joints.
2. **CPPD/haemochromatosis.**
3. **Ochronosis**—with internal disc calcification, disc space narrowing and osteopenia.

Nonmarginal osteophytes/paravertebral ossification

Bulky asymmetrical ossification of paravertebral tissues, which may connect with the sides of the vertebral bodies, but is separate from the margin of the endplate and disc.

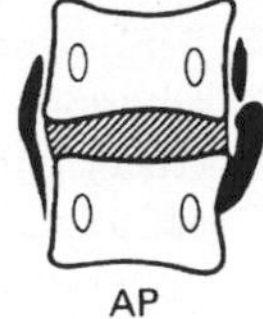

1. <u>Psoriatic arthropathy</u>.
2. <u>Chronic reactive arthropathy</u>—like psoriatic arthropathy, but less common.
3. <u>SAPHO</u>—nonmarginal osteophytes ± erosions, bony bridging or ankylosis.

Undulating anterior or posterior ossification

Undulating ossification of the anterior or posterior longitudinal ligament, disc annulus and paravertebral tissues.

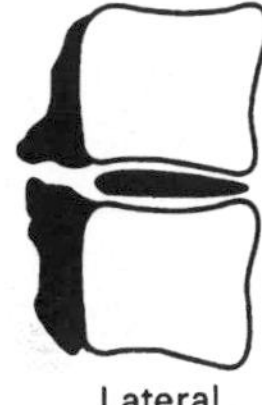

1. <u>DISH</u>—anterior ossification, most common in the thoracic spine with sparing of the left side due to aortic pulsations. Involves >3 contiguous vertebrae; disc height is usually preserved. Associated with enthesophytes elsewhere.
2. **Ossification of the posterior longitudinal ligament**—usually involves the cervical spine; most common in East Asians.

2.13 POSTERIOR SCALLOPING OF VERTEBRAL BODIES

Scalloping is most prominent: (a) at either end of the spinal canal; (b) with large and slow-growing lesions; and (c) with those lesions which originate during the period of active growth and bone modelling.

1. <u>Tumours in the spinal canal</u>—ependymoma (especially myxopapillary type), dermoid, lipoma, nerve sheath tumour and, less commonly, meningioma. Chronic raised intraspinal pressure distal to a tumour producing spinal block also causes extensive vertebral scalloping.
2. <u>Neurofibromatosis</u>—scalloping is due to mesodermal dysplasia and dural ectasia. Localized scalloping can also result from pressure resorption by a neurofibroma, ± enlargement of an intervertebral foramen and flattening of one pedicle ('dumbbell tumour'). However, multiple wide thoracic intervertebral foramina are more likely because of lateral meningocoeles rather than tumours.
3. <u>Acromegaly</u>—other spinal changes include increased axial diameters of the vertebral bodies giving a spurious impression of

decreased vertebral height, osteoporosis, spur formation and calcified discs.

4. Achondroplasia—with spinal stenosis (due to short pedicles) and anterior vertebral body beaks.
5. Other congenital syndromes—e.g. Ehlers-Danlos/Marfan (both cause dural ectasia), mucopolysaccharidosis, osteogenesis imperfecta.
6. **Communicating hydrocephalus**—if severe and untreated.
7. **Syringomyelia**—especially if the onset is <30 years.

2.14 ANTERIOR SCALLOPING OF VERTEBRAL BODIES

1. Aortic aneurysm—intervertebral discs remain intact. Well-defined anterior vertebral margin, ± calcification in aortic wall.
2. Lymphadenopathy—e.g. mycobacterial infection, malignancy. Pressure resorption of bone results in a well-defined anterior vertebral body margin unless there is bony infiltration.
3. **Delayed motor development**—e.g. Down's syndrome.

2.15 WIDENED INTERPEDICULAR DISTANCE

1. Myelomeningocoele—fusiform distribution of widened interpedicular distances with the greatest separation at the midpoint of the involved segment. Disc spaces are narrowed and bodies appear to be widened. Spinous processes and laminae are not identifiable. Facets may be fused into a continuous mass. Scoliosis in most cases ± kyphosis.
2. Intraspinal mass—especially ependymoma. See Section 2.17.
3. Diastematomyelia—50% occur between L1 and L3; 25% between T7 and T12. Widened interpedicular distances are common but not necessarily at the same level as the spur. The spur is visible in 33% of cases and extends from the neural arch anteriorly. Intersegmental laminar fusion + a neural arch defect at the same or adjacent level is highly suggestive. A meningocoele, neurenteric cyst or dermoid may also be seen.
4. Trauma—suggests a burst fracture.

2.16 DIFFUSE LOW MARROW T1 SIGNAL

In normal adults, the T1 signal of spinal bone marrow should be greater than the discs. Note that the conditions below also affect the proximal appendicular skeleton.

1. Red marrow reconversion—due to chronic anaemia (e.g. anaemia of chronic disease, sickle cell, thalassaemia, spherocytosis) or

increased oxygen demand (heavy smoking, endurance athletes), or in patients on marrow-stimulating therapy (GCSF).

2. **Diffuse malignant infiltration**—e.g. metastases (most commonly from prostate or breast), myeloma, lymphoma, leukaemia. Marrow signal is often hyperintense to skeletal muscle on STIR/T2 fatsat (isointense in red marrow reconversion).
3. **Haemosiderosis**—e.g. due to haemolytic anaemia or recurrent blood transfusions. Diffuse low T1 and T2 signal due to haemosiderin deposition in the marrow. Low signal is also present in the liver and spleen, confirming the diagnosis.
4. **Disorders causing diffuse bony sclerosis**—e.g. myelofibrosis, mastocytosis, osteopetrosis.
5. **Gaucher disease**—diffuse marrow infiltration by Gaucher cells. Bone infarcts may also be seen.

2.17 INTRASPINAL MASSES

Extradural mass

1. **Disc herniation, extrusion or sequestration**—usually extradural space, but can occasionally penetrate dura, especially in the thoracic spine. Low/intermediate T2 signal ± rim enhancement. May calcify or be associated with posterior osteophytes.
2. **Metastases, myeloma and lymphoma**—usually extending from the adjacent vertebral body. Primary bone tumours may also extend into the epidural space.
3. **Synovial cyst**—related to facet joint arthrosis, located in the posterolateral epidural space. Unilocular cyst ± rim enhancement.
4. **Extradural meningeal cyst**—e.g. perineural cyst (located along a spinal nerve, usually within the neural foramen) or extradural arachnoid cyst (located within the spinal canal, usually posterior). Perineural cysts are often multiple and bilateral and are common, especially in the sacrum (Tarlov cysts). Unilocular, no enhancement.
5. **Epidural phlegmon/abscess**—lobulated tissue/collection typically associated with spondylodiscitis. Phlegmon enhances uniformly; abscess enhances only peripherally. Paravertebral abscess may also be present.
6. **Epidural fibrosis**—postoperative scar/fibrosis in the surgical bed related to intervention, which demonstrates internal enhancement (unlike recurrent disc material).
7. **Neurofibroma**—nodular or plexiform-enhancing mass related to nerve root ± dumbbell configuration due to transforaminal extension. T2 hyperintense, often with central hypointensity (target sign). May be multiple in NF1.

8. Schwannoma—more commonly intradural, but may also be transforaminal with a dumbbell appearance. Similar appearance to neurofibroma, but the target sign is less common, and internal cystic change, haemorrhage or fatty degeneration is more common. May be multiple in NF2.
9. Epidural haematoma—typically extends over multiple vertebral segments; caused by trauma, intervention or coagulopathy. Signal characteristics relate to chronicity of blood products, but often T1 hyperintense.
10. Epidural lipomatosis—diffuse proliferation of epidural fat, most common in the lower thoracic and lumbar spine, causing mass effect on the thecal sac. Most commonly due to steroids or obesity.
11. **Discal cyst**—arises from the posterior disc margin via an annular fissure. Usually found in young Asian men.
12. **Other facet joint related lesions**—e.g. tumoural calcinosis (lobulated densely calcified mass) or gouty tophi (erosive juxta articular soft tissue mass ± calcification).
13. **Extramedullary haematopoiesis**—can be epidural and/or paravertebral in location, usually multifocal. Typically associated with widespread T1 hypointensity of bone marrow due to red marrow reconversion.
14. **Angiolipoma**—can mimic epidural lipomatosis but contains nonfatty vascular components, which show intermediate T1 signal + avid enhancement.
15. **Neuroblastoma and ganglioneuroma**—tumours of childhood arising in adrenal or paravertebral sympathetic chain. Direct extension through the neural foramina into the spinal canal may occur.
16. **Hydatid cyst**—usually epidural or intraosseous in location. Can be uni- or multilocular.
17. **Sarcoidosis**—rare, usually related to vertebral involvement.

Intradural extramedullary mass

NB: beware of CSF flow artefact mimicking a mass lesion.

1. Schwannoma—most common tumour in this location. T2 hyperintense + enhancement ± cystic change, etc.
2. Meningioma—typically solitary with a dural tail. Usually T2 isointense to cord (in contrast to nerve sheath tumours). Uniform enhancement, may be calcified. Can rarely be extradural. May be multiple in NF2.
3. Neurofibroma—purely intradural location is less common.
4. Arachnoid cyst—follows CSF signal on all sequences. No perceptible wall; its presence is usually inferred by focal deviation of the cord.

5. Leptomeningeal metastases—may present as discrete enhancing nodules or diffuse leptomeningeal enhancement coating the cord and cauda equina. Can be haematogenous (e.g. from lung, breast, melanoma, lymphoma, leukaemia) or 'drop' metastases from a CNS tumour (e.g. glioblastoma in adults, medulloblastoma in children).
6. Other leptomeningeal processes—sarcoidosis can cause nodular leptomeningeal enhancement mimicking malignancy, although the presence of disease elsewhere helps make the diagnosis. Meningitis can cause smooth leptomeningeal enhancement.
7. Dilated vessels—tortuous flow voids within CSF space. Most commonly due to a dural arteriovenous fistula (AVF); cord oedema is typically also present due to venous congestion. Other causes include AVM (intramedullary nidus/flow void also present—absent in AVF), hypervascular tumours with feeding vessels, and collateral vessels from IVC occlusion.
8. **Lipoma**—fat signal, most common posteriorly in the thoracic region.
9. **Epidermoid cyst**—either congenital (± dysraphism) or acquired secondary to lumbar puncture. Usually in the lumbosacral region, similar to arachnoid cyst on MRI but shows restricted diffusion.
10. **Dermoid cyst**—young patients; usually in lumbosacral region (± dysraphism), often contains fat ± calcification.
11. **Neurenteric cyst**—usually in the thoracic or cervical region anterior to the cord, ± vertebral anomalies. May contain T1 hyperintense proteinaceous material.
12. **Malignant peripheral nerve sheath tumour**—infiltrative heterogeneous enhancing mass ± bone destruction. Most are associated with NF1.
13. **Melanocytoma**—rare benign tumour. Typically small, T1 hyperintense, T2 hypointense, enhances. Mimics melanoma metastasis.
14. **Cysticercosis**—rare, usually associated with cerebral disease. Well-defined cyst(s) + eccentric mural nodule (scolex). Can rarely be intramedullary or epidural.

Intramedullary mass or swelling

1. Tumours.
   (a) Ependymoma—most common intramedullary tumour in adults. Cervical > thoracic location. Well-defined, T2 hyperintense + avid enhancement + peritumoural oedema ± necrosis or haemorrhage (hypointense haemosiderin rim). Cysts are often seen internally or adjacent to the upper/lower poles of the tumour. Arises from ependymal cells within the central canal, so is located centrally within the cord ± associated syrinx.
   (b) Astrocytoma—most common intramedullary tumour in children and young adults. Thoracic > cervical location.

Ill-defined, T2 hyperintense + patchy enhancement + peritumoural oedema. Can be eccentric, exophytic or involve the whole diameter of the cord. Often longer than ependymoma (>4 segments). Cystic change, haemorrhage and syrinx are less common compared to ependymoma.

(c) **Haemangioblastoma**—small, well-defined, avidly enhancing mass + extensive cord oedema, cystic change/syrinx, tortuous feeding vessels (flow voids) in subarachnoid space ± haemorrhage. Usually in the posterior cord, eccentric or exophytic; multiple in vHL.

(d) **Metastases**—small well-defined enhancing lesions + prominent cord oedema. Most commonly from lung or breast.

(e) **Lymphoma**—non-Hodgkin lymphoma is more common. Poorly defined, variable homogenous enhancement.

(f) **Ganglioglioma**—rare. Similar age group and imaging features to astrocytoma, but tumoural cysts are more common; adjacent cord oedema is less common, and cervical > thoracic location.

2. **Demyelination**—cord inflammation (T2 hyperintense) ± swelling ± variable enhancement (reflects disease activity); can mimic astrocytoma.
   (a) **Multiple sclerosis**—cord lesions are variable but usually multifocal, small (<2 vertebral segments) and involve <1/2 of the cross-sectional area of the cord. Most common in the cervical region, typically in the presence of brain involvement.
   (b) **ADEM**—acute monophasic postinfective autoimmune disorder, typically in children and adolescents. Multifocal or confluent cord lesions, nearly always in the presence of brain ± brainstem involvement.
   (c) **Neuromyelitis optica**—single very long cord lesion (>3 vertebral segments) typically involving the whole cross-sectional area, with optic nerve involvement. The brain is usually spared.
   (d) **Transverse myelitis**—many causes (e.g. infective, autoimmune, paraneoplastic), but often idiopathic. Single long cord lesion (>2 vertebral segments) involving >2/3 of the cross-sectional area, usually in the thoracic region. No brain or optic nerve involvement.
   (e) **Other myelopathies**—e.g. vasculitis (often multifocal), radiation (limited to treatment field), vitamin B12 deficiency (involves dorsal columns only), schistosomiasis (usually involves conus, history of travel to endemic area).
3. **Acute cord infarction**—often associated with aortic dissection or surgery. Central grey matter T2 hyperintensity ('owl's eye' appearance) and restricted diffusion extending >1 vertebral segment ± cord expansion, typically involving the thoracic cord.

May also involve adjacent white matter (especially anterior spinal artery territory) or whole cord cross-section.

4. Vascular malformations.
   (a) Cavernoma—well-defined T2 hyperintense lesion + hypointense foci (haemosiderin) giving a 'popcorn' appearance. Minimal enhancement. If small, may be purely T2 hypointense.
   (b) AVM—intramedullary nidus of vessels (flow voids) + multiple tortuous vessels in subarachnoid space + adjacent cord oedema ± haemorrhage. The vessels may enhance but there is no discrete enhancing mass.
5. **Spinal cord abscess**—may be due to haematogenous spread of infection (adults) or direct infection via dysraphism (children). Small ring-enhancing mass with central T2 hyperintensity and restricted diffusion, with extensive surrounding cord oedema.
6. **Dermoid/epidermoid/neurenteric cysts**—can be intramedullary.
7. **Sarcoidosis**—enhancing nodules typically in the cervical or upper thoracic cord, usually located peripherally. Intracranial and systemic disease is usually also present.

Lesions related to cauda equina

1. Any intradural extramedullary mass—see earlier.
2. Myxopapillary ependymoma (ME)—represents 90% of tumours arising from the filum terminale. Well-defined, T2 hyperintense + avid enhancement ± peripheral haemosiderin rim due to haemorrhage. Usually large, filling the spinal canal ± posterior vertebral scalloping because of slow growth.
3. Paraganglioma—usually arises from filum terminale; much less common than ME and schwannoma. Similar appearance to ME, but tends to be smaller and typically has prominent flow voids inside and outside the mass.
4. Filum terminale lipoma—fatty thickening of the filum ± cord tethering.
5. Guillain-Barré syndrome (GBS)—smooth enhancement of cauda equina ± slight thickening. Acute clinical presentation with ascending paralysis.
6. **Chronic inflammatory demyelinating polyneuropathy (CIDP)**—chronic equivalent of GBS. Similar MRI findings but nerve thickening is usually more pronounced and involves both intra- and extradural portions of the spinal nerves.
7. **Hereditary polyneuropathies**—e.g. Charcot-Marie-Tooth disease. Similar MRI findings to CIDP, but usually presents in younger patients.
8. **Other radiculopathies**—e.g. viral (CMV if immunocompromised), chemo- or radiotherapy induced. Similar appearance to GBS.

Joints

Syed Babar Ajaz, Hifz-ur-Rahman Aniq,
Andoni Toms, James MacKay

3.1 MONOARTHRITIS

Common

1. <u>**Septic arthritis**</u>—including tuberculosis. Marked juxtaarticular osteopenia with loss of definition of subchondral bone plate.
2. <u>**Trauma**</u>—evidence of fracture or lipohaemarthrosis.
3. <u>**Osteoarthritis (OA)**</u>—marginal osteophytes, subchondral sclerosis and/or cysts, joint space narrowing. Commonly involves weight-bearing joints.
4. <u>**Calcium pyrophosphate deposition disease (CPPD)**</u>—chondrocalcinosis is characteristic; most commonly seen in knee, wrist, symphysis pubis and intervertebral discs. Arthropathy mimics OA but has a characteristic distribution: radiocarpal, patellofemoral, C1/2. Large clustered subchondral cysts are common.
5. <u>**Gout**</u>—well-defined juxtaarticular erosions + periarticular soft tissue mass ± calcification (tophi—highly suggestive). The joint space and bone density are relatively preserved. Most commonly involves the hallux MTPJ; other sites include intertarsal, ankle and knee.

Less common

6. <u>**Neuropathic (Charcot) arthropathy**</u>—seven Ds: joint **d**egeneration, **d**estruction, **d**islocation, **d**eformity, **d**ebris (loose bodies), **d**istension (effusion) and increased **d**ensity (subchondral sclerosis). Due to reduced pain sensation and proprioception, most commonly seen in diabetics. The joint involved suggests the underlying cause:
   (a) <u>**Ankle/foot**</u>—<u>diabetes</u>, alcoholism, dysraphism, leprosy, congenital insensitivity to pain (young patients, multiple involved joints), amyloidosis, neurosyphilis.
   (b) **Knee**—steroid injection, alcoholism, congenital insensitivity to pain, neurosyphilis.
   (c) **Hip**—alcoholism, steroid injection, neurosyphilis.

(d) **Spine**—spinal cord injury, diabetes, syrinx (C-spine), neurosyphilis (L-spine).
(e) **Shoulder/elbow**—syrinx.
(f) **Wrist**—diabetes, syrinx.
(g) **Small joints of hand/feet**—diabetes, leprosy, congenital insensitivity to pain.

7. **Avascular necrosis**—e.g. in hip. Can mimic OA but changes mainly involve one side of the joint with relative preservation of the joint space.
8. **Monoarticular presentation of a usually polyarticular arthritis**—see Section 3.2.
9. **Viral**—typically hips in children, a.k.a. 'transient synovitis'.
10. **Pigmented villonodular synovitis (PVNS)**—well-defined erosions + synovial nodules on MRI showing low T2 signal and blooming on the gradient echo due to haemosiderin. Most cases occur in the knee; less commonly other large joints. A localized form limited to Hoffa's fat pad can also occur.
11. **Synovial osteochondromatosis**—multiple intraarticular loose bodies + calcification. Can be primary (uniform in size) or secondary (different sizes + coexistent OA).

3.2 THE MAJOR POLYARTHRITIDES

Synovial

1. **Rheumatoid arthritis***—proximal and symmetric distribution, especially MCPJs and carpus; other sites include feet (especially 5th MTPJ), knees, ankles, elbows and shoulders. Features include synovitis, juxtaarticular osteopenia, joint space narrowing, periarticular erosions, subluxation and ankylosis.
2. **Juvenile idiopathic arthritis***—presents in childhood. Common joints include hips, knees, ankles, elbows, hands and feet, C-spine. Features include soft tissue swelling, juxtaarticular osteopenia, periostitis, epiphyseal overgrowth, joint effusions and subluxation (e.g. carpus, hip, C1/2). Periarticular erosions, joint space narrowing and ankylosis are late features.

Entheseal

1. **Seronegative spondyloarthropathies**—enthesitis + proliferative entheseal erosions with preserved bone density; classically asymmetrical, oligoarticular involvement of peripheral joints.
   (a) **Psoriatic arthritis**—usually asymmetric and distal (especially distal interphalangeal joints). Can present with dactylitis ('sausage digit'). Occasionally symmetrical, resembling rheumatoid arthritis. Pencil-in-cup appearance and arthritis mutilans in severe disease. Acroosteolysis and interphalangeal joint ankylosis may be seen and are suggestive.

(b) Chronic reactive arthritis*—usually seen in young adults, following an STI or gut infection. Similar in appearance to psoriatic arthritis but the hands are typically spared. Commonly involves the feet, SIJs and spine. Calcaneal enthesitis (+ erosions) is suggestive. Dactylitis may also be seen.
(c) Ankylosing spondylitis*—typically involves SIJs and the spine. Other joints include hips, shoulders and knees.
(d) Enteropathic arthritis—associated with IBD. Distribution is similar to ankylosing spondylitis.

Degenerative

1. Osteoarthritis—e.g. hands; involves interphalangeal joints, thumb carpometacarpal and triscaphoid joints. The erosive form causes central erosions resulting in a 'gull-wing' deformity ± ankylosis.
2. Neuropathic arthropathy.

Depositional

1. Gout.
2. CPPD.
3. Haemochromatosis*—resembles CPPD but has a predilection for the index and middle finger MCPJs with hook-like osteophytes.

3.3 ARTHRITIS WITH OSTEOPENIA

1. Rheumatoid arthritis*—typically polyarticular.
2. Septic arthritis—typically monoarticular.
3. SLE*—typically causes symmetric osteopenia and joint subluxation (especially MCPJs) without erosions.
4. Systemic sclerosis—joint contractures, acroosteolysis and well-defined soft tissue calcifications (calcinosis).
5. Reactive arthritis*—juxtaarticular osteopenia in early phase.
6. Juvenile idiopathic arthritis*.
7. Haemophilic arthropathy—epiphyseal overgrowth, periarticular erosions, diffuse T2 hypointense synovial thickening + blooming on gradient echo MRI, due to recurrent haemarthrosis. Males only.

3.4 ARTHRITIS WITH PRESERVATION OF BONE DENSITY

1. Osteoarthritis.
2. CPPD.
3. Gout.
4. Seronegative spondyloarthropathies.
5. Neuropathic arthropathy.

3.5 ARTHRITIS WITH PERIOSTEAL REACTION

1. Seronegative spondyloarthropathy—mainly psoriatic arthritis (hands) and chronic reactive arthritis (feet). Fluffy appearance, represents entheseal bony proliferation.
2. Septic arthritis—associated bone destruction and/or abscess.
3. Juvenile idiopathic arthritis*—most often seen around metacarpals/metatarsals.
4. **HIV-associated arthritis**—similar to chronic reactive arthritis.

3.6 ARTHRITIS WITH PRESERVED OR WIDENED JOINT SPACE

1. Any early arthritis.
2. Gout.
3. Acromegaly*—'spade-like' terminal phalanges, enlarged sesamoids, thickened soft tissues, e.g. heel pad.
4. **SLE***.
5. **PVNS and primary synovial osteochondromatosis.**
6. **Multicentric reticulohistiocytosis**—symmetric erosive arthritis involving PIPJs and DIPJs + acroosteolysis; mimics psoriatic arthritis but with nodular soft tissue swelling.

3.7 ARTHRITIS WITH SOFT TISSUE NODULES

1. Rheumatoid arthritis*—subcutaneous rheumatoid nodules; typically on extensor surface of the forearm and other pressure points; more common in seropositive individuals. Intraarticular T2 hypointense rice bodies may also be present (also seen in infection especially TB).
2. Gout—tophi: eccentric, lobulated juxtaarticular soft tissue masses, typically around extensor tendons ± characteristic foci of calcification. Heterogeneous T2 signal on MRI.
3. PVNS—synovial nodules that bloom on gradient echo sequences ± extraarticular extension, e.g. into tendon sheath (giant cell tumour of tendon sheath).
4. Synovial chondromatosis—nonossified variant of osteochondromatosis. T2 hyperintense chondroid nodules on MRI.
5. Sarcoidosis*—periarticular granulomas causing characteristic lace-like lytic bone lesions, especially in finger phalanges.
6. **Amyloidosis***—large well-defined erosions + soft tissue swelling. On MR: low T1/T2 signal thickening of capsule, ligaments and tendons. Can involve wrists, shoulders, hips or knees; usually bilateral. History of primary/secondary amyloidosis or dialysis.
7. **Multicentric reticulohistiocytosis**—mainly involves hands.

3.8 ARTHRITIS MUTILANS

Destructive arthritis of hands and feet with resorption of bone ends and telescoping joints (*main-en-lorgnette*). Represents end-stage disease; determining the underlying cause can be difficult without supporting clinical information.

Common causes

1. **Rheumatoid arthritis***.
2. **Psoriatic arthritis**.
3. **Neuropathic arthropathy**—diabetes, leprosy or congenital insensitivity to pain. Leprosy causes distal bone resorption giving a 'licked candy stick' appearance.
4. **Juvenile idiopathic arthritis***.

Less common causes

5. **Chronic reactive arthritis***.
6. **Gout**—typically hallux MTPJ/IPJ.
7. **Mixed connective tissue disease**—acroosteolysis and sheet-like soft tissue calcification.
8. **Multicentric reticulohistiocytosis.**

3.9 ACROOSTEOSCLEROSIS

1. **Normal variant**—most common in middle-aged women.
2. **Psoriatic arthritis**—ivory phalanx.
3. **Rheumatoid arthritis***—in association with erosive disease.
4. **Systemic sclerosis**—osteosclerosis may precede or coexist with osteolysis.
5. **Any cause of sclerotic bone lesion affecting terminal phalanx**—see Sections 1.2 and 1.3.

3.10 INTRAARTICULAR LOOSE BODY

1. **Trauma**—osteochondral or avulsion fracture.
2. **Synovial osteochondromatosis**—more commonly secondary, due to OA with loose chondral bodies of different sizes ± calcification. Primary form is rare, due to synovial metaplasia with multiple uniform loose bodies (no significant OA unless late in disease).
3. **Osteochondritis dissecans**—characteristic age (adolescents) and location (femoral condyles, capitellum, talar dome).
4. **Neuropathic arthropathy**.

3.11 CALCIFICATION OF ARTICULAR CARTILAGE (CHONDROCALCINOSIS)

Common causes

1. Osteoarthritis.
2. CPPD.
3. Hyperparathyroidism*.
4. Gout.

Rare causes

5. Haemochromatosis*—similar distribution to CPPD.
6. Acromegaly*.
7. Wilson's disease.
8. Alkaptonuria*.

3.12 SACROILIITIS

The differential diagnosis depends on the distribution, but there is considerable overlap.

Bilateral symmetric

1. Ankylosing spondylitis*—associated with fine, vertical intervertebral syndesmophytes.
2. Osteoarthritis (mimic)—sclerosis ± marginal bridging osteophytes, no erosions.
3. Enteropathic arthritis—identical to ankylosing spondylitis.
4. Hyperparathyroidism (mimic)*—subchondral bone resorption, joint space widening.
5. Osteitis condensans ilii (mimic)—sclerosis on iliac side of SIJs. Seen in parous women.
6. Late manifestation of bilateral asymmetric disease.

Bilateral asymmetric

1. Psoriatic arthritis—associated with bulky, asymmetrical intervertebral syndesmophytes.
2. Chronic reactive arthritis*—identical to psoriatic arthritis.
3. Gout.
4. Early manifestation of bilateral symmetric disease.

Unilateral

1. Septic arthritis.
2. Early manifestation of bilateral disease.

3.13 WIDENING OF THE SYMPHYSIS PUBIS

>10 mm in early childhood, >6 mm in young adults, >3 mm in older adults.

Common causes

1. **Pregnancy (3rd trimester)**—usually resolves by third month postpartum.
2. **Trauma**.
3. **Osteitis pubis**—especially athletes. Subchondral bone irregularity and sclerosis.
4. **Septic arthritis**—with irregular bone destruction.

Less common causes

5. **Inflammatory arthritis**—rheumatoid arthritis or seronegative spondyloarthropathy.
6. **Hyperparathyroidism***—subperiosteal bone resorption, usually no sclerosis.
7. **Neoplasia**—direct invasion by bladder cancer, or lytic metastases.
8. **Osteonecrosis**—following radiotherapy for pelvic cancer.

3.14 PROTUSIO ACETABULI

Acetabular line projects medial to ilioischial line by >3 mm (men) or >6 mm (women).

Common causes

1. **Idiopathic**.
2. **Trauma**—typically unilateral.
3. **Rheumatoid arthritis***.
4. **Bone softening**—e.g. Paget's disease, osteomalacia, fibrous dysplasia.
5. **Chronic septic arthritis**—typically unilateral.

Less common causes

6. **Marfan* and Ehlers-Danlos* syndromes.**
7. **Osteogenesis imperfecta.**

3.15 ABNORMAL PROXIMAL FEMORAL MORPHOLOGY

Coxa magna—widened, flattened (toadstool) femoral head

1. **Developmental hip dysplasia (DDH)**—shallow acetabulum.
2. **Slipped capital femoral epiphysis (SCFE)**—medial position of femoral head relative to femoral neck.

3. Perthes' disease—normal position of femoral head and acetabulum.
4. Juvenile idiopathic arthritis*.
5. **Previous trauma.**
6. **Previous septic arthritis.**

Coxa plana—flattened, sclerotic femoral head

1. Any cause of avascular necrosis—especially Perthes' disease. See Section 1.26.

Coxa valga—femoral angle increased (femoral neck more vertical)

1. Neuromuscular disorders—most commonly cerebral palsy, resulting from abductor muscle weakness or adductor spasticity.
2. **Previous femoral neck fracture.**
3. **Juvenile idiopathic arthritis*.**
4. **Hereditary multiple exostoses.**
5. **Skeletal dysplasias**—e.g. mucopolysaccharidoses, diastrophic dwarfism.

Coxa vara—femoral angle reduced (femoral neck more horizontal)

Common causes

1. Developmental hip dysplasia.
2. Slipped capital femoral epiphysis.
3. Perthes' disease.
4. Previous femoral neck fracture.
5. Previous septic arthritis.
6. Bone softening—e.g. osteomalacia, rickets (metaphyseal fraying), Paget's disease, fibrous dysplasia (characteristic shepherd's crook deformity).
7. Idiopathic—coxa vara of childhood.

Less common causes

8. **Skeletal dysplasias**—e.g. osteogenesis imperfecta, multiple epiphyseal dysplasia, cleidocranial dysplasia.
9. **Proximal focal femoral deficiency**—congenital, usually unilateral. Rudimentary or absent femoral head/neck + variable shortening of shaft ± pseudarthrosis.

3.16 ENLARGEMENT OF THE DISTAL FEMORAL INTERCONDYLAR NOTCH

Common causes

1. Juvenile idiopathic arthritis*.
2. Haemophilia—males only; can look identical to juvenile idiopathic arthritis. A dense joint effusion (haemarthrosis), if present, favours haemophilia.

3. **Rheumatoid arthritis*.**
4. **Psoriatic arthritis.**
5. **Postoperative**—notchplasty common as part of anterior cruciate ligament reconstruction.

Less common causes

6. **Septic arthritis**—especially indolent (e.g. mycobacterial) infection.
7. **Gout.**
8. **PVNS.**
9. **Synovial osteochondromatosis.**
10. **Synovial haemangioma**—large feeding vessels on cross-sectional imaging.

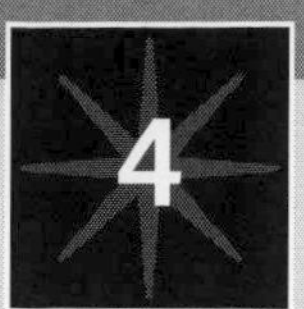

Soft tissues

Hifz-ur-Rahman Aniq, Syed Babar Ajaz, Andoni Toms, James MacKay

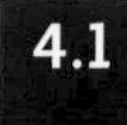

4.1 LINEAR AND CURVILINEAR SOFT TISSUE CALCIFICATION

Common causes

1. Arterial—i.e. atherosclerosis. If seen in the hands or feet, this suggests underlying diabetes or hyperparathyroidism (secondary > primary). Calcification can also be seen in aneurysms (e.g. popliteal).
2. Cartilage—i.e. chondrocalcinosis; suggests CPPD.
3. Ligament/tendon.
   - (a) **Calcific tendonitis**—i.e. hydroxyapatite deposition disease (HADD). Commonly involves supraspinatus and gluteus medius tendons.
   - (b) **Seronegative spondyloarthropathy**—entheseal calcification.
   - (c) **Alkaptonuria***—rare.
   - (d) **Fluorosis**—rare.

Less common causes

4. **Neural**—characteristic of leprosy.
5. **Parasites.**

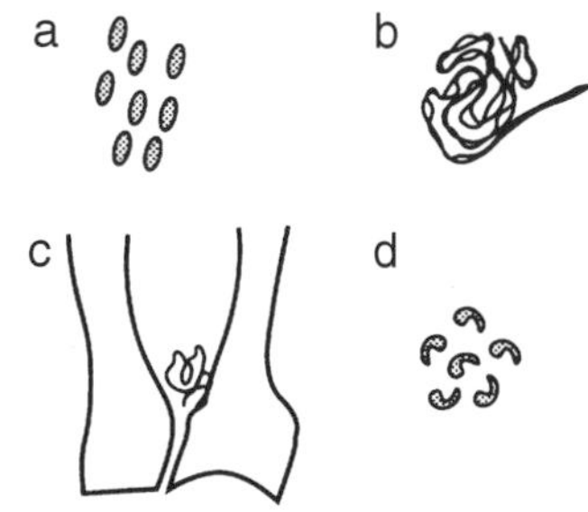

   - (a) **Cysticercosis***—oval with lucent centre. Often arranged in direction of muscle fibres.
   - (b) **Guinea worm**—irregular, coiled appearance.
   - (c) **Loa loa**—thread-like coil, in web spaces of hand.
   - (d) **Armillifer**—comma-shaped, in trunk muscles.

4.2 SOFT TISSUE CALCIFICATION

Common causes

1. Dystrophic calcification—calcification in abnormal tissue in the presence of normal calcium metabolism.
   (a) Previous trauma.
      (i) Injection granuloma—typically in gluteal region.
      (ii) Haematoma.
      (iii) **Calcific myonecrosis**—may occur without history of trauma, especially in diabetics. Amorphous calcification.
      (iv) **Burn injury.**
   (b) Connective tissue disease.
      (i) Systemic sclerosis—nodular, periarticular or subcutaneous calcification especially in the hands.
      (ii) Dermatomyositis/polymyositis—typically bilateral and symmetrical sheet-like calcification in skin and muscles, most common around the hips and in the thighs.
      (iii) **SLE***—can be nodular or sheet-like.
      (iv) **Mixed connective tissue disease**—nodular or sheet-like.
      (v) **Ehlers-Danlos syndrome***—nodular subcutaneous calcification over bony prominences.
      (vi) **Pseudoxanthoma elasticum.**
   (c) Arthropathy.
      (i) Tophi—gout; also rarely CPPD.
      (ii) **Rheumatoid nodules**—may calcify.
   (d) Venous (phleboliths)—oval with lucent centre, associated with venous insufficiency (± lacy subcutaneous calcification), but also seen in soft tissue haemangiomas. A deep vein thrombosis (DVT) may also calcify.

Less common causes

2. 'Metastatic' calcification—calcification in normal tissues in the presence of abnormal calcium metabolism. May be the result of chronic hypercalcaemia from any cause, particularly in dialysis patients. It has an identical appearance to tumoural calcinosis, but other features of secondary hyperparathyroidism are often present.
3. Tumoural calcinosis—rare, autosomal dominant, usually in Afro-Caribbeans. Well-defined lobulated calcified masses occur on the extensor surfaces of large joints. Internal fluid levels, if present, are highly suggestive (also seen in metastatic calcification).
4. Neoplasia.
   (a) Benign.
      (i) Haemangioma—multiple clustered phleboliths in an unusual distribution.
      (ii) **Chondroma**—chondroid calcification, often periarticular.

(iii) **Nerve sheath tumours**—e.g. ancient schwannoma.
(iv) **Pilomatricoma**—most common in the head or neck of children and adolescents. Benign tumour of the hair follicle, so located at the deep margin of the dermis.

(b) Malignant—most sarcomas can contain calcification; the commonest are:
(i) **Synovial sarcoma**—typically found in young adults in the lower limb close to a joint (especially the knee). 30% contain calcification.
(ii) **Liposarcoma**—may contain variable amounts of dystrophic calcification.
(iii) **Chondrosarcoma**—chondroid calcification. Can mimic chondroma but usually larger + adjacent bone erosion.

4.3 SOFT TISSUE OSSIFICATION

1. **Trauma.**
   (a) **Myositis ossificans**—posttraumatic soft tissue ossification (usually intramuscular) that evolves over weeks to months. Starts as an ill-defined osteoid matrix, which matures to bone with a dense periphery and a less dense centre. In the early stage this can mimic an aggressive lesion on plain film or MRI—follow-up imaging may be required.
   (b) **Postsurgical**—especially after hip replacement.
2. **Paralysis**—usually around large joints.
3. **Parosteal osteosarcoma**—arises from the outer periosteum. May mimic myositis ossificans, except density is highest centrally rather than peripherally. Extraskeletal osteosarcomas (arising within soft tissues) can also rarely occur.
4. **Fibrodysplasia ossificans progressiva**—hereditary; progressive mature ossification of muscles, ligaments and tendons. Sternocleidomastoid is often the first site of involvement.

4.4 SOFT TISSUE MASSES—DIFFERENTIATION ON MRI

Most soft tissue masses are T1 hypo- to isointense and T2 hyper- to isointense relative to skeletal muscle, so these features are usually not helpful in narrowing the differential diagnosis. In contrast, lesions that are T1 hyperintense, T2 hypointense or T2 bright (i.e. cyst-like) have a relatively limited list of differentials.

T1 hyperintense

1. Mass containing fat—these will show signal suppression on fat-sat sequences.
   (a) Lipomatous tumours.
      (i) Lipoma—benign, very common. Composed of pure fat with no solid elements apart from thin septa. The signal suppresses completely on fat-sat sequences. Usually subcutaneous in location, but can occur anywhere. Beware of lipomas deep to the subcutaneous fascia—biopsy is often required to exclude a well-differentiated liposarcoma, especially in the mediastinum or retroperitoneum (lipomas are rare here).
      (ii) Atypical lipomatous tumour/well-differentiated liposarcoma—predominantly fatty mass containing thick septa or small nonfatty nodules (<1 cm).
      (iii) Dedifferentiated liposarcoma—fatty mass with a large nonfatty nodular component (>1 cm) representing an area of dedifferentiation.
      (iv) **Myxoid liposarcoma**—often contains little fat. T2 bright, mimicking a cyst (see later section).
      (v) **Pleomorphic liposarcoma**—high grade; usually contains minimal fat, mimicking other sarcomas.
      (vi) **Lipoma variants**—e.g. lipoblastoma (young children only), angiolipoma, myolipoma, spindle cell lipoma, chondroid lipoma. These are benign but contain enhancing solid elements, mimicking liposarcoma.
   (b) Fat necrosis—subcutaneous fatty lesion + a thick hypointense capsule ± calcification. Most common in the gluteal region.
   (c) Haemangioma—contains streaky or lace-like areas of fat ± hypointense phleboliths.
   (d) Elastofibroma—classic location between the scapula and ribcage. Contains fibrous tissue and streaks of fat; may mimic the striated appearance of skeletal muscle.
   (e) **Hibernoma**—benign tumour of brown fat. T1 signal is usually not as high as normal fat. Well-defined, usually contains prominent feeding vessels (unlike liposarcoma), and often enhances avidly. High uptake on PET.
   (f) **Lipomatosis of nerve**—diffuse fatty infiltration along nerve fibres; most common in the median nerve. May be associated with macrodactyly (localised gigantism of one or more digits) due to overgrowth of fat and bone.
   (g) **Myositis ossificans**—when mature, contains fatty marrow elements.
2. Mass containing haemorrhage—e.g. subacute haematoma (no enhancement), haemorrhagic tumour (usually has enhancing components).

3. **Mass containing proteinaceous fluid**—e.g. ganglion, abscess, chronic seroma.
4. **Melanoma**—including melanoma metastases.

T2 hypointense

1. **Fibrotic mass**.
   (a) **Fibroma of tendon sheath**—typically found on tendons in the hand or wrist. Small T2 hypointense nodule, variable enhancement.
   (b) **Nodular fasciitis**—usually <4 cm, attached to subcutaneous or muscle fascia. Early lesions are cellular and T2 hyperintense, more mature lesions are collagenous and T2 hypointense. Usually shows diffuse enhancement. Tender and rapidly growing; can be well- or ill-defined. Most common benign lesion mistaken for sarcoma.
   (c) **Desmoid tumour**—usually painless (unlike nodular fasciitis). Typically very infiltrative (more so than sarcomas), with variable diffuse enhancement and no internal necrosis or haemorrhage (unlike sarcomas). Can be T2 hyperintense (early and cellular), hypointense (mature and collagenous) or mixed. Occurs in three locations:
      (i) **Anterior abdominal wall**—commonest tumour of the abdominal wall, typically associated with pregnancy. Often occurs at caesarean-section scar.
      (ii) **Intraabdominal**—usually in the mesentery but can be retroperitoneal or pelvic. Often associated with Gardner syndrome.
      (iii) **Intramuscular**—e.g. shoulder and hip girdles, chest wall, back, neck. Can be sporadic or associated with Gardner syndrome (especially if multiple).
   (d) **Elastofibroma**—may be mainly fibrotic with minimal fat.
   (e) **Fibrosarcoma**—lobulated mass with heterogeneous signal and enhancement ± areas of necrosis or haemorrhage. Can contain T2 hypointense bands of collagen.
2. **Mass containing calcium**—any cause of soft tissue calcification or ossification.
3. **Mass containing haemosiderin**.
   (a) **Endometrioma**—especially in caesarean-section scar. Can mimic desmoid tumour.
   (b) **Giant cell tumour of tendon sheath**—extraarticular form of pigmented villonodular synovitis (NB: can also occur in bursae). May mimic fibroma of the tendon sheath, but demonstrates blooming on gradient echo sequences.
4. **Mass containing flow voids**—e.g. aneurysm, AVM.
5. **Mass containing gas**—e.g. abscess.

Homogenously T2 bright (cyst-like)

No enhancement/rim enhancement only post IV gadolinium

1. **Degenerative/idiopathic**—e.g. epidermal inclusion cyst (aka sebaceous cyst, attached to dermis), ganglion cyst (associated with a joint, especially the wrist), bursa (e.g. iliopsoas bursa and many others), paralabral cyst (shoulder/hip), meniscal cyst (knee).
2. **Traumatic**—e.g. haematoma, seroma, lymphocele (related to lymphadenectomy) or Morel-Lavallée lesion (subcutaneous shearing injury resulting in a fluid collection ± fat globules, typically located over the greater trochanter, knee or scapula).
3. **Abscess**—usually has thick, irregular rim enhancement with surrounding oedema (except tuberculous 'cold' abscess).
4. **Lymphangioma**—multiloculated, often traverses compartments. Usually presents in childhood.
5. **Cysticercosis***—small intramuscular cyst + hypointense scolex; often multiple.
6. **Hydatid cyst**—rare in soft tissues.

Internal enhancement post IV gadolinium

1. **Peripheral nerve sheath tumour**—arises from nerve, either eccentric (schwannoma) or central/fusiform (neurofibroma). A peripheral rim of fat (split fat sign) is typical. Can occasionally be homogenously T2 bright without the characteristic central hypointensity (target sign). Large schwannomas can undergo cystic degeneration.
2. **Haemangioma**—T2 bright + streaks of fat ± hypointense phleboliths. Usually shows avid or delayed internal enhancement depending on speed of internal blood flow.
3. **Glomus tumour**—characteristic location under nailbed. Enhances avidly.
4. **Myxoma**—benign, typically intramuscular + a thin rim of fat. Mimics a cyst on T1/T2, but usually shows mild to moderate internal enhancement. Flame-shaped oedema is often seen extending along the muscle fibres at the poles of the mass.
5. **Myxoid sarcomas**—e.g. myxofibrosarcoma (older adults), fibromyxoid sarcoma (young adults), myxoid liposarcoma (small foci of fat), extraskeletal myxoid chondrosarcoma. Can mimic myxoma but often more heterogeneous with no rim of fat.
6. **Synovial sarcoma**—can be well-defined and homogenously T2 bright when small, mimicking a benign lesion, but usually shows avid enhancement and may contain hypointense calcification, haemorrhage or fluid-fluid levels.
7. **Other necrotic/cystic malignancies**—e.g. undifferentiated pleomorphic sarcoma, cystic or mucinous metastases.
8. **Hidradenoma**—arises from the dermis (sweat glands), usually benign. Often contains enhancing nodular components.

Chest

Patrick Wong, Thomas Semple

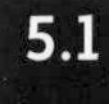

5.1 TRACHEAL/BRONCHIAL NARROWING, MASS OR OCCLUSION

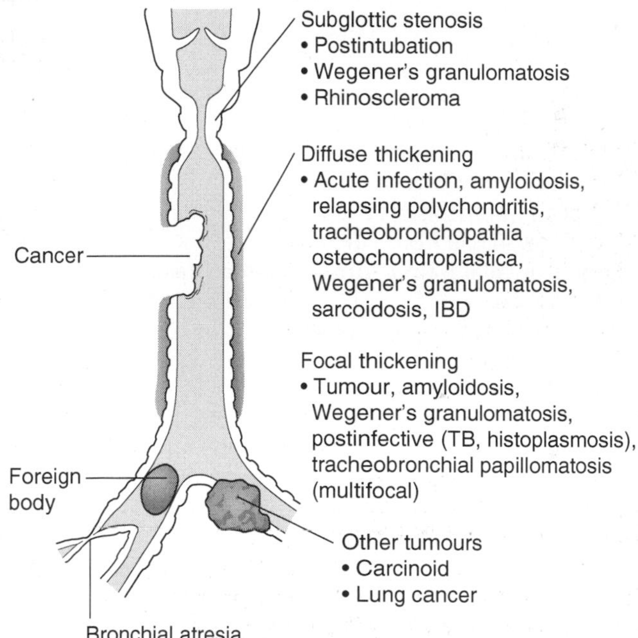

Airway narrowing may occur at any site from below the level of the vocal cords down to the segmental/subsegmental airways.

In the lumen

1. **Mucous plug**—e.g. asthma, cystic fibrosis, ABPA. Low density, usually contains gas bubbles.
2. **Foreign body**—air trapping is more common than atelectasis. Most frequently affects the lower lobes. The foreign body may be opaque. The column of air within the bronchus may be discontinuous ('interrupted bronchus sign').

3. Misplaced endotracheal tube.
4. **Broncholithiasis**—usually caused by a calcified lymph node (e.g. from previous TB or histoplasmosis) eroding into the adjacent bronchus.

Arising from the wall

1. Tracheal/bronchial tumours.
   (a) **Squamous cell carcinoma**—commonest tumour in the trachea and bronchi, associated with smoking. Irregular polypoid mass or focal wall thickening and narrowing. Small cell lung cancer can also be endobronchial.
   (b) **Carcinoid tumour**—second most common bronchial tumour. Usually a smooth, rounded enhancing mass ± calcification. Main tumour bulk may lie outside the lumen.
   (c) **Adenoid cystic carcinoma**—second most common tracheal tumour. Low grade, usually in young adults. Focal or diffuse mass, often extending beyond the tracheal wall. Typically extends longitudinally along the submucosa of the trachea.
   (d) **Metastasis**—e.g. from melanoma, RCC, colon, breast. Rare.
   (e) **Mucoepidermoid carcinoma**—rare, usually in lobar or segmental bronchi, most common in young adults. Indistinguishable from carcinoid.
   (f) **Endobronchial hamartoma**—often contains fat and calcification.
   (g) **Tracheobronchial papillomatosis**—due to HPV infection. Multiple small polyps in the larynx > trachea > bronchi ± cavitating lung nodules.
   (h) **Other rare tumours**—e.g. inflammatory myofibroblastic tumour (especially in children), lymphoma/PTLD, sarcomas, lipoma, leiomyoma, haemangioma, fibroma, granular cell tumour.
2. Inflammation/infiltration/fibrosis
   (a) **Wegener's granulomatosis**—typically causes focal subglottic stenosis, usually with concurrent lung involvement.
   (b) **Infection**—e.g. previous TB (look for calcified granulomas and nodes), fungal infection (in immunocompromised patients) and rhinoscleroma (tropical granulomatous infection, typically involves the nasal passages, but can spread to larynx and trachea).
   (c) **Amyloidosis***—irregular focal or circumferential tracheal thickening ± calcification, does not spare the posterior wall.
   (d) **Relapsing polychondritis**—diffuse smooth tracheal thickening, narrowing ± calcification, spares the posterior (noncartilaginous) tracheal wall. Also involves cartilage of ears, nose and larynx.

(e) **Tracheobronchopathia osteochondroplastica**—diffuse nodular tracheal thickening + coarse calcification, spares the posterior tracheal wall.
(f) **Sarcoidosis***—tracheal involvement rare, usually in the presence of lung and nodal disease.
(g) **Inflammatory bowel disease***—can rarely cause tracheal inflammation and narrowing. Ulcerative colitis > Crohn's.

3. **Bronchial atresia**—most commonly in the apicoposterior segment of the left upper lobe. Surrounding hyperlucent lung; mucus plug often seen distal to the atretic bronchus.
4. **Tracheobronchomalacia**—manifests as a normal/dilated trachea on inspiration with excessive dynamic airway collapse (EDAC) on expiration—AP diameter of trachea reduced by >50%. Most common causes are ageing, COPD and prolonged intubation; others include connective tissue diseases, chronic inflammation and Mounier-Kuhn syndrome.
5. **Tracheobronchial injury**—e.g. due to prolonged intubation, tracheostomy, inhaled toxins, burns, radiotherapy or trauma. Results in a smooth stenosis.
6. **Congenital tracheal stenosis**—due to complete cartilage rings (as opposed to normal C-shaped cartilage). Usually presents in childhood.

Outside the wall

1. **Lymphadenopathy**—e.g. due to malignancy, sarcoidosis, TB.
2. **Mediastinal masses**—e.g. retrosternal goitre, primary tumours, duplication cysts, mediastinal invasion by lung cancers. Smooth, eccentric airway narrowing due to extrinsic compression. Narrowing may be irregular if the airway is directly invaded by tumour.
3. **Fibrosing mediastinitis**—idiopathic or resulting from histoplasmosis, radiotherapy, autoimmune diseases, etc.
4. **Enlarged left atrium or grossly enlarged pulmonary arteries**—e.g. in Eisenmenger's syndrome or absent pulmonary valve.
5. **Aortic aneurysm**—indents left side of distal trachea.
6. **Left pulmonary artery sling**—due to the anomalous origin of the left pulmonary artery (LPA) from the right pulmonary artery (RPA), compressing the right main bronchus as it passes between the trachea and oesophagus to reach the left hilum. PA CXR shows right-sided tracheal indentation, and the vessel is seen end-on between the trachea and oesophagus on the lateral view. LPA sling is often associated with complete cartilage rings, causing further narrowing. Other vascular rings and slings (e.g. double aortic arch) can also cause tracheal narrowing.

Further reading

Chung, J.H., Kanne, J.P., Gilman, M.D., 2011. Structured review article – CT of diffuse tracheal diseases. AJR Am. J. Roentgenol. 196, W240–W246.

Semple, T., Calder, A., Owens, C.M., Padley, S., 2017. Current and future approaches to large airways imaging in adults and children. Clin. Radiol. 72, 352–374.

5.2 BRONCHIECTASIS

Bronchiectasis is permanent (localized or diffuse) airway dilatation, and is more reliably identified on CT than CXR, particularly with mild disease. On CT, dilated bronchi manifest as either nontapering airways ('tramlines'—airways imaged in longitudinal section) or 'signet-ring' opacities (i.e. a bronchus of increased diameter compared to its adjacent pulmonary artery branch). In severe disease, large cystic airway dilatations ± air–fluid levels may be present. Ancillary signs of bronchiectasis include volume loss, mucus plugging (including distal small airways resulting in a tree-in-bud pattern) and mosaic attenuation.

Causes of bronchiectasis

1. **Postinfective**
   (a) **TB***—upper lobes, look for calcified granulomas and nodes.
   (b) ***Mycobacterium avium* complex**—middle lobe and lingula, usually in older women (Lady Windermere syndrome).
   (c) **Chronic aspiration**—typically in lower lobes.
   (d) **Swyer-James syndrome**—secondary to childhood infection, e.g. measles, pertussis. Affected lung is hyperlucent with a paucity of vessels and may be small.
   (e) **Immunodeficiency**—e.g. HIV, post transplant, hypogammaglobulinaemia, severe combined immunodeficiency, common variable immunodeficiency, Chédiak-Higashi syndrome.
2. **Traction bronchiectasis**—in areas of lung fibrosis.
3. **Cystic fibrosis***—widespread bronchiectasis.
4. **Idiopathic**—no apparent cause in up to one-third of patients.
5. **Secondary to bronchial obstruction**—foreign body, neoplasm, broncholithiasis or bronchial stenosis.
6. **Congenital/genetic anomalies**
   (a) **Primary ciliary dyskinesia**—results in poor mucociliary clearance, recurrent infection and bronchiectasis (especially lower lobes). Associated chronic sinusitis, recurrent otitis media and fertility problems. ~50% have situs abnormalities, hence the classical triad of Kartagener syndrome (bronchiectasis, dextrocardia, chronic sinusitis).

(b) Mounier-Kuhn syndrome—also known as tracheobronchomegaly. Grossly dilated trachea (often >3 cm) and bronchi with diverticulosis between cartilage rings.
(c) **Williams-Campbell syndrome**—bronchial cartilage deficiency. Similar appearance to Mounier-Kuhn except trachea and proximal bronchi are spared.
(d) **Alpha-1 antitrypsin deficiency***—basal predominant panlobular emphysema is characteristic.

7. Immunological—ABPA (focal central bronchiectasis in an asthmatic patient, usually mucous-filled), obliterative bronchiolitis (look for mosaic attenuation due to air trapping).
8. **Collagen vascular diseases**—especially rheumatoid arthritis, Sjögren's syndrome.
9. **Gastrointestinal disorders**—ulcerative colitis, coeliac disease.

5

Upper zone predominant	• Cystic fibrosis • Post TB • Sarcoidosis
Middle zone predominant	• ABPA • *Mycobacterium avium* complex infection
Lower zone predominant	• Postinfective—staphyloccocal, whooping cough, measles, influenza, chronic aspiration, immunodeficiency • Primary ciliary dyskinesia • Alpha-1 antitrypsin deficiency • Obliterative bronchiolitis

Further reading

Hansell, D.M., Lynch, D.A., McAdams, H.P., Bankier, A.A., 2010. Diseases of the airways. In: Imaging of Diseases of the Chest, fifth ed. Elsevier Mosby, Philadelphia, PA.

Semple, T., Calder, A., Owens, C.M., Padley, S., 2017. Current and future approaches to large airways imaging in adults and children. Clin. Radiol. 72, 352–374.

5.3 UNILATERAL HYPERTRANSRADIANT HEMITHORAX

A paucity or decrease in the number of vessels on one side indicates an abnormal lung. Discrepancy in density despite an approximately equal number and calibre of vessels in both lungs suggests that the contralateral hemithorax is of increased density, e.g. caused by a pleural effusion (in a supine patient) or pleural thickening. Note that a rotated film will make the side to which the patient is turned appear hyperlucent.

Chest wall

1. **Mastectomy**—absent breast ± absent pectoral muscle shadows.
2. **Poliomyelitis**—atrophy of pectoral muscles ± atrophic changes in the shoulder girdle and humerus.
3. **Poland syndrome**—unilateral congenital absence of pectoral muscles ± rib defects. Seen in 10% of patients with syndactyly.

Pleura

Pneumothorax—note the visceral pleural edge and absent vessels peripherally. In supine patients look for the deep sulcus sign or abnormally well-defined mediastinal and diaphragmatic contours.

Lung

1. **Compensatory hyperexpansion**—e.g. following lobectomy (look for rib defects and sutures indicating previous surgery) or lobar collapse.
2. **Airway obstruction**—air trapping on expiration results in increased lung volume and contralateral mediastinal shift.
3. **Unilateral bullae**—vessels are absent rather than attenuated. May mimic pneumothorax.
4. **Swyer-James syndrome**—the late sequela of bronchiolitis in childhood (usually viral). Normal or reduced lung volume with air trapping on expiration. Ipsilateral hilar vessels are small. CT often shows bilateral disease with mosaic attenuation and bronchiectasis.
5. **Congenital lobar overinflation**—previously known as congenital lobar emphysema. One-third present clinically at birth, the remainder later in life. Marked overinflation of a lobe (left upper > right middle > right upper). The ipsilateral lobes are compressed ± contralateral mediastinal shift.

Pulmonary vessels

Pulmonary embolus—to a main/lobar pulmonary artery. In addition to the area of hyperlucency (Westermark sign), the pulmonary artery is dilated proximally ± ipsilateral loss of volume. NB: this sign is only present in 2% of PEs, and small emboli are unlikely to result in any disparity.

5.4 BILATERAL HYPERTRANSRADIANT HEMITHORACES

With overexpansion of the lungs

1. Emphysema—± bullae; centrilobular emphysema typically in mid/upper zones, whereas panlobular emphysema commonly affects lower zones.
2. Asthma—during an acute episode or in chronic disease with 'fixed' airflow obstruction due to airway remodelling.
3. Acute bronchiolitis—particularly in infants. Overexpansion is due to small airways (bronchiolar) obstruction. May be associated with bronchial wall thickening on CXR. Collapse and consolidation are not primary features of bronchiolitis.
4. **Tracheal, laryngeal or bilateral bronchial stenoses**—see Section 5.1.

With normal or small lungs

1. Bilateral anterior pneumothoraces—seen in postoperative patients imaged supine, most commonly neonates/infants.
2. Pulmonary oligaemia—due to cyanotic heart disease.

Further reading

Engelke, C., Schaefer-Prokop, C., Schirg, E., et al., 2002. High-resolution CT and CT angiography of peripheral pulmonary vascular disorders. Radiographics 22, 739–764.

Frazier, A.A., Galvin, J.R., Franks, T.J., Rosado-De-Christenson, M.L., 2000. Pulmonary vasculature: hypertension and infarction. Radiographics 20, 491–524.

5.5 INCREASED DENSITY OF ONE HEMITHORAX

With an undisplaced mediastinum

1. Consolidation—see Section 5.6.
2. Pleural effusion—on a supine CXR, an uncomplicated effusion gravitates to the dependent part of the chest, producing a generalized increased density ± an apical 'cap' of fluid. Note that pulmonary vessels will be visible through the increased density (cf. consolidation). Erect or decubitus CXRs or US may confirm the diagnosis.
3. Malignant pleural mesothelioma—often associated with a pleural effusion that obscures the tumour ± calcified pleural plaques (better seen on CT). Encasement of the lung limits mediastinal shift; the affected hemithorax may even be smaller.

With mediastinal displacement away from the dense hemithorax

1. **Large pleural effusion**—NB: a large effusion with no mediastinal shift indicates significant lung collapse (and central obstruction) or relative 'fixation' of the mediastinum (e.g. caused by malignant pleural mesothelioma).
2. **Very large intrathoracic tumour**—e.g. solitary fibrous tumour of pleura (older adults), Ewing sarcoma of chest wall (children and young adults). These can be large enough to fill the entire hemithorax.
3. **Diaphragmatic hernia**—on the right side with herniated liver; on the left side the hemithorax is not usually opaque because of air within the herniated bowel (except in the early neonatal period when air may not yet have reached the herniated bowel).

With mediastinal displacement towards the dense hemithorax

1. **Lung collapse**.
2. **Post pneumonectomy**—look for surgical clips and rib defects.
3. **Lymphangitis carcinomatosa**—bilateral and symmetrical infiltration is most common; unilateral lymphangitis occurs more often with lung cancer. Linear and nodular opacities + septal lines ± ipsilateral hilar and mediastinal lymphadenopathy. Pleural effusions are common.
4. **Pulmonary agenesis, aplasia or hypoplasia**—usually asymptomatic. Absent or hypoplastic pulmonary artery. Agenesis is the absence of lung and bronchus; aplasia is absence of lung with rudimentary bronchus, and hypoplasia is the presence of a bronchial tree with variable underdevelopment of lung volume.
5. **Malignant pleural mesothelioma**—see earlier.

5.6 AIR-SPACE OPACIFICATION/ CONSOLIDATION

Results in increased parenchymal density obscuring visibility of vessels and bronchial walls ± air bronchograms. Note that any of the following may be unilateral or confined to a single lobe.

1. **Oedema**—air spaces filled with fluid. See Section 5.12.
2. **Infection**—air spaces filled with pus.
3. **Diffuse pulmonary haemorrhage**—e.g. Goodpasture's syndrome, Wegener's granulomatosis, idiopathic pulmonary haemosiderosis, microscopic polyangiitis, SLE, Behçet's disease, contusion, bleeding diatheses, pulmonary infarction.

4. **Malignancy**—adenocarcinoma and lymphoma can both appear as an area (or areas) of consolidation.
5. **Sarcoidosis***—an 'air-space' pattern can be seen in up to 20%, due to filling of air spaces by macrophages and granulomatous infiltration.
6. **Chronic eosinophilic pneumonia**—characteristically nonsegmental, upper zone predominant and peripheral, paralleling the chest wall.
7. **Organizing pneumonia**—may be cryptogenic or as a response to another 'insult', e.g. infection, drug toxicity, connective tissue disease. Typically there are multifocal air-space opacities in the periphery of mid/lower zones. Occasionally unifocal. A characteristic perilobular distribution may be seen. Another pattern is the 'reverse halo' or atoll sign (a ring of consolidation surrounding a central area of GGO).
8. **Lipoid pneumonia**—due to aspiration of ingested or inhaled oils. Consolidation tends to be basal and has an attenuation close to fat on CT.

5

5.7 NONRESOLVING OR RECURRENT CONSOLIDATION

1. **Bronchial obstruction**—e.g. caused by a tumour or foreign body.
2. **Inappropriate antimicrobial therapy**—e.g. in unsuspected TB, *Klebsiella* or fungal infection.
3. **Malignancy**—adenocarcinoma, lymphoma.
4. **Recurrent aspiration**—due to a pharyngeal pouch/cleft, achalasia, systemic sclerosis, hiatus hernia, paralytic/neuromuscular disorders, chronic sinusitis or 'H' type tracheooesophageal fistula (in infants).
5. **Preexisting lung pathology**—e.g. bronchiectasis.
6. **Impaired immunity**—e.g. prolonged steroid or other immunosuppressive therapy, immunoglobulin deficiency, diabetes, cachexia, HIV.
7. **Organizing pneumonia.**
8. **Sarcoidosis*.**
9. **Vasculitis**—e.g. Wegener's, Churg-Strauss.

Further reading

Franquet, T., Giménez, A., Rosón, N., et al., 2000. Aspiration diseases: findings, pitfalls and differential diagnosis. Radiographics 20, 673–685.

5.8 MIGRATORY CONSOLIDATION

Transient air-space opacities that change in location over time.

1. **Organizing pneumonia**—peripheral mid-lower zone distribution.
2. **Recurrent aspiration**—typically in lower zones.

3. **Pulmonary eosinophilia**—both simple pulmonary eosinophilia (Löffler syndrome, resolves spontaneously within 1 month) and chronic eosinophilic pneumonia (persists for several months). Peripheral upper zone distribution.
4. **Pulmonary haemorrhage/infarcts/vasculitis.**
5. **Alveolar proteinosis.**

5.9 CONSOLIDATION WITH AN ENLARGED HILUM

Hilar lymphadenopathy may be secondary to pneumonia, or pneumonia may be secondary to bronchial obstruction caused by a hilar mass. Signs suggestive of a secondary pneumonia include segmental or lobar consolidation, slow resolution, local recurrence and associated volume loss/lobar collapse.

Secondary pneumonias

See Section 5.1, but note particularly lung cancer/other tumours.

Primary pneumonias

1. **Primary TB***—lymphadenopathy is unilateral in 80% and involves hilar ± paratracheal nodes.
2. **Viral pneumonias.**
3. ***Mycoplasma* pneumonia**—lymphadenopathy is common in children but rare in adults. May be unilateral or bilateral.
4. **Primary histoplasmosis**—in endemic areas. Hilar lymphadenopathy is common, particularly in children. Upon healing lymph nodes calcify and may obstruct bronchi (broncholith) causing distal infection.
5. **Coccidioidomycosis**—in endemic areas. The pneumonic type consists of predominantly lower lobe consolidation frequently associated with hilar lymphadenopathy.

5.10 PNEUMONIA INVOLVING ALL OR PART OF ONE LOBE

Segmental or lobar consolidation (± a degree of collapse) is most often caused by the following organisms:

1. **Streptococcal pneumonia**—most common cause. Usually unilobar. Cavitation is rare; pleural effusion uncommon. Little or no collapse.
2. ***Klebsiella* pneumonia** – often multilobar. High propensity for cavitation and lobar enlargement (bulging the adjacent fissure).
3. **Staphylococcal pneumonia**—especially in children, 40% to 60% of whom develop pneumatocoeles. Parapneumonic effusion,

empyema and pneumothorax are common complications. Bronchopleural fistula may develop.
4. TB*—primary > postprimary; right lung > left lung. Associated collapse is common. Primary TB has a predilection for the anterior segment of upper lobes or medial segment of the middle lobe.
5. ***Streptococcus pyogenes* pneumonia**—mainly affects the lower lobes. Often associated with pleural effusion or empyema.

5.11 CONSOLIDATION WITH BULGING OF FISSURES

1. Infection with abundant exudates—pneumonia caused by *Klebsiella pneumoniae, Streptococcus pneumoniae, Mycobacterium tuberculosis* or *Yersinia pestis* (plague).
2. **Abscess**—when an area of consolidation breaks down. Organisms that commonly produce abscesses include *Staphylococcus aureus, Klebsiella* spp. and other gram-negative organisms.
3. **Lung cancer**—adenocarcinoma can fill and expand a lobe.

5.12 PULMONARY OEDEMA

Defined as an increase in extravascular pulmonary fluid due to cardiogenic or noncardiogenic causes. See Section 5.13 for unilateral causes.

Cardiogenic pulmonary oedema

Any cause of mitral valve dysfunction or impaired LV function.

Noncardiogenic pulmonary oedema

1. Fluid overload—excess IV fluids, renal failure, excess hypertonic fluids (e.g. contrast media).
2. Acute respiratory distress syndrome—may be primary (e.g. caused by severe pneumonia, aspiration) or secondary (e.g. following nonthoracic sepsis or trauma); CXR may be normal in the first 24 hours but shows progressive widespread opacification due to interstitial and then alveolar oedema and haemorrhagic fluid.
3. Cerebral disease—stroke, head injury, raised intracranial pressure or large shunt (e.g. vein of Galen malformation).
4. Near drowning—no significant radiological difference between freshwater and seawater drowning.
5. Aspiration—of acidic gastric contents causing a chemical pneumonitis (Mendelson's syndrome).
6. Liver disease—and other causes of hypoproteinaemia.

7. <u>Transfusion-related acute lung injury (TRALI)</u>—most common cause of transfusion-related mortality in the UK. Onset of oedema is either during transfusion or within 1–2 hours.
8. <u>Drug-induced</u>—includes those which induce cardiac arrhythmias or depress myocardial contractility, and those which alter pulmonary capillary wall permeability, e.g. overdoses of heroine, morphine, methadone, cocaine, dextropropoxyphene and aspirin. Hydrochlorothiazide, phenylbutazone, aspirin and nitrofurantoin can cause oedema as an idiosyncratic response; interleukin-2 and tumour necrosis factor may cause increased permeability by an unknown process. Contrast media can induce arrhythmias, alter capillary wall permeability and produce a hyperosmolar load.
9. <u>Poisons</u>
   (a) Inhaled—e.g. nitrogen dioxide (NO_2), sulphur dioxide (SO_2), carbon monoxide (CO), phosgene, hydrocarbons and smoke.
   (b) Circulating—paraquat and snake venom.
10. **Mediastinal tumours**—producing pulmonary venous or lymphatic obstruction.
11. **Radiotherapy**—several weeks following treatment. Ultimately it has a characteristic straight edge as fibrosis ensues.
12. **Altitude sickness**—following rapid ascent to >3000 metres.

Further reading

Asrani, A., 2011. Urgent findings in portable chest radiography. AJR Am. J. Roentgenol. 196, WS37–WS46.

Desai, S.R., Wells, A.U., Suntharalingam, G., et al., 2001. Acute respiratory distress syndrome caused by pulmonary and extrapulmonary injury: a comparative CT study. Radiology 218, 689–693.

Desai, S.R., 2002. Acute respiratory distress syndrome: imaging the injured lung. Clin. Radiol. 57, 8–17.

Gluecker, T., Capasso, P., Schnyder, P., et al., 1999. Clinical and radiologic features of pulmonary edema. Radiographics 19, 1507–1531.

5.13 UNILATERAL PULMONARY OEDEMA

Pulmonary oedema ipsilateral to the underlying abnormality

1. <u>Prolonged lateral decubitus position</u>.
2. <u>Rapid lung reexpansion post thoracocentesis</u>.
3. <u>Unilateral aspiration</u>.
4. <u>Pulmonary contusion</u>.
5. **Mitral regurgitation**—rarely, the regurgitant jet flows into the right upper pulmonary vein, causing isolated right upper lobe oedema.
6. **Bronchial obstruction.**
7. **Reperfusion injury postpulmonary vascular surgery or stenting.**

8. **Large systemic artery to pulmonary artery shunts**—e.g. Waterston (ascending aorta to RPA), Blalock–Taussig (right or left subclavian artery to RPA or LPA) and Pott (descending aorta to LPA).

Pulmonary oedema contralateral to the underlying abnormality (typically a perfusion defect).

1. **Congenital absence or hypoplasia of a pulmonary artery.**
2. **Swyer-James syndrome.**
3. **Thromboembolism.**
4. **Unilateral emphysema.**
5. **Lobectomy.**
6. **Pleural disease.**

5

Further reading

Calenoff, L., Kruglik, G.D., Woodruff, A., 1978. Unilateral pulmonary oedema. Radiology 126, 19–24.

5.14 SEPTAL (KERLEY B) LINES

Pulmonary lobules are the smallest lung units bounded by interlobular septa (see illustration). Any pathological process involving the lymphatics, pulmonary veins or interstitium may thicken the interlobular septa, making them visible. On CXR these are best seen in the costophrenic angles, but they are more apparent on CT (NB: a few normal interlobular septa are commonly seen on CT).

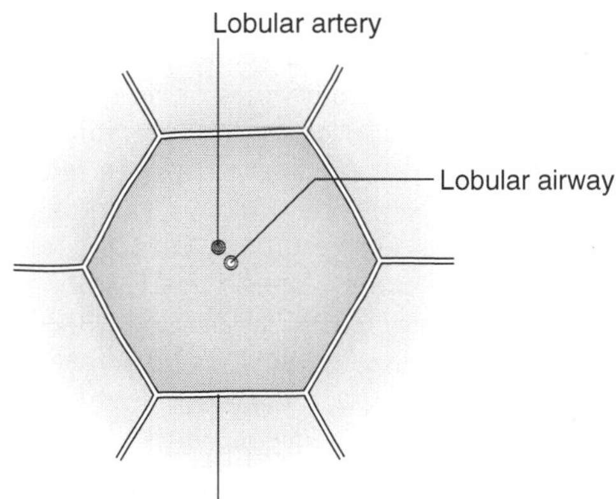

Schematic illustration of a pulmonary lobule.

Pulmonary venous hypertension/engorgement

This causes smooth interlobular septal thickening due to interstitial oedema. NB: noncardiogenic causes of pulmonary oedema (see Section 5.12) can also cause smooth septal thickening.

1. **Left ventricular failure**.
2. **Mitral stenosis**.
3. **Pulmonary venoocclusive disease**—smooth septal thickening, centrilobular ground-glass nodularity and signs of pulmonary arterial hypertension, but with a normal left heart.
4. **Pulmonary vein stenosis**—e.g. post left atrial ablation (for atrial fibrillation), or associated with sarcoidosis or malignancy.

Lymphatic/interstitial infiltration

1. **Lymphangitis carcinomatosa/lymphomatosa**—most often caused by lymphatic infiltration in patients with cancer of the lung, breast, stomach, pancreas, Kaposi sarcoma or lymphoma. Septal lines may be bilateral or unilateral (most other causes tend to be bilateral). Nodular interlobular septal thickening is the characteristic finding on CT. Leukaemia can also infiltrate interlobular septa, usually causing smooth thickening.
2. **Interstitial lung diseases**—e.g. NSIP, LIP, UIP. Other features are also present.
3. **Sarcoidosis***—nodular septal thickening may be seen.
4. **Pneumoconioses**—widespread nodularity may involve interlobular septa.
5. **Acute eosinophilic pneumonia**—similar to pulmonary oedema on imaging.
6. **Alveolar proteinosis**—smooth thickening of interlobular and intralobular septa in geographic areas of GGO ('crazy-paving' pattern). Infiltration of air spaces and interstitium by surfactant proteins due to impaired alveolar macrophage function.
7. **Erdheim-Chester disease***—infiltration of pulmonary interstitium by histiocytes of non-Langerhans type. On CXR, reticulonodular infiltrate is seen in mid/upper zones. On CT, smooth interlobular septal thickening is characteristic, associated with GGO, centrilobular nodules and often chylous pleural effusions ± thickening.
8. **Idiopathic bronchiectasis**—thickened interlobular septa are a feature in around one-third of patients.
9. **Recurrent diffuse pulmonary haemorrhage (haemosiderosis)**—smooth septal thickening may be seen on CT.
10. **Diffuse pulmonary lymphangiomatosis**—proliferation of lymphatic channels in pleura, interlobular septa and peribronchovascular connective tissue.

11. **Congenital lymphangiectasia**—abnormal dilatation of lymphatic channels without an increase in their number (cf. lymphangiomatosis). May be associated with extrathoracic congenital anomalies (e.g. renal, cardiac); commonly seen in Noonan and Turner syndromes.
12. **Lysosomal storage diseases**—Niemann-Pick, Gaucher disease. Smooth or nodular.
13. **Amyloidosis***—rare manifestation; usually nodular.
14. **Alveolar microlithiasis**—calcified interlobular septal thickening.

Smooth interlobular septal thickening	Nodular interlobular septal thickening
Any cause of interstitial oedema	Lymphangitis carcinomatosa
Acute eosinophilic pneumonia	Sarcoidosis
Alveolar proteinosis	Pneumoconioses
Erdheim-Chester disease	Amyloidosis
Recurrent pulmonary haemorrhage	Alveolar microlithiasis (calcified)
Lymphangiomatosis/lymphangiectasia	

Further reading

Webb, W.R., 2006. Thin-section CT of the secondary pulmonary lobule: anatomy and the image – the 2004 Fleischner Lecture. Radiology 239, 322–338.

5.15 MULTIPLE LUNG NODULES

A nodule is a roughly rounded, well- or ill-defined opacity measuring <3 cm in diameter. Nodules <3 mm are called 'micronodules' and those >3 cm are termed 'masses'. Further characterization of nodules (e.g. solid versus ground-glass versus mixed; centrilobular versus random distribution) is possible with CT; see also Section 5.23.

Multiple micronodules less than 2 mm

Soft-tissue or ground-glass attenuation

1. Miliary TB*—widespread, secondary to haematogenous dissemination. Uniform size, random distribution. Indistinct margins, but discrete. No septal lines. Normal hila unless superimposed on primary TB.
2. Fungal infection—histoplasmosis, coccidioidomycosis, blastomycosis and cryptococcosis. Similar appearance to miliary TB.

3. Coal worker's pneumoconiosis—predominantly midzones, sparing the extreme bases and apices. Ill-defined, may be arranged in a circle or rosette. Septal lines.
4. Sarcoidosis*—predominantly upper/midzones and strikingly bronchocentric, causing 'bronchovascular beading' ± hilar lymphadenopathy.
5. **Berylliosis**—indistinguishable from sarcoidosis.

Greater than soft-tissue density

1. Post varicella infection—multiple tiny calcific nodules throughout both lungs.
2. Haemosiderosis—secondary to chronic raised venous pressure (seen in 10%–15% of patients with mitral stenosis), repeated pulmonary haemorrhage (e.g. Goodpasture's syndrome) or idiopathic (see also Section 5.6). Septal lines. Smaller than miliary TB.
3. Silicosis—relative sparing of bases and apices. Very well-defined and dense when caused by inhalation of pure silica; ill-defined and of lower density when due to mixed dusts. Septal lines.
4. Post lymphangiography—ethiodized oil (lipiodol) emboli. Contrast medium may be visible in the terminal thoracic duct.
5. **Siderosis**—due to inhalation of iron particles. Lower density than silica. Widely disseminated. Asymptomatic.
6. **Stannosis**—inhalation of tin oxide. Even distribution throughout the lungs + septal lines.
7. **Barytosis**—inhalation of barium dust. Very dense, discrete opacities. Generalized distribution but bases and apices usually spared.
8. **Limestone and marble workers**—inhalation of calcium.
9. **Alveolar microlithiasis**—rare familial disorder. Lung detail obscured by widespread miliary calcifications. Few symptoms but may progress to cor pulmonale. Pleura, heart and diaphragm may be seen as 'negative' shadows on CXR.

Multiple nodules 2–5 mm

Soft-tissue or ground-glass attenuation and remaining discrete

1. Disseminated cancer—breast, thyroid, sarcoma, melanoma, prostate, pancreas or lung (eroding a pulmonary artery). Variable sizes, progressive increase in size, ± lymphatic obstruction.
2. Subacute hypersensitivity pneumonitis—centrilobular nodules, GGO, lobular air trapping (on expiratory CT), ± scattered thin-walled cysts. Smoking has a 'protective' effect (cf. respiratory bronchiolitis).
3. Respiratory bronchiolitis—similar CT appearances to hypersensitivity pneumonitis, but invariably linked to smoking. May also see thickened interlobular septa and limited emphysema.

4. Sarcoidosis*.
5. **Lymphoma***—usually with hilar or mediastinal lymphadenopathy.

Tending to confluence and/or varying in appearance over hours to days

1. Multifocal pneumonia—including aspiration pneumonia and TB.
2. Pulmonary oedema—rapid fluid shifts can occur over a few hours, in contrast to many other air-space diseases.
3. Diffuse pulmonary haemorrhage.

Multiple nodules greater than 5 mm

Neoplastic

1. Metastases—most commonly from breast, thyroid, kidney, GI tract and testes. In children: Wilms tumour, Ewing sarcoma, neuroblastoma and osteosarcoma. Predilection for lower lobes, more common peripherally. Range of sizes. Well-defined. Ill definition suggests prostate, breast or gastric metastases. Hilar lymphadenopathy and effusions are uncommon.
2. **Multiple synchronous lung cancers.**
3. **Kaposi sarcoma**—multiple bilateral perihilar and peribronchovascular ill-defined nodules ('flame-shaped') with thoracic lymphadenopathy, interlobular septal thickening ± pleural effusions.
4. **Benign metastasizing tumours**—most commonly seen with uterine leiomyomas, but also reported with meningiomas, pleomorphic adenomas of the salivary glands, chondroblastomas and giant cell tumours of bone.

Infections

1. Abscesses—widespread distribution but asymmetrical. Commonly *Staphylococcus aureus.* Cavitation common. No calcification.
2. **Coccidioidomycosis**—in endemic areas. Well-defined; predilection for the upper lobes. Calcification and cavitation may be present.
3. **Histoplasmosis**—in endemic areas. Round, well-defined, few in number. Sometimes calcify. Usually unchanged for many years.
4. **Hydatid**—more common on the right side and in the lower zones. Well-defined unless there is surrounding pneumonia. Often ≥10 cm. May rupture and show the 'water lily' sign on CT.

Immunological

1. Wegener's granulomatosis*—bilateral nodules or masses ± cavitation, or uni/multifocal consolidation. Widespread distribution. Round, well-defined. No calcification.
2. Rheumatoid nodules—peripheral, more common in the lower zones. Round, well-defined. No calcification. Cavitation common. May be associated with pneumoconiosis (Caplan syndrome).
3. Progressive massive fibrosis—large conglomerate masses, typically in both mid-upper zones, usually symmetrical; starts

5

peripherally and migrates centrally over years. Caused by chronic silicosis, coal worker's pneumoconiosis, talcosis or sarcoidosis. Associated traction bronchiectasis and background widespread nodularity are also present.

4. **Organizing pneumonia.**
5. **Amyloidosis***—multiple nodules of varying size, calcified in up to 50%.
6. **Hyalinizing granulomas**—rare, unknown aetiology but can be associated with fibrosing mediastinitis, IgG4-related disease and other autoimmune disorders. Multiple (or occasionally solitary) lung nodules mimicking metastatic disease.

Vascular

<u>Arteriovenous malformations</u>—33% are multiple, especially in hereditary haemorrhagic telangiectasia. Well-defined and lobulated; may see feeding and draining vessels on CXR (best seen on CT). Calcification is rare.

Further reading

Kim, K.I., Kim, C.W., Lee, M.K., et al., 2001. Imaging of occupational lung disease. Radiographics 21, 1371–1391.

5.16 SOLITARY PULMONARY NODULE OR MASSLIKE LESION

Granulomatous

1. <u>Tuberculoma</u>—more common in upper lobes, R>L. Well-defined; 0.5–4 cm. Calcification frequent. 80% have satellite lesions. Cavitation is uncommon, and if present, is small and eccentric. Usually persists unchanged for years.
2. <u>Histoplasmoma</u>—in endemic areas (Mississippi and Atlantic coast of USA). More frequent in lower lobes. Well-defined; seldom >3 cm. Calcification is common and may be central ('target' appearance). Cavitation is rare. Satellite lesions are common.
3. **Others**—e.g. coccidioidomycosis, cryptococcosis.

Malignant tumours

1. <u>Lung cancer</u>—features suggesting malignancy include: recent appearance or rapid growth (review previous imaging); size >4 cm; lesion crossing a fissure (also seen in some fungal infections); ill-defined, notched or spiculated margins; peripheral line shadows. Calcification is rare. Most appear 'solid' on CT ± foci of fluid attenuation (necrosis). Pure ground-glass/part-solid ground-glass nodules >5 mm may represent premalignant lesions (atypical adenomatous hyperplasia), adenocarcinoma in situ or invasive adenocarcinoma.

2. **Solitary metastasis**—accounts for 3%–5% of asymptomatic nodules. 25% of lung metastases may be solitary. Most likely primary tumours are breast, sarcoma, seminoma and RCC. Predilection for the lung periphery. Calcification is rare, but if present suggests metastatic osteosarcoma or chondrosarcoma.
3. **Rare malignant lung tumours**—pleuropulmonary blastoma, pleural and pulmonary sarcomas, plasmacytoma, atypical carcinoid (see below).

Benign tumours

1. **Carcinoid tumour**—'typical' carcinoids (90% of cases) are generally central and tend to be more benign than atypical tumours (10%), which tend to be peripheral. However, malignant potential varies from benign to frank small cell carcinoma. May calcify (often peripheral) and may be associated with ectopic ACTH production (Cushing's syndrome).
2. **Hamartoma**—96% occur >40 years of age. 90% are intrapulmonary and usually <2 cm from the pleura. 10% cause bronchial stenosis. Usually <4 cm. Well-defined, lobulated. 60% contain fat visible on CT. May calcify, especially if large. Calcification may have a 'popcorn', craggy or punctate configuration.

Infectious/inflammatory

1. **Pneumonia**—especially pneumococcal.
2. **Rounded atelectasis**—typically the sequela of an exudative pleural effusion. Peripheral mass + adjacent smooth pleural thickening and parenchymal bands giving a 'comet tail' appearance.
3. **Hydatid**—in endemic areas. Most common in lower lobes, R>L. Well-defined; 1–10 cm. Solitary in 70%. May have a bizarre shape. Rupture results in the 'water lily' sign.
4. **Wegener's granulomatosis***—solitary nodules in up to one-third of patients, but more commonly multiple. May cavitate.
5. **Sarcoidosis***—a solitary lung nodule is rare, but reported.
6. **Organizing pneumonia**—can mimic a (malignant) solitary pulmonary nodule.

Congenital

1. **Intrapulmonary lymph node**—usually solitary, small (<2 cm), peripheral (<2 cm from pleura) and well-defined. Common incidental finding on CT in mid/lower zones. Typically triangular in shape with a thin tether to the pleural surface. Usually benign, even when detected in the context of a known malignancy.
2. **Sequestration**—intralobar (more common; no separate pleural covering; venous drainage into pulmonary veins) or extralobar (rare; separate pleural covering; venous drainage into systemic

veins). Nearly always in a lower lobe (L>R), contiguous with the diaphragm. Well-defined, round or oval. Diagnosis confirmed by identifying its systemic arterial supply on CT/MRI.
3. **Bronchogenic cyst**—usually mediastinal or hilar, but occasionally intrapulmonary. Round or oval; smooth thin nonenhancing wall (enhancement implies infection or alternative diagnosis).

Vascular

1. **Haematoma**—peripheral, smooth and well-defined. Slow resolution over several weeks.
2. **Arteriovenous malformation**—66% are single. Well-defined, lobulated. Feeding and draining vessels may be seen on CXR, confirmed on CT. Calcification rare.

Further reading

Winer-Muram, H., 2006. The solitary pulmonary nodule. Radiology 239, 34–49.

5.17 APICAL MASS

1. **Pancoast tumour**—look for adjacent rib destruction.
2. **Tortuous/aneurysmal subclavian artery**—R>L, usually in older patients. Well-defined inferolateral margin, merges with mediastinum medially. Can be hard to differentiate from tumour on CXR—compare with previous imaging.
3. **Apical scarring/fibrosis**—usually in older patients (bilateral) or post infection (e.g. TB) or radiotherapy (uni- or bilateral).
4. **Mycetoma in a preexisting apical cavity**—look for air crescent sign.
5. **Metastasis**—more common in lower zones.
6. **Pleural/chest wall tumours**—mesothelioma, chondrosarcoma, Ewing sarcoma, metastasis, myeloma, lymphoma, neurogenic tumour.
7. **Plombage**—historical treatment for cavitating TB. Apical density + multiple rounded lucencies.
8. **Meningocoele.**

5.18 PULMONARY CAVITIES

A cavity is any gas-filled space within a nodule, mass or area of consolidation (cf. a pulmonary cyst that has a very thin wall).

Infective

1. ***Staphylococcus aureus***—thick-walled with a ragged inner lining. Usually multiple; no lobar predilection. Associated with effusion or empyema ± pneumothorax, especially in children.

2. ***Klebsiella pneumoniae***—thick-walled with a ragged inner lining. More common in the upper lobes. Usually single but may be multilocular ± effusion.
3. **TB***—thick-walled and smooth. Upper lobes and apical segment of lower lobes mainly. Usually surrounded by consolidation ± fibrosis.
4. **Septic emboli**—e.g. in IV drug users, tricuspid/pulmonary valve infective endocarditis, infected IV catheters/wires, septic thrombophlebitis or following oropharyngeal infection (Lemierre syndrome).
5. **Aspiration**—look for a foreign body, e.g. tooth.
6. **Infection of a preexisting lung abnormality**—e.g. emphysematous bulla, sequestration, bronchogenic cyst. Internal air–fluid level and surrounding consolidation may be present.
7. **Others**—gram-negative organisms, actinomycosis, nocardiosis, histoplasmosis, coccidioidomycosis, aspergillosis, hydatid, amoebiasis.

Neoplastic

1. **Lung cancer**—thick-walled with an eccentric cavity. Predilection for upper lobes. Found in 2%–10% of carcinomas, especially if peripheral. More common in SCC (may be thin-walled).
2. **Metastases**—especially in squamous cell, colonic and sarcoma metastases. Thin- or thick-walled. May involve only a few of the nodules.
3. **Tracheobronchial papillomatosis**—see Section 5.1. Parenchymal involvement gives rise to multiple nodules that can cavitate. Typically in children or young adults.
4. **Lymphoma***—including lymphomatoid granulomatosis. Cavitation is uncommon, may be thin- or thick-walled, typically in an area of infiltration + hilar/mediastinal lymphadenopathy.

Vascular

Infarction—secondary infection of an initially sterile infarct can occur. An aseptic cavitating infarct may also become infected. Aseptic cavitation is usually solitary and arises in a large area of consolidation after ~2 weeks; most common sites are apical or posterior segments of an upper lobe or apical segment of a lower lobe (cf. lower lobe predominance of noncavitating infarction). Majority have scalloped inner margins and crosscavity band shadows ± effusion.

Inflammatory

1. **Wegener's granulomatosis***—cavitation in some of the nodules. Thick-walled, becoming thinner with time. Can be transient.
2. **Rheumatoid nodules**—especially in lower lobes and peripherally. Well-defined, thick-walled with a smooth inner lining; become thin-walled with time.

3. **Progressive massive fibrosis**—mid and upper zones. Thick-walled and irregular. Background nodularity.
4. **Sarcoidosis***—thin-walled, usually in early disease. May later develop mycetoma within cavity resulting in wall thickening.

Traumatic

1. **Haematoma**—peripheral. Air–fluid level if it communicates with a bronchus.
2. **Traumatic lung cyst**—thin-walled and peripheral. Single or multiple, unilocular or multilocular. Distinguished from cavitating haematomas that present early, within hours of the injury.

Further reading

Vourtsi, A., Gouliamos, A., Moulopoulos, L., et al., 2001. CT appearance of solitary and multiple cystic and cavitary lung lesions. Eur. Radiol. 11, 612–622.

5.19 CYSTIC LUNG DISEASE

A pulmonary air cyst is defined as a rounded parenchymal lucency with a thin well-defined wall (generally <2 mm thick); cf. cavities (thicker wall) and emphysema (no discrete wall). Cysts may contain solid material or fluid (implying secondary infection).

Postinfective

1. **Bacterial pneumonia**—e.g. *Staphylococcus aureus* (a characteristic feature in children, seen in 40%–60% of cases), *Streptococcus pneumoniae, Escherichia coli, Klebsiella pneumoniae, Haemophilus influenzae, Legionella pneumophila*. Cysts can appear during the first 2 weeks of infection and may resolve over several months.
2. ***Pneumocystis jirovecii***—usually multiple and in the upper zones; cysts increase the risk of pneumothorax.
3. **Hydatid cyst**—initially fluid-filled, can contain air if they communicate with the bronchial tree.

Posttraumatic

Lung laceration—cyst within an area of contusion; resolves over time.

Congenital

1. **Congenital pulmonary airway malformation (CPAM)**—single multiloculated cyst.
2. **Bronchogenic cyst**—if communicating with the bronchial tree (generally following secondary infection).

Neoplastic

1. **Following treatment of lung metastases**—e.g. bladder cancer and germ cell tumours. May only be visible on CT.
2. **Cystic lung metastases**—rare. Can occur with colonic adenocarcinoma, epithelioid sarcoma and endometrial stromal sarcoma.

Diffuse lung diseases

1. Langerhans cell histiocytosis (LCH)*—cysts, sometimes bizarre (noncircular) in shape, mid/upper zone predominance. In 'early' disease there are multiple nodules, which later cavitate. Relative sparing of lower zones and medial tips of the middle lobe and lingula. Usually presents in young adults, strongly linked to cigarette smoking.
2. Lymphangioleiomyomatosis (LAM)*—exclusively in women of childbearing age. Smooth muscle proliferation around vessels, lymphatics and airways. Multiple cysts, relatively uniform in size with no zonal predilection (cf. LCH).
3. Tuberous sclerosis*—lung disease almost identical to LAM.
4. **Lymphocytic interstitial pneumonia**—usually occurs in the context of dysproteinaemias, connective tissue disorders (especially Sjögren's syndrome and rheumatoid arthritis) or HIV infection. Basal-predominant ill-defined centrilobular nodules, GGO and lung cysts are characteristic ± septal thickening. May have associated calcified nodules in the cyst walls due to amyloid deposition.
5. **Neurofibromatosis***—cystic lung disease and interstitial fibrosis are reported.
6. **Birt-Hogg-Dubé syndrome***—autosomal dominant multisystem disorder characterized by lower zone predominant lung cysts (typically 'cigar-shaped' ± recurrent pneumothoraces), cutaneous fibrofolliculomas and increased risk of renal tumours.
7. **Hypersensitivity pneumonitis**—a few cysts may be seen in the subacute or chronic fibrotic phase, but not a dominant feature.
8. **End-stage fibrotic diffuse interstitial lung diseases**—e.g. idiopathic pulmonary fibrosis, sarcoidosis. Peripheral honeycombing.
9. **Desquamative interstitial pneumonia**—typically in heavy smokers, at the severe end of the smoking related interstitial lung disease spectrum. Also seen in connective tissue disease and genetic disorders of surfactant protein dysfunction. Small cysts may be seen but basal predominant GGO ± reticulation are the major features.

5

Further reading

Biyyam, D.R., Chapman, T., Ferguson, M.R., et al., 2010. Congenital lung abnormalities: embryologic features, prenatal diagnosis, and postnatal radiologic–pathologic correlation. Radiographics 30, 1721–1738.

Seaman, D.M., Meyer, C.A., Gilman, M.D., McCormack, F.X., 2011. Pictorial essay: diffuse cystic lung disease at high-resolution CT. AJR Am. J. Roentgenol. 196, 1305–1311.

5.20 PULMONARY CALCIFICATION OR OSSIFICATION

Localized

1. <u>TB</u>*—small nidus of calcification. Calcification ≠ healed.
2. <u>Histoplasmosis</u>—in endemic areas. Calcification may be laminated, producing a target lesion ± multiple punctate splenic calcifications.
3. **Coccidioidomycosis.**
4. **Blastomycosis**—rare.

Calcification in a solitary nodule

This usually suggests a benign nature. The exceptions are:

(a) Lung cancer 'engulfing' a preexisting calcified granuloma (eccentric calcification).

(b) Solitary calcifying/ossifying metastasis—osteosarcoma, chondrosarcoma, mucinous adenocarcinoma of the colon or breast, papillary carcinoma of the thyroid, cystadenocarcinoma of the ovary, carcinoid.

(c) Primary peripheral squamous cell or papillary adenocarcinoma.

Diffuse or multiple calcifications

1. <u>Infections</u>—healed miliary TB, histoplasmosis or varicella (chicken pox) pneumonia. The latter results in numerous 1–3mm calcifications.
2. <u>Chronic pulmonary venous hypertension</u>—especially mitral stenosis. Up to 8 mm in size ± ossification; most prominent in mid and lower zones.
3. <u>Silicosis</u>—in up to 20% of those showing nodular opacities.
4. <u>Metastases</u>—as earlier.
5. **Alveolar microlithiasis**—often familial. Myriad minute calcifications in alveoli that obscure all lung detail. Due to the increased lung density, the heart, pleura and diaphragm may be seen as negative shadows on plain film.
6. **Metastatic due to hypercalcaemia**—chronic renal failure, secondary hyperparathyroidism and multiple myeloma. Predominantly in upper zones.

7. **Talcosis**—usually in IV drug users due to injected talc. Numerous very dense micronodules ± progressive massive fibrosis in late stage.
8. **Lymphoma* following radiotherapy.**

Interstitial ossification

1. **Dendriform/disseminated pulmonary ossification**—branching or nodular calcific densities extending along the bronchovascular distribution of the interstitial space. Seen in long-term busulphan therapy, chronic pulmonary venous hypertension (e.g. due to mitral stenosis), idiopathic pulmonary fibrosis, asbestosis, following ARDS, chronic bronchitis and chronic aspiration.
2. **Idiopathic.**

Further reading

Lara, J.F., 2005. Dendriform pulmonary ossification, a form of diffuse pulmonary ossification: report of a 26-year autopsy experience. Arch. Pathol. Lab. Med. 129, 348–353.

5.21 NONTHROMBOTIC PULMONARY EMBOLI

1. <u>Septic embolism</u>—associated with indwelling venous catheters, pacemaker leads, tricuspid or pulmonary valve endocarditis and peripheral septic thrombophlebitis. Ill-defined nodules of varying sizes, predominantly in lower lobes ± cavitation.
2. <u>Iatrogenic embolism</u>—common examples include cement post vertebroplasty and catheter tips or guidewires. Rarer causes include iodinated oil embolism post lymphangiography, cotton adherent to intravascular lines and air from pump injectors.
3. **Phlebolith embolism**—most commonly from a pelvic vein ± additional thrombotic emboli.
4. **Fat embolism**—1–2 days post trauma. Predominantly peripheral, associated with geographic areas of GGO ± septal thickening ± small nodules. Resolves in 1–4 weeks. Normal heart size. Pleural effusions uncommon.
5. **Amniotic fluid embolism**—rare. The majority suffer cardiopulmonary arrest and the CXR shows pulmonary oedema.
6. **Tumour embolism**—common sources are liver, breast, stomach, kidney, prostate and choriocarcinoma. CXR is usually normal.
7. **Talc embolism**—in IV drug abusers. May result in pulmonary hypertension.
8. **Hydatid embolism.**

Further reading

Han, D., Lee, K.S., Franquet, T., et al., 2003. Thrombotic and non-thrombotic pulmonary arterial embolism: spectrum of imaging findings. Radiographics 23, 1521–1539.

Rossi, S.E., Goodman, P.C., Franquet, T., 2000. Nonthrombic pulmonary emboli. AJR Am. J. Roentgenol. 174, 1499–1508.

5.22 FIBROSING LUNG DISEASES ON HRCT

Diffuse interstitial lung diseases can be divided into two groups: fibrosing and nonfibrosing. Radiologic signs of fibrosis include traction bronchiectasis, parenchymal distortion and volume loss (look for displacement of fissures). NB: if emphysema is also present (as in combined pulmonary fibrosis with emphysema [CPFE]), volume loss may be masked by adjacent overinflation of emphysematous lung. Honeycombing is defined by clustered, subpleural, thick-walled cystic spaces of similar diameters, generally measuring 3–5 mm (occasionally up to 25 mm), and is synonymous with usual interstitial pneumonia. Whereas the list of nonfibrosing lung diseases is long (N>150), the list of fibrosing lung diseases is short (N=5).

1. **Usual interstitial pneumonia (UIP)**—may be primary (idiopathic pulmonary fibrosis [IPF]) or secondary to connective tissue disease, asbestos exposure, medications. Typically affects men >50 years. Predominantly has a basal and subpleural reticular pattern + honeycombing. Often follows a 'propeller blade' distribution with disease more anterior toward the apices and more posterior at the bases. Atypical findings can occur, e.g. GGO (suggests an acute exacerbation). Increased risk of lung cancer.
2. **Nonspecific interstitial pneumonia (NSIP)**—may be idiopathic, but more commonly is associated with other conditions, especially collagen vascular disease, drugs and immunological conditions. Typically affects middle-aged women. Predominantly basal, diffuse GGO ± evidence of fibrosis (fibrotic versus cellular NSIP).
3. **Fibrotic organizing pneumonia**—many causes and associations, mirroring NSIP. Typical features include perilobular opacities, peripheral consolidation ± air bronchograms, and, in contrast to NSIP, more focal peribronchovascular GGO. Rarely the 'reverse halo' sign.
4. **Chronic (fibrotic) hypersensitivity pneumonitis**—due to repeated or prolonged exposure to a wide variety of antigens originating from animals, plants, drugs, bacteria or fungi. Typical features include a reticular pattern ± honeycombing, GGO ± traction bronchiectasis, with lobular areas of 'spared' lung and air trapping. Upper/mid zone predominance (cf. UIP/NSIP).
5. **Sarcoidosis***—typically causes a symmetrical, bronchocentric reticular pattern in upper zones, seemingly 'streaming' from the hila. Calcified mediastinal and hilar nodes.

Upper zone predominant fibrosis	Lower zone predominant fibrosis
Sarcoidosis	UIP
Old TB (usually unilateral)	NSIP
Silicosis/pneumoconiosis/PMF	DIP
Chronic hypersensitivity pneumonitis	Fibrotic organizing pneumonia
Radiation fibrosis	Asbestosis
Ankylosing spondylitis	Chronic aspiration pneumonitis
Pleuroparenchymal fibroelastosis	

Further reading

Jacob, J., Hansell, D., 2015. HRCT of fibrosing lung disease. Respirology 20, 859–872.

5.23 NODULAR PATTERNS ON HRCT

These may be centrilobular, perilymphatic or random in distribution.

Centrilobular

The most peripheral nodules are >5 mm from pleural surfaces; often seen close to small vessels, related to endobronchial and small airway disease. A 'tree-in-bud' appearance suggests endobronchial disease—the opacified bronchioles are the 'branches' of the tree, and the centrilobular nodules are the 'buds'.

1. **Infective bronchiolitis**
   (a) **TB***—look for calcified granulomas and nodes, lung cavities (spillage of cavity contents into bronchial tree results in distant tree-in-bud). Nontuberculous mycobacterial (NTM) infection can look similar.
   (b) **Aspiration**—basal predominance.
   (c) **Other infections**—bacterial (e.g. mycoplasma), viral (e.g. influenza), fungal (e.g. invasive aspergillosis).
2. **Hypersensitivity pneumonitis**—due to an allergic reaction to a variety of inhaled particles. Causes centrilobular nodularity in the subacute phase, typically without tree-in-bud. Lobular air trapping and GGO can also be seen.

3. **Other causes of bronchiolitis**
   (a) **Respiratory bronchiolitis**—almost exclusively in smokers. Upper zone predominance.
   (b) **Follicular bronchiolitis**—associated with autoimmune disorders, e.g. rheumatoid arthritis, Sjögren's syndrome. Basal predominance.
   (c) **Diffuse panbronchiolitis**—typically seen in East Asia. Basal predominance.
4. **Diseases associated with bronchiectasis**—e.g. cystic fibrosis, primary ciliary dyskinesia, NTM infection (Lady Windermere syndrome).
5. **Endobronchial spread of tumour**—e.g. adenocarcinoma.
6. **Metastatic pulmonary calcification**—fluffy 'cotton-ball' centrilobular nodules, often dense/calcified, with an upper zone predominance. Most commonly due to chronic renal failure.

Perilymphatic

Nodules are seen closely related (i.e. <5 mm) to the pleural surfaces, interlobular septa, large vessels and bronchi.

1. **Sarcoidosis***—characteristic feature.
2. **Lymphangitis carcinomatosa**—nodular thickening of interlobular septa.
3. **Silicosis and coal worker's pneumoconiosis.**
4. **Lymphoma*.**
5. **Amyloidosis*.**

Random

1. **Miliary TB*.**
2. **Miliary metastases.**
3. **Silicosis and coal worker's pneumoconiosis.**
4. **Other miliary infections**—e.g. histoplasmosis, blastomycosis.
5. **Langerhans cell histiocytosis***—nodules often cavitate, forming irregular cysts. Upper zone predominance.
6. **Lymphocytic interstitial pneumonia**—nodules may be centrilobular or subpleural. Lower zone predominance.
7. **Fungal infection**—e.g. candidiasis, blastomycosis.

5.24 GROUND-GLASS OPACIFICATION ON HRCT

Defined as a hazy increase in lung parenchymal attenuation that does not obscure bronchial and vascular margins. This is wholly nonspecific and can reflect partial air-space filling, interstitial infiltration, collapse of air spaces or increased capillary blood volume. The clinical presentation (acute or chronic) aids differentiation of the causes.

Acute illnesses

1. **Pulmonary oedema**—with smooth septal thickening and effusions.
2. **Infection**—e.g. PCP, CMV. Both occur in immunocompromised patients. Cysts ± pneumothoraces may also be seen in PCP.
3. **Pulmonary haemorrhage**—e.g. due to vasculitis (Wegener's granulomatosis, Goodpasture's syndrome), SLE, coagulopathy.
4. **ARDS and acute interstitial pneumonia (AIP)**—both are characterized by widespread consolidation and GGO that may increase in density towards dependent areas, representing diffuse alveolar damage (DAD). ARDS has many causes (e.g. sepsis and other causes of systemic inflammatory response syndrome [SIRS]), AIP is idiopathic.
5. **Acute hypersensitivity pneumonitis**—centrilobular ground-glass nodules, upper zone predominance. Many allergic triggers.
6. **Acute eosinophilic pneumonia**—mimics pulmonary oedema on imaging. Usually in young adults.

Subacute/chronic illnesses

1. **Diffuse interstitial lung diseases**
   (a) **Nonspecific interstitial pneumonia**—with reticulation and traction bronchiectasis. Basal predominance.
   (b) **Organizing pneumonia**—consolidation and GGO, occasionally with a 'reverse halo' morphology.
   (c) **Respiratory bronchiolitis-interstitial lung disease (RB-ILD)**—centrilobular ground-glass nodules and GGO, upper zone predominance. Almost exclusively in smokers (cf. hypersensitivity pneumonitis where smoking is protective).
   (d) **Desquamative interstitial pneumonia**—bilateral GGO ± reticulation ± cysts, lower zone predominance. Almost exclusively in smokers (more advanced stage of RB-ILD).
   (e) **Lymphocytic interstitial pneumonia**—with ill-defined nodules and lung cysts.
2. **Chronic hypersensitivity pneumonitis**—bilateral GGO with an upper zone predominance + lobular 'sparing' due to air trapping + areas of fibrosis.
3. **Chronic eosinophilic pneumonia**—peripheral migratory consolidation ± GGO.
4. **Drug-induced**—amiodarone causes peripheral GGO and consolidation that is often hyperdense (due to iodine content); the liver ± myocardium may also be hyperdense, suggesting the diagnosis. Other causes of GGO include methotrexate, nitrofurantoin and chemotherapy agents.

5. **'Alveolar' sarcoidosis***—uncommon form of the disease. Multifocal areas of GGO, mid/upper zone distribution. Small nodules may coexist, creating the 'sarcoid galaxy' sign.
6. **Alveolar proteinosis**—with interlobular septal thickening, resulting in 'crazy-paving'.
7. **Adenocarcinoma**—can present as a solid/ground-glass nodule or a larger area of GGO/consolidation. Can be multifocal and bilateral.

Further reading

Hansell, U.D.M., Bankier, A.A., MacMahon, H., et al., 2008. Fleischner Society: glossary of terms for thoracic imaging. Radiology 246, 697–722.

Travis, W.D., King, T.E., Bateman, E.D., et al., 2002. ATS/ERS international multidisciplinary consensus classification of idiopathic interstitial pneumonias. General principles and recommendations. Am. J. Respir. Crit. Care Med. 165, 277–304.

Webb, W.R., Müller, N.L., Naidich, D.P., 2000. High Resolution CT of the Lung. Lippincott Williams & Wilkins, Philadelphia, PA.

5.25 MOSAIC ATTENUATION PATTERN ON HRCT

Defined as regions of differing lung density ('black' and 'grey'), usually conforming to the geographic boundaries of secondary pulmonary lobules. Causes can be split into three categories. Note that differentiating between these is not always easy.

Small airways diseases (obliterative bronchiolitis)

The 'black' lung is abnormal, with smaller or fewer vessels compared to the 'grey' areas and air trapping on expiratory phase CT.

1. **Postinfective**—i.e. Swyer-James syndrome.
2. **Posttransplantation**—heart ± lung, bone marrow. Termed bronchiolitis obliterans syndrome (BOS) in chronic lung allograft dysfunction.
3. **Connective tissue diseases**—especially rheumatoid arthritis, Sjögren's syndrome.
4. **Drugs**—penicillamine, *Sauropus androgynus* (Katuk leaves).
5. **Toxic fume inhalation.**
6. **Diffuse idiopathic pulmonary neuroendocrine hyperplasia (DIPNECH)**—mosaic attenuation + small well-defined lung nodules (representing neuroendocrine tumourlets).
7. **Bronchiectasis.**
8. **Sarcoidosis*.**

Pulmonary vascular diseases

The 'black' lung is abnormal, with smaller or fewer vessels compared to the 'grey' areas, but without air trapping.

1. Chronic thromboembolic disease—usually with other features, e.g. laminar thrombus, webs, stenoses, pulmonary hypertension. NOT a feature of acute PE.
2. **Pulmonary arterial hypertension.**
3. **Pulmonary artery tumours**—e.g. sarcoma.

Infiltrative lung diseases

The 'grey' lung is abnormal, with no disparity in vessel size between 'grey' and 'black' areas. See Section 5.24, especially chronic hypersensitivity pneumonitis (although note that this does cause air trapping and can mimic small airways disease).

Further reading

Grosse, C., Grosse, A., 2010. CT findings in diseases associated with pulmonary hypertension: a current review. Radiographics 30, 1753–1777.

Sibtain, N.A., Padley, S.P., 2004. HRCT in small and large airways diseases. Eur. Radiol. 14 (Suppl. 4), L31–L43.

5.26 UNILATERAL HILAR ENLARGEMENT

Lymph nodes

1. Lung cancer—hilar enlargement may be the tumour itself or malignant lymph nodes.
2. Infection—e.g. primary TB, histoplasmosis, coccidioidomycosis, *Mycoplasma*, pertussis.
3. **Unicentric Castleman disease**—benign lymph node hyperplasia, presents as localized mediastinal or hilar lymphadenopathy that classically enhances avidly on CT.
4. **Lymphoma***—unilateral involvement is unusual.
5. **Sarcoidosis***—unilateral disease in only 1%–5%.

Pulmonary artery

1. Poststenotic dilatation—on the left side.
2. Aneurysm—in severe chronic pulmonary arterial hypertension, Behçet's and Hughes-Stovin syndromes, ± vessel wall calcification.
3. **Pulmonary embolus**—massive embolus to one lung; short dilated ipsilateral proximal pulmonary artery. Peripheral oligaemia.

Others

1. Carcinoid tumour—most commonly arises from a central bronchus ± distal collapse.

2. Mediastinal mass—involving the hilum, e.g. bronchogenic cyst.
3. Perihilar pneumonia—ill-defined ± air bronchogram.

See also Section 5.9.

5.27 BILATERAL HILAR ENLARGEMENT

Lymph nodes

NB: there are many causes of small volume reactive mediastinal and hilar lymph node enlargement on CT, e.g. interstitial lung diseases, hypersensitivity pneumonitis, etc., but these do not usually cause appreciable hilar enlargement on CXR.

1. **Sarcoidosis***—symmetrical and lobulated. Hilar ± unilateral or bilateral paratracheal lymphadenopathy ± calcification.
2. **Lymphoma***—typically asymmetrical.
3. **Lymph node metastases**—often accompanied by lymphangitis carcinomatosa.
4. **Multicentric Castleman disease**—usually related to HIV.
5. **Infective**—e.g. viruses (most common in children), histoplasmosis, coccidioidomycosis. Primary TB is rarely bilateral and symmetrical.
6. **Silicosis**—symmetrical ± egg-shell calcification. May also be seen in other inhalational diseases, e.g. berylliosis.

Vascular

Pulmonary arterial hypertension—tubular hilar enlargement (cf. lobulated enlargement seen in lymphadenopathy). Note that small-volume lymphadenopathy may also be seen on CT. See also Sections 6.20 and 6.21.

5.28 'EGG-SHELL' CALCIFICATION OF LYMPH NODES

Defined as shell-like peripheral calcifications <2 mm thick within ≥2 lymph nodes, in at least one of which the ring of calcification must be complete and one of the affected lymph nodes must be ≥1 cm in maximum diameter. Calcifications may be solid or broken ± central calcifications.

1. **Silicosis**—seen in ~5%. Predominantly affects hilar nodes. Calcification is more common in complicated pneumoconiosis. Lungs show multiple small nodular shadows or areas of massive fibrosis.
2. **Coal worker's pneumoconiosis**—seen in only 1%. Associated lung changes are identical to silicosis.

3. Sarcoidosis*—nodal calcification in ~5%. Classically described as 'icing-sugar-like' but occasionally 'egg-shell' in appearance. Calcification appears ~6 years after disease onset and is nearly always associated with advanced lung disease and in some cases with steroid therapy.
4. Lymphoma* following radiotherapy—1–9 years after therapy.

Differential diagnosis

Note that identifying the anatomical location of calcification is generally not problematic on CT. Beware of IV contrast pooling in the azygos vein on valve leaflets; this can mimic a calcified node.

1. Aortic calcification—especially in the wall of a saccular aneurysm.
2. **Pulmonary artery calcification**—a rare feature of severe pulmonary hypertension, common in Eisenmenger's syndrome.
3. **Anterior mediastinal tumours**—teratodermoids and thymomas may occasionally exhibit rim calcification.
4. **Fibrosing mediastinitis**—often calcifies.

Further reading

Gross, B.H., Schneider, H.J., Proto, A.V., 1980. Eggshell calcification of lymph nodes: an update. AJR Am. J. Roentgenol. 135, 1265.

Jacobsen, G., Felson, B., Pendergress, E.P., et al., 1967. Eggshell calcification in coal and metal miners. Semin. Roentgenol. 2, 276–282.

5.29 PLEURAL EFFUSION

Transudate (protein <30 g/l)

These usually cause bilateral effusions.

1. Cardiac failure.
2. Hepatic failure.
3. Renal failure—especially nephrotic syndrome.

Exudate (protein >30 g/l)

1. Infection.
2. Malignancy—primary or metastatic.
3. Collagen vascular diseases—e.g. SLE, rheumatoid arthritis.
4. Pulmonary infarction—may also be haemorrhagic.

Haemorrhagic

1. Lung cancer.
2. Trauma—look for rib fractures.
3. Coagulopathy.
4. **Pleural endometriosis**—R>>L side.

Chylous

Obstructed or leaking thoracic duct—due to surgery, trauma, malignant invasion, lymphangiomatosis or filariasis.

5.30 PLEURAL EFFUSION DUE TO EXTRATHORACIC DISEASE

1. **Pancreatitis**—acute, chronic or relapsing. Effusions are predominantly left-sided. Elevated amylase content.
2. **Subphrenic abscess**—with elevation and restricted motion of the ipsilateral diaphragm and basal atelectasis or consolidation.
3. **Post abdominal surgery**—especially after upper abdominal surgery, most often on the side of the surgery. Resolves after 2 weeks.
4. **Meigs syndrome**—usually right-sided, with ascites and a benign ovarian tumour (usually fibroma).
5. **Nephrotic syndrome.**
6. **Fluid overload**—e.g. due to renal disease.
7. **Cirrhosis.**

5.31 PLEURAL EFFUSION DUE TO INTRATHORACIC DISEASE

Effusion may be the only abnormality or may obscure other signs.

Infective

1. **Parapneumonic effusion or empyema**—can occur as an isolated pleural infection without pneumonia. Presence of scoliosis concave to the side of the fluid suggests empyema.
2. **Primary TB***—in adults > children. Rarely bilateral.
3. **Viruses and mycoplasma**—effusions are usually small.

Neoplastic

1. **Lung cancer**—effusion may hide a peripheral carcinoma.
2. **Metastases**—most commonly from breast; less commonly pancreas, stomach, ovary and kidney. Look for evidence of surgery.
3. **Mesothelioma**—effusion in 90%; often massive and obscures the underlying pleural disease.
4. **Lymphoma***—effusion is usually associated with lymphadenopathy or pulmonary infiltrates.
5. **Primary adenocarcinoma of the pleura.**

Immunological

1. **Systemic lupus erythematosus***—effusion is usually small, but may be massive or bilateral. Cardiomegaly may also be present.

2. Rheumatoid arthritis*—almost exclusively in males. Usually unilateral and may predate joint disease. Tends to remain unchanged for a long time.

Others

1. Pulmonary embolus—effusion is common and may obscure an underlying area of infarction.
2. Trauma—effusion may contain blood, lymph or food (due to oesophageal rupture, e.g. Boerhaave syndrome). The latter is almost always left-sided.
3. **Asbestosis**—mesothelioma and lung cancer should be excluded, but an effusion may be present in their absence. Frequently bilateral and recurrent.

Further reading

Ayres, J., Gleeson, F., 2010. Imaging of the pleura. Semin. Respir. Crit. Care Med. 31, 674–688.

5.32 PLEURAL CALCIFICATION

1. Asbestos exposure—pleural plaques most commonly form adjacent to the anterior rib ends and over the diaphragm. Usually bilateral.
2. Prior infection—especially previous tuberculous pleuritis/ empyema. Usually a unilateral large calcified plaque.
3. Talc pleurodesis—NB: the resulting calcified pleural thickening can remain PET avid for years and should not be mistaken for malignancy.
4. **Prior haemothorax**—may leave a residual calcified haematoma.

5.33 FOCAL PLEURAL MASS

Pleural and chest wall masses characteristically form an obtuse angle with the chest wall and have a well-defined medial margin on CXR, fading out laterally.

1. Loculated pleural effusion—or empyema.
2. Metastases—e.g. from lung or breast. Often multiple ± effusion.
3. Malignant mesothelioma—usually causes diffuse thickening, but can be focal. Nearly always related to asbestos exposure. May be obscured by an effusion.
4. Solitary fibrous tumour of the pleura (SFT)—benign in most cases. Usually a smooth lobular mass, up to 15 cm in diameter (may opacify entire hemithorax). May change position due to pedunculation. Patients are usually >40 years of age and asymptomatic. High rate of hypertrophic osteoarthropathy.

5. **Extrapleural haematoma**—in the setting of trauma.
6. **Chest wall masses**—e.g. lipoma, nerve sheath tumour, rib lesions, sarcoma. Look for scalloping or destruction of ribs.

5.34 DIFFUSE PLEURAL THICKENING

1. **Exudative pleural effusion**—including empyema. Mild smooth pleural thickening + associated effusion. The thickening is best seen on postcontrast CT (in the portal phase). Pleural thickening often persists after resolution of an empyema.
2. **Benign asbestos-related pleural thickening**—often bilateral, usually smooth, does not extend over the mediastinal pleural surface. Associated pleural plaques are typically present.
3. **Malignant mesothelioma**—typically unilateral, lobulated contour, extends over mediastinal pleural surface. Often associated with a small hemithorax.
4. **Extrapleural fat proliferation**—bilateral and symmetrical, smooth, usually seen in midzones. Associated with increased mediastinal and pericardial fat.
5. **Pleural metastases**—can be diffuse, usually lobulated + effusion.
6. **Post haemothorax.**
7. **Post thoracotomy or pleurodesis.**
8. **Related to peripheral lung fibrosis**—e.g. pleuroparenchymal fibroelastosis (apical and bilateral).

5.35 PNEUMOTHORAX

1. **Spontaneous**—M >> F, especially in tall, thin patients, usually due to ruptured blebs or bullae. ± Small pleural effusion. Association with Marfan and Loeys-Dietz syndromes.
2. **Iatrogenic**—following chest aspiration, positive pressure ventilation, lung biopsy or central line/pacemaker insertion.
3. **Trauma**—± rib fractures, haemothorax, surgical emphysema or pneumomediastinum.
4. **Secondary to lung disease**—e.g. emphysema, cystic fibrosis, cystic lung diseases (LAM, LCH, PCP, etc.), bronchopleural fistula (e.g. due to lung abscess or carcinoma), lung metastases (e.g. from osteosarcoma and other sarcomas).
5. **Extension of pneumomediastinum**—see Section 5.36.
6. **Extension of pneumoperitoneum**—air passage through a pleuroperitoneal foramen.

5.36 PNEUMOMEDIASTINUM

Radiographic signs depend on air outlining normal anatomical structures, e.g. continuous diaphragm sign, pneumopericardium, gas in cervical soft tissues. May be associated with a pneumothorax.

1. Extension of pulmonary interstitial emphysema (PIE)—a sudden rise in intraalveolar pressure, often with airway narrowing, causes air to dissect through the interstitium to the hilum and then to the mediastinum.
   (a) **Spontaneous**—most common cause, may follow coughing or strenuous exercise.
   (b) **Positive pressure ventilation.**
   (c) **Chest trauma.**
   (d) **Vaginal delivery**—due to repeated Valsalva manoeuvres.
   (e) **Asthma**—but usually not <2 years of age.
   (f) **Foreign body aspiration**—especially if <2 years.
2. Perforation of oesophagus, trachea or bronchus—a ruptured oesophagus is often associated with a hydrothorax or hydropneumothorax, usually on the left side.
3. Perforation of a hollow abdominal viscus—with extension of gas via the retroperitoneal space and diaphragmatic hiatus.

Further reading

Katabathina, V.S., Restrepo, C.S., Martinez-Jimenez, S., Riascos, R.F., 2011. Nonvascular, nontraumatic mediastinal emergencies in adults: a comprehensive review of imaging findings. Radiographics 31, 1141–1160.

Zylak, C.M., Standen, J.R., Barnes, G.R., Zylak, C.J., 2000. Pneumomediastinum. Radiographics 20, 1043–1057.

5

5.37 DIAPHRAGMATIC HUMPS

At any site

1. Collapse/consolidation of adjacent lung.
2. Localized eventration.
3. Subpulmonary effusion—often moves apex of 'diaphragm' shadow laterally on erect CXR. If on the left side, the distance between lung and stomach bubble is increased.
4. Pulmonary infarct—Hampton's hump.
5. Subphrenic abscess.
6. Hepatic abscess, metastasis or hydatid cyst—may extend through the diaphragm.

Medially

1. Pericardial fat pad.
2. Hiatus hernia.
3. Aortic aneurysm.
4. Pleuropericardial cyst.
5. Pulmonary sequestration.

Anteriorly

Morgagni hernia.

Posteriorly

1. Bochdalek hernia.
2. Neurogenic tumour—e.g. schwannoma, paraganglioma, plexiform neurofibroma, etc.

Further reading

Nason, L.K., Walker, C.M., McNeeley, M.F., et al., 2012. Imaging of the diaphragm: anatomy and function. Radiographics 32, E51–E70.

5.38 UNILATERAL ELEVATED HEMIDIAPHRAGM

Causes above the diaphragm

1. Phrenic nerve palsy—smooth hemidiaphragm. No movement on respiration. Paradoxical movement on sniffing. The mediastinum is usually central. The cause may be evident on the X-ray.
2. Lung collapse.
3. Pleural disease—e.g. old haemothorax, empyema, thoracotomy.
4. Splinting of the diaphragm—due to pain associated with rib fractures, pleurisy or subphrenic abscess.
5. **Hemiplegia**—upper motor neuron lesion, e.g. stroke.

Diaphragmatic causes

1. Eventration—left > right. The heart is often displaced to the contralateral side. Limited movement on normal respiration.
2. Herniation—right-sided may result in liver herniation with no gas above the diaphragmatic defect. Left-sided is generally more obvious with aerated bowel in the thoracic cavity. May be congenital or traumatic (rupture); both are more common on the left.

Causes below the diaphragm

1. Subphrenic inflammation—e.g. subphrenic abscess, hepatic or splenic abscess, pancreatitis.
2. Marked hepatomegaly or splenomegaly—e.g. extensive liver metastases.
3. **Gaseous distension of the stomach or splenic flexure**—left side only. May be transient.

Scoliosis

The raised hemidiaphragm is on the side of the concavity.

Decubitus film

The raised hemidiaphragm is on the dependent side.

5.39 BILATERAL ELEVATED HEMIDIAPHRAGMS

General causes

1. **Poor inspiratory effort**.
2. **Obesity**.
3. **Muscular weakness and myopathy**—myotonia, SLE.
4. **Lordotic projection**—causes apparent elevation of the diaphragm. The clavicles will also appear abnormally high.

Causes above the diaphragm

1. **Bilateral basal lung collapse**—e.g. due to infarction, obstructive atelectasis or poor inspiratory excursion.
2. **Small lungs**—congenital (e.g. hypoplastic lung) or acquired (e.g. fibrotic lung disease).

Causes below the diaphragm

1. **Ascites**.
2. **Pneumoperitoneum**.
3. **Pregnancy**.
4. **Hepatosplenomegaly**.
5. **Large intraabdominal tumour**.
6. **Bilateral subphrenic abscesses.**

5.40 ANTERIOR MEDIASTINAL MASSES IN ADULTS

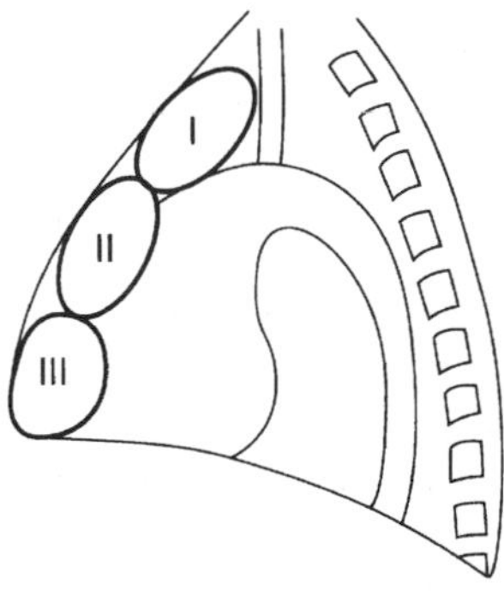

Anterior to the pericardium and trachea. On a lateral CXR, the retrosternal air space is obliterated. On a frontal CXR, anterior mediastinal masses do not have visible margins above the level of the clavicles; if these margins are visible this suggests a middle or posterior mediastinal mass. The anterior mediastinum can be divided into three regions.

Region I

1. Retrosternal goitre—on a PA CXR it appears as an inverted truncated cone with its base uppermost. It is well-defined, smooth or lobulated, without a visible upper margin. The trachea may be displaced posteriorly and laterally and may be narrowed. Calcification is common. CT shows the connection with the thyroid. Relatively high attenuation compared with other mediastinal structures and tumours. Uptake by iodine-123 is diagnostic when positive, but the thyroid may be nonfunctioning.
2. Lymphadenopathy—due to lymphoma, metastases, Castleman disease or granulomatous disorders.
3. Thymic tumours/enlargement
   (a) Thymoma—usually in middle-aged patients; occurs in 15% of those with myasthenia gravis and 40% of these will be malignant. If malignant it is usually locally invasive and can spread along pleura to involve the diaphragm and even into the abdomen. Can contain calcification.
   (b) **Thymic hyperplasia**—lymphoid hyperplasia most commonly occurs in myasthenia gravis but can be seen in other autoimmune disorders. True hyperplasia can occur post chemotherapy ('rebound' hyperplasia), steroid therapy, radiotherapy, burns and other systemic stressors. Thymus is diffusely enlarged but normal in shape.
   (c) **Thymic germ cell tumour**—teratodermoid, benign and malignant teratomas.
   (d) **Thymic lymphoma**—thymus can be infiltrated in Hodgkin disease but there is always associated lymphadenopathy.
   (e) **Thymolipoma**—usually children or young adults. Asymptomatic. Contains fat on CT.
   (f) **Thymic cyst**—can develop after radiotherapy for lymphoma.
4. **Ectopic parathyroid adenoma**—typically small (only visible on CT), often avidly enhancing, may mimic a lymph node.

Region II

1. Germ cell neoplasms—including dermoids, teratomas, seminomas, choriocarcinomas, embryonal carcinomas and endodermal sinus tumours. Most are benign. Usually larger than thymomas (but not thymolipomas) and peak in a younger age group. Round/oval, smooth, ± calcification especially rim calcification or fragments of bone/teeth, the latter being diagnostic. Fat may be seen within teratodermoids.
2. Thymic tumours—see earlier.

3. Sternal tumours—metastases (breast, lung, kidney and thyroid) are the most common. Of the primary tumours, malignant (chondrosarcoma, myeloma, lymphoma) are more common than benign (chondroma, aneurysmal bone cyst, giant cell tumour).

Region III (anterior cardiophrenic angle masses)

1. Pericardial fat pad—especially in the obese. A triangular opacity in the cardiophrenic angle on the PA view, less dense than expected due to the fat content. CT is diagnostic. Excessive mediastinal fat can be the result of steroid therapy.
2. Diaphragmatic eventration—commonest in the anteromedial portion of the right hemidiaphragm.
3. Morgagni hernia—through a defect between the septum transversum and costal portion of the diaphragm. Almost invariably on the right side, but occasionally extends across the midline. Often contains a knuckle of colon ± stomach. Appears solid if it contains omentum and/or liver.
4. Pericardial cysts—either a true pericardial cyst or a pericardial diverticulum. Oval or spherical, usually situated in the right cardiophrenic angle. Fluid attenuation on CT.

5

Further reading

Drevelegas, A., Palladas, P., Scordalaki, A., 2001. Mediastinal germ cell tumours: a radiologic–pathologic review. Eur. Radiol. 11, 1925–1932.

Frank, L., Quint, L.E., 2012. Chest CT incidentalomas: thyroid lesions, enlarged mediastinal lymph nodes, and lung nodules. Cancer Imaging 12, 41–48.

Landwehr, P., Schulte, O., Lackner, K., 1999. MR imaging of the chest: mediastinum and chest wall. Eur. Radiol. 9, 1737–1744.

Quint, L.E., 2007. Imaging of anterior mediastinal masses. Cancer Imaging 7 (SpecA), S56–S62.

Takahashi, K., Al-Janabi, N.J., 2010. Computed tomography and magnetic resonance imaging of mediastinal tumors. J. Magn. Reson. Imaging 32, 1325–1339.

5.41 MIDDLE MEDIASTINAL MASSES IN ADULTS

These occur between the anterior and posterior mediastinum, containing the heart, great vessels and pulmonary roots. Causes of cardiac enlargement are not described here. Note that if a mediastinal mass overlaps one or both hila on a frontal CXR, but the hilar margins are still visible ('hilum overlay' sign), this suggests the mass is not in the middle mediastinum.

1. Lymphadenopathy—paratracheal, tracheobronchial, bronchopulmonary and/or subcarinal nodes may be enlarged. This may be due to metastases (most frequently from lung cancer), lymphoma (most frequently Hodgkin disease), infection (e.g. TB,

histoplasmosis or coccidioidomycosis), sarcoidosis or Castleman disease.
2. Bronchogenic carcinoma—arising from a major bronchus.
3. Tortuous subclavian artery—common finding in the elderly; R>L. Can mimic a Pancoast tumour.
4. Aortic aneurysm—peripheral rim calcification is a useful sign if present.
5. Bronchogenic cyst—usually subcarinal or right paratracheal site. 50% homogeneous water density, 50% hyperattenuating due to protein or milk of calcium content. May contain air if communicating with the airway (generally due to prior infection).
6. **Fibrosing mediastinitis**—infiltrative mass that can encase and narrow mediastinal vessels and airways. Causes include histoplasmosis (most common, usually focal and calcified), IgG4-related disease (usually diffuse and noncalcified), TB, fungal infection and radiotherapy.

5.42 POSTERIOR MEDIASTINAL MASSES IN ADULTS

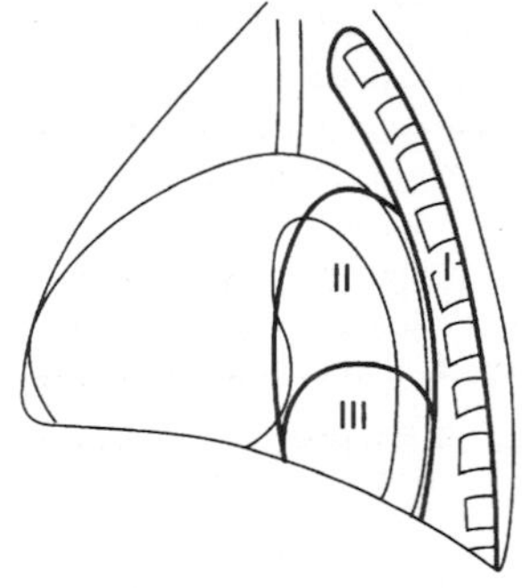

For ease of discussion it can be divided into three regions.

Region I (paravertebral)

1. Lymphoma*, myeloma and metastases—bone destruction with preserved discs.
2. Abscess—with disc space and/or vertebral body destruction.
3. Extramedullary haematopoiesis—with splenomegaly ± bone changes of the underlying haematological disorder.
4. Neurogenic tumours—e.g. neurofibroma, ganglioneuroma (young adults). Often extends through neural foramina into the spinal canal ± vertebral remodelling.
5. **Meningocoele**—with associated vertebral remodelling.
6. **Pancreatic pseudocyst**—fluid can extend into the mediastinum through a diaphragmatic hiatus and form a pseudocyst.
7. **Neurenteric cyst**—with an associated congenital spinal anomaly.

Region II

1. Dilated oesophagus—especially in achalasia. Contains mottled gas shadows ± an air–fluid level. Confirmed on barium swallow.
2. Descending aorta—unfolded, dilated or ruptured.
3. Oesophageal duplication cyst.

Region III

Hiatus hernia—often contains an air–fluid level that is projected through the cardiac shadow on a penetrated PA view.

Further reading

Takahashi, K., Al-Janabi, N.J., 2010. Computed tomography and magnetic resonance imaging of mediastinal tumors. J. Magn. Reson. Imaging 32, 1325–1339.

5.43 MEDIASTINAL MASS CONTAINING FAT

1. Hernia containing fat—e.g. hiatal (adjacent to oesophagus), Morgagni (anterior), Bochdalek (posterior).
2. Teratodermoid—usually also contains cystic and/or calcified components.
3. Thymolipoma—in anterior mediastinum, contains fat and soft-tissue strands, and can be very large. No cystic or calcified elements (cf. teratodermoid).
4. **Mediastinal lipomatosis**—generalized increase in mediastinal fat; related to obesity and steroids (endogenous or exogenous).
5. **Lipoma/liposarcoma**—discrete fatty mass; the latter contains soft-tissue elements that are typically more irregular than thymolipoma.
6. **Extramedullary haematopoiesis**—paravertebral mass or masses that may contain fat + signs of an underlying haematological disorder.
7. **Myelolipoma**—rare in the mediastinum, usually paravertebral in location.
8. **Epipericardial fat necrosis**—focal area of fat necrosis in pericardial fat pad resulting in focal fat stranding. Resolves spontaneously.
9. **Haemangioma**—often contains phleboliths, may show heterogeneous enhancement.
10. **Hibernoma**—very rare in the mediastinum.

5.44 AVIDLY ENHANCING MEDIASTINAL MASS

1. Saccular aneurysm.
2. Retrosternal thyroid goitre.

3. Varices—may be 'uphill' (found around distal oesophagus, due to portal hypertension) or 'downhill' (found around upper oesophagus, due to SVC obstruction).
4. Hypervascular nodal metastases—e.g. from RCC, melanoma, thyroid cancer.
5. Castleman disease—avidly enhancing hyperplastic lymph nodes.
6. Ectopic parathyroid adenoma—usually small and in the upper mediastinum.
7. **Paraganglioma**—usually in posterior mediastinum or pericardial.
8. **Haemangioma**—may contain phleboliths.
9. **Bacillary angiomatosis**—in AIDS patients; avidly enhancing nodes due to *Bartonella* infection.
10. **Kaposi sarcoma**—also in AIDS patients; nodes may enhance avidly and are usually accompanied by ill-defined lung nodules.

5.45 FOCAL RIB LESION (SOLITARY OR MULTIPLE)

1. Healed rib fracture.
2. Rib metastases—e.g. from lung, kidney, prostate or breast.
3. Fibrous dysplasia—most common benign rib lesion. Expansile, ground-glass density.
4. Paget's disease*—rib expansion + cortical thickening.
5. Rib destruction by an adjacent invasive mass.
   (a) Neoplastic—e.g. lung cancer, mesothelioma, lymphoma.
   (b) Infective—e.g. TB (tuberculous empyema), actinomycosis (lung mass), blastomycosis, nocardiosis.
6. Primary malignant tumours.
   (a) Multiple myeloma/plasmacytoma*—plasmacytoma is solitary and expansile, myeloma is multiple and punched-out.
   (b) Chondrosarcoma—most common primary malignant rib neoplasm.
   (c) Ewing sarcoma of chest wall—in children or young adults. Large soft-tissue mass, may fill hemithorax.
7. Benign tumours.
   (a) Osteochondroma—usually in multiple hereditary exostosis, at costochondral junction.
   (b) Enchondroma—lucent ± endosteal scalloping ± chondroid matrix.
   (c) **Langerhans cell histiocytosis***—lytic, variable appearance. Young patients.
   (d) **Aneurysmal bone cyst**—lytic and expansile, usually in posterolateral rib.
   (e) **Osteoblastoma**—lytic + sharp sclerotic margins, usually in posterolateral rib.

(f) **Osteoid osteoma**—rare. Lucent nidus + surrounding sclerosis that may involve adjacent ribs. Usually posterior ± painful scoliosis if close to the spine.
(g) **Giant cell tumour**—rare. Lytic and expansile.

8. **Nonneoplastic.**
   (a) **Brown tumour**—well-defined and lytic ± other features of hyperparathyroidism.
   (b) **Infection**—tuberculous (most common, well-defined margins), bacterial (usually at costochondral or costovertebral junction), fungal (e.g. aspergillosis) or parasitic (e.g. hydatid—well-defined expansile multiloculated cystic lesion).
   (c) **Radiation osteitis.**
   (d) **Lymphangiomatosis**—rare, involves multiple bones.

5

Further reading

Mullan, C.P., Madan, R., Trotman-Dickenson, B., et al., 2011. Radiology of chest wall masses. AJR Am. J. Roentgenol. 197, W460–W470.
Restrepo, R., Lee, E.Y., 2012. Updates on imaging of chest wall lesions in pediatric patients. Semin. Roentgenol. 47, 79–89.

5.46 RIB NOTCHING—INFERIOR SURFACE

Enlarged collateral vessels

1. **Coarctation of the aorta**—third to eighth ribs, usually bilateral, but may be right-sided if coarctation is proximal to the left subclavian artery, or left-sided if there is an anomalous right subclavian artery distal to the coarctation. Prominent ascending aorta, small descending aorta with an intervening notch.
2. **Proximal subclavian artery occlusion**—e.g. in Takayasu arteritis or after a Blalock shunt for tetralogy of Fallot (upper two ribs).
3. **Interrupted aortic arch.**
4. **Abdominal aortic occlusion**—notching of lower ribs bilaterally.
5. **Lung/chest wall arteriovenous malformation.**
6. **SVC obstruction**—venous collaterals less likely to cause notching.

Neurogenic

1. **Neurofibromatosis***—intercostal neurofibromas may scallop the inferior rib margin. Dysplastic 'ribbon ribs' may also be seen.
2. **Schwannoma**—single notch.

5.47 RIB NOTCHING—SUPERIOR SURFACE

1. **Connective tissue disorders**—e.g. rheumatoid arthritis, SLE, scleroderma, Sjögren's syndrome, Marfan syndrome.
2. **Hyperparathyroidism***—subperiosteal bone resorption. Can also involve inferior surface.

3. **Iatrogenic**—chest drains, thoracotomy retractors, radiotherapy.
4. **Osteogenesis imperfecta.**
5. **Neurofibroma/vascular collaterals**—if large enough, can cause superior + inferior notching.
6. **Intercostal muscle atrophy**—e.g. due to paralysis, poliomyelitis or restrictive lung disease. Reduced mechanical stress leads to bone loss.
7. **Progeria**—thin slender osteoporotic ribs.

5.48 WIDE OR THICK RIBS

1. **Fibrous dysplasia**.
2. **Healed fractures with callus**.
3. **Chronic anaemias**—e.g. thalassaemia. Due to marrow hyperplasia.
4. **Paget's disease***.
5. **Tuberous sclerosis*.**
6. **Achondroplasia***—short, wide ribs.
7. **Mucopolysaccharidoses***—ribs are widened distally.

5.49 CXR FOLLOWING CHEST TRAUMA

NB: CT is the modality of choice for assessment of major trauma.

Soft tissues

1. **Surgical emphysema**.
2. **Foreign bodies**—e.g. glass fragments.

Ribs

1. **Simple fracture**—± surgical emphysema, pneumothorax, haemothorax or extrapleural haematoma. First rib fractures have a high incidence of other associated injuries.
2. **Flail chest**—defined as ≥ 2 contiguous ribs fractured in two places. Suggests severe trauma and usually associated with other injuries, e.g. pneumothorax, haemothorax, lung contusion or laceration.

Sternum

1. **Fracture**—may be associated with a clinically unsuspected thoracic spine fracture.
2. **Sternoclavicular dislocation**.

Clavicles and scapulae

Fracture—scapular fractures are usually associated with other bony or intrathoracic injuries.

Spine

1. Fractures—when present, are multiple in 10% and noncontiguous in 80% of these. Thoracic spine injuries have a much higher incidence of neurological deficit than cervical or lumbar spine injuries.
2. Cord trauma.
3. Nerve root trauma—especially to the brachial plexus.

Pleura

1. Pneumothorax—simple or tension. Signs of a small pneumothorax on a supine CXR include a deep costophrenic sulcus, basal hyperlucency, a 'double' diaphragm, unusually clear definition of the right cardiophrenic angle or left cardiac apex and visualization of apical pericardial fat tags. CT is more sensitive than plain film.
2. Haemothorax—more common with penetrating trauma.

Lung

1. Contusion—nonsegmental alveolar opacities that resolve in a few days.
2. Laceration—a shearing injury results in a parenchymal tear that may fill with blood or air and result in a rounded opacity or lucency. Usually resolves spontaneously.
3. Haematoma—usually appears following resolution of a contusion. Round, well-defined nodule. Resolution in several weeks.
4. Aspiration pneumonia.
5. Pulmonary oedema—following blast injuries or head injury (neurogenic oedema).
6. ARDS—widespread consolidation appearing 1–3 days after injury.
7. Fat embolism—1–2 days post trauma. Resembles pulmonary oedema, but normal heart size and pleural effusions are uncommon. Resolves in 1–4 weeks. Neurological symptoms and skin abnormalities may be seen.
8. **Foreign body.**

Trachea and bronchi

Laceration or fracture—initially pneumomediastinum and surgical emphysema followed by collapse of the affected lung or lobe + pneumothorax. Indicates severe trauma. The pneumothorax does not usually resolve with tube drainage. May heal with stenosis.

Diaphragm

Rupture—left > right, more common with penetrating thoracoabdominal trauma. Diagnosis may be delayed for months or years, especially with right-sided rupture. CXR findings include herniated stomach or bowel above the diaphragm, pleural effusion, a supradiaphragmatic mass or a poorly visualized or abnormally contoured diaphragm. Often associated with liver and splenic injuries.

Mediastinum

1. **Aortic injury/rupture**—90% occur just distal to the origin of the left subclavian artery. The majority die before radiological evaluation, especially if the rupture involves the ascending aorta. Plain film signs of aortic rupture include mediastinal widening, abnormal aortic contour, left apical cap, tracheal displacement to the right, nasogastric (NG) tube displacement to the right of the T4 spinous process, thickening of the right paraspinal stripe, depression of the left main bronchus >40 degrees below the horizontal and loss of definition of the aortopulmonary window.
2. **Mediastinal haematoma**—blurred mediastinal outline. Most cases are not due to aortic rupture but are related to other large or small vessel bleeds.
3. **Pneumomediastinum**.
4. **Haemopericardium**—suggests pericardial, myocardial or ascending aortic injury.
5. **Oesophageal rupture**.

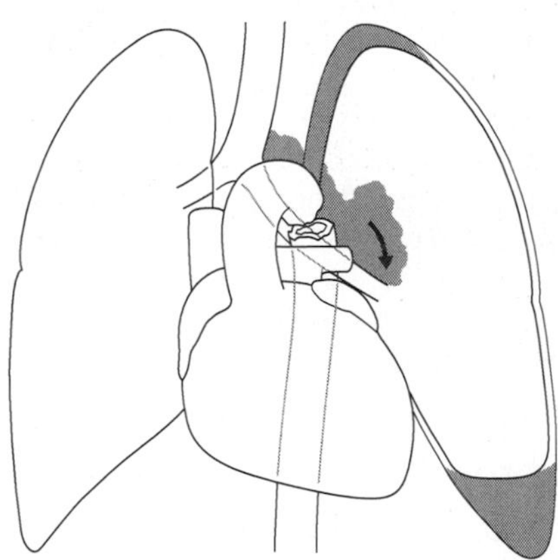

Aortic rupture. Haematoma widens mediastinum, causes apical capping, displaces the trachea to the right, depresses the left main bronchus and causes a pleural effusion.

Further reading

Desai, S.R., 2002. Acute respiratory distress syndrome: imaging of the injured lung. Clin. Radiol. 57, 8–17.

Peters, S., Nicolas, V., Heyer, C.M., 2010. Multidetector computed tomography-spectrum of blunt chest wall and lung injuries in polytraumatized patients. Clin. Radiol. 65, 333–338.

Cardiovascular system

Swamy Gedela, Jeremy Rabouhans, Alessandro Ruggiero

6.1 GROSS CARDIOMEGALY ON CXR

1. Ischaemic heart disease—and other cardiomyopathies.
2. Pericardial effusion—globular (supine radiograph) or flask-shaped heart (erect radiograph), crisp cardiac outline (as the effusion masks ventricular wall motion).
3. Multivalve disease—particularly regurgitation.
4. Congenital heart disease—ASD is the most common to present in adults. Eisenmenger's syndrome may develop in longstanding untreated ASD, resulting in chronic pulmonary hypertension, shunt reversal and gross cardiomegaly.

6.2 RIGHT ATRIAL ENLARGEMENT

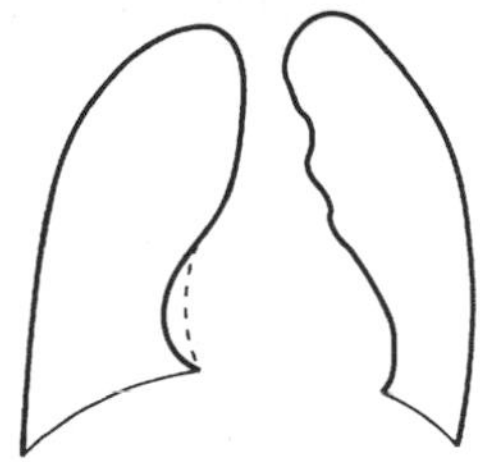

PA
Prominent right heart border

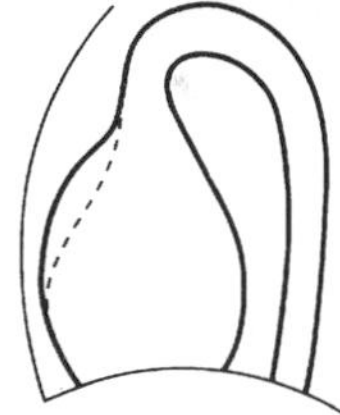

Lateral
Prominent anterosuperior part of cardiac shadow

Secondary to RV failure—most common cause.

Volume loading

1. Tricuspid regurgitation.
2. ASD or AVSD.
3. Chronic atrial fibrillation (AF).
4. Anomalous pulmonary venous return—partial type if presents in adulthood.
5. **Ebstein's anomaly**—congenitally abnormal tricuspid valve, which is displaced into the RV, resulting in a large RA and a small RV ±

tricuspid regurgitation. Usually presents in childhood. May be associated with other congenital heart defects, particularly ASD.

Pressure loading

1. **Tricuspid stenosis**.
2. **Constrictive pericarditis or restrictive cardiomyopathy**—both usually cause biatrial enlargement with small/normal ventricles. In constrictive pericarditis there is usually pericardial calcification/ thickening >3 mm and often a diastolic septal 'bounce' on MRI. In restrictive cardiomyopathy these features are absent and there may be myocardial thickening/LGE on MRI depending on the cause (e.g. amyloidosis, HCM, systemic sclerosis).
3. **Tricuspid valve obstruction**—by tumour or thrombus.

6.3 RIGHT VENTRICULAR ENLARGEMENT

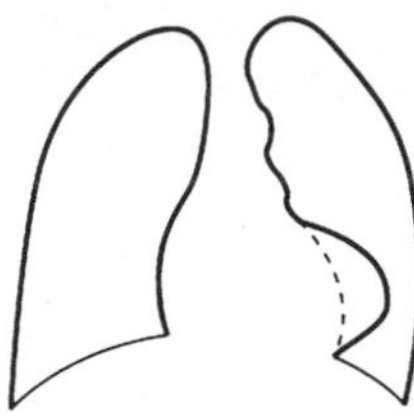

PA
Prominent left heart border
Elevated apex

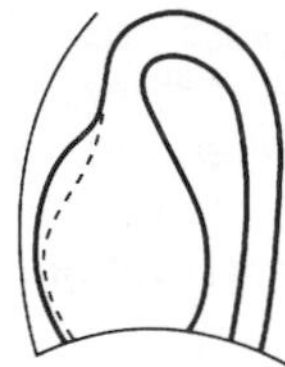

Lateral
Prominent anterior part of cardiac shadow

Volume loading

1. **Tricuspid or pulmonary regurgitation**.
2. **ASD, VSD or AVSD**.
3. **Anomalous pulmonary venous return**—partial type if presents in adulthood.
4. **Cardiomyopathy**—ARVC (fibrofatty replacement of the RV myocardium + dilatation + hypokinesis ± small RV aneurysms ± LGE, usually presents in young adults) or Uhl's anomaly (absence of the RV myocardium resulting in a paper-thin RV wall but no intramural fat, usually presents in infancy).

Pressure loading (which may lead to increased RV volume)

1. **Pulmonary hypertension**—see Section 6.21.
2. **Pulmonary stenosis**—including Tetralogy of Fallot.
3. **Acute PE**—right heart strain.

6.4 LEFT ATRIAL ENLARGEMENT

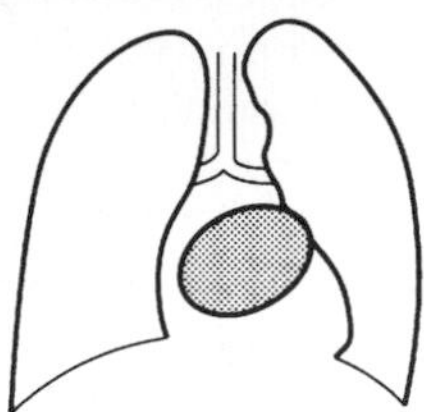

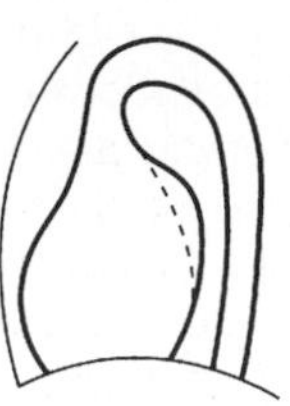

PA

1 Prominent left atrial appendage
2 'Double' right heart border
3 Increased density due to left atrium
4 Splaying of carina and elevated left main bronchus

Lateral

1 Prominent posterosuperior part of cardiac shadow
2 Prominent left atrial impression on oesophagus during barium swallow

Volume loading

1. Mitral regurgitation.
2. Chronic atrial fibrillation.
3. VSD or PDA.

Pressure loading

1. Left ventricular failure.
2. Mitral stenosis.
3. Hypertrophic cardiomyopathy—via LV diastolic dysfunction, outflow obstruction and mitral regurgitation.
4. Constrictive pericarditis or restrictive cardiomyopathy—both usually cause biatrial enlargement (see Section 6.2).
5. **Mitral valve obstruction due to tumour**—e.g. myxoma.

6.5 LEFT VENTRICULAR ENLARGEMENT

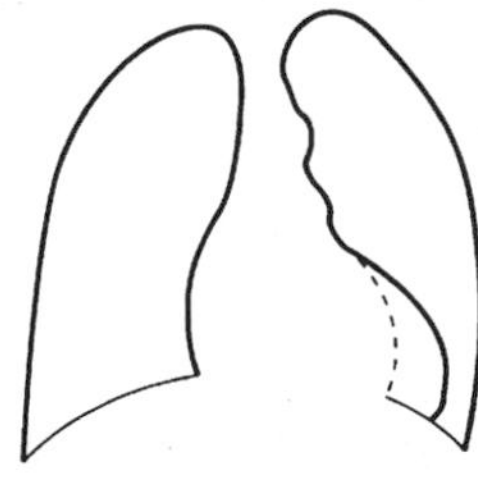

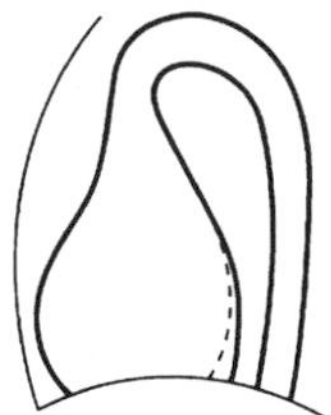

PA

1 Prominent left heart border
2 Rounding of left heart border
3 Apex displaced inferiorly

Lateral

Prominent posteroinferior part of cardiac shadow

Myocardial disease

1. Ischaemic heart disease—evidence of significant coronary artery disease on CT. Old myocardial infarcts are seen on MRI as focal areas of subendocardial/transmural LGE ± wall thinning/ calcification/fat deposition conforming to a vascular territory.
2. Cardiomyopathy
   (a) DCM—dilated LV + systolic dysfunction without evidence of IHD/valve disease. Linear midwall/subepicardial LGE is common and a poor prognostic indicator. Many different causes, though idiopathic is most common and often shows LGE in the septum. Some causes have suggestive features on MRI:
      (i) **Haemochromatosis***—diffusely reduced T2/T2* signal throughout the myocardium (as well as the liver).
      (ii) **Sarcoidosis***—patchy areas of myocardial thinning and midwall/subepicardial LGE ± aneurysms. Lung and nodal involvement is usually also present.
      (iii) **Chagas disease***—focal myocardial thinning typically involving the apex and inferolateral wall with midwall/ subepicardial LGE ± apical aneurysm.
   (b) **ARVC**—can be biventricular; LV-dominant forms also exist. Diagnosis is based on task force criteria; MRI cannot make the diagnosis alone. Intramural fat may be present.
3. LV aneurysm/pseudoaneurysm—focal thin-walled saccular dilatation ± mural thrombus ± calcification. True aneurysms usually develop weeks to months after myocardial infarction (MI) and typically arise from the apex/anterolateral wall, with a broad neck and a low risk of rupture. Pseudoaneurysms usually represent a contained LV rupture (developing soon after a transmural MI) and typically arise from the basal inferolateral wall, with a narrow neck and a high risk of rupture. Cardiac surgery/trauma are less common causes. If visible on CXR (due to calcification), true aneurysms are best seen on the frontal view, whereas pseudoaneurysms are best seen on the lateral view (arising from the posterior margin of the cardiac shadow). A congenital LV diverticulum may mimic an aneurysm on MRI, but is usually found in younger patients and often demonstrates contractility.

Volume loading

1. Aortic or mitral regurgitation.
2. PDA—the pulmonary arteries and ascending aorta are also usually dilated.
3. VSD—this shunts blood directly into the right ventricular outflow tract (RVOT) leading to LV dilatation even in large defects.
4. **Athlete's heart**—depending on the type of athletic activity, can lead to increased LV/RV volumes and/or LV hypertrophy (which

rarely exceeds 15 mm in thickness). Mild LA dilatation may also be seen. Cardiac function is normal.

5. **High-output cardiac failure**—e.g. due to severe anaemia (e.g. sickle cell), hyperthyroidism, systemic arteriovenous shunting.

Pressure loading (usually causes diffuse concentric hypertrophy but may increase LV volume)

1. **Hypertension.**
2. **Aortic stenosis.**

Further reading for 6.1–6.5

Baron, M.G., Book, W.M., 2004. Congenital heart disease in the adult: 2004. Radiol. Clin. North Am. 42, 675–690.

Gross, G.W., Steiner, R.M., 1991. Radiographic manifestations of congenital heart disease in the adult patient. Radiol. Clin. North Am. 29, 293–318.

6.6 CARDIAC CALCIFICATION

Valves (if visible on CXR, suggests clinically significant stenosis)

1. **Aortic valve calcification**—bicuspid aortic valve (especially in patients <65 years), degenerative aortic sclerosis (usually >65 years), previous rheumatic fever. A calcified ring with a central bar (calcified commissure) suggests a bicuspid valve. Rarer causes include previous infective endocarditis, end-stage renal failure, Paget's disease and ochronosis.
2. **Mitral calcification**—degenerative annular calcification (involves valve annulus only; curvilinear/J-shaped), previous rheumatic fever (involves valve leaflets; amorphous/nodular).
3. **Pulmonary valve calcification**—rare; pulmonary stenosis, chronic pulmonary hypertension, rheumatic fever.
4. **Tricuspid valve calcification**—rare; rheumatic fever, previous infective endocarditis, ASD. Degenerative annular calcification can also occur (curvilinear, C-shaped).
5. **Homograft calcification.**

Intracardiac (intraluminal)

1. **Calcified thrombus**—e.g. in the LV (post MI) or LA appendage. Often thick and laminated.
2. **Papillary muscle calcification**—associated with coronary artery disease, dilated cardiomyopathy, mitral valve disease and disorders of calcium metabolism.
3. **Calcified tumour**—mostly myxomas, although rare intracardiac tumours such as haemangiomas, paragangliomas and primary cardiac osteosarcomas can also calcify.

4. **Postinfective calcification**—valve vegetations, tuberculomas and hydatid cysts may all calcify.

Myocardium

On CXR the calcification is usually located in the LV with a rim of soft tissue between it and the margin of the cardiac shadow.

1. **Postinfarction**—usually involves LV. Myocardial thinning ± fat also present on CT/MR.
2. **Previous rheumatic fever**—usually involves the posterior LA wall. Curvilinear, may be extensive ('porcelain atrium'—ring shape on frontal CXR, C shape on lateral view).
3. **Calcified tumour**—cardiac fibromas often contain dystrophic calcification. Some metastases can also calcify.
4. **Metastatic calcification**—due to chronic renal failure/ hypercalcaemia/oxalosis. Usually diffuse throughout myocardium.
5. **Severe sepsis/myocarditis**—can rarely cause diffuse myocardial calcification in the acute setting, which may slowly resolve after recovery.

Pericardium

On CXR the calcification is usually located at the margin of the cardiac shadow, particularly overlying the RV on the lateral view. Pericardial calcification is strongly associated with constrictive pericarditis.

1. **Previous pericarditis**—idiopathic, uraemic, viral, TB, pyogenic infection. Calcification related to previous TB is usually thick, irregular and located along the atrioventricular groove.
2. **Following radiotherapy.**
3. **Previous trauma**—e.g. haemopericardium, cardiac surgery.
4. **Chronic renal failure/hypercalcaemia.**
5. **Asbestos-related pleural plaques**—overlying the pericardium.
6. **Calcified pericardial mass**—e.g. pericardial cyst or teratoma.

Coronary arteries

1. **Atheroma**—Agatston score obtained by an unenhanced low-dose CT assesses the extent of coronary artery calcification (not soft-tissue plaques). It allows for a risk stratification for major adverse cardiac events.
2. **Chronic renal failure**—often heavy diffuse calcification that is partly related to advanced atheroma.

Further reading

Ferguson, E.C., Berkowitz, E.A., 2010. Cardiac and pericardial calcifications on chest radiographs. Clin. Radiol. 65, 685–694.

Gowda, R.M., Boxt, L.M., 2004. Calcifications of the heart. Radiol. Clin. North Am. 42, 603–617.
Greenland, P., Bonow, R.O., Brundage, B.H., et al., 2007. ACCF/AHA 2007 Clinical expert consensus document on coronary artery calcium scoring by CT in global cardiovascular risk assessment and in evaluation of patients with chest pain. J. Am. Coll. Cardiol. 49, 378–402.

6.7 MYOCARDIAL DISEASES

LV generalized (concentric) myocardial wall thickening ≥12 mm (measured at end-diastole)

1. Hypertension—LV wall usually <15 mm. Typically no LGE.
2. Aortic stenosis—LV wall usually <15 mm. Typically no LGE.
3. Athlete's heart—LV wall usually <15 mm. No LGE. Normal cardiac function.
4. Hypertrophic cardiomyopathy (concentric subtype)—LV wall usually >15 mm. Patchy midwall areas of LGE, particularly at the anterior and posterior insertion points of the RV.
5. Myocardial infiltration
   (a) Amyloid—usually in older patients. Concentric myocardial hypertrophy, diastolic dysfunction and restrictive filling. Global subendocardial LGE is pathognomonic. Difficult to achieve myocardial nulling on the TI scout. Often involves both ventricles and atria; thickening of the RA free wall >6 mm is suggestive. Pericardial and pleural effusions are common.
   (b) **Fabry disease**—younger patients, M>F (X-linked). Concentric LV hypertrophy with focal LGE typically in the basal inferolateral midwall.
   (c) **Danon disease**—younger patients, X-linked, rare. Marked concentric LV thickening (up to 60 mm) ± RV thickening. Subendocardial LGE not conforming to a vascular territory.

RV generalized myocardial wall thickening

1. Pulmonary hypertension.
2. **RV outflow tract obstruction**—e.g. tumour, myocardial infiltration or congenital bands.
3. **Pulmonary valve stenosis.**

Focal myocardial thickening

1. Hypertrophic cardiomyopathy—many subtypes depending on region of LV myocardium involved. Thickness usually >15 mm. LGE is usually present in a patchy midwall distribution, often involving the thickest segments.

6

(a) Classical (asymmetric)—most common (70% of patients). Hypertrophy involves the basal anteroseptal and anterior segments, which can obstruct the LV outflow tract and cause systolic anterior motion of the mitral valve.
(b) **Apical (Yamaguchi syndrome)**—more common in East Asian patients. 'Ace of spades' appearance of LV due to apical thickening ± thin-walled apical aneurysm with LGE ('burned-out apex'). RV apex may also be involved.
(c) **Midventricular**—thickened mid-third of LV myocardium ± apical aneurysm, resulting in a dumbbell configuration. Rare.
(d) **Mass-like**—focal myocardial thickening, which may mimic a neoplasm, but can be differentiated based on T1/T2 signal (isointense to normal myocardium), contractility on myocardial tagging sequences and the typical LGE pattern.
(e) **Noncontiguous**—separate focal areas of LV wall thickening ± patchy LGE.

2. Sarcoidosis* (acute phase)—focal nodular areas of myocardial thickening, most commonly in the basal septum and LV free wall, demonstrating increased T2 signal and midwall/transmural LGE, representing active granulomatous inflammation.
3. **Eosinophilic myocarditis/endomyocardial fibrosis**—both conditions have similar and characteristic features on MRI: obliteration of the RV and/or LV apex with subendocardial LGE and overlying mural thrombus. Differentiation between the two is based on the presence of eosinophilia (absent in endomyocardial fibrosis). The appearances may mimic apical HCM, but the apical obliteration is due to fibrosis rather than true hypertrophy.
4. **Friedreich ataxia**—young patients. Focal thickening of LV septum and posterior wall. Diagnosis usually known due to earlier onset of neurological abnormalities.

Myocardial thinning

1. Generalized—in LV dilatation due to IHD or DCM. The presence/absence of coronary artery disease and pattern of LGE helps differentiate the two—subendocardial in IHD, midwall (or no LGE) in DCM.
2. Focal
   (a) Previous infarction—most common cause. May be associated with focal fat deposition, calcification and aneurysm/pseudoaneurysm formation. Subendocardial or transmural LGE on MRI. Conforms to coronary artery territory.
   (b) LV noncompaction—congenital arrest of the normal compaction process of LV trabeculae resulting in characteristic focal myocardial thinning and hypertrabeculation, most commonly involving the midapical myocardium ± subendocardial/trabecular LGE ± small mural thrombi. The

ratio of noncompacted to compacted myocardium is usually >2:1 at end systole on short-axis views.

(c) Sarcoidosis* (chronic/fibrotic phase)—typically involves the basal septum and LV free wall with focal thinning and patchy subepicardial/midwall LGE ± aneurysms.

(d) **Myocardial crypt**—narrow U/V-shaped clefts within the LV myocardium most commonly found in the inferobasal region, without evidence of noncompaction. Usually a normal variant but can also be associated with HCM mutations.

(e) **Takotsubo cardiomyopathy**—transient LV dysfunction caused by severe emotional/physical stress, most common in postmenopausal women, although it can also rarely be due to an underlying phaeochromocytoma. Typically causes hypokinesis of the midapical LV with apical ballooning and thinning in systole ± myocardial oedema, but characteristically no LGE. An 'inverted' pattern of hypokinesis involving the basal/midventricular myocardium has also been described.

(f) **Burned-out HCM**—e.g. at the LV apex in the apical/midventricular subtypes.

(g) **Chagas disease* (chronic)**—protozoan infection (*Trypanosoma cruzi*) endemic in areas of Central/South America. Causes focal thinning, akinesis and fibrosis of the LV myocardium typically involving the apex and inferolateral wall with midwall/subepicardial LGE. Apical aneurysms are common.

6

Fatty lesions of the myocardium

1. Lipomatous hypertrophy of the interatrial septum—normal variant associated with increasing age, obesity and steroid use. Typically dumbbell-shaped and spares the fossa ovalis. Often demonstrates increased uptake on PET due to brown fat content.
2. Fatty replacement of an old myocardial infarct—usually linear and subendocardial in the LV, with evidence of coronary artery disease ± myocardial calcification/thinning.
3. **Lipoma**—well-defined purely fatty mass, usually endocardial (protruding into lumen) or epicardial (protruding into pericardial space).
4. **Fatty infiltration of the RV free wall**—typically seen in ARVC, but may also be seen incidentally in older patients (usually in the RVOT). In ARVC there is also RV enlargement + hypokinesis ± LGE ± small aneurysms. The LV is affected less frequently.
5. **Tuberous sclerosis***—unencapsulated fatty deposits (often multiple), typically midmyocardial in the septum/LV. Cardiac angiomyolipomas have also been reported.
6. **Teratoma**—rare, usually intrapericardial, typically presents in infancy. Soft-tissue, fluid and calcified components also present.

7. **Liposarcoma**—very rare. Often large, infiltrative + soft-tissue component ± metastases.

Further reading

Bogaert, J., Olivotto, I., 2014. MR imaging in hypertrophic cardiomyopathy: from magnet to bedside. Radiology 273 (2), 329–348.

Chun, E.J., Choi, S.I., Jin, K.N., et al., 2010. Hypertrophic cardiomyopathy: assessment with MR imaging and multidetector CT. Radiographics 30, 1309–1328.

Hansen, M.W., Merchant, N., 2007. MRI of hypertrophic cardiomyopathy: part 1, MRI appearances. AJR Am. J. Roentgenol. 189, 1335–1343.

Hansen, M.W., Merchant, N., 2007. MRI of hypertrophic cardiomyopathy: part 2, differential diagnosis, risk stratification and posttreatment MRI appearances. Radiographics 189, 1344–1352.

Pruente, R., Restrepo, C.S., Ocazionez, D., et al., 2015. Fatty lesions in and around the heart: a pictorial review. Br. J. Radiol. 88 (1051), 20150157.

Seward, J.B., 2010. Casaclang-Verzosa G. Infiltrative cardiovascular diseases: cardiomyopathies that look alike. J. Am. Coll. Cardiol. 55, 1769–1779.

6.8 PERICARDIAL DISEASES

Pericardial thickening (>3 mm)

NB: always look for evidence of pericardial constriction especially if calcification is present. Signs include normal/small/tubular ventricles with biatrial enlargement, a diastolic septal 'bounce' and inspiratory diastolic septal flattening/bowing towards the LV (D-shaped on short-axis MRI) due to increased RV diastolic pressure on inspiration.

1. **Previous pericarditis**—idiopathic, infection (viral, TB, pyogenic), connective tissue diseases (most commonly seen in SLE and rheumatoid arthritis).
2. **Post cardiac surgery or mediastinal radiotherapy.**
3. **Previous trauma/haemopericardium.**
4. **Malignancy**—e.g. metastases (most common by far), pericardial mesothelioma, lymphoma, sarcoma, direct invasion from lung/oesophageal cancer. Nodular pericardial thickening + enhancement ± effusion. Lymphoma and sarcomas may present as a large infiltrative pericardial mass.

Pericardial effusion

Globular heart on frontal CXR if effusion is large. 'Oreo cookie' sign may be seen on lateral CXR. May cause tamponade if fluid accumulates quickly—features on MRI include diastolic collapse of the RA and RV free wall, and IVC dilatation without inspiratory collapse.

1. Transudate—e.g. cardiac failure, hypoalbuminaemia, renal failure. No pericardial thickening, enhancement or septations. Fluid attenuation close to water (<20 HU).
2. Exudate—e.g. infection (viral, TB, empyema), uraemic pericarditis, collagen vascular diseases (SLE, rheumatoid arthritis, scleroderma), malignancy, Dressler syndrome. Smooth pericardial thickening + enhancement may be present. Fluid attenuation is often higher than in transudate. Septations may be present in empyema.
3. Haemopericardium—acute aortic dissection, trauma, following cardiothoracic surgery, acute MI, tumour (metastases, lymphoma, local tumour invasion, primary pericardial malignancy). High attenuation fluid on CT, high T1 signal on MRI.
4. **Chylous**—e.g. malignancy, cardiothoracic surgery, pericardial lymphangioma. Fluid may be of low attenuation.

Further reading

Bogaert, J., Francone, M., 2013. Pericardial disease: value of CT and MR imaging. Radiology 267 (2), 340–356.

Peebles, C.R., Shambrook, J.S., Harden, S.P., 2011. Pericardial disease – anatomy and function. Br. J. Radiol. 84 (Spec3), S324–S337.

6

6.9 CARDIAC MASSES

1. Thrombus—most common intracardiac mass, often broad-based/crescent-shaped, may mimic a tumour but does not enhance. Usually occurs in aneurysms or in areas of hypokinesis, e.g. post MI (ventricles) or in AF (LA appendage). Also seen at ventricle apices in endomyocardial fibrosis/eosinophilic myocarditis, and around trabeculae in LV noncompaction. Can occur in RA around indwelling venous catheters with insufficient anticoagulation. May contain calcification if chronic.
2. Benign tumours—typically well-defined and noninfiltrative.
   - (a) Myxoma—most common primary cardiac tumour, typically within the LA arising from the interatrial septum close to the fossa ovalis. Lobular/oval shape, low attenuation on CT, usually pedunculated and mobile (can prolapse through the AV valve), ± calcification. Patchy LGE on MRI. If multiple/recurrent, consider a familial syndrome, e.g. Carney complex.
   - (b) **Papillary fibroelastoma**—typically small (<15 mm), pedunculated, arising from a valve (usually aortic/mitral). May mimic valve vegetation but can usually be differentiated based on clinical history and presence of other features seen in infective endocarditis, e.g. valve perforation, perivalvular abscess, pseudoaneurysm.
   - (c) **Lipoma**—purely fatty on CT/MRI. See Section 6.7.

(d) **Fibroma**—typically located within ventricle myocardium (LV>RV), usually presents in infancy/childhood but occasionally is seen in adults. Homogenous, low attenuation on CT, T2 hypointense on MRI + intense LGE. Dystrophic calcification is common. Associated with Gorlin-Goltz syndrome and Gardner variant FAP.

(e) **Rhabdomyoma**—most common cardiac neoplasm in children, presents in infancy or prenatally in most cases. Located within the myocardium (LV/RV>atria), often multiple. Strongly associated with tuberous sclerosis, particularly if multiple. Homogenous, T2 hyperintense on MRI, no LGE or calcification. Most regress spontaneously in childhood.

(f) **Haemangioma**—can arise from any location. May contain phleboliths. Diffuse high T2 signal on MRI with intense heterogenous first pass and delayed enhancement.

(g) **Teratoma**—usually in children, typically arises from the pericardium.

(h) **Solitary fibrous tumour**—rare, typically arises from pericardium. Well-defined, heterogenous enhancement.

(i) **Paraganglioma**—very rare. Arises from neuroendocrine cells located in the interatrial/AV grooves or root of the great vessels, therefore typically epicardial in location. Very high T2 signal, intense first pass and delayed enhancement.

(j) **Cystic tumour of the AV node**—very rare. Small (<2 cm), arises from the AV node region at the base of the interatrial septum. High T1/T2 signal + LGE. Causes arrhythmias ± sudden death.

(k) **Tumour mimics**—caseous calcification of the mitral valve annulus: mass-like variant of mitral annulus calcification, which may be uniformly dense on CT (putty-like) or have a low attenuation centre with a calcified rim. Other tumour mimics include a prominent crista terminalis (lateral RA wall) or Eustachian valve (RA–IVC junction).

3. <u>Malignant tumours</u>—typically ill-defined, infiltrative, enhance on MRI, often involve >1 chamber and/or pericardium (pericardial effusion suggests malignancy).

   (a) <u>Metastasis</u>—e.g. from lung, breast, lymphoma, melanoma. Much more common than primary tumours. Often multiple; usually seen in the presence of metastases elsewhere. Pericardial > epicardial > myocardial > endocardial. Melanoma metastases are often T1 hyperintense. RCC/HCC may extend into the RA directly via the IVC.

   (b) **Primary sarcoma**—angiosarcoma is most common; typically arises from the lateral RA wall and often infiltrates the AV groove (± right coronary artery aneurysm) and tricuspid valve. Other sarcomas usually arise from the LA. Calcification suggests osteosarcoma, fat suggests liposarcoma. Pulmonary vein invasion suggests leiomyosarcoma. Pericardial involvement and metastases are common in all sarcomas.

   (c) **Primary lymphoma**—typically involves RA/RV and encases the right coronary artery in the AV groove. Often multifocal/diffuse with a homogenous signal on MRI + pericardial effusion. Primary cardiac lymphoma usually occurs in immunocompromised patients, particularly with HIV.

4. **Mass-forming infections**
   (a) **Tuberculosis***—most commonly involves the pericardium but can rarely involve the myocardium (usually right heart). Tuberculoma may be single or multiple. T1/T2 iso/hypointense, heterogenous LGE.
   (b) **Hydatid cyst**—cardiac involvement is rare but has a characteristic multiloculated cystic appearance due to multiple daughter cysts. May rupture and embolize to other sites.
   (c) **Cysticercosis***—cardiac involvement is rare, usually in the presence of disseminated disease elsewhere. Multiple small cystic lesions throughout the heart, each containing a focus of low T2 signal representing the scolex.

6

Further reading

Hoey, E.T., Mankad, K., Puppala, S., et al., 2009. MRI and CT appearances of cardiac tumours in adults. Clin. Radiol. 64 (12), 1214–1230.

Hoey, E.T., Shahid, M., Ganeshan, A., et al., 2014. MRI assessment of cardiac tumours: part 1, multiparametric imaging protocols and spectrum of appearances of histologically benign lesions. Quant. Imaging Med. Surg. 4 (6), 478–488.

Hoey, E.T., Shahid, M., Ganeshan, A., et al., 2014. MRI assessment of cardiac tumours: part 2, spectrum of appearances of histologically malignant lesions and tumour mimics. Quant. Imaging Med. Surg. 4 (6), 489–497.

Kassop, D., Donovan, M.S., Cheezum, M.K., et al., 2014. Cardiac masses on cardiac CT: a review. Curr. Cardiovasc. Imaging Rep. 7 (8), 9281.

Motwani, M., Kidambi, A., Herzog, B.A., et al., 2013. MR imaging of cardiac tumors and masses: a review of methods and clinical applications. Radiology 268 (1), 26–43.

6.10 LATE GADOLINIUM ENHANCEMENT ON CARDIAC MRI

The concept is based on the delayed washout of gadolinium in tissues with an increased extracellular space, caused by either cellular necrosis + oedema (acute MI, myocarditis), cell infiltration + oedema (myocarditis, infiltrative processes) or myocardial fibrosis (chronic infarcted tissue or fibrous scar tissue from previous myocarditis). LGE is demonstrated on T1-weighted imaging 8–10 min after contrast administration. In most cardiomyopathies the presence of LGE is associated with a worse prognosis. The pattern of LGE in the LV myocardium can indicate the likely diagnosis. Note that cardiac masses can also demonstrate LGE—see Section 6.9.

Subendocardial or transmural LGE

1. **Myocardial infarction**—conforms to a coronary artery territory. In the chronic phase there is usually myocardial thinning ± intramural fat/calcification.
2. **Amyloidosis***—typically global subendocardial LGE and diffuse myocardial thickening in an older patient. LGE may also be diffuse throughout the myocardium.
3. **Sarcoidosis***—commonly midwall or subepicardial, but can be subendocardial or transmural. Does not conform to a coronary artery territory.
4. **Eosinophilic myocarditis/endomyocardial fibrosis**—characteristic subendocardial LGE at RV/LV apex + overlying mural thrombus.
5. **Danon disease**—marked concentric myocardial thickening and subendocardial LGE in a young patient.
6. **LV noncompaction**—subendocardial LGE can sometimes be seen at the LV apex or within the prominent trabeculae.

Subepicardial or midmyocardial LGE

1. **Myocarditis**—typically subepicardial but may be midmyocardial or transmural. Commonly involves inferolateral LV wall but may be concentric in severe cases. Associated with myocardial oedema and hyperaemia, i.e. increased T2 signal relative to skeletal muscle (>1.9x) and increased early gadolinium enhancement relative to skeletal muscle (>4×). Usually viral, but can be bacterial, tuberculous, inflammatory (e.g. SLE), iatrogenic (drugs, radiotherapy) or idiopathic.
2. **Sarcoidosis***—commonly involves the basal septum and LV free wall. Associated with myocardial oedema (acute phase) or myocardial thinning ± aneurysms (chronic phase).
3. **HCM**—typically patchy, most marked at regions of maximal myocardial thickening and at RV insertion points.
4. **DCM**—typically midmyocardial, particularly in the septum, with LV dilatation.
5. **Systemic sclerosis**—typically midwall in the septum and RV insertion points.
6. **Chagas disease***—typically involves the apex and inferolateral wall ± aneurysm.
7. **ARVC**—in cases with LV involvement. In LV-dominant forms, LGE is seen as a circumferential band in the outer third of the

myocardium and right side of the interventricular septum. LGE of the RV myocardium can be hard to appreciate as the RV wall is thin, but tends to appear transmural if present.

8. **Fabry disease**—commonly basal inferolateral midwall LGE + concentric left ventricular hypertrophy.

Further reading

Doltra, A., Amundsen, B.H., Gebker, R., et al., 2013. Emerging concepts for myocardial late gadolinium enhancement MRI. Curr. Cardiol. Rev. 9 (3), 185–190.

Vermes, E., Carbone, I., Friedrich, M.G., Merchant, N., 2012. Patterns of myocardial late enhancement: typical and atypical features. Arch. Cardiovasc. Dis. 105 (5), 300–308. 2012 Mar 14.

6.11 MALIGNANT CORONARY ARTERY ANOMALIES IN THE ADULT

1. **Myocardial bridging**—common; possible increased risk of ischaemia (controversial). Typically involves the mid-left anterior descending artery. The vessel dives into the myocardium over a short distance ± narrowing in systole. Depth and length of bridge is linked to risk of ischaemia.
2. **Interarterial course of an aberrant coronary artery**—increased risk of sudden cardiac death due to a combination of a slit-like ostium, an acute angle of take-off and an intramural course through the ascending aorta.
   (a) **Aberrant right coronary artery**—arising from the left coronary sinus and passing between the aorta and main pulmonary artery.
   (b) **Aberrant left main coronary artery**—arising from the right coronary sinus and passing between the aorta and main pulmonary artery. Less common than (a), but has a higher risk of sudden death.
3. **Anomalous left coronary artery from the pulmonary artery (ALCAPA)**—rare, can present in infancy or adulthood. Causes ischaemia of the left coronary artery territory with dilatation of the right coronary artery + multiple collaterals. Eventually results in a left-to-right shunt due to reversal of flow in the anomalous left coronary artery. ARCAPA is a rarer variant involving the right coronary artery.
4. **Coronary artery fistula**—rare abnormal communication between a coronary artery and another vessel or cardiac chamber (commonest being RV or RA). Usually congenital but can rarely be traumatic/iatrogenic. The involved coronary artery is dilated and tortuous but has a normal origin from its coronary sinus.

Further reading

Kim, S.Y., Seo, J.B., Do, K.H., et al., 2006. Coronary artery anomalies: classification and ECG-gated multidetector row CT findings with angiographic correlation. Radiographics 26 (2), 317–333.

6.12 CAUSES OF A PERFUSION DEFECT ON CARDIAC STRESS PERFUSION MRI

This technique acquires first-pass postcontrast images, both at rest and under adenosine stress. Adenosine causes vasodilatation and hyperaemia within the myocardium—areas of ischemia will show less hyperaemia/enhancement relative to normal myocardium on stress images, resulting in a perfusion defect.

1. **Inducible ischaemia**—perfusion defect present on stress but absent at rest. No LGE to suggest infarction. Will benefit from revascularization.
2. **Infarction**—perfusion defect present on both stress and rest images (may not be appreciable on rest images due to enhancement from residual gadolinium), with associated subendocardial/transmural LGE. Unlikely to benefit from revascularization if LGE involves >50% of myocardial thickness.
3. **Microvascular disease**—tends to be circumferential.
4. **Hibernating myocardium**—mild perfusion defect present on both stress and rest images (may be hard to appreciate on rest images, as above) with an associated wall motion abnormality but no LGE to suggest infarction. Indicates chronic ischaemia that will benefit from revascularization. Myocardial stunning can have a similar appearance, but occurs in the context of an acute transient ischaemic event, and perfusion is usually nearly normal.
5. **Susceptibility artefact**—appears as a dark rim in the subendocardium as the gadolinium bolus arrives in the LV cavity and lasts until the bolus leaves the LV cavity.

6.13 ACUTE AORTIC SYNDROMES

This term relates to three main pathologies (1-3 below), all of which present with similar clinical features and are traditionally classified on CT as type A (if there is any involvement of the aorta proximal to the left subclavian artery; treated surgically) or type B (if only the aorta distal to the left subclavian artery is involved). Recent research suggests classifying dissections involving the arch but not the ascending aorta as type B, since these are usually treated medically or with endovascular stents. CXR may be normal, but may show predisposing factors (atherosclerosis, thoracic aortic aneurysm) ± evidence of mediastinal haemorrhage (widened mediastinum >8 cm, indistinct contours, rightward tracheal deviation, depressed left main bronchus, widened paratracheal/paravertebral stripe, left apical pleural cap) ± pleural effusion/haemothorax. Haemopericardium may be seen on CT in type A syndromes. On non-ECG-gated CT beware of pulsation artefact in the ascending aorta mimicking a dissection flap or intramural haematoma; an ECG-gated CT is preferred.

1. Aortic dissection—on CXR, medial displacement of intimal calcification may be seen. CT demonstrates the dissection flap with flow in the true ± false lumen. The dissection flap may extend into (and occlude) branches of the aorta ± end-organ infarction. A chronic dissection with a thrombosed false lumen may mimic an aortic aneurysm with mural thrombus, but the location of intimal calcification helps differentiate the two—along the inner margin of the thrombus in dissection, along the outer margin of the thrombus in an aneurysm.
2. Intramural haematoma—blood collects in the media of the aortic wall due to rupture of the vasa vasorum (usually no visible intimal tear). Tends to occur in hypertensive patients or in blunt trauma. Characteristic crescentic hyperattenuation within the aortic wall on unenhanced CT, which does not fill with contrast, although sometimes contrast-filled ulcer-like projections (communicating with lumen) or intramural blood pools (not communicating with lumen) may be seen. May resolve or progress to dissection, rupture or aneurysm—higher risk of progression if ulcer-like projections are present.
3. Penetrating aortic ulcer—focal deep ulceration of the aortic wall at a site of intimal atherosclerosis, usually in descending aorta. May be hard to differentiate from an ulcerated plaque, but a penetrating ulcer should extend beyond the expected margin of the aortic wall ± adjacent stranding/haemorrhage. May progress to intramural haematoma, dissection, rupture or pseudoaneurysm. Mycotic pseudoaneurysm should be considered in the differential if there are clinical features of infection and no atherosclerosis.
4. Traumatic aortic injury—usually due to rapid deceleration injury. Typically occurs at the aortic isthmus due to tethering by the ligamentum arteriosum. May be subtle on CT (best seen on sagittal reformats), particularly in minimal aortic injury where there is only intimal irregularity ± a small (<1 cm) intimal flap ± an adherent intraluminal thrombus ± intramural haematoma, with an otherwise normal aortic contour and no mediastinal haemorrhage. More severe injuries will demonstrate an irregular aortic pseudoaneurysm ± mediastinal haemorrhage. The differential diagnosis includes a chronic traumatic pseudoaneurysm (nearly

always rim-calcified) and a congenital ductus diverticulum (usually smooth with obtuse margins).

Further reading

Gutschow, S.E., Walker, C.M., Martínez-Jiménez, S., et al., 2016. Emerging concepts in intramural hematoma imaging. Radiographics 36 (3), 660–674.

Lempel, J.K., Frazier, A.A., Jeudy, J., et al., 2014. Aortic arch dissection: a controversy of classification. Radiology 271 (3), 848–855.

6.14 THORACIC AORTIC ANEURYSM

Dilatation >50% of expected diameter. Surgical intervention is recommended for ascending aneurysms >5.5 cm and descending aneurysms >6.5 cm (earlier in some conditions, e.g. Marfan syndrome). Note that there is some overlap between the categories below.

Isolated sinus of Valsalva aneurysm

1. **Mycotic**—usually due to infective endocarditis of the aortic valve (perivalvular pseudoaneurysm), but can rarely be due to TB or tertiary syphilis. Irregular shape, often also involves aortic annulus with valve thickening/vegetations. High risk of rupture/fistulation.
2. **Congenital**—smooth contour, usually involves the right coronary sinus, may be associated with VSD. May rupture into RV.

Annuloaortic ectasia

Dilated aortic root and annulus with effacement of the sinotubular junction, creating a 'tulip-bulb' appearance. Pathology usually shows cystic medial necrosis.

1. **Marfan syndrome***—classically linked to this aneurysm type.
2. **Other genetic disorders**—e.g. Ehlers-Danlos syndrome, Loeys-Dietz syndrome, homocystinuria, osteogenesis imperfecta, Shprintzen-Goldberg syndrome.
3. **Bicuspid aortic valve**—aneurysm formation can occur regardless of aortic stenosis.

Ascending aortic aneurysm

1. **Poststenotic dilatation from aortic stenosis**.
2. **Previous aortic dissection**—fusiform aneurysm + chronic dissection flap.
3. **Atherosclerosis/hypertension**—descending > arch > ascending aorta. Usually in older patients, fusiform morphology in most cases, but can be saccular.

4. **Aortitis**—e.g. Takayasu arteritis, giant cell arteritis, rheumatoid arthritis, seronegative spondyloarthropathies, relapsing polychondritis, SLE, Behçet's disease, Cogan syndrome.
5. **Congenital heart disease**—as well as PDA and aortic coarctation.
6. **Mycotic pseudoaneurysm**—usually due to *Staphylococcus aureus* or *Salmonella* spp. Irregular, lobulated, noncalcified saccular aneurysm + adjacent fat stranding/abscess, can occur at any site but descending > ascending aorta. Rapidly progressive, high risk of rupture. In TB, pseudoaneurysms are usually due to extrinsic erosion of the aorta from an adjacent involved lymph node. HIV is also associated with aortitis and fusiform aneurysms.
7. **Tertiary syphilis***—rare, usually causes saccular aneurysms of the ascending aorta. Associated with extensive confluent 'tree-bark' calcification of the aortic wall.

Descending aortic aneurysm

1. **Atherosclerosis/hypertension**—often together with an AAA.
2. **Previous aortic dissection or penetrating ulcer**—postdissection aneurysms are usually fusiform, whereas penetrating ulcers progress to saccular aneurysms.
3. **Previous trauma with missed rupture**—focal saccular pseudoaneurysm at the anterior margin of the isthmus. Look for other signs of old trauma, e.g. healed rib fractures.
4. **Mycotic pseudoaneurysm**—see above. More common in descending aorta, including TB.
5. **Kommerell diverticulum**—saccular bulge at the origin of an aberrant subclavian artery.

6

Further reading

Isselbacher, E.M., 2005. Thoracic and abdominal aortic aneurysms. Circulation 111, 816–828.

6.15 INCREASED AORTIC WALL THICKNESS

1. **Intramural haematoma**—characteristic crescentic hyperattenuation within the wall on unenhanced CT, which does not fill with contrast.
2. **Vasculitis**—particularly Takayasu arteritis (<50 years) and giant cell arteritis (>50 years). Circumferential wall thickening ± mild periaortic stranding. Can involve both thoracic and abdominal aorta ± major branches. Increased uptake on PET. Takayasu arteritis typically causes stenoses/occlusions. Other vasculitides (see Section 6.14) can also occasionally cause aortitis, but are usually limited to the ascending aorta.
3. **IgG4-related disease***—can manifest as periaortitis, inflammatory AAA or RPF (ill-defined periaortic soft-tissue thickening ± IVC involvement/narrowing ± ureteric tethering/obstruction). Typically

does not extend posterior to the aorta (cf. malignancy and Erdheim-Chester disease). Treated lymphoma can mimic RPF.

4. **Infectious aortitis**—usually associated with mycotic pseudoaneurysm, periaortic fat stranding ± abscess. Infection may be related to an indwelling stent/graft or could have spread from an adjacent source, e.g. discitis.
5. **Erdheim-Chester disease***—ill-defined periaortic soft-tissue thickening sparing IVC and not displacing ureters. If perirenal soft-tissue thickening is also present this is almost pathognomonic.

Further reading

Restrepo, C.S., Ocazionez, D., Suri, R., Vargas, D., 2011. Aortitis: imaging spectrum of the infectious and inflammatory conditions of the aorta. Radiographics 31 (2), 435–451.

6.16 FOCAL NARROWING OF THE AORTA

1. **Atherosclerosis**—lumen narrowed by calcified and/or noncalcified plaque. In severe cases can lead to occlusion of the infrarenal aorta (aortoiliac occlusive disease).
2. **Coarctation**—in adults, usually just distal to the aortic isthmus + multiple collaterals. May be visible on CXR as a 'figure 3' aortic knuckle with inferior rib notching. Beware of pseudocoarctation, which is kinking of the aorta at the isthmus without true stenosis or collateral formation.
3. **Takayasu arteritis**—typically causes multifocal arterial stenoses. In the aorta the arch is the commonest site of stenosis. Aortitis and aneurysms may also be present.
4. **Narrowing due to mass lesion or retroperitoneal fibrosis.**
5. **Midaortic syndrome**—young patients, relatively long smooth narrowing of the suprarenal abdominal aorta ± involvement of renal arteries, SMA or coeliac axis ± multiple collaterals. Associated with NF1, Williams syndrome and Alagille syndrome.
6. **Supravalvular aortic stenosis**—focal smooth stenosis of the ascending aorta just distal to the sinuses of Valsalva, characteristic of Williams syndrome.

Further reading

Sebastia, C., Quiroga, S., Boyé, R., et al., 2003. Aortic stenosis: spectrum of diseases depicted at multisection CT. Radiographics 23 (Suppl 1), S79–S91.

6.17 SYSTEMIC DISORDERS ASSOCIATED WITH NONAORTIC ANEURYSMS

Excluding atherosclerosis and inflammatory/mycotic/traumatic/iatrogenic pseudoaneurysms.

1. Vasculitis
   (a) Kawasaki disease—characteristically produces coronary artery aneurysms ± stenoses.
   (b) Behçet's disease*/Hughes-Stovin syndrome—both cause pulmonary artery aneurysms.
   (c) Takayasu arteritis—more commonly causes multifocal stenoses, but aneurysms of the arch vessels can also occur.
   (d) Polyarteritis nodosa*—classically causes multiple microaneurysms of the renal, hepatic and/or mesenteric arteries ± occlusions/infarcts. Best seen on angiography, may be occult on CT. A similar appearance may also be seen in SLE, Wegener's granulomatosis and IV drug abuse-related necrotizing vasculitis.
2. Connective tissue disorders—Marfan syndrome, Ehlers-Danlos syndrome type 4 and Loeys-Dietz syndrome can all cause arterial aneurysms at any location, although the ascending aorta is most commonly involved. Loeys-Dietz syndrome classically also causes marked arterial tortuosity.
3. Fibromuscular dysplasia/segmental arterial mediolysis—both conditions are noninflammatory, nonatherosclerotic arteriopathies causing a characteristic 'string of beads' appearance in involved arteries due to alternating aneurysms and stenoses. FMD usually occurs in adults <50 years and most commonly involves the renal and carotid arteries. SAM usually occurs in adults >50 years and most commonly involves the mesenteric arteries, coeliac axis and branches. Dissection and haemorrhage is more common in SAM.
4. **Neurofibromatosis***—can rarely cause arterial stenoses and aneurysms involving the aorta, arch vessels, renal arteries, intracranial arteries and visceral arteries.

Further reading

Baker-LePain, J.C., Stone, D.H., Mattis, A.N., et al., 2010. Clinical diagnosis of segmental arterial mediolysis: differentiation from vasculitis and other mimics. Arthritis Care Res. 62 (11), 1655–1660.

6.18 INTRAVASCULAR LESIONS

1. Atheroma—in arteries only, may be noncalcified or calcified. Noncalcified atheroma is irregular in shape and of low attenuation on CT. Aortic occlusion/stenosis caused by a large endoluminal calcification is known as a 'coral reef aorta'.
2. Thrombus/embolus—thrombus is much more common in veins (e.g. DVT or superficial thrombophlebitis), but can occur in abnormal arteries, e.g. at sites of atherosclerosis or intimal damage (e.g. aortic injury), in aneurysms (crescentic mural thrombus) and

in vasculitis. Emboli are found almost exclusively in arteries (and occasionally in hepatic portal veins), usually lodging at branching points ± signs of end-organ ischaemia. Acute thrombus is often hyperattenuating on unenhanced CT. MRI signal varies widely: acute thrombus (<7 days) is usually T1 isointense and T2 hypointense, subacute thrombus (7–14 days) is usually T1 and T2 hyperintense and chronic thrombus is usually T1 isointense and T2 hyperintense. Acute and subacute thrombus often shows high signal on DWI and low signal on T2*. Thrombus does not enhance on CT/MRI and does not show internal flow on Doppler US—any enhancement or internal vascularity suggests tumour thrombus.

3. <u>**Tumour thrombus**</u>—direct intravenous extension of a tumour, most commonly from RCC or HCC, but can also be seen with adrenal carcinoma, pancreatic NET and leiomyosarcoma. Tumour thrombus usually shows internal flow on Doppler US, enhances on CT/MRI and often expands the vein. Rarely, intravenous extension can occur from uterine fibroids (intravenous leiomyomatosis)—this usually involves the pelvic veins and IVC, but can extend into the right heart.
4. **Nonthrombotic pulmonary emboli**—see Section 5.21.
5. **Cystic adventitial disease**—rare, typically presents in young adult males as a benign multiloculated cystic mass arising from the adventitia of the popliteal artery causing luminal narrowing. Can occasionally involve other arteries (and rarely veins) adjacent to joints.
6. **Intravascular lipoma**—rare. Most commonly arises from the IVC; characteristic fatty appearance on CT/MRI.
7. **Intravenous lobular capillary haemangioma**—rare. Most commonly arises from veins in the neck/arms. Hypervascular on Doppler US, enhances on CT/MRI.
8. **Primary vascular sarcomas**—rare. Typically involve large veins or, less commonly, large arteries. Usually demonstrate internal flow on Doppler US and enhancement on CT/MRI ± extravascular invasion. Pulmonary artery sarcomas may mimic pulmonary emboli. Arterial sarcomas may mimic focal atheroma, particularly on CT where internal enhancement may be difficult to appreciate. Venous sarcomas often cause vessel expansion and associated thrombosis. Leiomyosarcoma is the most common subtype (most arising from the IVC); other subtypes include intimal sarcoma (most arising from the descending aorta or central pulmonary arteries), angiosarcoma, synovial sarcoma and epithelioid haemangioendothelioma.

6.19 ENDOLEAK APPEARANCES ON MULTIPHASIC CT FOLLOWING ENDOVASCULAR ANEURYSM REPAIR

High density contrast present within the excluded aneurysm sac. Unenhanced CT is essential to exclude preexisting sac calcifications (very common). Also beware of Nellix stent grafts, which have 'endobags' filled with high attenuation fluid around the stent—this is a normal appearance.

1. Type I—from the graft attachment site. **Type Ia** proximal. **Type Ib** distal. Contrast present in sac, usually on arterial phase. High pressure, high risk; requires treatment.
2. Type II—retrograde sac filling from collateral vessels (inferior mesenteric and lumbar arteries). Most common type; best depicted on delayed phase. 50% spontaneously resolve. Serial surveillance and treatment if sac expands.
3. Type III—structural failure of stent graft, including junctional separations, fractures or perforations of the graft. High pressure, high risk; requires treatment.
4. **Type IV**—sac filling through graft fabric due to graft porosity after placement. By definition not detected on follow-up imaging.
5. **Type V**—endotension; sac expansion without visible endoleak. Controversial, usually occult Type I–IV endoleak or ultrafiltration of blood.

Further reading

Rand, T., Uberoi, R., Cil, B., et al., 2013. Quality improvement guidelines for imaging detection and treatment of endoleaks following endovascular aneurysm repair (EVAR). Cardiovasc. Intervent. Radiol. 36 (1), 35–45.
Stavropoulos, S.W., Charagundla, S.R., 2007. Imaging techniques for detection and management of endoleaks after endovascular aortic aneurysm repair. Radiology 243 (3), 641–655.

6.20 PULMONARY ARTERIAL ENLARGEMENT

Diffuse MPA enlargement (MPA > adjacent ascending aorta)

1. Pulmonary hypertension—dilated MPA and bilateral central PAs with peripheral pruning. See Section 6.21.
2. Left-to-right shunt—dilated MPA, central and peripheral PAs (plethora).
3. **Pulmonary valve stenosis**—dilated MPA only (± left PA).
4. **Marfan syndrome***—can rarely cause MPA root dilatation.

Focal pulmonary artery aneurysm

1. **Vasculitis**—typically in Behçet's disease, but consider Hughes-Stovin syndrome if there are no oral/genital ulcers. Often multiple ± thrombosis ± pulmonary infarcts. High risk of rupture.
2. **Chronic pulmonary hypertension**—particularly in left-to-right shunts, e.g. PDA, due to shear stresses. Associated mural thrombus/calcification is common. Aneurysms may be very large.
3. **Mycotic pseudoaneurysm**—e.g. due to lung abscess, septic emboli, TB (Rasmussen aneurysm), invasive fungal infection or tertiary syphilis.
4. **Traumatic pseudoaneurysm**—most commonly due to Swan-Ganz catheters.
5. **Malignancy**—a lung tumour/metastasis may erode into an adjacent pulmonary artery, causing a pseudoaneurysm. Primary sarcoma of the pulmonary artery can also cause focal aneurysmal dilatation with an intraluminal mass ± extraluminal extension.
6. **AVM**—look for dilated feeding pulmonary artery and draining vein.

Further reading

Nguyen, E.T., Silva, C.I., Seely, J.M., et al., 2007. Pulmonary artery aneurysms and pseudoaneurysms in adults: findings at CT and radiography. AJR Am. J. Roentgenol. 188 (2), W126–W134.

6.21 PULMONARY HYPERTENSION

Characterized by enlarged central pulmonary arteries with peripheral pruning and RV dilatation/hypertrophy ± pulmonary artery calcification (in severe cases). Causes include:

1. **Pulmonary venous hypertension**—due to left heart failure (e.g. LVF, mitral valve disease). Pulmonary oedema and pleural effusions may be present.
2. **Chronic lung disease**—e.g. emphysema, interstitial lung disease, cystic fibrosis, LCH, LAM, hypoventilation.
3. **Chronic thromboembolic pulmonary hypertension (CTEPH)**—signs on CT include laminar thrombus (usually seen in larger arteries), intraluminal webs, pulmonary artery stenoses/occlusions (may be very subtle in smaller vessels—look for bronchi without accompanying arteries), peripheral lung scarring due to previous infarcts, dilated bronchial arteries (due to collateralization) and mosaic attenuation in the lungs with smaller pulmonary arteries in the more lucent areas.
4. **Chronic left-to-right shunt**—e.g. ASD, VSD, PDA, partial anomalous pulmonary venous return (PAPVR).
5. **Vasculitis**—Takayasu arteritis often involves the pulmonary arteries, causing multifocal stenoses/occlusions, which can mimic CTEPH. Behçet's disease and Hughes-Stovin syndrome can also cause

pulmonary artery stenoses/occlusions due to thrombosis/emboli in addition to the characteristic PA aneurysms. Small vessel vasculitides can also cause pulmonary hypertension ± areas of pulmonary haemorrhage ± nodules/cavities, but the pulmonary arteries visible on CT typically appear normal.

6. **Pulmonary venoocclusive disease**—usually young adults. HRCT features are similar to LVF with interlobular septal thickening, pleural effusions and ground-glass opacities, but with a normal left heart. Centrilobular nodules are usually absent (cf. below).
7. **Pulmonary capillary haemangiomatosis**—usually young adults. Widespread ill-defined centrilobular nodules on HRCT. Interlobular septal thickening is rare. Normal left heart.
8. **Idiopathic pulmonary arterial hypertension**—typically young adult women. Usually no other imaging features apart from those of pulmonary hypertension.
9. **Other causes**—sarcoidosis, connective tissue diseases (e.g. scleroderma), fibrosing mediastinitis, portal hypertension, NF1, HIV, schistosomiasis, drugs/toxins and others.

Further reading

Ley, S., Grunig, E., Kiely, D.G., et al., 2010. Computed tomography and magnetic resonance imaging of pulmonary hypertension: pulmonary vessels and right ventricle. J. Magn. Reson. Imaging 32 (6), 1313–1324.

Peña, E., Dennie, C., Veinot, J., Muñiz, S.H., 2012. Pulmonary hypertension: how the radiologist can help. Radiographics 32 (1), 9–32.

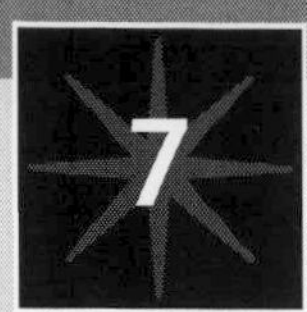

Abdomen and gastrointestinal tract

Hameed Rafiee, Stuart Taylor, Andrew Plumb

7.1 PNEUMOPERITONEUM

Plain film signs include:

- **Erect CXR**—free gas under diaphragm or liver. Can detect 10 ml of gas. Takes 10 minutes for all gas to rise.
- **Supine AXR**—most sensitive signs are often in the right upper quadrant. Gas outlines both sides of bowel wall, which appears as a white line (Rigler sign). The liver may appear hyperlucent or have an overlying oval gas shadow. The falciform ligament may also be outlined by free gas. In infants, a large volume of gas collects centrally, producing a rounded translucency over the central abdomen ('football' sign).

CT is more sensitive for detecting extraluminal gas and can also show focal bowel wall thickening ± mural discontinuity at the site of perforation with adjacent gas bubbles ± extraluminal oral contrast (if given). The distribution of free gas on CT may suggest the site of perforation:

- **Large volume**—usually stomach, duodenum, colonic diverticulum, post endoscopy or secondary to obstruction.
- **Lesser sac**—usually gastric or duodenal (rarely oesophagus or transverse colon).
- **Under left lobe of liver**—often gastric or duodenal.
- **Mesenteric folds**—usually small bowel or colon.
- **Retroperitoneal**—duodenum, ascending/descending colon, rectum.

Causes

1. Perforation
   (a) Peptic ulcer—gastric or duodenal.
   (b) Inflammation—e.g. diverticulitis, appendicitis, toxic megacolon, necrotizing enterocolitis (neonates).
   (c) Obstruction—especially closed loop or large bowel obstruction.
   (d) Infarction.
   (e) Malignant neoplasms.
   (f) Trauma—blunt or penetrating.
   (g) Stercoral—due to hard faeces, usually in rectum/sigmoid.
   (h) Foreign body—e.g. fish bone.
   (i) Pneumatosis coli—the cysts may rupture, or gas may dissect through the bowel wall without a discrete site of perforation.
2. **Iatrogenic**—e.g. recent surgery or endoscopy, peritoneal dialysis. Free gas may be seen on CT up to 18 days after laparotomy (though free gas >10 days post-op should be treated with suspicion). Resolves faster in the obese, children and following laparoscopy (insufflated with CO_2—free gas >3 days after laparoscopy is suspicious).
3. **Pneumomediastinum**—see Section 5.36.
4. **Introduction per vaginam**—e.g. douching.
5. **Pneumothorax**—via a congenital pleuroperitoneal fistula.
6. **Idiopathic.**

Further reading

Chiu, Y.H., Chen, J.D., Tiu, C.M., et al., 2009. Reappraisal of radiographic signs of pneumoperitoneum at emergency department. Am. J. Emerg. Med. 27 (3), 320–327.

Hainaux, B., Agneessens, E., Bertinotti, R., et al., 2006. Accuracy of MDCT in predicting site of gastrointestinal tract perforation. AJR Am. J. Roentgenol. 187 (5), 1179–1183.

7.2 GASLESS ABDOMEN

1. Ascites.
2. **Fluid-filled bowel**—closed-loop obstruction, active pancolitis, early mesenteric infarction, bowel washout.
3. **Acute pancreatitis**—due to excessive vomiting.
4. **High obstruction**—e.g. gastric outlet obstruction, congenital atresia (neonates).
5. **Large abdominal mass**—pushes bowel laterally.
6. **Normal.**

7

7.3 PHARYNGEAL/OESOPHAGEAL POUCHES AND DIVERTICULA

Upper third

1. **Zenker's diverticulum**—posterior, usually on left side, between the fibres of inferior constrictor and cricopharyngeus ± an air–fluid level.
2. **Lateral pharyngeal pouch and diverticulum**—through the unsupported thyrohyoid membrane in the anterolateral wall of the upper hypopharynx. Pouches (transient) are common and usually asymptomatic. Diverticula (persistent) are uncommon and seen in patients with chronically elevated intrapharyngeal pressure, e.g. glass-blowers and trumpeters.
3. **Lateral cervical oesophageal pouch and diverticulum**—through the Killian-Jamieson space, below the level of cricopharyngeus. Usually asymptomatic.

Middle third

1. **Traction**—at level of carina, due to tethering of the oesophagus to adjacent granulomatous (often calcified) nodes, e.g. due to TB; sinus tracts may also be seen.
2. **Developmental**—failure to completely close a tracheo-oesophageal fistula.
3. **Intramural pseudodiverticulosis**—rare. Multiple tiny flask-shaped outpouchings. 90% have associated oesophageal strictures, mainly in the upper third.

Lower third

1. **Epiphrenic**—mimics a hiatus hernia.
2. **Ulcer**—peptic or related to steroids, immunosuppression or radiotherapy.
3. **Mucosal tears**—Mallory-Weiss syndrome, post oesophagoscopy.
4. **After Heller's operation.**

Mimics

1. **Contained oesophageal perforation.**
2. **Oesophageal anastomosis**—may have a small outpouching.
3. **Oesophageal duplication cyst communicating with oesophagus.**

Further reading

Grant, P.D., Morgan, D.E., Scholz, F.J., Canon, C.L., 2009. Pharyngeal dysphagia: what the radiologist needs to know. Curr. Prob. Diagn. Radiol. 38 (1), 17–32.

7.4 OESOPHAGEAL ULCERATION

There may also be nonspecific signs of oesophagitis, e.g. thickening of longitudinal and transverse folds, reduced or absent peristalsis.

Inflammatory

1. **Reflux oesophagitis**—± hiatus hernia. Characteristic signs are:
   (a) A gastric fundal fold crossing the gastrooesophageal junction (GOJ) and ending as a polypoid protuberance in the distal oesophagus.
   (b) Erosions—dots or linear streaks of barium in the distal oesophagus.
   (c) Ulcers—may be linear, serpiginous or round.
2. **Barrett's oesophagus**—especially if ulceration is midoesophageal, though strictures are more common distally. The background mucosa typically has a reticular pattern. Hiatus hernia in 75%–90%. Increased risk of adenocarcinoma.
3. **Corrosive ingestion**—ulceration is most marked at sites of anatomical hold-up (e.g. aortic arch, GOJ) + diffuse spasm and oedema. Progresses to a long, smooth stricture.
4. **Intramural pseudodiverticulosis**—can mimic ulceration.
5. **Graft-versus-host disease***—rare in the oesophagus.

Infective

1. ***Candida* oesophagitis**—mostly in immunosuppressed patients. Early: small plaque-like filling defects, often orientated in the long axis of the oesophagus. Advanced: cobblestone or 'shaggy' mucosal surface ± luminal narrowing. Ulceration is uncommon. There may be tiny bubbles on top of the barium column ('foamy' oesophagus). Patients with mucocutaneous candidiasis or oesophageal stasis due to achalasia, scleroderma, etc. may develop chronic infection, which is characterized by a lacy or reticular appearance of the mucosa ± nodular filling defects.
2. **Viral**—herpes and CMV, mostly in immunocompromised patients, e.g. HIV (which itself can cause ulcers). May manifest as discrete ulcers (which may be large) or ulcerated plaques, or mimic *Candida* oesophagitis. Discrete ulcers on an otherwise normal background mucosa are strongly suggestive.

Iatrogenic

1. **Oral drug-induced**—due to prolonged contact with tetracycline, quinidine or potassium tablets, at sites of anatomical hold-up.
2. **Longstanding nasogastric (NG) tube.**
3. **Radiotherapy**—ulceration is rare. Dysmotility is often the only abnormality.

7

Related to systemic diseases

1. Crohn's disease*—aphthoid ulcers and, in advanced cases, undermining ulcers, intramural tracking and fistulae.
2. **Behçet's disease***—discrete superficial ulcers + history of oral and genital ulceration.
3. **Bullous skin disorders**—e.g. epidermolysis bullosa, pemphigus.

Neoplastic

In the presence of a mass or stricture.

1. Carcinoma.
2. **Leiomyosarcoma and leiomyoma.**
3. **Lymphoma*.**
4. **Melanoma.**

Further reading

Levine, M.S., Rubesin, S.E., 2005. Diseases of the esophagus: diagnosis with esophagography. Radiology 237, 414–427.

7.5 OESOPHAGEAL MUCOSAL NODULARITY

1. Reflux oesophagitis and Barrett's—granular appearance, usually mid-distal oesophagus.
2. Glycogenic acanthosis—multiple small well-defined nodules, often in upper-mid oesophagus. Seen incidentally in elderly patients, or in young patients with Cowden syndrome.
3. Advanced *Candida*/viral oesophagitis—cobblestone mucosa.
4. **Superficial spreading oesophageal carcinoma.**
5. **Eosinophilic oesophagitis**—diffuse narrowing with a corrugated or ringed appearance.
6. **Oesophageal papillomatosis**—due to HPV infection. Laryngeal or tracheobronchial papillomatosis may coexist.

7.6 OESOPHAGEAL STRICTURES—SMOOTH

Inflammatory

1. Peptic—the stricture develops relatively late, ± ulceration. Usually distal if associated with reflux and hiatus hernia; midoesophageal if associated with Barrett's.
2. Corrosives—caustic stricture; typically long and symmetrical; may take years to develop. More likely with alkalis than acids.
3. **Scleroderma***—reflux through an open GOJ may produce a distal stricture. The oesophagus is dilated with poor peristalsis.

4. **Iatrogenic**—prolonged use of an NG tube (distal stricture, probably due to reflux). Also radiotherapy (typically midoesophageal) and drugs, e.g. bisphosphonates.
5. **Crohn's disease***—rare, suggests severe disease.
6. **Eosinophilic oesophagitis**—strictures may be short ('ringed' oesophagus) or long.

Neoplastic submucosal and extrinsic masses

Typically have a smooth contour but focal mucosal ulceration may be seen.

1. **Squamous carcinoma**—may infiltrate submucosally. The absence of a hiatus hernia and the presence of an extrinsic soft-tissue mass should differentiate it from a peptic stricture, but tumours arising around the cardia may predispose to reflux.
2. **Mediastinal tumours**—e.g. lung cancer, lymphadenopathy. Extrinsic soft-tissue mass ± obstruction.
3. **Leiomyoma**—focal narrowing due to a smooth, eccentric submucosal mass. Calcification is highly suggestive if present. Most common benign oesophageal tumour; most are in the distal third. May be diffuse (leiomyomatosis), e.g. in Alport syndrome.
4. **Rare submucosal tumours**—e.g. fibrovascular polyp (pedunculated, arises from upper oesophagus, can be very large, ± fat on CT), lipoma (purely fatty on CT), granular cell tumour (small, usually distal), nerve sheath tumours, haemangioma, glomus tumour, paraganglioma, solitary fibrous tumour, salivary gland-type tumours.
5. **GIST**—the oesophagus is the least common location. Much less common than leiomyoma (cf. the rest of the GI tract where GIST is much more common).
6. **Metastasis**—rare.

7

Nonneoplastic submucosal and extrinsic masses

1. **Oesophageal varices**—smooth tubular filling defects; can be distal ('uphill' varices due to portal hypertension) or proximal ('downhill' varices due to SVC obstruction).
2. **Other vascular impressions**—aberrant subclavian or pulmonary artery; right or double aortic arch; aortic aneurysm or tortuosity.
3. **Intramural haematoma**—associated with coagulopathy, protracted vomiting or instrumentation. Acute chest pain, dysphagia and haematemesis. Focal submucosal mass, high attenuation on unenhanced CT.
4. **Oesophageal duplication cyst**—smooth indentation of oesophagus. Cystic and nonenhancing on CT.

5. **Other rare lesions**—e.g. sarcoidosis, fibrosing mediastinitis, amyloidosis, malakoplakia, actinomycosis.

Others

1. **Achalasia**—'rat-tail' tapering may mimic a stricture; this occurs below the diaphragm. Marked oesophageal dilatation with food in the lumen.
2. **Oesophageal webs**—typically in cervical oesophagus; very short (shelf-like), arise perpendicularly from the anterior wall. Can be associated with Plummer-Vinson syndrome. Increased risk of carcinoma.
3. **Bullous skin disorders**—epidermolysis bullosa, pemphigus. Short web-like strictures, may be multiple.
4. **Graft-versus-host disease***—rare; short web-like strictures, may be multiple.

Further reading

Lewis, R.B., Mehrotra, A.K., Rodriguez, P., Levine, M.S., 2013. From the radiologic pathology archives: esophageal neoplasms: radiologic-pathologic correlation. Radiographics 33 (4), 1083–1108.

Luedtke, P., Levine, M.S., Rubesin, S.E., et al., 2003. Radiologic diagnosis of benign esophageal strictures: a pattern approach. Radiographics 23 (4), 897–909.

7.7 OESOPHAGEAL STRICTURES—IRREGULAR

Neoplastic

1. **Oesophageal carcinoma**—increased incidence in achalasia, Plummer-Vinson syndrome, Barrett's oesophagus, coeliac disease, asbestosis, lye ingestion and tylosis. Squamous carcinomas are most common in the midoesophagus; adenocarcinomas are most common distally and arise from underlying Barrett's. Appears as an irregular filling defect (annular or eccentric) ± shouldering, ulceration and upstream dilatation. May create a 'pseudoachalasia' appearance if very distal. An associated soft-tissue mass or focal thickening is typically seen on CT.
2. **Gastric carcinoma**—can directly invade oesophagus.
3. **Carcinosarcoma**—big polypoid tumour ± stalk arising from the mid-distal oesophagus, often without obstruction.
4. **Leiomyosarcoma**—bulky mass, often without obstruction.
5. **Lymphoma***—usually extension from gastric involvement.
6. **Other rare tumours**—neuroendocrine tumours, melanoma, Kaposi sarcoma, other sarcomas.

Inflammatory

1. **Reflux**—rarely irregular.
2. **Crohn's disease***—rare.

Iatrogenic

Radiotherapy—rare, unless treating an oesophageal carcinoma. Dysphagia after radiotherapy is usually due to dysmotility. Acute oesophagitis may occur with a dose of 50–60 Gy (5000–6000 rad).

7.8 DILATED OESOPHAGUS

1. **Obstructing tumour or stricture**—see Sections 7.6 and 7.7.
2. **Achalasia**—patients are often younger than those with carcinoma. The oesophagus is often markedly dilated (more so than with malignancy) with a smooth 'beaked' tapering at the GOJ. Normal peristaltic waves should be absent (though some contractility may be present)—if not, consider pseudoachalasia due to tumour.
3. **Scleroderma***—dilated oesophagus with poor peristalsis and contractility. Look for associated lung fibrosis and bowel features.
4. **Post oesophagectomy**—the gastric pull-up can mimic a dilated oesophagus.
5. **Iatrogenic**—e.g. over-tight gastric band or fundoplication wrap.
6. **Chagas disease***—mimics achalasia. Small and large bowel (especially sigmoid) may also be dilated. Cardiomegaly is often present due to associated cardiomyopathy. Endemic in Central and South America.
7. **Oesophageal amyloidosis**—rare; can mimic achalasia.

7.9 TERTIARY CONTRACTIONS IN THE OESOPHAGUS

Uncoordinated, nonpropulsive contractions.

1. **Reflux oesophagitis**.
2. **Presbyoesophagus**—impaired motor function due to muscle atrophy in the elderly. Seen in 25% of people >60 years.
3. **GOJ obstruction**—from any cause.
4. **Neuropathy**—e.g. early achalasia (before dilatation occurs), diabetes, alcoholism, malignant infiltration, Chagas disease.

Further reading

Levine, M.S., Rubesin, S.E., Laufer, I., 2008. Barium esophagography: a study for all seasons. Clin. Gastroenterol. Hepatol. 6 (1), 11–25.

7

7.10 GASTRIC MASSES AND FILLING DEFECTS

Malignant neoplasms

1. Carcinoma—most polypoid carcinomas are 1–4 cm in diameter; any polyp >2 cm is suspicious for malignancy especially if it has a central depression (ulcer). Local adenopathy is common; metastasizes most often to liver and peritoneum.
2. GIST—stomach is the most common location. Variable size and malignant potential. Typically a discrete endophytic or exophytic mass ± central ulcer. Can be large with heterogeneous enhancement on CT/MRI ± cystic, necrotic or haemorrhagic areas. Metastasizes most frequently to liver and peritoneum, but lymphadenopathy is very uncommon and would suggest an alternative diagnosis if present. May enlarge with treatment; reduced enhancement suggests response. Can be associated with Carney triad or NF1.
3. Lymphoma*—1–5% of gastric malignancies. Usually NHL. May be ulcerative, infiltrative and/or polypoid; often involves the whole stomach. May mimic carcinoma, but extension across the pylorus (without causing obstruction) and/or marked wall thickening (mean 3–5 cm) suggests lymphoma. Most have adjacent lymphadenopathy. MALT lymphoma is strongly associated with *Helicobacter pylori* infection.
4. Metastases—frequently ulcerate. Usually melanoma, but lung, breast, lymphoma, carcinoid, Kaposi sarcoma and any adenocarcinoma may metastasize to stomach. Breast metastases are often infiltrative, mimicking linitis plastica.
5. **Sarcoma**—rare. Many subtypes.

Polyps

1. **Hyperplastic**—usually multiple, small (<1 cm) and scattered throughout the stomach (predilection for the body/fundus). Associated with chronic gastritis. Can rarely be large (3–10 cm).
2. **Fundic gland polyps**—usually multiple, small (<5 mm) and found mainly in the fundus. Can be sporadic or associated with FAP.
3. **Adenomatous**—usually solitary, 1–4 cm, sessile and typically in antrum. High risk of malignant transformation, esp. if >2 cm and if carcinomas are present elsewhere in the stomach (due to dysplastic epithelium). Associated with pernicious anaemia and FAP.
4. **Hamartomatous**—characteristically multiple, small and relatively sparing of the antrum. Associated with FAP (including Gardner variant), Peutz-Jeghers, Cowden and Cronkhite-Canada syndromes.

Benign submucosal neoplasms

Smooth, well-defined mass with an obtuse angle to the gastric wall.

1. **Leiomyoma**—much less common than gastric GIST but similar in appearance (including the tendency for central ulceration if large), though often more homogeneous in appearance.
2. **Lipoma**—fat attenuation on CT.
3. **Neurofibroma**—may be multiple. NB: leiomyomas and lipomas are more common, even in patients with NF1.
4. **Other rare neoplasms**—e.g. NET (often hypervascular), haemangioma (may be hypervascular ± phleboliths), glomus tumour (hypervascular), plexiform fibromyxoma (myxoid appearance), schwannoma.

Extrinsic indentation

1. **Pancreatic tumour/pseudocyst**.
2. **Splenomegaly/hepatomegaly.**
3. **Retroperitoneal tumours.**
4. **Duplication cyst.**
5. **Splenosis.**

Others

1. **Gastric fundoplication**—may mimic a distorted mass in the fundus. Scarring following gastric band removal can also cause mass-like distortion.
2. **Bezoar**—mass of undigestible material in the stomach; contains mottled gas on CT. Types include tricho- (hair, nearly always young women), phyto- (fruit or vegetable matter), lacto- (milk curds, most common in infants), pharmaco- (medication) and foreign body (e.g. tissue paper) bezoars.
3. **Pancreatic 'rest'**—small mass of ectopic pancreatic tissue, usually in the inferior wall of the antrum, resembling a submucosal tumour. Homogeneous enhancement similar to normal pancreas. On MRI, signal characteristics follow normal pancreas; often has a primitive duct remnant which may be visible on MRCP. May become inflamed and undergo necrosis/cystic change. There may be an adjacent stripe of submucosal fat due to recurrent inflammation. Can also occur in duodenum, jejunum, Meckel's diverticulum, liver, gallbladder and spleen.
4. **Intramural haematoma**—e.g. traumatic, iatrogenic. Hyperattenuating on unenhanced CT.
5. **Lymphoid hyperplasia**—innumerable 1–3 mm round nodules in the antrum and/or body. Associated with *H. pylori*.

7.11 GASTRIC FOLD THICKENING

Increased prominence of gastric folds. CT assessment is aided by gas or water distension.

Inflammatory

Characterized by submucosal thickening/oedema, which is near fluid attenuation on CT, ± mucosal hyperaemia.

1. Gastritis—e.g. due to NSAIDs, alcohol, corrosive ingestion, *H. pylori*, CMV, or radiotherapy. Localized or generalized fold thickening ± ulcers and inflammatory nodules (<1 cm, mostly in the antrum).
2. Zollinger-Ellison syndrome—due to a gastrinoma causing excess acid secretion, resulting in multiple and recurrent gastric and duodenal ulcers. Ulceration in both D1 and D2 is suggestive; ulceration distal to D2 is virtually diagnostic. Thick hyperaemic rugal folds ± small bowel dilatation (in response to excess acid). The underlying gastrinoma is best seen on arterial phase CT.
3. Acute pancreatitis—reactive oedema of gastric wall.
4. **Crohn's disease***—mild fold thickening especially in antrum, aphthoid ulceration ± conical stricture of antrum.
5. **Acute eosinophilic gastroenteritis**—oedematous folds, most commonly involves the gastric antrum but rest of the GI tract can also be involved.

Infiltrative/neoplastic

Fold thickening is of soft-tissue attenuation on CT with enhancement.

1. Carcinoma—can manifest as focal irregular fold thickening.
2. **Lymphoma***—usually NHL, may be primary or secondary.
3. **Pseudolymphoma**—benign reactive lymphoid hyperplasia. Most have an ulcer near the centre of the area affected.
4. **Amyloidosis***—wall thickening and dysmotility.
5. **Sarcoidosis***—focal or diffuse thickening, most common in antrum. May mimic linitis plastica or Ménétrier disease.

Others

1. Gastric ischaemia—e.g. due to gastric volvulus, arterial embolization or occlusion, vasculitis or systemic hypotension. Results in submucosal oedema with reduced or absent mucosal enhancement ± intramural gas.
2. Ménétrier disease—huge 'cerebriform' rugal folds, especially fundus and body; involvement of antrum is less common. No rigidity or ulcers. 'Weeps' protein sufficient to cause

hypoproteinaemia (effusions, ascites, oedema e.g. of the small bowel). Commonly achlorhydric: cf. Zollinger-Ellison syndrome.
3. Portal hypertension—e.g. due to cirrhosis or portal vein thrombosis. Oedematous stomach ± varices in fundus and oesophagus if chronic.
4. Emphysematous gastritis—intramural gas due to gas-forming infections.

Further reading

Hargunani, R., Maclachlan, J., Kaniyur, S., et al., 2009. Cross-sectional imaging of gastric neoplasia. Clin. Radiol. 64 (4), 420–429.

7.12 LINITIS PLASTICA

Diffuse gastric wall thickening and rigidity with effacement of rugal folds.

Neoplastic

1. Gastric carcinoma—signet ring cell adenocarcinoma.
2. Lymphoma*—thickening is typically more marked than with carcinoma.
3. Metastases—especially lobular breast cancer.
4. **Local invasion**—e.g. from pancreatic carcinoma.

Inflammatory

1. **Chronic corrosive ingestion**—can cause rigid stricture of body/antrum extending to the pylorus.
2. **Radiotherapy**—can cause rigid stricture of antrum with some deformity. Mucosal folds may be thickened or effaced ± large antral ulcers.
3. **Granulomatous inflammation**—Crohn's disease, TB. Conical antral stricture.
4. **Chronic eosinophilic gastroenteritis**—commonly involves gastric antrum (causing narrowing and nodularity) + small bowel, often with blood eosinophilia.
5. **Sarcoidosis***—predilection for antrum, usually in the presence of disease elsewhere.

7.13 GASTRIC OR DUODENAL OBSTRUCTION

1. Benign peptic stricture—most common.
2. Gastric or duodenal tumour—carcinoma, GIST, large polyp prolapsing into pylorus. NB: lymphoma does not usually cause obstruction.
3. Extrinsic compression/infiltration—e.g. by adjacent pancreatitis, pseudocyst, pancreatic cancer, annular pancreas (compressing

D2) or SMA syndrome (compression of D3 by proximal SMA, usually seen in very thin patients especially those who have recently lost weight).
4. Gastric volvulus—can be organoaxial (most common in adults, typically associated with a large hiatus hernia) or mesenteroaxial (most common in children).
5. **Other causes of pyloric stricturing**—e.g. metastases (especially breast), corrosives, Crohn's, TB, sarcoidosis, amyloid, syphilis.
6. **Obstructing bezoar.**
7. **Bouveret syndrome**—a proximal form of gallstone ileus where the calculus obstructs the pylorus or proximal duodenum.
8. **Iatrogenic**—e.g. slipped gastric band (often obstructs gastric body), fundoplication (can restrict burping, resulting in 'gas bloat' syndrome).
9. **Ileus/gastroparesis**—e.g. postsurgical, diabetes, opioids.
10. **Gastric antral web**—very short prepyloric ring or 'diaphragm' of mucosa; more common in childhood.
11. **Midgut malrotation**—with either obstructing Ladd's bands or midgut volvulus. Rare in adults, typically presents in infancy.
12. **Idiopathic hypertrophic pyloric stenosis**—nearly always presents in infancy, but has rarely been described in adults.

7.14 DECREASED/ABSENT DUODENAL FOLDS

1. Scleroderma*—often with dilatation.
2. **Coeliac disease***—especially in distal duodenum and jejunum.
3. **Crohn's disease*.**
4. **Strongyloides.**
5. **Cystic fibrosis*.**
6. **Amyloidosis*.**

7.15 DUODENAL WALL/FOLD THICKENING OR MASS

Neoplastic

1. Primary adenocarcinoma—most small bowel carcinomas occur in the duodenum or proximal jejunum. Polypoid mass or asymmetric wall thickening on CT ± obstruction. Often metastatic at presentation.
2. Infiltration by adjacent tumour—e.g. pancreatic, gallbladder, colonic, renal or adrenal carcinoma.
3. Ampullary adenoma/carcinoma—usually obstructs CBD/PD.
4. **Lipoma**—fat attenuation on CT.

5. **Polyps**—adenoma (malignant potential, associated with FAP) or hamartoma (benign, associated with many polyposis syndromes).
6. **Brunner's gland hamartoma**—benign polypoid mass of variable size, usually in D1, often pedunculated. May contain fat or cystic spaces. Can be multiple.
7. **GIST**—uncommon in duodenum, usually D2/3. Discrete endophytic or exophytic mass.
8. **Leiomyoma**—and other rare mesenchymal tumours, e.g. nerve sheath tumour.
9. **Lymphoma***—usually NHL; nonobstructing mural thickening or extrinsic mass ± aneurysmal dilatation.
10. **Neuroendocrine tumour**—avidly enhancing polyp or mass on CT. Usually nonfunctional; nearly all functional duodenal NETs are gastrinomas.
11. **Metastasis**—most commonly melanoma, breast and lung. Can cause obstruction.

Inflammatory

1. <u>Duodenitis/ulcer</u>—usually D1, related to *H. pylori*. Focal oedematous wall thickening and avid mucosal enhancement on CT ± large ulcer cavity.
2. <u>Reactive oedema</u>—due to adjacent pancreatitis or cholecystitis. Mucosal enhancement is less pronounced than in duodenitis.
3. **Cystic dystrophy**—due to heterotopic pancreatic tissue in the duodenal wall (D2) which becomes recurrently inflamed, resulting in intramural cystic change, often with delayed mural enhancement due to fibrosis ± signs of chronic pancreatitis. See also Section 7.10 (pancreatic 'rest').
4. **Paraduodenal ('groove') pancreatitis**—focal inflammation between the head of pancreas and duodenum ± cystic change. Closely related to cystic dystrophy.
5. **Crohn's disease***—mural thickening mainly in D1/2 ± layered contrast enhancement. Uncommon.
6. **Infiltration**—e.g. eosinophilic gastroenteritis, mastocytosis (dense bones), Whipple's disease (low-density mesenteric nodes), amyloid.
7. **Infections**—e.g. *Giardia*, *Strongyloides*, worms.

Vascular

1. **Varices**—due to portal hypertension or thrombosis.
2. **Intramural haematoma**—e.g. post trauma, coagulopathy.
3. **Ischaemia**—diffuse submucosal oedema ± poor or absent mucosal enhancement. Can be widespread in vasculitis secondary to radiotherapy, collagen diseases and Henoch-Schönlein purpura.

Congenital/developmental

1. Choledochocele—cystic protrusion of distal CBD into ampullary region.
2. Annular pancreas—may mimic annular duodenal thickening; enhancement and MRI signal identical to normal pancreas.
3. **Duplication cyst**—<5% of intestinal duplications; thin-walled cyst on CT/MRI often with no luminal communication.

Further reading

Wei, C.J., Chiang, J.H., Lin, W.C., et al., 2003. Tumor and tumor-like lesions of duodenum: CT and barium imaging features. Clin. Imaging 27, 89–96.

7.16 DILATED SMALL BOWEL

Calibre: proximal jejunum >3.5 cm (4.5 cm if small bowel enema)
mid-small bowel >3.0 cm (4.0 cm if small bowel enema)
ileum >2.5 cm (3.0 cm if small bowel enema).

Normal folds

1. Mechanical obstruction—± dilated large bowel depending on level of obstruction. Discrete transition point at the site of obstruction; small bowel faeces sign can help to find this. Always check for a closed loop as this will require urgent surgery due to risk of strangulation/ischaemia. Causes of obstruction include:
   (a) Extrinsic—e.g. adhesions (most common cause, look for 'hairpin' angulations ± small amount of trapped fat within an adhesive band), hernias (both external and internal), volvulus, congenital bands (e.g. Ladd's bands, persistent omphalomesenteric duct), compression or infiltration by an adjacent mass or abscess.
   (b) Mural—e.g. strictures (Section 7.17), masses (Section 7.18), intussusception (usually ileocolic), intramural haematoma.
   (c) Luminal—e.g. gallstone ileus (look for chronically inflamed gallbladder adherent to duodenum ± pneumobilia), enterolith (often related to jejunal diverticulosis), foreign body, bezoar, mass of parasitic worms (especially ascariasis), distal intestinal obstruction syndrome (DIOS, due to thick secretions in a patient with cystic fibrosis).
2. Paralytic ileus—dilated small ± large bowel, no discrete transition point. Most commonly seen postoperatively but can also be caused by trauma, sepsis, drugs and metabolic disturbances.
3. Early arterial ischaemia—dilatation is the earliest sign on CT and reflects an ischaemic ileus. Other signs (e.g. reduced mural enhancement and pneumatosis) develop as ischaemia progresses. NB: mural thickening is not a common feature of acute arterial ischaemia.

4. **Scleroderma***—dilated small bowel with crowded valvulae conniventes ('hidebound' appearance) ± antimesenteric pseudodiverticula (NB: true diverticula are on the mesenteric border).
5. **Coeliac disease* and tropical sprue**—can produce identical signs. Dilated fluid-filled small bowel ± effaced jejunal folds and prominent ileal folds (reversed fold pattern) ± 'hidebound' appearance ± mesenteric adenopathy.
6. **Chronic intestinal pseudo-obstruction**—many causes including collagen vascular diseases (e.g. SLE), endocrine disorders (e.g. diabetes), CNS disorders (e.g. Parkinson's), enteric neuropathies, myopathies, Ehlers-Danlos syndrome, amyloidosis, drugs (e.g. opioids) and infections (e.g. Chagas). Resembles paralytic ileus on imaging; dilatation can be marked.
7. **Small bowel diverticulosis (mimic)**—especially in the jejunum. Diverticula can be large and numerous, mimicking small bowel dilatation, but these do not contain valvulae conniventes.
8. **Iatrogenic**—vagotomy and gastrectomy may produce dilatation due to rapid emptying of stomach contents. A side-to-side small bowel anastomosis may appear as a focally dilated small bowel segment. Extensive small bowel resection results in compensatory dilatation of the remaining small bowel ± mild fold thickening.
9. **Duplication cyst**—can contain gas if it communicates with the small bowel, mimicking a dilated small bowel segment.

7

Thick folds

1. **Venous ischaemia**—especially with closed-loop obstruction. Dilatation + oedematous thickening is typical (cf. arterial ischaemia). Reduced mural enhancement suggests progressive ischaemia.
2. **Crohn's disease***—alternating segments of narrowed thick-walled small bowel (strictures) and dilated thin-walled small bowel ('skip' segments).
3. **Lymphoma***—aneurysmal dilatation of a thickened small bowel segment.
4. **Metastases**—especially from melanoma. Can mimic lymphoma.
5. **Radiotherapy.**
6. **Zollinger-Ellison syndrome**—ileus ± thickening due to excess acidity.
7. **Amyloidosis***—diffuse thickening + dilatation.

Further reading

Masselli, G., Gualdi, G., 2012. MR imaging of the small bowel. Radiology 264 (2), 333–348.

Silva, A.C., Pimenta, M., Guimaraes, L.S., 2009. Small bowel obstruction: what to look for. Radiographics 29 (2), 423–439.

7.17 SMALL BOWEL STRICTURES

See also Section 7.18.

1. **Crohn's disease***—either acute inflammatory strictures (longer segment, prominent thickening and submucosal oedema, avid enhancement, surrounding fat stranding ± inflammatory mass) or chronic fibrotic strictures (shorter segment, only mild thickening and enhancement, no surrounding inflammation). The presence of mesenteric 'fat wrapping' around a strictured small bowel segment is almost pathognomonic for Crohn's.
2. **NSAID-induced**—typically short or very short (diaphragm-like); usually multiple in mid-distal small bowel ± ascending colon. Also look for papillary necrosis in kidneys.
3. **Ischaemic**—may be short or long; look for atherosclerotic narrowing of the mesenteric arteries. Can also occur in microvascular disease and vasculitis (especially Behçet's).
4. **Radiation-induced**—typically involves pelvic ileal loops after pelvic radiotherapy. Strictures can be long.
5. **Anastomotic**—especially after resections for Crohn's.
6. **Metastases**—usually with metastatic disease elsewhere.
7. **Adenocarcinoma**—see Section 7.18. The thickening can be subtle and mimic a benign stricture, especially in patients with Crohn's (who are at increased risk).
8. **Endometriosis***—serosal small bowel deposits can cause stricturing. Look for other features of the disease in the pelvis.
9. **Mycobacterial infection**—TB (terminal ileum) or *Mycobacterium avium* complex (jejunum), often with mesenteric adenopathy.
10. **Cryptogenic multifocal ulcerous stenosing enteritis**—rare disease characterized by multiple idiopathic short strictures typically in the ileum, usually without obstruction. No fistulation or abscess.
11. **Sarcoidosis***—rare.

7.18 SMALL BOWEL MASSES

Malignant

1. **Metastases**—either haematogenous (melanoma, lung, breast) or via peritoneal spread (ovary, stomach, pancreas, colon, uterus). Usually multiple + metastases elsewhere ± ascites (if via peritoneal spread).
2. **Neuroendocrine tumour (carcinoid)**—most common primary small bowel malignancy beyond the duodenojejunal flexure, usually in the distal ileum. May be multifocal ± associated with MEN 1. Avidly enhancing discrete intramural nodule; may cause obstruction. Mesenteric lymphadenopathy is usually present ± calcification and desmoplastic reaction. Carcinoid syndrome only develops with liver metastases.

3. **Adenocarcinoma**—most common primary small bowel malignancy in the duodenum. Ileal lesions are rare (except in Crohn's). Short thick-walled annular stricture, usually presenting with obstruction and commonly with nodal and metastatic disease. High incidence of second primary tumours.
4. **Lymphoma***—secondary > primary. Long segment of small bowel thickening + aneurysmal dilatation + mesenteric adenopathy; obstruction is uncommon. Increased risk in coeliac disease.
5. **GIST**—second most common location after the stomach. Discrete exophytic heterogeneous soft-tissue mass, often large at presentation ± central ulceration. Its large size can make it difficult to ascertain its exact site of origin. No associated lymphadenopathy. Metastasizes most commonly to the liver and peritoneum. Associated with Carney triad and NF1.
6. **Sarcoma**—e.g. leiomyosarcoma (may see tumour thrombus invading SMV branches), MPNST (in NF1). Similar appearance to GIST, but much less common.

Benign

1. **Polyps**—these can act as a lead point for intussusception and are associated with polyposis syndromes especially if multiple.
   (a) **Adenoma**—associated with FAP (including Gardner syndrome) especially in the duodenum. Has malignant potential.
   (b) **Hamartoma**—associated with Peutz-Jeghers, Cowden, Cronkhite-Canada and juvenile polyposis syndromes. No malignant potential in itself, but the syndromes are associated with increased risk of various malignancies.
   (c) **Inflammatory fibroid polyp**—no malignant potential.
2. **Crohn's disease***—an inflammatory mass can mimic a tumour.
3. **Intramural haematoma**—high attenuation on unenhanced CT.
4. **Mesenchymal lesions**—e.g. lipoma (fat attenuation), leiomyoma (mimics GIST but is less common), haemangioma (avid nodular enhancement), neurogenic tumours (e.g. schwannoma, neurofibroma and ganglioneuroma, especially in NF1), angiomyolipoma, inflammatory myofibroblastic tumour.
5. **Amyloidoma**—rare manifestation; mimics adenocarcinoma.
6. **Mesenteric tumours**—e.g. desmoid tumour; can mimic an exophytic small bowel GIST if large.
7. **Duplication cyst**—cystic, on serosal surface of small bowel, most commonly distal ileum.

Further reading

Anzidei, M., Napoli, A., Zini, C., et al., 2011. Malignant tumours of the small intestine: a review of histopathology, multidetector CT and MRI aspects. Br. J. Radiol. 84 (1004), 677–690.

Fletcher, J.G., 2009. CT enterography technique: theme and variations. Abdom. Imaging 34 (3), 283–288.

7

7.19 SMALL BOWEL WALL THICKENING

	Focal (<6 cm)	Segmental (6–40 cm)	Diffuse (>40 cm)
Soft-tissue attenuation wall thickening	Neoplasm Active Crohn's disease Chronic fibrotic strictures	Active Crohn's disease Intramural haemorrhage Lymphoma Diffuse serosal metastases	Intramural haemorrhage Diffuse serosal metastases
Submucosal oedema, avid mucosal enhancement	Active Crohn's disease Focal ulceration/perforation Low-grade ischaemia	Active Crohn's disease Low-grade ischaemia Infectious enteritis Postobstructive oedema Acute radiation enteritis Angioedema Zollinger-Ellison syndrome	Low-grade ischaemia Shock bowel CMV enteritis Chemotherapy-induced enteritis Graft-vs-host disease Eosinophilic enteritis Mastocytosis
Submucosal oedema, normal mucosal enhancement	Reactive oedema Closed-loop SBO	PV/SMV thrombosis Portal hypertension Closed-loop SBO Coeliac disease/tropical sprue Whipple's disease Lymphatic obstruction	Hypoalbuminaemia PV/SMV thrombosis Portal hypertension Amyloidosis Lymphatic obstruction Primary intestinal lymphangiectasia
Submucosal oedema, reduced mucosal enhancement	Venous/arterial ischaemia	Venous/arterial ischaemia Vasculitis	Venous/arterial ischaemia

Normal mural thickness: 1–2 mm (distended); 3–4 mm (collapsed). Causes can be differentiated based on the attenuation and enhancement of the wall and the length of involvement: focal (<6 cm), segmental (6–40 cm) or diffuse (>40 cm).

Soft-tissue attenuation wall thickening

Submucosal attenuation >25 HU on portal venous phase CT.

1. Neoplasm—see Section 7.18, especially metastases, adenocarcinoma and lymphoma. Thickening is typically short in length (except lymphoma and diffuse serosal metastases) and irregular/eccentric, with obliteration of the normal bowel layers.
2. Active Crohn's disease*—florid transmural inflammation causes marked segmental thickening, avid mucosal and patchy transmural enhancement + surrounding fat stranding and vascular engorgement (comb sign), often with an inflammatory mass or abscess. Most commonly involves terminal ileum (TI) but can occur anywhere in the GI tract. Fat wrapping is almost pathognomonic. Also look for other features, e.g. fibrotic strictures, relative sparing of the antimesenteric border and fistulation, e.g. with other bowel loops, skin surface or bladder.
3. Chronic fibrotic strictures—of any cause (see Section 7.17). Typically short and only mildly thickened + mild homogeneous enhancement.
4. Intramural haemorrhage—e.g. due to trauma (most common in duodenum), coagulopathy (most common in jejunum), vasculitis (e.g. Henoch-Schönlein purpura) or haemolytic uraemic syndrome (caused by *E. coli* in children). The thickening is often segmental ± upstream obstruction. The high mural attenuation is due to intramural blood rather than enhancement; this can be confirmed on unenhanced CT (mural attenuation >60 HU). Intraluminal blood and haemorrhagic ascites may also be present.

7

Submucosal oedema with avid mucosal enhancement

Homogeneous submucosal attenuation of <25 HU on CT and T2 hyperintensity on MRI suggests oedema, and avid mucosal enhancement (relative to normal bowel loops) suggests inflammation, infection or hyperaemia.

1. Active Crohn's disease*—less florid than the transmural inflammation above.
2. Focal ulceration or perforation—e.g. peptic ulceration (typically in duodenum but can occur more distally), small bowel diverticulitis (jejunal or Meckel's), fish-bone perforation. Focal small bowel inflammation + surrounding fat stranding.

3. **Low-grade ischaemia**—arterial, venous or vasculitic. The mucosal hyperenhancement is due to vasodilatation. Often seen at the border zones of a segment of high-grade ischaemia, but can also be seen in isolation especially in vasculitis. May be focal, segmental or diffuse.
4. **Shock bowel**—due to acute severe hypotension or hypovolaemia (e.g. major trauma). Diffuse small bowel involvement. Look for other signs, e.g. IVC collapse, hyperenhancing adrenals.
5. **Infectious enteritis**—common condition but uncommonly seen on CT as imaging is usually not indicated. Mild segmental small bowel thickening + mesenteric adenitis; ileocaecal involvement suggests *Salmonella, Shigella, Yersinia* or *Campylobacter*; duodenojejunal involvement suggests *Giardia* or *Strongyloides*. In immunocompromised patients with opportunistic infections (e.g. CMV enterocolitis) the inflammation is often diffuse.
6. **Postobstructive oedema**—due to recent spontaneous resolution of SBO, resulting in transient mucosal hyperaemia and submucosal oedema in a segmental pattern upstream of the point of obstruction. Check for a recent AXR—if this shows SBO but the subsequent CT shows normal calibre oedematous small bowel, this implies the diagnosis.
7. **Iatrogenic enteritis**
   (a) **Acute radiation enteritis**—usually involves pelvic small bowel loops; extent depends on number of loops within the radiation field.
   (b) **Chemotherapy-induced enteritis**—diffuse small bowel involvement.
   (c) **Graft-versus-host disease***—diffuse small bowel and/or colonic involvement; occurs after bone marrow transplant. Mimics opportunistic infection on imaging.
8. **Angioedema**—due to C1 esterase inhibitor deficiency, may be hereditary (younger patients) or acquired (older patients, e.g. due to ACE inhibitors, lymphoma or autoimmune disorders). Recurrent transient episodes of segmental submucosal oedema, mucosal hyperenhancement and ascites.
9. **Zollinger-Ellison syndrome**—duodenal ± proximal jejunal inflammation due to acid secretions.
10. **Eosinophilic enteritis**—diffuse thickening of proximal small bowel + gastric antrum is most common. Peripheral eosinophilia is usually present.
11. **Mastocytosis***—diffuse small bowel thickening + splenomegaly, lymphadenopathy, ascites and sclerotic bones.

Submucosal oedema with normal mucosal enhancement

Normal mucosal enhancement suggests passive submucosal oedema. NB: there is some overlap with mucosal hyperenhancement above.

1. Reactive oedema—focal thickening secondary to adjacent inflammation, e.g. appendicitis, diverticulitis, pancreatitis, cholecystitis, abscess.
2. Hypoalbuminaemia—e.g. renal/liver failure, protein-losing enteropathy. Diffuse submucosal oedema + ascites, pleural effusions and subcutaneous oedema.
3. Portal venous system congestion
   (a) PV/SMV thrombosis—the extent of submucosal oedema is proportional to the proximity of a thrombus to the bowel; isolated thrombosis around the portal confluence is less likely to cause significant oedema, whereas thrombosis extending into multiple peripheral SMV branches can cause diffuse oedema.
   (b) Portal hypertension—usually due to cirrhosis. Often the right colon is most affected. Look for varices, splenomegaly, ascites.
   (c) Closed loop SBO—dilated cluster of small bowel loops with two adjacent transition points and variable submucosal oedema and mucosal enhancement depending on the severity of venous ischaemia. The mesenteric veins usually appear focally narrowed adjacent to the point of obstruction—this reflects extrinsic venous compression by either an adhesive band (most common cause), neck of an internal hernia or torted mesentery.
4. Coeliac disease* and tropical sprue—dilated and fluid-filled jejunum with mild segmental submucosal oedema, reversal of jejunoileal fold patterns and mesenteric lymphadenopathy.
5. **Whipple's disease**—most commonly segmental involvement of jejunum and distal duodenum + mesenteric lymphadenopathy with central fat attenuation.
6. **Amyloidosis***—diffuse small bowel thickening and dilatation ± diffuse mesenteric infiltration and adenopathy.
7. **Lymphatic obstruction**—e.g. by malignancy (including the desmoplastic reaction associated with carcinoids), sclerosing mesenteritis, retroperitoneal fibrosis or sarcoidosis. Segmental or diffuse oedema upstream of the obstruction + chylous ascites.
8. **Primary intestinal lymphangiectasia**—children and young adults, due to congenital maldevelopment of lacteals resulting in leakage of lymph into bowel; presents with protein-losing enteropathy, peripheral oedema and lymphopenia. Diffuse submucosal oedema, mesenteric oedema and chylous ascites on imaging.

Submucosal oedema with reduced mucosal enhancement

Reduced mucosal enhancement (relative to other bowel loops) suggests acute high-grade ischaemia. Often accompanied by haemorrhagic ascites (look for dependent layering of dense blood products, e.g. in pelvis).

1. Venous ischaemia—e.g. due to closed-loop SBO or acute extensive SMV thrombosis. Submucosal and mesenteric oedema occurs earlier and more prominently than in arterial ischaemia.
2. Arterial ischaemia—either thrombotic or embolic SMA occlusion. Look for splenic/renal infarcts and thrombus in the left atrial appendage (suggests embolic shower). Reduced mucosal enhancement occurs earlier than in venous ischaemia.
3. Vasculitis—segmental area or areas of ischaemia, usually in young patients. Mucosal hyperenhancement is more common than hypoenhancement. Examples include SLE (± thrombotic bowel infarction due to antiphospholipid syndrome), polyarteritis nodosa (look for renal microaneurysms and infarcts), Henoch-Schönlein purpura (children and young adults, classic skin rash) and Behçet's disease (usually TI, can mimic Crohn's).

7.20 ILEOCAECAL REGION THICKENING

Inflammatory

1. Acute appendicitis—inflammation can secondarily involve the caecal pole and TI, especially in the presence of an abscess, potentially mimicking Crohn's.
2. Crohn's disease*—the presence of fat wrapping is almost pathognomonic and aids differentiation from complicated appendicitis. Also, abscesses related to Crohn's typically have a thick rind of enhancing inflammatory tissue around them (cf. the thin-walled abscesses in appendicitis). In addition, look for other sites of disease distant from the ileocaecal region.
3. Ulcerative colitis*—terminal ileal 'backwash' ileitis can be seen for up to 25 cm, in the presence of pancolitis.
4. Neutropenic colitis—also known as typhlitis. Inflammation typically involves the caecum ± ascending colon and TI. Clinical context (neutropenia due to chemotherapy or other cause of immunocompromise) clarifies the diagnosis.
5. Right-sided colonic diverticulitis—focal inflammation centred on a diverticulum + adjacent fat stranding.
6. Pelvic inflammatory disease—in patients with a low-lying caecum, a right-sided tubo-ovarian abscess can involve the ileocaecal region, mimicking complicated appendicitis.
7. **Radiation enterocolitis**—in patients with a low-lying caecum in the pelvis.
8. **Portal hypertension**—most commonly causes oedema of the right colon.
9. **Behçet's disease***—most commonly involves TI, mimicking Crohn's.

10. **Dropped gallstone**—post cholecystectomy. Gallstone can migrate to the right iliac fossa via the right paracolic gutter and cause recurrent abscesses around the ileocaecal region.

Infective

1. **TB***—can mimic Crohn's; TI and caecum are predominantly involved with stricturing and caecal contraction ± fistulae ± necrotic ileocolic nodes. Caecal involvement is more prominent than in Crohn's. <50% have pulmonary TB.
2. ***Salmonella, Shigella, Yersinia, Campylobacter***—typically involve the ileocaecal region causing mild inflammation and mesenteric adenitis.
3. **CMV colitis**—right-sided ± TI involvement, may be extensive. Seen in the immunocompromised—overlaps with neutropenic colitis.
4. **Amoebic colitis**—typically involves the caecum and ascending colon, with characteristic sparing of the TI. Can cause marked colonic thickening and narrowing, mimicking a tumour. Look for associated amoebic liver abscess.
5. **Actinomycosis**—rare; most commonly involves the ileocaecal region with an associated strikingly infiltrative soft-tissue mass + abscess, often invading abdominal wall ± fistulae. Occasionally pelvic bowel is secondarily involved from the gynaecological tract.
6. **Histoplasmosis**—very rare.

7

Neoplastic

1. **Adenocarcinoma**—caecal and ascending colon tumours can invade the TI and can mimic inflammation, especially if mucinous—the presence of mucinous ileocolic nodes aids differentiation. Caecal tumours can also occlude the appendix orifice and cause secondary appendicitis—always have a high index of suspicion in an elderly patient presenting with acute appendicitis, since the acute inflammation may mask the underlying tumour; consider follow-up imaging.
2. **Carcinoid**—appendix is the most common site (generally benign and often too small to see on CT). Most small bowel carcinoids originate in the distal ileum and are invariably malignant if >2 cm. Discrete hypervascular mural nodule with mesenteric adenopathy ± calcification. The desmoplastic reaction may cause lymphatic or venous obstruction resulting in segmental ileal oedema, mimicking an inflammatory process.
3. **Lymphoma***—TI is the most common site.
4. **Appendix mucocoele**—grossly dilated appendix filled with mucin ± mural calcification. Caused by a low-grade mucinous appendiceal neoplasm. Results in pseudomyxoma peritonei if it ruptures into the peritoneal space.
5. **Metastases.**

Ischaemia

1. **Isolated caecal necrosis**—the caecum is an uncommon but recognized site for ischaemic colitis. Focal mural thickening and reduced mucosal enhancement ± pneumatosis in the caecal pole, usually in an elderly vasculopath without a discrete arterial filling defect.
2. **Exercise-induced ischaemic colitis**—seen in marathon runners. Caused by catecholamine-induced splanchnic vasoconstriction and dehydration, resulting in watershed ischaemia, which can affect the caecum.

Further reading

Silva, A.C., Beaty, S.D., Hara, A.K., et al., 2007. Spectrum of normal and abnormal CT appearances of the ileocecal valve and cecum with endoscopic and surgical correlation. Radiographics 27 (4), 1039–1054.

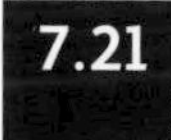

7.21 COLITIS ON CROSS-SECTIONAL IMAGING

Signs of inflammatory colitis on CT/MRI are often nonspecific; the following is a guide only. On AXR, colitis typically appears as an absence of colonic faeces (earliest sign) ± 'thumbprinting' due to haustral thickening. Always check for signs of toxic megacolon (see Section 7.24). Beware of inflammatory carcinomas mimicking colitis; irregular thickening and marked lymphadenopathy are suggestive.

Diffuse

1. Ulcerative colitis (UC)*.
2. Pseudomembranous colitis—*Clostridium difficile* toxin. Marked colonic wall oedema (mean 15 mm, more than other causes of colitis) with mucosal hyperenhancement + 'accordion' sign due to grossly thickened haustra (suggestive but not pathognomonic) ± ascites. Often diffuse but may be right or left sided.
3. CMV—in immunocompromised patients, ± TI involvement.
4. *E. coli*—diffuse or segmental, nearly always involving transverse colon. Can cause haemolytic uraemic syndrome in children, resulting in intramural haemorrhage and enlarged hyperechoic kidneys.
5. **Graft-versus-host disease***—often with diffuse small bowel involvement. Colonic thickening is typically mild—thickness >7 mm strongly suggests an alternative diagnosis, e.g. CMV, *C. difficile* or neutropenic colitis.

Predominantly right-sided

1. Reactive oedema—e.g. secondary to appendicitis (caecum), cholecystitis (hepatic flexure), omental infarction (ascending) or postobstructive oedema.
2. Crohn's disease*—TI involvement usually present and often more marked than colonic involvement (cf. TB), but isolated Crohn's colitis can occur. Skip segments and fat wrapping are characteristic features.
3. Neutropenic colitis—see Section 7.20. Overlaps with CMV.
4. ***Salmonella*, *Yersinia* and *Campylobacter***—usually with TI involvement.
5. **TB***—see Section 7.20. Necrotic ileocolic nodes are suggestive. No fat wrapping (cf. Crohn's).
6. **Amoebiasis**—usually right-sided but may be diffuse; TI typically spared. May cause toxic megacolon, mass-like amoeboma or liver abscess.
7. **Portal hypertension**—submucosal oedema + other features (varices, ascites, splenomegaly).
8. **Ischaemic colitis**—hypovolaemic states in young patients, cocaine users or elderly vasculopaths (isolated caecal necrosis).
9. **Angioedema**—more common in small bowel.
10. **Phlebosclerotic colitis**—rare (mostly seen in Japan); involves caecum and ascending colon ± extension distally. Caused by sclerotic occlusion of mesenteric veins—thread-like calcification of small SMV branches close to or within the colonic wall is almost pathognomonic. May result in ischaemia/obstruction.

7

Predominantly left-sided

1. Ulcerative colitis*—nearly always involving the rectum and extending proximally in a contiguous fashion (cf. skip segments in Crohn's). Proliferation of mesorectal fat is suggestive, but can also be seen in Crohn's and radiation proctitis.
2. Diverticulitis—may be focal thickening around a single inflamed diverticulum (look for adjacent fat stranding) or involving a longer segment of diverticulosis + surrounding fat stranding ± abscess. May occasionally be right-sided.
3. Ischaemic colitis—either involving the inferior mesenteric artery territory (distal transverse to rectosigmoid) or watershed areas near the rectosigmoid junction and splenic flexure (especially the elderly). Rectum usually spared. Submucosal oedema and mucosal hyperenhancement in low-grade ischaemia. In high-grade ischaemia the mucosa enhances poorly and there may be minimal wall thickening; associated pneumatosis suggests infarction.
4. Epiploic appendagitis—usually left-sided but can occur anywhere. Well-defined oval or round area of fat with a 'halo' of fat stranding

± central dense 'dot' (thrombosed vessel). Located adjacent to the colon ± mild mural oedema.
5. *Shigella*—can also affect ileocaecal region.
6. **Schistosomiasis***—mural calcification is highly suggestive if present.
7. **Hermansky-Pudlak syndrome**—rare autosomal recessive disorder characterized by granulomatous colitis, pulmonary fibrosis, bleeding diatheses and oculocutaneous albinism.

Predominantly rectal (proctitis)

1. Ulcerative colitis*—proctitis is rare in Crohn's.
2. Radiation colitis—rectum ± sigmoid.
3. Reactive inflammation—e.g. secondary to perianal sepsis (especially in immunocompromised) or prostatic abscess.
4. **Sexually transmitted infections**—due to receptive anal intercourse; e.g. gonorrhoea, HSV, lymphogranuloma venereum (LGV), syphilis. Rectum ± sigmoid involvement. LGV also typically presents with large necrotic inguinal nodes.
5. **Solitary rectal ulcer syndrome**—due to recurrent rectal prolapse. Diffuse thickening with ulceration of the anterior wall ± inflammatory cystic mass (proctitis cystica profunda).
6. **Stercoral colitis**—due to hard impacted faeces in the rectum. Usually in the elderly.
7. **Chemical colitis**—e.g. hydrogen peroxide enema. Rectosigmoid.
8. **Eosinophilic colitis**—may be primary or secondary (parasites, drugs, autoimmune disorders). The primary form has two peaks in infancy and young adults; most commonly involves rectum.

Further reading

Barral, M., Boudiaf, M., Dohan, A., et al., 2015. MDCT of acute colitis in adults: an update in current imaging features. Diagn. Interv. Imaging 96 (2), 133–149.

Thoeni, R.F., Cello, J.P., 2006. CT imaging of colitis. Radiology 240 (3), 6236–6238.

7.22 COLONIC POLYPS ON CT COLONOGRAPHY

See also polyposis syndromes in Part 2.

1. Tubular, tubulovillous and villous adenomas—these form a spectrum both in size and degree of dysplasia. Villous adenoma is the largest with the most severe dysplasia and highest risk of malignancy—these are typically fronded and sessile with a surface layer of mucus. Polyps <6 mm have minimal risk of malignancy; larger polyps require endoscopic biopsy if clinically appropriate.

Polyps >2 cm are more likely to be malignant than benign. An irregular or ulcerated surface and puckering of the colonic wall at the polyp base are also suggestive of malignancy. Polyps may be pedunculated, sessile or flat (plaque-like, <3 mm height, most difficult to see—a coating of oral contrast can aid identification). Adenomas are associated with FAP (including Gardner variant) and Turcot syndrome.

2. **Inflammatory**—benign, seen in IBD (UC > Crohn's). Polyps can be seen at all stages of activity of the colitis: acute—pseudopolyps (i.e. mucosal hyperplasia); chronic—sessile polyp (resembles villous adenoma); quiescent—filiform polyp (worm-like ± branching pattern).
3. **Hamartomatous**—seen in various syndromes (see Part 2). Although the polyps themselves are benign, the syndromes are associated with an increased risk of various malignancies.
4. **Hyperplastic**—often multiple and small, typically in younger patients. Associated with hyperplastic polyposis syndrome.
5. **Nodular lymphoid hyperplasia**—in children and adolescents; very small, usually in the right colon.
6. **Infective**—e.g. tuberculoma, amoeboma and schistosomiasis (mainly rectosigmoid ± strictures or calcification).

Polyp mimics

1. **Untagged faecal matter**—often heterogeneous with tiny gas bubbles.
2. **Thick folds**—especially at the ileocaecal valve (fat attenuation), due to spasm (triangular shape on 3D intraluminal view, often only seen on one view due to transient nature) or in diverticular disease. Typically linear with a smooth surface.
3. **Lipoma**—fat attenuation may be masked by streak artefact from luminal contrast.
4. **Other mesenchymal neoplasms**—e.g. haemangioma (most commonly rectosigmoid ± phleboliths), leiomyoma (usually rectosigmoid), fibroma, desmoid tumour, schwannoma, neurofibroma, ganglioneuroma, granular cell tumour. Submucosal location, smooth overlying mucosa.
5. **Metastases**—location may be serosal (if via peritoneal spread) or submucosal (if haematogenous, e.g. melanoma, lung, breast), usually with disease elsewhere ± ascites.
6. **Carcinoid tumour**—most commonly rectal and small in size.
7. **Endometriosis***—serosal deposits especially on rectosigmoid can mimic a polyp or mass. Smooth overlying mucosal surface. Look for disease elsewhere in the pelvis.
8. **Intramural haemorrhage**—may mimic a submucosal mass; hyperattenuating on unenhanced CT.
9. **Internal haemorrhoid or varix**—in distal rectum abutting the anorectal junction. Varices are typically linear.

10. **Inverted diverticulum**—may contain a focus of indrawn fat.
11. **Inverted appendix stump**—following appendectomy.
12. **Cystic lymphangioma**—rare. Fluid attenuation.

7.23 COLONIC STRICTURES AND MASSES

Neoplastic

1. **Carcinoma**—irregular mural thickening with 'shouldering'. May be a sessile or semiannular mass or annular stricture. Often <6 cm in length. Usually of soft-tissue attenuation except if mucinous (fluid attenuation ± calcification). Necrotic or mucinous mesenteric nodes are suggestive.
2. **Metastasis**—via peritoneal or haematogenous spread, usually with disease elsewhere ± ascites. Peritoneal metastases most commonly deposit on the rectosigmoid. Some primaries (e.g. linitis plastica, lobular breast cancer) can cause long smooth thick-walled strictures mimicking benign pathology.
3. **Direct invasion by adjacent tumours**—e.g. transverse colon invasion by gastric cancer, rectal invasion by prostate or gynaecological tumours.
4. **Lymphoma***—long segment irregular thickening, typically without obstruction. Usually right colon, may be multifocal.
5. **GIST**—rare in the colon, most located in the rectum. Large endophytic or exophytic mass without lymphadenopathy (cf. carcinoma).
6. **Sarcoma**—e.g. leiomyosarcoma. Rare, often bulky and aggressive, indistinguishable from carcinoma. Can occur in the rectum years after pelvic radiotherapy.

Inflammatory and ischaemic

Tend to be symmetrical, smooth and tapered.

1. **Diverticular stricture**—differentiation from cancer is not always possible. Features suggesting diverticulitis: >10 cm involvement, tapered margins, presence of gas-filled diverticula within thickened segment, pericolic stranding or fluid, engorged mesenteric vessels. Features suggesting cancer: focal shouldered mass, straightening of thickened segment, large or necrotic pericolic nodes.
2. **Ulcerative colitis***—usually requires extensive involvement for >5 years; look for associated haustral effacement, submucosal fat deposition and mesorectal fat proliferation. Strictures are commonest in the sigmoid and may be multiple. Beware of malignant complications—these are often irregular annular strictures. Risk factors: total colitis, length of history (risk starts at 10 years and increases with time), epithelial dysplasia especially DALM (dysplasia-associated lesion or mass).

3. Crohn's disease*—single or multiple with skip segments.
4. Ischaemic—infarction heals by stricture formation relatively rapidly. Most common at splenic flexure. Tapered margins, may be long.
5. Radiotherapy—occurs several years after treatment, usually in rectosigmoid.
6. **Anastomotic stricture**—especially if there is a history of anastomotic leak.
7. **Caustic stricture**—rectosigmoid.
8. **Cathartic colon**—due to chronic laxative abuse. Results in narrow-calibre ahaustral colon with long pseudostrictures due to spasm. Most commonly involves ascending and transverse colon, spares rectum (cf. chronic UC).
9. **Sarcoidosis***—rare, usually in the presence of thoracic disease.

Infective

1. Tuberculosis*—most common in the ileocaecal region with contraction of caecum.
2. **Amoeboma**—rare mass-like form of amoebiasis. Rapid improvement after treatment with metronidazole.
3. **Actinomycosis**—markedly infiltrative mass, most common in ileocaecal region.
4. **Schistosomiasis***—commonly rectosigmoid. Granulation tissue forming after the acute stage (oedema, fold thickening and polyps) may cause a stricture.
5. **Lymphogranuloma venereum**—sexually transmitted *Chlamydia*. Strictures are a late complication, characteristically long and tubular, affecting the rectosigmoid ± fistulae.

Extrinsic masses

Pericolic abscess, endometriosis (usually rectosigmoid), desmoid tumour, solitary fibrous tumour, amyloidoma, duplication cyst. Also, an adhesive band may focally distort/narrow the colon, mimicking a stricture.

7.24 MEGACOLON IN AN ADULT

Colonic dilatation >6 cm.

Nontoxic (without mural abnormalities)

1. Distal obstruction—e.g. carcinoma, chronic intermittent sigmoid volvulus.
2. Paralytic ileus—many causes (see Section 7.16). Dilated thin-walled colon ± gradual tapering at the splenic flexure without a visible obstructing cause. Small bowel is also often dilated.

3. Chronic pseudoobstruction—symptoms and signs of large bowel obstruction but without an obstructing cause on CT. Many causes (see Section 7.16). Dilated thin-walled gas-filled colon. High risk of caecal necrosis and perforation despite the lack of mechanical obstruction.
4. **Faecal impaction**—markedly dilated rectum ± sigmoid due to impacted faeces, ± mural thickening due to stercoral colitis.
5. **Hirschsprung's disease and hypoganglionosis**—can present in adults. Dilated colon with a transition in the sigmoid region.
6. **Laxative abuse**—dilated ahaustral colon ± spasm.
7. **Amyloidosis***—dilatation is the most common manifestation of colonic involvement.

Toxic (with severe mural abnormalities)

Mural abnormalities include thickening, loss of haustral folds ± pneumatosis or free gas.

1. IBD*—UC > Crohn's.
2. Infectious colitis—especially pseudomembranous colitis.
3. Ischaemic colitis.

7.25 PNEUMATOSIS INTESTINALIS

Gas in the bowel wall, best seen on CT. Differential diagnosis depends on the clinical state of the patient.

Benign causes (well patient)

1. Idiopathic—also known as pneumatosis cystoides intestinalis; usually involves the colon. Appears as clusters of gas-filled intramural cysts.
2. Drug-induced—corticosteroids, chemotherapy.
3. Intestinal—pyloric stenosis, intestinal pseudoobstruction, ileus, bowel obstruction, IBD.
4. Pulmonary – asthma, emphysema, PEEP, cystic fibrosis.
5. Connective tissue disease—e.g. scleroderma.
6. Iatrogenic—following endoscopy, CT colonography, jejunostomy tube, bowel anastomosis.
7. **Organ transplants**—including small-bowel transplants and graft-versus-host disease.

Life-threatening causes (unwell patient)

1. Intestinal ischaemia—including closed-loop bowel obstruction.
2. Toxic megacolon—due to IBD or severe enterocolitis. Suggests imminent perforation.
3. Trauma—suggests significant bowel injury.
4. **Stevens-Johnson syndrome**—with skin and mucosal involvement.

Further reading

Ho, L.M., Paulson, E.K., Thompson, W.M., 2007. Pneumatosis intestinalis in the adult: benign to life-threatening causes. AJR Am. J. Roentgenol. 88, 1604–1613.

7.26 BOWEL WALL CALCIFICATION

1. **Mucinous adenocarcinoma**—calcification can be seen in the primary tumour or involved mesenteric nodes.
2. **TB***—ileocaecal region.
3. **Schistosomiasis***—usually left colon. Also look for hepatic calcification.
4. **Metastatic calcification**—due to renal failure; look for other sites.
5. **Calcification within other masses**—e.g. GIST, haemangioma.
6. **Amyloidosis***.
7. **Phlebosclerotic colitis**—thread-like calcification of small SMV branches close to or within the colonic wall is almost pathognomonic.

7.27 BOWEL WALL FAT DEPOSITION

1. **Normal variant**—especially in the undistended colon of obese patients. Tends to disappear when the colon is distended.
2. **Chronic IBD**—UC (favours rectum and colon) and Crohn's (favours distal ileum). The submucosal fat layer tends to be thicker than in normal obese patients and often persists even when the bowel is distended; ± mesenteric or mesorectal fatty proliferation.
3. **Post chemotherapy or graft-versus-host disease***—may be diffuse.
4. **Post radiotherapy**—in the rectum.
5. **Coeliac disease***—in the duodenum and jejunum.

7.28 RECTAL MASS OR THICKENING ON MRI

Malignant neoplasms

1. **Adenocarcinoma**—intermediate T2 signal mass or irregular annular thickening. Loss of underlying mural stratification, extramural extension and mesorectal lymphadenopathy suggest malignancy. Foci of high T2 signal suggest mucinous histology. Signet ring cell tumours can appear like linitis plastica.
2. **Squamous cell carcinoma**—usually extending from the anus.
3. **Rectal invasion by an adjacent tumour**—e.g. prostate and gynaecological tumours.
4. **Carcinoid tumour**—discrete nodule, usually <1 cm, with homogeneous enhancement. Usually well-differentiated; poorly differentiated tumours mimic adenocarcinoma.

5. **GIST**—large heterogeneous endophytic or exophytic mass ± central ulceration; no lymphadenopathy (cf. adenocarcinoma).
6. **Lymphoma***—infiltrative homogeneous nonobstructing mass with marked restricted diffusion and lymphadenopathy. The mass infiltrates through muscularis without obliterating the muscle layers (cf. adenocarcinoma).
7. **Metastasis**—e.g. from bladder, breast, lung, stomach. May be a submucosal mass or may resemble linitis plastica.
8. **Sarcoma**—e.g. leiomyosarcoma; can occur years after pelvic radiotherapy.
9. **Melanoma**—primary or metastatic. May be T1 bright.
10. **Kaposi sarcoma**—rare; seen in immunosuppressed patients, e.g. AIDS. Diffuse T2 hypointense rectal thickening.

Benign neoplasms

1. <u>Adenoma</u>—villous adenomas are often large and appear fronded with a cap of T2 bright mucin. A fibrovascular stalk may also be visible and is highly suggestive. Underlying rectal wall stratification is preserved unless there is malignant transformation.
2. **Leiomyoma**—discrete T2 hypointense mass, smaller and often more homogeneous than GIST but may undergo necrosis or calcification. An overlying T2 bright submucosal stripe may be seen, confirming origin from muscularis.
3. **Lipoma**—T1 bright with suppression on fatsat sequences.
4. **Nerve sheath tumour**—e.g. schwannoma, plexiform neurofibroma (in NF1: diffuse lobulated grape-like mass infiltrating rectum and surrounding fat).

Inflammatory and infective

See Section 7.21. Usually causes diffuse thickening and oedema, except proctitis cystica profunda, which appears as a focal multicystic mass.

Others

1. **Endometriosis***—T2 hypointense fibrosis obliterating the pouch of Douglas ± rectosigmoid deposits. Serosal endometriomas may be seen, containing T1 hyperintensity (which does not suppress on fatsat sequences) + peripheral T2 hypointense haemosiderin.
2. **Haemangioma**—T2 bright ± phleboliths ± feeding vessels. May diffusely infiltrate rectum.
3. **Extrinsic masses of peritoneal origin**—e.g. solitary fibrous tumour. See Section 7.33.
4. **Infiltrative disorders**—e.g. amyloidosis, malakoplakia, Rosai-Dorfman disease. Can rarely produce rectal masses.

Further reading

Kim, H., Kim, J.H., Lim, J.S., et al., 2011. MRI findings of rectal submucosal tumours. Korean J. Radiol. 12 (4), 487–498.

Virmani, V., Ramanathan, S., Virmani, V.S., et al., 2014. What is hiding in the hindgut sac? Looking beyond rectal carcinoma. Insights Imaging 5 (4), 457–471.

7.29 RETRORECTAL/PRESACRAL MASS

1. **Abscess**—e.g. due to rectal perforation, anastomotic leak or supralevator collection related to perianal sepsis.
2. **Presacral fibrosis**—due to previous radiotherapy or chronic sepsis, e.g. previous rectal anastomotic leak. Ill-defined, poorly enhancing presacral soft tissue ± tethering of adjacent structures.
3. **Local tumour recurrence**—of rectal cancer after surgery. Usually appears as a discrete soft-tissue nodule with some restricted diffusion on MRI.
4. **Retrorectal developmental cysts**—congenital, associated with sacral anomalies. Can be complicated by infection (internal gas), haemorrhage or malignant degeneration (nodular mural thickening is suspicious).
   (a) **Tailgut cyst**—multilocular, thin-walled retrorectal cyst ('honeycomb' appearance), typically sited just above levator plate ± a small extension into the intersphinteric plane of the anal canal. May contain proteinaceous material (hyperattenuating on CT, T1 hyperintense on MRI).
   (b) **Duplication cyst**—unilocular cyst with its own mucosa, submucosa and muscularis. Adherent to rectum ± fistula to rectum or anus.
   (c) **Epidermoid cyst**—unilocular T2 hyperintense cyst ± linear hypointensities (keratin strands) + restricted diffusion.
   (d) **Dermoid cyst**—contains fat and calcification.
   (e) **Sacrococcygeal teratoma**—typically in neonates, very rare in adults.
5. **Sacral tumours**—especially lymphoma, which may extend into the presacral space without causing significant bone destruction. Other tumours (e.g. metastases, plasmacytoma, chordoma) usually cause bone destruction, making it easier to confirm the sacral origin of the mass.
6. **Subperitoneal adenomucinosis**—well-defined, slow-growing septated cystic mass ± calcification. Usually seen after resection of a mucinous appendiceal tumour or after proctocolectomy performed for UC.
7. **Myelolipoma**—most common extraadrenal location is presacral. Benign, well-defined mass containing fat and soft-tissue elements, usually in older patients.

8. **Extramedullary haematopoiesis**—presacral mass containing soft tissue and often fat; can mimic myelolipoma. Look for signs of marrow failure, e.g. bone sclerosis/splenomegaly.
9. **Nerve sheath tumours**—arising from sacral nerve roots, e.g. schwannoma, plexiform neurofibroma in NF1. Extension of a mass into an enlarged sacral foramen is characteristic.
10. **Anterior sacral meningocoele**—a CSF-containing sac protruding anteriorly through a defect in the sacrum.
11. **Ectopic prostate**—rare.
12. **Other lesions not specific to the presacral space**—e.g. sarcomas, solitary fibrous tumour, extraintestinal GIST, leiomyoma, lymphangioma, vascular malformations, endometrioma.

Further reading

Dahan, H., Arrivé, L., Wendum, D., et al., 2001. Retrorectal developmental cysts in adults: clinical and radiologic–histopathologic review, differential diagnosis, and treatment. Radiographics 21, 575–584.

Shanbhogue, A.K., Fasih, N., Macdonald, D.B., et al., 2012. Uncommon primary pelvic retroperitoneal masses in adults: a pattern-based imaging approach. Radiographics 32 (3), 795–817.

7.30 ANAL AND PERIANAL MASSES

See also Section 10.11 for vulval and vaginal masses.

1. **Squamous cell carcinoma**—intermediate T2 signal mass, often infiltrates internal and external anal sphincters, may spread onto perianal skin or extend cranially into rectum.
2. **Adenocarcinoma**—usually from a distal rectal tumour invading the anal canal.
3. **Perianal sepsis, fistulae and abscesses**.
   (a) **Cryptoglandular anal fistula**—originates from blockage and infection of anal glands located in the intersphincteric plane, resulting in a small abscess that drains to the skin surface forming a fistula. Classified as intersphincteric, transphincteric or suprasphincteric depending on the path of the fistula tract relative to the external anal sphincter. Associated perianal abscesses are common. Anterior transphincteric fistulae may open onto the vagina or posterior scrotum. There is a risk of malignant transformation of anal fistula tracts—irregular soft-tissue thickening within a tract is suspicious.
   (b) **Crohn's disease***—typically causes multiple complex anal fistulae, as well as extrasphincteric fistulae, which originate from the distal rectum and course to the skin surface outside of the anal sphincter complex.

(c) **Pilonidal sinus**—blind-ending sinus tract originating in the natal cleft ± subcutaneous abscess. Inflammation may involve the coccyx. No communication with anal canal.

(d) **Hidradenitis suppurativa**—recurrent infection of sweat glands typically in the axillae, groins and perineum. MRI shows diffuse subcutaneous oedema with a network of multiple sinus tracts and abscesses, which do not communicate with the anal canal.

(e) **Neutropenic perianal sepsis**—in immunocompromised patients; often manifests initially as diffuse perianal inflammation without a discrete abscess or fistula tract.

4. **Haematoma**—e.g. due to pelvic trauma.
5. **Condyloma acuminatum**—due to HPV infection. Large, irregular, superficial, carpet-like perianal mass. Can be invasive and transform to SCC.
6. **Aggressive angiomyxoma**—typically in women of reproductive age. Arises from perineal soft tissues, often large and extends through the pelvic floor without invading pelvic viscera. Heterogeneously T2 hyperintense with a characteristic swirled appearance + avid enhancement. Similar but less invasive variants can occur, e.g. cellular angiofibroma (in men) and angiomyofibroblastoma—these are usually smaller (<5 cm) without extending through the pelvic floor and may be more homogeneous on MRI.
7. **Cyclist's nodule**—seen in keen cyclists and horse riders. Benign subcutaneous fibrous mass caused by repetitive perineal microtrauma.
8. **Metastasis**—e.g. from prostate, colon, bladder, lymphoma. Rare.
9. **Melanoma**—primary or metastatic. May be T1 bright.
10. **Sacrococcygeal tumours**—metastases, plasmacytoma, chordoma.
11. **Proximal-type epithelioid sarcoma**—rare, usually in young adults. Perineum is a common location. Heterogeneous soft-tissue mass within subcutaneous fat, often with calcification.
12. **Other masses not specific to the perianal region**—e.g. lipoma, liposarcoma, angiolipoma, solitary fibrous tumour, extramedullary plasmacytoma, lymphoma.

Further reading

Tappouni, R.F., Sarwani, N.I., Tice, J.G., Chamarthi, S., 2011. Imaging of unusual perineal masses. AJR Am. J. Roentgenol. 196 (4), W412–W420.

7

7.31 MESENTERIC AND OMENTAL FAT STRANDING

Focal

1. **Local inflammation**—e.g. appendicitis, diverticulitis, cholecystitis, mild pancreatitis, gastritis, duodenitis, enteritis (of any cause, e.g. Crohn's), colitis, adjacent to a site of perforation or abscess (e.g. tuboovarian, postsurgical). Fat stranding is localized around the inflamed organ ± ascites.
2. **SMV branch occlusion**—e.g. due to thrombosis, closed-loop SBO or soft-tissue infiltration (including the desmoplastic reaction seen with carcinoid tumours). Fat stranding within the involved mesenteric folds due to venous congestion ± bowel wall oedema or ischaemia. Ascites is common.
3. **Mesenteric panniculitis**—idiopathic fibroinflammatory disorder of the small bowel mesentery, occasionally associated with IgG4-related disease. Characteristic appearance on CT: focal area of 'misty' mesentery with discrete borders formed by the visceral peritoneum, containing prominent lymph nodes which retain their elongated shape. The stranding spares a 'halo' of fat around the mesenteric vessels and nodes. The inflamed mesenteric folds appear focally expanded—this is not usually seen in other causes of mesenteric stranding. NB: ascites is not a feature of panniculitis and suggests an alternative diagnosis.
4. **Epiploic appendagitis**—small 'halo' of inflammation around a fatty epiploic appendage ± a central dense 'dot' (thrombosed vessel). Usually affects the left colon.
5. **Omental infarct**—discrete area of fat stranding in the greater omentum usually involving its free edge (R>L). There may be some reactive oedema in the adjacent colon (mimicking colitis), but the stranding is centred on the omentum itself. The area of stranding is usually >5 cm, larger than in epiploic appendagitis. NB: the greater omentum typically lies anterior to all of the bowel loops and its blood supply arises from gastroepiploic rather than mesenteric vessels. Infarction of the lesser omentum is rare.
6. **Mesenteric contusion**—post trauma. Look carefully for an associated bowel injury.
7. **Lymphoma***—can mimic mesenteric panniculitis, but the lymph nodes tend to be larger (>1 cm) and more rounded, and the stranded mesentery is not usually focally expanded.
8. **Whipple's disease, coeliac disease* and tropical sprue**—stranding in the jejunal mesentery + low density nodes.
9. **Liposarcoma**—rare; internal soft-tissue elements may resemble fat stranding. Look for mass effect displacing adjacent mesenteric vessels (cf. panniculitis where mesenteric vessels are undisplaced).

Diffuse

1. Oedema—e.g. cardiac, hepatic or renal failure, hypoalbuminaemia, angioedema.
2. Severe acute pancreatitis—can cause widespread fat necrosis throughout mesenteric and retroperitoneal fat, which initially appears as diffuse fat stranding, later consolidating into nodular fat necrosis, which can mimic malignancy, but resolves over time.
3. Diffuse peritonitis—e.g. due to perforated peptic ulcer, faecal peritonitis, TB.
4. Main SMV/PV occlusion—e.g. due to thrombosis, soft-tissue infiltration (especially pancreatic cancer) or midgut volvulus.
5. Portal hypertension—due to cirrhosis. Look for varices, splenomegaly and ascites.
6. Disseminated peritoneal malignancy—can appear as diffuse fat stranding or ill-defined nodularity, especially in omentum.
7. **Diffuse enteritis**—e.g. due to chemotherapy, graft-versus-host disease, CMV, eosinophilic enteritis, mastocytosis. See Section 7.19.
8. **Lymphatic obstruction or lymphangiectasia**—see Section 7.19.
9. **Amyloidosis***—can cause diffuse infiltration and stranding throughout intraabdominal fat. Calcification is suggestive if present. Ascites is often absent (cf. the other causes in this list).
10. **Familial Mediterranean fever***—see Section 7.34.
11. **Sarcoidosis***—rare; usually with lymphadenopathy and disease elsewhere.
12. **Erdheim-Chester disease***—very rare; typically with periaortic and perinephric soft-tissue thickening.
13. **Post small bowel transplantation**—a normal postsurgical finding, but if severe or persistent can suggest lymphoedema, venous thrombosis, transplant rejection, graft-versus-host disease or opportunistic infection (CMV).

Further reading

Johnson, P.T., Horton, K.M., Fishman, E.K., 2009. Nonvascular mesenteric disease: utility of multidetector CT with 3D volume rendering. Radiographics 29 (3), 721–740.

McLaughlin, P.D., Filippone, A., Maher, M.M., 2013. The "misty mesentery": mesenteric panniculitis and its mimics. AJR Am. J. Roentgenol. 200 (2), W116–W123.

7.32 MESENTERIC LYMPHADENOPATHY

1. Reactive lymphadenopathy—due to mesenteric adenitis, infectious mononucleosis (+ splenomegaly) or any cause of bowel inflammation. Nodes are usually only mildly enlarged and retain their elongated shape. Can also be seen in systemic autoimmune

disorders (e.g. SLE, RA, vasculitis) as part of generalized lymphadenopathy.

2. **Lymphoma***—enlarged rounded homogeneous mesenteric nodes with a tendency to form confluent masses, which encase but do not occlude mesenteric vessels. The nodes may cause lymphatic obstruction resulting in mesenteric stranding, which can mimic panniculitis, but usually the nodal enlargement is a more prominent feature than the stranding.
3. **Metastatic lymphadenopathy**—most commonly from large or small bowel, e.g. adenocarcinoma (nodes are typically close to the primary tumour, ± central mucin) or carcinoid (+ calcification and desmoplastic reaction). Advanced gastric, pancreatic and hepatobiliary malignancies can also spread to mesenteric nodes, as well as more distant primaries such as melanoma, lung, breast and Kaposi sarcoma (often hypervascular). Note that GISTs do not typically spread to lymph nodes.
4. **Mesenteric panniculitis**—lymph nodes tend to retain their elongated shape and are a less prominent feature than the degree of mesenteric stranding.
5. **Mycobacterial infection**—e.g. TB (typically necrotic, most commonly ileocolic) and *Mycobacterim avium* complex (solid or necrotic, most commonly jejunal).
6. **HIV**—due to the infection itself, or opportunistic infection (especially mycobacterial) or as part of immune reconstitution inflammatory syndrome (IRIS, typically seen <3 months after initiation of highly active antiretroviral therapy).
7. **Sarcoidosis***—usually in the presence of thoracic disease ± liver and spleen involvement.
8. **Coeliac disease* and tropical sprue**—low density (fatty) nodes that may be markedly enlarged ± fat-fluid levels (cavitating mesenteric lymph node syndrome). Look for jejunoileal fold reversal and mild jejunal thickening and dilatation. There is also an increased risk of lymphoma with coeliac disease.
9. **Whipple's disease**—low density (fatty) nodes ± mild jejunal thickening.
10. **Aseptic abscesses**—rare extraintestinal manifestation of IBD (especially Crohn's). More commonly involves the spleen, but can present with necrotic mesenteric lymphadenopathy.
11. **Familial Mediterranean fever***—see Section 7.34.
12. **Castleman disease**—enlarged hypervascular lymph nodes.
13. **Amyloidosis***—with mesenteric stranding ± calcification.
14. **Mastocytosis***—with bowel wall thickening, splenomegaly and sclerotic bones.
15. **Neurofibromatosis***—multiple mesenteric neurofibromas can mimic lymphadenopathy, though neurofibromas tend to be of lower attenuation on CT.

Further reading

Lucey, B.C., Stuhlfaut, J.W., Soto, J.A., 2005. Mesenteric lymph nodes seen at imaging: causes and significance. Radiographics 25 (2), 351–365.

7.33 PERITONEAL, OMENTAL OR MESENTERIC MASS

Solid

See also Section 7.32 for causes of mesenteric lymphadenopathy and Section 7.34 for causes of nodular peritoneal thickening.

Neoplasms

1. **Metastasis**—either via peritoneal spread (e.g. ovary, stomach, pancreas, colon, uterus, bladder; often with ascites) or haematogenous (e.g. melanoma, lung, breast). Metastases from GISTs or sarcomas are not usually associated with ascites.
2. **GIST**—can be large and very exophytic, making it difficult to identify the site of bowel origin. Can rarely be extraintestinal. Large heterogeneous mass ± peritoneal or liver metastases.
3. **Solitary fibrous tumour**—usually benign and slow-growing, more common in pleura than peritoneum. Well-defined, hyperenhancing mass ± internal necrosis, haemorrhage, calcification or cystic change. Often has internal vessels (flow voids on MRI). Tends to displace rather than invade adjacent structures.
4. **Desmoplastic small round cell tumour**—rare, highly aggressive malignant peritoneal tumour usually seen in males aged 15–25 years. Single or multiple peritoneal masses usually arising from pelvis + internal necrosis, haemorrhage or calcification. Often metastatic at presentation. Adenopathy is common (cf. GIST).
5. **Malignant mesothelioma**—see Section 7.34; can rarely present as a focal mass.
6. **Sarcomas**—rare, many types; nonspecific heterogeneous mass, often invading adjacent structures. Leiomyosarcoma may invade mesenteric veins, creating tumour thrombus.
7. **Benign mesenchymal tumours**—rare, typically well-defined, e.g. neurofibroma, schwannoma, leiomyoma, fibroma, haemangioma (often contains phleboliths).
8. **Ectopic gastrinoma**—most arise from the pancreas or duodenum, but rarely gastrinomas can be ectopic, usually arising within the 'gastrinoma triangle' close to the pancreas, duodenum, pylorus or common bile duct. Typically well-defined and hypervascular + gastric fold thickening (Zollinger-Ellison syndrome).
9. **Extramedullary plasmacytoma**—rarely occurs in the mesentery.

Fibroinflammatory and infiltrative processes

1. **Desmoid tumour**—well- or ill-defined mesenteric mass, variable enhancement; often related to previous surgery, trauma or Gardner syndrome. Local recurrence is common after resection.
2. **Retractile mesenteritis**—end-stage of mesenteric panniculitis. Spiculated fibrotic mesenteric mass ± calcification, usually occluding vessels and lymphatics ± ascites. Mimics carcinoid lymphadenopathy + desmoplastic reaction.
3. **Inflammatory pseudotumour**—nonspecific well- or ill-defined mass. Associated with IgG4-related disease.
4. **Actinomycosis**—markedly infiltrative mass, usually originating from the uterus (associated with an IUD) or ileocaecal region.
5. **Amyloidoma**—rare mass-like form of amyloidosis. Usually contains calcification.

Others

1. **Haematoma**—due to trauma, surgery, coagulopathy, aneurysm or bleeding neoplasm. High attenuation on unenhanced CT; no enhancement—look for pseudoaneurysm or active contrast extravasation to suggest site of bleeding. Haemorrhagic ascites is often present. Blood-fluid levels within the haematoma suggest coagulopathy ('haematocrit' sign).
2. **Splenosis/wandering splenunculus**—the former is seen post splenic trauma or surgery, due to discrete peritoneal implants of splenic tissue (no vascular pedicle). The latter is a congenital splenunculus which has a long vascular pedicle and can be located anywhere in the peritoneal cavity (or even herniate into the chest via diaphragmatic foramina). Both enhance similarly to the spleen with identical signal characteristics on MRI. Diagnosis can be confirmed on sulphur colloid scan or heat-damaged red blood cell scan.
3. **Endometriosis***—most common in the pelvis, but deposits can be seen anywhere in the peritoneal cavity. Low T2 signal (± foci of high T1 signal) on MRI with susceptibility artefact on T2*.
4. **Dropped gallstones**—post cholecystectomy, often located close to liver. Variable attenuation on CT, may be calcified. Often small and multiple. Usually T1 and T2 hypointense on MRI (except pigment stones that may be T1 hyperintense). No enhancement. Can act as a nidus for recurrent abscess formation.
5. **Peritoneal loose body**—due to a torted and detached epiploic appendage, which develops concentric outer layers of homogeneous fibrous tissue. Round or oval mass with a smooth surface; typically contains a central focus of calcification, giving a 'boiled egg' appearance. Usually mobile, can be large.
6. **Parasitic leiomyoma**—due to a detached uterine fibroid which adheres to the peritoneum, most often in the pelvis. Well-defined, typically T2 hypointense on MRI.

7. **Foreign body granuloma**—usually due to retained surgical materials. May be calcified.
8. **Osseous metaplasia**—secondary to trauma or recurrent abdominal surgery. Multiple linear or branching ossified masses.

Cystic

1. **Loculated fluid collection/abscess**—e.g. due to perforation, peritonitis, pancreatitis, foreign bodies (e.g. fish or chicken bones that have penetrated the bowel) or postsurgical collections (including those related to dropped gallstones or gossypibomas—retained surgical materials). Internal gas bubbles suggest infection or perforation, except in the case of gossypibomas which often contain gas; these also contain a curvilinear radiopaque marker which aids diagnosis. Beware of haemostatic packing materials; these are deliberately left inside the abdomen post-op to stop bleeding and can mimic an abscess.
2. **Pseudocyst**—most commonly due to subacute pancreatitis (>4 weeks old, most commonly in lesser sac), but can also be seen post trauma due to incomplete resolution of a haematoma. Smooth fibrotic wall, which may be thick; no internal enhancement.
3. **Cystic metastasis**—from a mucinous primary, e.g. ovary, stomach.
4. **Pseudomyxoma peritonei**—most commonly due to a low grade mucinous tumour of the appendix which perforates into the peritoneal cavity. Large volume of multiloculated mucinous fluid, which may mimic ascites on CT—look for surface scalloping of the liver or spleen suggesting mass effect (not seen in simple ascites). Curvilinear septal calcification may be seen.
5. **Lymphangioma**—congenital lymphatic anomaly, most common true cyst. Multicystic mass that tends to be elongated, insinuating between organs without much mass effect. Thin septa ± mild enhancement or calcification. The fluid may be of low attenuation (chylous).
6. **Enteric duplication cyst**—unilocular, usually attached to bowel. Thin wall containing normal bowel wall layers, which may be appreciable on US or MRI.
7. **Enteric/mesothelial cyst**—indistinguishable on imaging. Both present as a simple unilocular cyst.
8. **Benign multicystic mesothelioma**—benign cystic neoplasm arising from the peritoneum, typically in young women. Usually a multilocular cyst on imaging with thin walls ± mild septal enhancement.
9. **Peritoneal inclusion cyst**—typically located in the pelvis in premenopausal women who have adhesions related to surgery, trauma, pelvic inflammatory disease or endometriosis. Caused by

the accumulation of fluid released during ovulation which is not reabsorbed due to the adhesions, resulting in cysts which often have unusual shapes, conforming to adjacent structures without mass effect. No discrete wall.

10. **Omphalomesenteric duct cyst**—congenital, due to a persistent omphalomesenteric duct with focal cyst formation. The persistent duct may be seen connecting the cyst to the umbilicus and/or distal ileum.
11. **Hydatid cyst**—unilocular or multilocular depending on stage. Usually caused by rupture of a hepatic hydatid. May be multiple. No internal septal enhancement.
12. **Cystic change in a solid lesion**—e.g. necrotic mesenteric nodes, GIST, schwannoma.

Fat-containing

1. Fat necrosis.
   (a) Omental infarct—see Section 7.31; can appear mass-like. Involutes over time. Can become infected.
   (b) Epiploic appendagitis—see Section 7.31; typically <5 cm. Infarcted appendages may detach, becoming peritoneal loose bodies, which are often rim-calcified with central fat.
   (c) Acute pancreatitis—can cause widespread nodular fat necrosis mimicking peritoneal carcinomatosis; resolves over time.
   (d) **Encapsulated fat necrosis**—can occur anywhere, often due to trauma or surgery. Fatty mass with a smooth fibrous capsule ± internal stranding and calcification; can mimic liposarcoma, but will involute over time.
   (e) **Idiopathic nodular panniculitis**—typically causes multifocal nodular necrosis of subcutaneous fat, but can rarely also involve the mesentery.
2. Mesenteric panniculitis—see Section 7.31; the discrete margins and focal mesenteric expansion can mimic a mass lesion, but the undisplaced centrally located mesenteric vessels within the lesion aid diagnosis.
3. Postsurgical omental flaps—e.g. following liver surgery or duodenal repair, or for pelvic floor reconstruction following abdominoperineal resection. These flaps can undergo infarction especially in the pelvis, thereby developing internal soft-tissue elements which may mimic local tumour recurrence.
4. **Pseudolipoma of Glisson's capsule**—small fatty lesion attached to the liver capsule; represents a detached epiploic appendage.
5. **Liposarcoma**—rare; more common in the retroperitoneum, but these are often large and it can be difficult to categorize their origin. Fatty mass containing soft-tissue components.
6. **Lipoma**—purely fatty, usually very difficult to see as it blends in with the surrounding mesenteric fat. Sometimes the local

mass effect can be appreciated, and if there is generalized mesenteric oedema this usually spares the lipoma, making it easier to see.

7. **Hibernoma**—benign tumour of brown fat, rare in the abdominal cavity. See Section 7.35.
8. **Fat-containing metastases**—e.g. from teratoma or recurrent liposarcoma.
9. **Fatty mesenteric lymph nodes**—in coeliac disease, tropical sprue and Whipple's disease (see Section 7.32).
10. **Extramedullary haematopoiesis**—can rarely involve the mesentery, creating soft-tissue masses containing a variable amount of soft tissue and fat.
11. **Haemangioma/lymphangioma**—can rarely contain foci of fat.
12. **Hydatid cyst**—can rarely contain foci of fat if chronic.
13. **Failed renal transplant**—thinned poorly enhancing cortex + hypertrophy of renal sinus fat can mimic a fat-containing mass. Iliac fossa location.

Further reading

Kamaya, A., Federle, M.P., Desser, T.S., 2011. Imaging manifestations of abdominal fat necrosis and its mimics. Radiographics 31 (7), 2021–2034.

Levy, A.D., Arnáiz, J., Shaw, J.C., Sobin, L.H., 2008. From the archives of the AFIP: primary peritoneal tumors: imaging features with pathologic correlation. Radiographics 28 (2), 583–607.

Levy, A.D., Shaw, J.C., Sobin, L.H., 2009. Secondary tumors and tumorlike lesions of the peritoneal cavity: imaging features with pathologic correlation. Radiographics 29 (2), 347–373.

Pickhardt, P.J., Bhalla, S., 2005. Unusual nonneoplastic peritoneal and subperitoneal conditions: CT findings. Radiographics 25 (3), 719–730.

Yoo, E., Kim, J.H., Kim, M.J., et al., 2007. Greater and lesser omenta: normal anatomy and pathologic processes. Radiographics 27 (3), 707–720.

7.34 PERITONEAL THICKENING

Nodular or irregular

1. Metastatic peritoneal carcinomatosis—e.g. from ovary, stomach, pancreas, colon, appendix, uterus, bladder. Peritoneal thickening may be subtle and is often best seen in the pelvis, paracolic gutters and subphrenic spaces. Usually associated with ascites, omental nodularity or caking ± obstruction of bowel, bile ducts or ureters.
2. Primary peritoneal carcinoma—identical appearance to peritoneal carcinomatosis, but without a visible primary tumour. Almost exclusively in women, usually postmenopausal. Psammomatous calcification is common.
3. Lymphomatosis—secondary peritoneal involvement is more common and typically associated with widespread

lymphadenopathy (more than with peritoneal carcinomatosis). Primary peritoneal lymphoma occurs in immunocompromised patients and is not usually associated with lymphadenopathy or disease elsewhere. Leukaemia can produce a similar appearance.
4. **Malignant mesothelioma**—of the peritoneum. Most commonly causes diffuse 'sheet-like' thickening throughout the peritoneum + ascites ± omental caking, usually with pleural plaques suggesting prior asbestos exposure. M>F. Lymphadenopathy is uncommon and would suggest an alternative diagnosis.
5. **Tuberculous peritonitis**—nodular peritoneal thickening ± ascites (in the 'wet' form), often with necrotic mesenteric nodes, calcification and ileocaecal involvement. Also look for thoracic disease.
6. **Leiomyomatosis peritonealis disseminata**—peritoneal dissemination of benign leiomyomas, typically in premenopausal women with uterine fibroids. On imaging the masses are well defined, of low T2 signal and often heterogeneously enhancing, similar to fibroids. Omental caking is absent, and ascites is minimal (cf. malignant peritoneal disease).
7. **Gliomatosis peritonei**—benign peritoneal implants of mature glial tissue, nearly always in the presence of an ovarian teratoma. Indistinguishable from peritoneal metastases on imaging.

Smooth

NB: causes of transudative ascites (cardiac, hepatic or renal failure, hypoalbuminaemia, fluid overload) typically produce ascites without peritoneal thickening or enhancement.

1. **Acute peritonitis**—e.g. due to bowel inflammation, perforation, postsurgical sepsis (e.g. anastomotic leak, collections), pancreatitis, bile leak, spontaneous bacterial peritonitis. Peritoneal thickening is usually mild, and ascites is typically present.
2. **Diffuse peritoneal malignancy**—e.g. carcinomatosis, lymphomatosis, mesothelioma. Thickening can sometimes appear smooth on imaging.
3. **Portal hypertension**—can cause mild peritoneal thickening (partly due to serpiginous subperitoneal shunts) with ascites and diffuse fat stranding.
4. **Tuberculous peritonitis**—thickening may be smooth, though usually thicker than in acute peritonitis. Ascites may be present ('wet' form) or absent ('dry' form). Look for other features of TB.
5. **Sclerosing encapsulating peritonitis**—usually in patients on long-term peritoneal dialysis. Smooth peritoneal thickening (often thicker than in acute peritonitis) encasing loops of bowel ± linear calcification.
6. **SLE peritonitis**—diffuse mild peritoneal thickening and ascites ± bowel wall oedema or vasculitis.

7. **Familial Mediterranean fever***—rare inherited disorder prevalent in the Mediterranean, characterized by recurrent self-limiting attacks of peritonitis ± pleurisy, synovitis and pericarditis. CT findings are nonspecific and may include peritoneal thickening, ascites and diffuse mesenteric or omental fat stranding.
8. **Sarcoidosis***—rare, usually in the presence of disease elsewhere.

7.35 ABDOMINAL WALL MASS

Lesions arising from the skin

NB: large or invasive masses arising from deeper tissues can also involve the overlying skin; the following lesions specifically arise from the skin itself.

1. **Epidermal inclusion cyst**—also known as a sebaceous cyst. Smooth and rounded contour, typically attached to skin surface. Usually of fluid attenuation on CT ± rim calcification, no internal enhancement. Variable signal on MRI. Can rupture or become infected.
2. **Dermatofibrosarcoma protuberans (DFSP)**—lobulated mass extending from the skin into subcutaneous fat.
3. **Melanoma**—arises from skin ± subcutaneous extension.
4. **Sweat gland tumours**—well-defined, solid-cystic mass extending from the skin into subcutaneous fat.
5. **Keloid scar**—focal cutaneous thickening at site of previous surgery or trauma.

Lesions containing fat

1. **Hernias**—e.g. inguinal, femoral, paraumbilical, epigastric, hypogastric, Spigelian, lumbar, incisional. Contain fat ± bowel or other abdominal organs. May mimic a lipoma if the hernial neck is very small and difficult to see.
2. **Lipoma**—encapsulated purely fatty mass ± thin septa. May be subcutaneous or intramuscular. May be multiple in familial multiple lipomatosis. Features concerning for liposarcoma include rapid growth, size >5 cm, location deep to subcutaneous fascia and internal soft-tissue elements.
3. **Liposarcoma**—fatty mass containing soft-tissue elements <1 cm (well-differentiated) or >1 cm (dedifferentiated). NB: myxoid and pleomorphic variants contain minimal or no fat.
4. **Fat necrosis**—ill-defined subcutaneous soft-tissue nodules with internal fat and without significant mass effect. Usually posttraumatic; occasionally secondary to warfarin. If widespread, consider idiopathic nodular panniculitis.

7

5. Haemangioma—lobulated mass, may extend through fascial planes. Often contains phleboliths and foci of fat. T2 hyperintense on MRI, variable enhancement.
6. **Hibernoma**—rare benign tumour of brown fat. Well-defined, slightly higher attenuation than normal fat on CT + internal septa ± enhancement. A prominent feeding vessel is almost pathognomonic. Typically shows high FDG uptake on PET.
7. **Other rare lipomatous tumours**—e.g. angiolipoma, chondroid lipoma, osteolipoma, lipoleiomyoma.

Iatrogenic or traumatic lesions

1. Haematoma—most common in rectus abdominis muscle. May be related to trauma, surgery, protracted coughing/vomiting or coagulopathy (internal blood-fluid levels suggest the latter). Hyperattenuating on unenhanced CT, no internal enhancement. Look for an associated pseudoaneurysm or active contrast extravasation.
2. Postsurgical seroma—encapsulated unilocular homogeneous fluid collection, often large. May become infected.
3. Injection site—e.g. insulin, heparin. Small subcutaneous focus of fluid/nodularity ± gas bubbles, most common in lower abdominal wall or buttocks. Can form a discrete injection granuloma over time (often calcified). Recurrent insulin injections can cause ill-defined subcutaneous soft-tissue thickening (lipohypertrophy).
4. **Foreign body granuloma**—e.g. related to sutures (stitch granuloma, typically located at one end of a surgical scar), wood splinters (very low attenuation on CT), shotgun pellets, dropped gallstones within the abdominal wall. Calcification is common.
5. **Heterotopic ossification**—at sites of prior surgery (most common along linea alba) or trauma.
6. **Skull bone flap**—stored in the abdominal wall after craniectomy to keep the bone viable.

Cystic lesions

See also epidermal inclusion cyst and postsurgical seroma above.

1. Abscess—e.g. postsurgical collection (± wound dehiscence), extension of intraabdominal sepsis into abdominal wall, penetrating Crohn's disease, infected haematoma, infected umbilical sinus, disseminated septic emboli, necrotizing fasciitis (look for gas dissecting along fascial planes), pyomyositis, TB, actinomycosis (ill-defined, often solid).
2. Lymphangioma—macrocystic or microcystic. Often extends through tissue planes.
3. **Cysticercosis***—multiple subcutaneous and intramuscular cysts or calcifications depending on stage of disease.

Malignant neoplasms

See also liposarcoma and DFSP above.

1. <u>Soft-tissue metastasis</u>—e.g. from lung, breast, ovary, uterus, colon, melanoma; usually in the presence of widespread disease. May be seen in isolation at surgical incisions or port/needle tracts. Irregular soft-tissue nodule ± central necrosis. Intramuscular metastases are often subtle on CT.
2. <u>Malignant invasion of abdominal wall</u>—by an intraabdominal tumour.
3. <u>Soft-tissue sarcomas</u>—many types. Often large, heterogeneous and invasive.
4. **Lymphoma*/leukaemia**—can present as a discrete homogeneous mass or ill-defined thickening.

Benign neoplasms

See also lipoma above.

1. <u>Neurofibroma</u>—multiple in NF1; may be cutaneous and pedunculated, subcutaneous or intramuscular. Well-defined round, tubular or plexiform mass oriented along a nerve. Low attenuation on CT, T2 hyperintense with 'target' sign on MRI.
2. **Schwannoma**—well-defined rounded mass arising from a nerve. T2 hyperintense on MRI ± cystic change. May be densely calcified ('ancient' schwannoma).
3. **Solitary fibrous tumour**—well-defined avidly enhancing mass, often with internal vessels (flow voids on MRI). Tends to displace rather than invade other structures.
4. **Leiomyoma**—rare, usually seen in young patients or those with HIV. Well-defined subcutaneous soft-tissue mass. May also occur in the inguinal canal in premenopausal women (round ligament leiomyoma).
5. **Inflammatory pseudotumour**—rare. Nonspecific well- or ill-defined mass, may be invasive.

Other lesions

1. <u>Desmoid tumour</u>—most commonly in rectus abdominis, related to previous surgical incision, trauma or Gardner syndrome. Can also be seen postpartum (± caesarean section), where the main differential is endometriosis. Well- or ill-defined mass. Early tumours are cellular, T2 hyperintense and avidly enhancing; longstanding tumours become collagenous, T2 hypointense and mildly enhancing. Internal T2 hypointense bands and a 'fascial tail' along the muscle fascia are highly suggestive features.
2. <u>Endometriosis*</u>—typically seen at a caesarean-section or hysterectomy scar, usually without evidence of pelvic disease. Small

spiculated mass, homogeneous on CT, slightly T2 hyperintense to muscle on MRI ± foci of T1 hyperintensity, mild enhancement.

3. **Abdominal wall varices**—due to portal hypertension. May be seen around stoma sites. Round ligament varicosities may be seen in the inguinal canal in pregnant women.
4. **Undescended testis**—in the inguinal canal. Increased risk of malignancy.
5. **Accessory breast tissue**—seen anywhere along the line of the embryologic mammary streak. 'Feathery' subcutaneous breast tissue that may be attached to skin surface ± accessory nipple.
6. **Muscle swelling/oedema**—e.g. due to myositis, rhabdomyolysis or angioedema.
7. **Rosai-Dorfman disease***—rare; can present with nonspecific subcutaneous soft-tissue nodules or thickening.

Further reading

Ahn, S.E., Park, S.J., Moon, S.K., et al., 2016. Sonography of abdominal wall masses and masslike lesions: correlation with computed tomography and magnetic resonance imaging. J. Ultrasound Med. 35 (1), 189–208.

Bashir, U., Moskovic, E., Strauss, D., et al., 2014. Soft-tissue masses in the abdominal wall. Clin. Radiol. 69 (10), e422–e431.

Gayer, G., Park, C., 2018. Abdominal wall masses: CT findings and clues to differential diagnosis. Semin. Ultrasound CT MR 39 (2), 230–246.

Virmani, V., Sethi, V., Fasih, N., et al., 2014. The abdominal wall lumps and bumps: cross-sectional imaging spectrum. Can. Assoc. Radiol. J. 65 (1), 9–18.

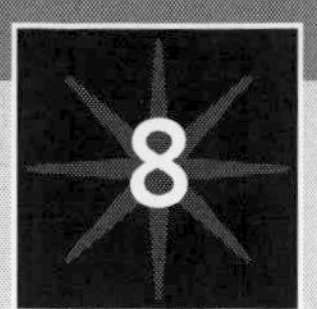

Hepatobiliary, pancreas and spleen

Hameed Rafiee

8.1 INTRALUMINAL GALLBLADDER LESIONS

1. Gallstones—single or multiple, small or large. ~80% are radiolucent on plain film, but ~80% are visible on CT. Often calcified, may contain central fat or gas. Typically mobile, but can be adherent to the GB wall. Typically show posterior acoustic shadowing, but calculi <5 mm may be nonshadowing and mimic a cholesterol polyp. Microlithiasis = multiple 1–3 mm calculi. A GB packed with calculi can mimic bowel gas on US (though gas shadows tend to be 'dirtier'). Two main types of calculi (NB: most contain a mixture):
   (a) **Cholesterol stones**—most common in middle-aged obese women. Variable size and number. Pure cholesterol stones are often invisible on CT. Typically T1 and T2 hypointense on MRI, but can be heterogeneous.
   (b) **Pigment stones**—usually seen in chronic liver disease and chronic haemolysis. Typically small, numerous and calcified. Often T1 hyperintense and T2 hypointense on MRI.
2. Sludge—often forms mobile 'balls' of nonshadowing avascular echogenic material. May fill GB.
3. Gallbladder polyps—polyps measuring 6–9 mm require follow-up; surgery is suggested for polyps ≥10 mm. In patients with PSC, polyps of any size should be followed up or considered for cholecystectomy.
   (a) Cholesterol polyps—usually small (<10 mm), multiple and avascular. Nonmobile, nonshadowing. Mildly enhancing, intermediate T1 and T2 signal on MRI. Numerous small cholesterol polyps = cholesterolosis. No malignant potential.
   (b) Adenoma—usually solitary, often >10 mm and sessile with internal vascularity on US. Associated with PSC and polyposis syndromes. Risk of progression to adenocarcinoma.
   (c) **Inflammatory polyps**—usually small (<10 mm) and multiple, seen in chronically inflamed GBs. No malignant potential.

(d) **Rare polypoid lesions**—e.g. leiomyoma, lipoma (fatty on CT/MR), fibroma, neurofibroma (usually in NF1), haemangioma, granular cell tumour, carcinoid tumour, and heterotopic gastric, hepatic or pancreatic tissue.

4. **Gallbladder empyema**—distended thick-walled tender GB filled with echogenic material, in a patient with sepsis.
5. **Haematoma**—due to trauma, surgery, biliary intervention, coagulopathy or cystic artery aneurysm (usually postinflammatory). Heterogeneous and avascular on US, hyperattenuating on unenhanced CT. Look for active contrast extravasation. Blood may fill and obstruct CBD or enter the duodenum, presenting with melaena.
6. **Gallbladder carcinoma**—may present as a solitary polypoid mass similar to an adenoma. Features suggesting malignancy: large size, wide polyp base, focal GB wall thickening adjacent to polyp, polyp enhancement > GB wall.
7. **Limy bile**—milk of calcium in GB; very dense on CT.
8. **Gallbladder parasites**—e.g. clonorchiasis, opisthorchiasis, fascioliasis, ascariasis. Endemic in Southeast Asia. Floating echogenic foci in the GB/bile ducts that may move spontaneously.

Further reading

Gore, R.M., Thakrar, K.H., Newmark, G.M., et al., 2010. Gallbladder imaging. Gastroenterol. Clin. North Am. 39 (2), 265–287.

Mellnick, V.M., Menias, C.O., Sandrasegaran, K., et al., 2015. Polypoid lesions of the gallbladder: disease spectrum with pathologic correlation. Radiographics 35 (2), 387–399.

8.2 GALLBLADDER WALL THICKENING

>3 mm in a well-distended gallbladder.

Diffuse

1. **Acute calculous cholecystitis**—caused by an obstructing gallstone in the GB neck or cystic duct. Distended thick-walled GB with adjacent fluid ± mucosal hyperenhancement on CT. Irregular or absent mucosal enhancement suggests gangrenous cholecystitis that may perforate, resulting in pericholecystic or intrahepatic collections. Intramural gas = emphysematous cholecystitis (usually in diabetics).
2. **Chronic cholecystitis**—thick-walled contracted GB containing gallstones, no adjacent fluid. Chronic cystic duct obstruction can also result in a grossly distended GB (hydrops). A chronically inflamed GB can become adherent to the duodenum or hepatic flexure ± erosion of calculi directly into the duodenum or colon, forming a fistula.

3. Passive mural oedema—seen in acute hepatitis, cirrhosis, portal hypertension, right heart failure, renal failure, fluid overload and hypoalbuminaemia. Diffuse mural oedema throughout GB with normal smooth mucosal enhancement, usually with periportal oedema and ascites. Reactive GB oedema can also be seen due to adjacent duodenitis or pancreatitis.
4. Acute acalculous cholecystitis—usually seen in critically ill patients due to hypoperfusion and ischaemia; the GB is usually distended (atonic) with sludge but no discrete calculi. Can also be caused by infectious mononucleosis and AIDS-related opportunistic infections, e.g. CMV, *Cryptosporidium.*
5. Diffuse adenomyomatosis—contracted, mildly thick-walled GB with echogenic intramural foci + comet-tail artefacts on US. Smooth mucosal hyperenhancement on CT with tiny enhancing foci extending into the thickened wall, representing Rokitansky-Aschoff sinuses—on MRI these appear as a string of small intramural cystic spaces.
6. **Xanthogranulomatous cholecystitis (XGC)**—chronic inflammatory disorder causing marked diffuse GB wall thickening with multiple intramural hypoattenuating nodules on CT, representing xanthogranulomas (mildly T2 hyperintense on MRI) or abscesses (T2 bright). Associated GB perforation or hepatic infiltration may be seen, mimicking adenocarcinoma; preservation of smooth mucosal enhancement suggests XGC.
7. **Gallbladder volvulus**—rare; markedly distended and thick-walled GB extending beyond fossa + reduced mural enhancement.
8. **Gallbladder carcinoma**—the rare signet ring variant can cause diffuse wall thickening similar to linitis plastica, mimicking benign thickening. Look for infiltration into adjacent structures.
9. **Lymphoma***—rare, can diffusely infiltrate GB wall.

8

Focal

1. Adenomyomatosis—can be focal (typically at GB fundus) or segmental (causing circumferential thickening of the GB body, giving it an hourglass shape). Characterized by intramural Rokitansky-Aschoff sinuses which appear on US as echogenic foci + 'comet-tail' artefact, and on CT/MRI as a string/cluster of small intramural cystic spaces. The sinuses may contain foci of calcification on CT.
2. Gallbladder carcinoma—most commonly presents as focal irregular thickening of the GB wall ± extension into the lumen or into adjacent structures (e.g. liver), ± lymphadenopathy or metastases. Risk factors include gallstones, polyposis, PSC and segmental GB wall calcification.
3. **Xanthogranulomatous cholecystitis**—can sometimes be focal.

4. **Gallbladder metastases**—via direct invasion (from liver tumours), haematogenous (e.g. melanoma) or peritoneal spread (e.g. gastric).
5. **Lymphoma***—rare, usually in the presence of disease elsewhere.
6. **Intramural haematoma**—due to trauma, liver biopsy, cystic artery aneurysm, coagulopathy. Hyperattenuating on unenhanced CT.
7. **Gallbladder varices**—due to portal hypertension. Serpiginous collateral veins.
8. **Cystic artery aneurysm**—usually due to severe or recurrent cholecystitis.

Further reading

Levy, A.D., Murakata, L.A., Abbott, R.M., Rohrmann, C.A., Jr., 2002. From the archives of the AFIP: benign tumors and tumorlike lesions of the gallbladder and extrahepatic bile ducts: radiologic-pathologic correlation. Radiographics 22 (2), 387–413.

Watanabe, Y., Nagayama, M., Okumura, A., 2007. MR imaging of acute biliary disorders. Radiographics 27 (2), 477–495.

Yeh, B.M., Liu, P.S., Soto, J.A., et al., 2009. MR imaging and CT of the biliary tract. Radiographics 29 (6), 1669–1688.

8.3 BILIARY DILATATION

CBD: >6 mm up to the age of 60 years, adding 1 mm for every decade thereafter. Postcholecystectomy: CBD >10 mm.

Intrahepatic ducts: >2 mm or >40% of the adjacent portal vein diameter.

On CT, beware of portal vein thrombosis mimicking intrahepatic biliary dilatation—with biliary dilatation, patent portal veins should be visible paralleling the dilated ducts. On MRCP, beware of pitfalls that can mimic a ductal lesion:

- Intraductal gas bubbles—antidependent signal voids (more common in left lobe), form gas–fluid levels in larger ducts.
- Biliary flow voids—located centrally within the duct (calculi sit dependently).
- Normal cystic duct folds—spiral valves of Heister.
- Extrinsic vascular impression of hepatic artery on CHD—common, no clinical significance.
- Susceptibility artefact from cholecystectomy clips.

Luminal causes (and nonobstructive dilatation)

1. <u>Obstructing ductal filling defect</u>—e.g. stone (most common, may be multiple), sludge (less discrete than a stone), blood clot (look for GB haematoma) or parasites (ascariasis, clonorchiasis, fascioliasis, opisthorchiasis). Obstruction leads to infection and

cholangitis—diffuse smooth mural thickening and enhancement of extrahepatic ducts.

2. Small bowel obstruction—duodenal dilatation can impair biliary drainage.
3. Choledochal cyst—focal or diffuse dilatation of common duct ± central intrahepatic ducts, caused by an anomalous pancreaticobiliary junction—CBD and PD form a long common channel upstream of the sphincter of Oddi, resulting in reflux of pancreatic juices into the CBD, degenerating the bile duct wall. Can be complicated by stone formation or cholangiocarcinoma.
4. Caroli disease—congenital DPM affecting the larger bile ducts, resulting in multifocal saccular dilatation of intrahepatic bile ducts, often containing a central 'dot' representing portal radicals. May be diffuse or segmental. Intraductal calculi are often seen. May be associated with congenital hepatic fibrosis (DPM affecting smaller ducts).
5. Choledochocoele—focal cystic dilatation of the distal CBD within the ampulla, bulging into the duodenum.
6. Bile duct diverticulum—solitary and saccular; usually extrahepatic but can also be intrahepatic (e.g. in PSC). May mimic a GB diverticulum or accessory GB if large.
7. **Intraductal papillary mucinous neoplasm (biliary IPMN)**—most common in Southeast Asia; usually arises from intrahepatic bile ducts. Results in marked segmental intrahepatic biliary dilatation (due to mucin hypersecretion) without a downstream obstructing stone or stricture. Slowly progressive premalignant lesion; causes lobar atrophy over time. Mural nodularity within the dilated ducts may be seen and suggests malignancy.
8. **Other rare polypoid neoplasms**—e.g. bile duct adenoma, inflammatory polyp, neurofibroma, primary melanoma.

Mural causes (strictures)

1. Papillary stenosis/sphincter of Oddi dysfunction—recurrent passage of small stones through the ampulla can cause papillary stenosis due to fibrosis—small nonobstructing calculi may also be seen within the dilated CBD. Sphincter of Oddi dysfunction is caused by functional dyskinesia/spasm and can be seen postcholecystectomy or due to opioids.
2. Cholangiocarcinoma—risk factors include gallstones, PSC, cirrhosis, recurrent pyogenic cholangitis, Caroli disease, choledochal cyst. Three main types:
   (a) **Mass-forming**—typically arise from peripheral ducts in the liver.
   (b) **Periductal infiltrating**—subtle enhancing stricture with upstream biliary dilatation; infiltrates along ducts, usually without a significant soft tissue mass. Most common at the

hilum (Klatskin tumour), where it causes complex stricturing with separation of intrahepatic ducts.

(c) **Intraductal**—rare, polypoid intraluminal mass; usually arises from biliary IPMN (see earlier).

3. **Primary sclerosing cholangitis (PSC)**—autoimmune disease usually associated with IBD (UC > Crohn's). Results in multifocal short intra- and extrahepatic strictures, giving a 'beaded' or discontinuous appearance to the ducts. Biliary dilatation is often only mild. Acute episodes of cholangitis can cause diffuse mural thickening and enhancement involving a longer ductal segment. Extrahepatic strictures may also be long. Eventually progresses to cirrhosis, often with peripheral atrophy and marked caudate hypertrophy. Increased risk of cholangiocarcinoma—a dominant stricture or progressive biliary dilatation is worrying.
4. **Iatrogenic stricture**—e.g. post biliary intervention, postsurgical anastomotic stricture, postcholecystectomy injury to bile duct (especially if there is variant anatomy, e.g. aberrant insertion of segment 6 duct close to the cystic duct), post radiotherapy.
5. **IgG4-related sclerosing cholangitis**—typically causes long strictures with mural thickening and enhancement (cf. the shorter strictures in PSC); most common in the CBD but can involve any part of biliary tree. Look for other features of IgG4-related disease, especially autoimmune pancreatitis.
6. **Recurrent pyogenic cholangitis**—endemic in Southeast Asia, related to parasitic (especially clonorchiasis) or bacterial infections. Recurrent cholangitis results in multifocal strictures and pigment stone formation in intra- and extrahepatic ducts (especially in the left lobe). Can be complicated by abscess formation, lobar atrophy or cholangiocarcinoma.
7. **Cystic fibrosis-related sclerosing cholangitis**—similar appearance to PSC.
8. **Chemotherapy-induced sclerosing cholangitis**—develops months after hepatic artery infusion chemotherapy or TACE. Typically involves the proximal CHD, hilum and central intrahepatic ducts ± GB and cystic duct; spares peripheral intrahepatic ducts and distal CBD. Mural thickening and enhancement on CT/MRI with mild upstream biliary dilatation.
9. **Ischaemic cholangiopathy**—most commonly seen <6 months after liver transplant; other causes include vasculitis (polyarteritis nodosa, giant cell arteritis), sickle cell disease and long-term ICU admissions. Typically involves the proximal CHD, hilum and central intrahepatic ducts initially, but can progress to involve the entire biliary tree. Intraluminal filling defects (sloughed mucosa) and associated bilomas are highly suggestive of ischaemia.
10. **AIDS cholangiopathy**—caused by opportunistic infections, e.g. *Cryptosporidium*, CMV, HSV. Multifocal strictures similar to PSC; also often causes papillary stenosis and can involve the GB.

11. **Eosinophilic cholangitis**—rare; can be related to parasites, fungi or drugs.
12. **Sarcoidosis***—can rarely cause a granulomatous cholangitis leading to stricture formation, typically in the presence of disease elsewhere.
13. **Rare neoplasms**—e.g. granular cell tumour, carcinoid, squamous cell carcinoma, heterotopia. These can present as single short strictures.

Extrinsic causes (arranged from distal to proximal)

1. Ampullary tumours—e.g. adenoma, carcinoma, carcinoid. Obstructs CBD ± PD. Often small and hard to see on imaging if the duodenum is not well-distended; ampullary soft tissue >1 cm in diameter is abnormal and warrants endoscopy.
2. **Lemmel's syndrome**—rare; extrinsic compression of the distal CBD by a periampullary duodenal diverticulum.
3. Pancreatic head tumour—especially adenocarcinoma. Abrupt CBD narrowing at the level of the tumour, usually with upstream PD dilatation and atrophy (cf. cholangiocarcinoma of distal CBD).
4. Pancreatitis—acute, chronic or autoimmune. Usually a smooth tapered CBD narrowing ± PD dilatation/calculi. Associated pseudocysts can also compress the CBD.
5. **Periportal lymphadenopathy**—compressing extrahepatic ducts.
6. **Cavernous transformation of portal vein**—following portal vein thrombosis. Venous collaterals around extrahepatic ducts can cause mild dilatation (portal biliopathy).
7. **Bile duct metastasis**—via direct invasion (e.g. from GB), haematogenous (e.g. melanoma) or peritoneal spread (e.g. gastric). Usually involves hilum or proximal common duct.
8. Mirizzi syndrome—extrinsic compression of the CHD by a large stone impacted in the GB neck. The stone may erode into the common duct.
9. Hepatic masses—primary or metastatic tumours, abscesses. Compress intrahepatic ducts causing focal or asymmetrical intrahepatic biliary dilatation.
10. **Hepatic hydatid cyst**—may rupture contents into the biliary tree, obstructing the lumen.

Further reading

Menias, C.O., Surabhi, V.R., Prasad, S.R., et al., 2008. Mimics of cholangiocarcinoma: spectrum of disease. Radiographics 28 (4), 1115–1129.

8

8.4 GAS IN THE BILIARY TREE

Within the bile ducts

Irregularly branching gas shadows which do not reach to the liver edge, probably because of the direction of bile flow. The gallbladder may also be outlined.

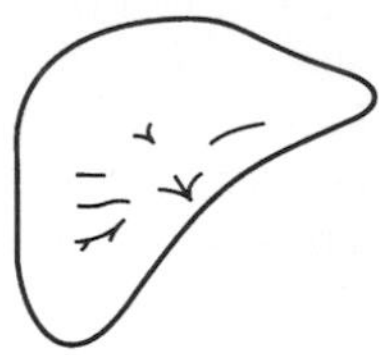

1. **Incompetent sphincter of Oddi**—e.g. following sphincterotomy or gallstone passage. A patulous sphincter can also be seen in the elderly.
2. **Spontaneous biliary fistula**—typically due to a large GB calculus eroding through a chronically inflamed GB wall into the duodenum (± gallstone ileus) or less commonly the hepatic flexure. Rarely, a fistula may be caused by trauma, malignancy or a duodenal ulcer eroding into the CBD.
3. **Postoperative**—e.g. hepaticojejunostomy for Whipple's procedure.

Within the gallbladder

1. **All of the above**.
2. **Gallstone containing gas**—often has a 'Mercedes-Benz' morphology.
3. **Emphysematous cholecystitis**—due to gas-forming organisms, often in elderly diabetics. Intramural and intraluminal gas, usually without gas in the bile ducts (due to cystic duct obstruction).

8.5 GAS IN THE PORTAL VEINS

Gas shadows which extend to within 2 cm of the liver capsule because of the direction of blood flow in the portal veins. Gas may also be present in the portal and mesenteric veins and the bowel wall.

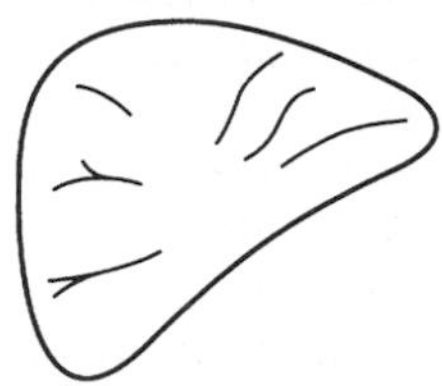

1. **Bowel infarction**—high mortality.
2. **Any other cause of bowel pneumatosis**—see Section 7.25.
3. **Acute gastric dilatation**—may resolve following decompression.
4. **Intraabdominal sepsis**—e.g. diverticulitis, appendicitis, pancreatitis, cholecystitis.
5. **Following liver transplant.**

Further reading

Shah, P.A., Cunningham, S.C., Morgan, T.A., Daly, B.D., 2011. Hepatic gas: widening spectrum of causes detected at CT and US in the interventional era. Radiographics 31 (5), 1403–1413.

8.6 HEPATOMEGALY WITHOUT DISCRETE LESIONS

Acute hepatitis

The liver is enlarged and often hypoechoic on US. Periportal oedema and GB oedema are often seen on CT/MR ± reactive periportal nodes.

1. Infective.
   (a) Viral—hepatitis, infectious mononucleosis.
   (b) **Protozoal**—malaria, African trypanosomiasis, visceral leishmaniasis.
2. Alcoholic.
3. Drug-induced—e.g. paracetamol overdose.
4. **Autoimmune**—can rarely present acutely.
5. **Sickle cell crisis**—look for other features of the disease.

Cardiovascular

These can all cause venous congestion in the liver, creating a mottled 'nutmeg' appearance on postcontrast CT/MR and signs of (postsinusoidal) portal hypertension.

1. Right heart failure—e.g. due to congestive cardiac failure, constrictive pericarditis or tricuspid valve disease. Distended hepatic veins and IVC ± ascites.
2. Acute Budd-Chiari syndrome—thrombosed hepatic veins.
3. **Hepatic venoocclusive disease**—seen following bone marrow transplant/chemotherapy. Small calibre but patent hepatic veins.

Neoplastic

Diffuse malignant infiltration can cause parenchymal heterogeneity without discrete lesions. The liver surface can be irregular, mimicking cirrhosis. The portal and hepatic veins may appear distorted.

1. Diffuse lymphoma—with lymphadenopathy and splenomegaly. Also seen in leukaemia.
2. Diffuse metastases—especially from breast or small-cell lung cancer.
3. Infiltrative HCC—can blend in with background cirrhosis.
4. **Angiosarcoma**—rare; often diffusely infiltrative.

Infiltrative/depositional

1. **Steatosis**—fat infiltration. Hyperechoic on US (relative to normal renal cortex), hypoattenuating on unenhanced CT (>10 HU less than spleen). On MRI, shows signal loss on opposed-phase T1-weighted sequence, in keeping with microscopic fat content. May be diffuse or geographic.
2. **Haemochromatosis***—iron deposition. Liver may appear hyperattenuating on unenhanced CT. T2 hypointense on MRI (especially on gradient echo sequences that are more prone to susceptibility effects), with signal loss on in-phase T1-weighted sequence (cf. steatosis).
3. **Wilson's disease**—copper deposition, often with coexisting steatosis.
4. **Sarcoidosis***—usually with splenic and thoracic involvement.
5. **Amyloidosis***—hypoattenuating liver on CT ± calcifications.

Storage disorders

1. **Glycogen storage diseases**—hyperechoic on US, hyperattenuating on CT; ± hepatic adenomas.
2. **Gaucher disease***.
3. **Niemann-Pick disease***—with interlobular septal thickening in the lungs (type B) or CNS involvement (type C). Type A is fatal in early childhood.
4. **Mucopolysaccharidoses***.

Myeloproliferative disorders

Usually accompanied by splenomegaly.

1. **Extramedullary haematopoiesis**—e.g. in myelofibrosis.
2. **Polycythaemia vera.**
3. **Mastocytosis***.

Congenital

1. **Riedel's lobe**—anatomical variant; tongue-like inferior extension of right lobe that can mimic hepatomegaly. Often associated with an accessory hepatic vein.

Further reading

Boll, D.T., Merkle, E.M., 2009. Diffuse liver disease: strategies for hepatic CT and MR imaging. Radiographics 29 (6), 1591–1614.

8.7 HEPATIC CALCIFICATION AND INCREASED DENSITY

Small and punctate calcification

1. Healed granulomas—TB, histoplasmosis; less commonly brucellosis or coccidioidomycosis. Small, punctate, usually multiple ± calcified granulomas elsewhere (lungs, nodes, spleen).
2. Intrahepatic ductal calculi—can be seen in PSC, Caroli disease and recurrent pyogenic cholangitis.
3. **Amyloidosis***—rare, can be numerous.

Curvilinear calcification

1. Hydatid cyst—calcification does not necessarily indicate death of the parasite, but extensive calcification favours an inactive cyst. Calcification of daughter cysts produces several calcified rings.
2. Simple cyst—wall calcification is uncommon but can occur following haemorrhage or infection. More common in polycystic liver disease.
3. Chronic haematoma or abscess.
4. Calcified (porcelain) gallbladder—possible association with GB carcinoma, especially if segmental rather than diffuse.
5. **Hepatic artery calcification**—atherosclerosis or aneurysm.
6. **Portal vein calcification**—chronic thrombus or portal hypertension.
7. **Schistosomiasis***—especially *S. japonicum*. Causes linear septal and capsular calcification creating a characteristic 'turtleback' appearance.

Calcification within a mass

1. Metastases—especially from mucinous primaries, e.g. colorectal and gastric; rarely from osteosarcoma or teratoma. Metastases can also calcify following radiotherapy or chemotherapy.
2. Fibrolamellar HCC—located within stellate central scar.
3. **Lipiodol**—component of TACE therapy, deposits in the treated tumour (e.g. HCC). Very dense on CT.
4. **Haemangioma**—cavernous and sclerosing subtypes may contain central foci of calcification, especially if large.
5. **Other tumours**—can occasionally contain calcification, e.g. adenoma and HCC (related to prior haemorrhage), cholangiocarcinoma, FNH (within central scar, rare), biliary cystadenoma/carcinoma (mural), epithelioid haemangioendothelioma, teratoma. Calcification is also common in certain paediatric liver tumours (hepatoblastoma, nested stromal–epithelial tumour).

8

Diffusely increased density

Assess by comparing the liver with the spleen (normally up to 12 HU > spleen). Also, intrahepatic vessels stand out as low-density against high-density background liver.

1. **Haemochromatosis***—due to iron deposition. Pancreas and heart may also be involved. NB: secondary haemosiderosis (due to chronic blood transfusions or iron therapy) usually affects the spleen and bone marrow more than the liver.
2. **Amiodarone therapy**—due to iodine content of the drug; ± lung infiltrates.
3. **Gold therapy.**
4. **Wilson's disease**—though findings may be confounded by coexistent fatty infiltration.
5. **Glycogen storage diseases.**
6. **Previous Thorotrast administration**—old radiographic contrast agent. Deposited in liver, spleen and lymph nodes, creating marked diffuse or reticular hyperdensity (as dense as calcium). Associated with hepatic angiosarcoma and other malignancies.

Focal increased density (noncalcified)

1. **Haematoma**—including haemorrhagic lesions such as adenoma, HCC and angiomyolipoma.
2. **Siderotic regenerative/dysplastic nodule**—seen in cirrhosis.

Further reading

Patnana, M., Menias, C.O., Pickhardt, P.J., et al., 2018. Liver calcifications and calcified liver masses: pattern recognition approach on CT. AJR Am. J. Roentgenol. 211 (1), 76–86.

8.8 DIFFUSELY HYPOECHOIC LIVER

1. **Acute hepatitis**—with prominent periportal echogenicity giving a 'starry-sky' appearance. Mild hepatitis has a normal echo pattern.
2. **Diffuse malignant infiltration**—e.g. leukaemia.

8.9 DIFFUSELY HYPERECHOIC LIVER

NB: liver echogenicity is normally similar to or slightly higher than that of a normal renal cortex.

1. **Fatty infiltration**—attenuates the US beam when severe, obscuring the deep portions of the liver. May see focal hypoechoic fatty sparing in typical locations, e.g. adjacent to GB or porta.
2. **Cirrhosis**—irregular contour ± signs of portal hypertension.

3. **Hepatitis**—particularly chronic.
4. **Glycogen storage disease**—associated with hepatic adenomas (often multiple).

8.10 DIFFUSELY HETEROGENEOUS LIVER

This applies to US, CT and MRI.

1. **Cirrhosis**—nodular liver contour ± signs of portal hypertension (splenomegaly, ascites, portosystemic shunts). The liver is often small with hypertrophy of the caudate and segments 2 and 3. It is usually difficult to ascertain the underlying cause on imaging, but some aetiologies can offer clues:
   (a) **PSC**—multifocal biliary strictures, peripheral distribution of fibrosis and volume loss, with hypertrophy of the caudate and central liver.
   (b) **Primary biliary cirrhosis**—typically in middle-aged women. Lace-like pattern of fibrosis ± characteristic periportal 'halo' of T2 hypointensity on MRI.
   (c) **Haemochromatosis***—diffuse iron deposition causes T2 hypointensity and signal loss on the in-phase T1-weighted sequence.
   (d) **Alpha-1 antitrypsin deficiency***—basal emphysema.
   (e) **Cystic fibrosis***—bronchiectasis and fatty replacement of pancreas.
   (f) **Cardiac cirrhosis**—dilated hepatic veins and right atrium.
   (g) **Congenital hepatic fibrosis**—congenital ductal plate malformation (DPM) involving small ducts, resulting in fibrosis and cirrhosis usually by early adulthood. Associated with ARPKD and other hepatic DPMs: multiple biliary hamartomas (small ducts), polycystic liver disease (medium ducts) and Caroli disease (large ducts).
2. **Diffuse malignancy**—primary (HCC, angiosarcoma) or metastatic (breast, small-cell lung cancer, lymphoma, leukaemia). The liver is typically enlarged ± a nodular contour, though breast cancer metastases can induce fibrosis and volume loss ('pseudocirrhosis').
3. **Fatty infiltration**—can be very patchy or bizarre in distribution, mimicking metastatic disease on US/CT. Diagnosis confirmed on in-/opposed-phase MRI, with signal loss on the opposed phase.
4. **Abnormal perfusion**—e.g. hepatic infarction (in severe shock, hypercoagulable states, sickle cell crisis or HELLP syndrome), hepatic artery occlusion (e.g. following TACE or liver transplant) or portal vein thrombosis. Also seen in:
   (a) **Venous congestion**—due to right heart failure, acute Budd-Chiari syndrome or venoocclusive disease; see Section 8.6. Chronic Budd-Chiari syndrome results in peripheral liver

atrophy and marked caudate hypertrophy; the normal hepatic veins are obliterated and replaced by tortuous intrahepatic venous shunts; multiple large regenerative nodules may also be seen.

(b) **Hereditary haemorrhagic telangiectasia***—markedly heterogeneous enhancement throughout the liver, especially on arterial phase CT/MR, due to innumerable intrahepatic telangiectasias and AVMs. Tends to equilibrate on later phases. Hepatic arteries and veins are often dilated with early venous filling due to shunting. FNH-like lesions can also be seen. Look for lung AVMs to confirm diagnosis.

5. **Acute fulminant hepatitis**—most commonly due to viral hepatitis or drugs/toxins (e.g. paracetamol overdose). Heterogeneous liver due to patchy necrosis.
6. **Sarcoidosis***—usually in the presence of disease elsewhere. Innumerable small (<1 cm) granulomas throughout the liver and spleen; hypovascular on CT/MR, usually T2 hypointense.
7. **Hepatic microabscesses**—in immunocompromised patients; most commonly due to candidiasis, but can be seen in other fungal infections and TB. Innumerable small abscesses (most <1 cm) throughout the liver ± spleen, T2 hyperintense on MRI with restricted diffusion.
8. **Schistosomiasis***—periportal fibrosis with a network of linear septal fibrosis and calcification giving a 'turtleback' appearance. Echogenic on US, dense on CT.
9. **Nodular regenerative hyperplasia**—microscopic regenerative nodules without fibrosis (cf. cirrhosis). Associated with organ transplantation, immunosuppression, pulmonary hypertension, autoimmune diseases, myeloproliferative disorders and other malignancies. The liver may appear normal or heterogeneous on imaging with signs of portal hypertension. The individual nodules are invisible and the liver surface is usually smooth (cf. cirrhosis).
10. **Amyloidosis***—enlarged heterogeneous liver, hypoattenuating on CT ± calcifications.

Further reading

Boll, D.T., Merkle, E.M., 2009. Diffuse liver disease: strategies for hepatic CT and MR imaging. Radiographics 29 (6), 1591–1614.

8.11 FOCAL HYPERECHOIC LIVER LESION

With posterior acoustic shadowing

1. **Calcified lesions**—see Section 8.7.
2. **Pneumobilia**—linear, periportal; see Section 8.4.
3. **Gas within an abscess**.
4. **Portal venous gas**—linear, usually peripheral; see Section 8.5.

5. Biliary hamartomas—small, numerous; cause posterior 'comet-tail' artefact rather than shadowing.

Nonshadowing

1. Focal fatty infiltration—most common adjacent to falciform ligament but can occur anywhere. Geographic margins, no distortion of vessels or liver contour. Can be multifocal.
2. Haemangioma—well-defined homogeneously hyperechoic lesion without a hypoechoic halo. May be heterogeneous if large.
3. Metastases—from GI tract (especially colon), ovary, pancreas, urogenital tract, thyroid, melanoma, NET, choriocarcinoma. Often multiple + hypoechoic halo.
4. HCC—especially if fatty. Usually well-defined + hypoechoic halo. Look for signs of cirrhosis.
5. Hepatic adenoma—especially if fatty or haemorrhagic, ± hypoechoic halo.
6. Mass-forming cholangiocarcinoma—especially if large. Usually ill-defined, no hypoechoic halo. Look for peripheral biliary dilatation and capsular retraction.
7. **Debris within a lesion**—e.g. abscess, haematoma, hydatid cyst (hydatid 'sand').
8. **Rare lesions containing fat**—e.g. angiomyolipoma, lipoma.
9. **Other lesions with variable echogenicity**—e.g. FNH, inflammatory pseudotumour, haemangioendothelioma.

8.12 FOCAL HYPOECHOIC LIVER LESION

Excluding anechoic cystic lesions (see Section 8.16). NB: lesions which are usually hyperechoic (e.g. haemangiomas) can appear hypoechoic in a fatty liver.

1. Focal fatty sparing—typically adjacent to GB or porta, with background steatosis. No distortion of vessels or liver contour.
2. Metastasis—including cystic or mucinous metastases (e.g. from GI tract, pancreas, NET, ovary).
3. HCC—most commonly hypoechoic ± internal vascularity. Look for signs of cirrhosis.
4. Abscess—± hyperechoic wall due to fibrosis, ± surrounding hypoechoic rim due to oedema. Look for echogenic foci of gas.
5. Haemorrhagic or infected cyst—contains internal floating echoes ± septations. No internal vascularity.
6. Mass-forming cholangiocarcinoma—especially if small.
7. Lymphoma*—may be markedly hypoechoic. Look for splenomegaly and adenopathy.
8. **Hydatid cyst**—can contain hydatid 'sand' or solid material.

9. **Other lesions with variable echogenicity**—e.g. FNH, adenoma, atypical haemangioma, haematoma.

Further reading

Jang, H.J., Kim, T.K., Wilson, S.R., 2006. Imaging of malignant liver masses: characterization and detection. Ultrasound Q. 22 (1), 19–29.

8.13 PERIPORTAL HYPERECHOGENICITY

1. **Pneumobilia**—with posterior acoustic shadowing; see Section 8.4.
2. **Portal venous gas**—see Section 8.5.
3. **Periportal fibrosis**—e.g. in cystic fibrosis, schistosomiasis infection (± 'turtleback' appearance) or vinyl chloride workers.
4. **Hepatic artery calcification**—e.g. diabetes, chronic renal failure.
5. **Intrahepatic duct calculi**—e.g. in PSC or recurrent pyogenic cholangitis.
6. **Inflammatory bowel disease***—echo-rich periportal cuffing can rarely be seen.
7. **Stents, drains and surgical clips.**
8. **Langerhans cell histiocytosis***—in children; periportal xanthomatous (fatty) deposits.

8.14 PERIPORTAL OEDEMA

Hypoechoic on US, hypoattenuating on CT, T2 hyperintense on MRI. Circumferential 'halo' around portal veins (cf. biliary dilatation and peribiliary cysts that are adjacent to portal veins).

Hepatic causes

1. **Acute hepatitis/cholangitis**—see Sections 8.3 and 8.6.
2. **Cirrhosis**.
3. **Regional inflammation**—e.g. cholecystitis, abscess, eosinophilic gastroenteritis.
4. **Following liver transplant**—can reflect lymphoedema, biliary necrosis or rejection.

Extrahepatic causes

1. **Raised central venous pressure/cardiac failure**.
2. **Hypoproteinaemia**.
3. **Systemic inflammation**—e.g. sepsis, trauma, acute pancreatitis.
4. **Lymphatic obstruction**—e.g. by malignant periportal adenopathy.

Further reading

Karcaaltincaba, M., Haliloglu, M., Akpinar, E., et al., 2007. Multidetector CT and MRI findings in periportal space pathologies. Eur. J. Radiol. 61 (1), 3–10.

8.15 PERIPORTAL LESIONS

Vascular

1. **Portal vein thrombosis**—either bland thrombus (e.g. related to portal hypertension, local inflammation or hypercoagulable states) or tumour thrombus (most commonly due to direct extension from HCC). Tumour thrombus tends to expand the portal vein and may contain internal vascularity or enhancement.
2. **Cavernous transformation of portal vein**—a tangle of periportal venous collaterals that develop after PV thrombosis.
3. **Aneurysm**—arterial (e.g. due to trauma, surgery, atherosclerosis, polyarteritis nodosa, fibromuscular dysplasia, mycotic) or portal venous (e.g. congenital or due to portal hypertension, trauma, surgery or pancreatitis).

Biliary

1. **Cholangiocarcinoma**—periductal infiltrating or intraductal forms. Both cause severe biliary dilatation ± PV narrowing or occlusion.
2. **Cholangitis/strictures**—see Section 8.3.
3. **Bile duct stones**.
4. **Choledochal cyst**—see Section 8.3.
5. **Biliary cystadenoma**—can rarely arise from extrahepatic ducts.

Haematological/lymphatic

1. **Reactive/inflammatory lymphadenopathy**—e.g. due to acute hepatitis, cirrhosis (especially Hep C, PBC and PSC), TB (necrotic), sarcoidosis. Nodes tend to be discrete, homogeneous (except TB) and small volume.
2. **Metastatic lymphadenopathy**—e.g. from HPB/GI malignancies.
3. **Lymphoma***—confluent homogeneous periportal adenopathy. PTLD also commonly involves the periportal region, manifesting as a homogeneous soft tissue mass encasing but not occluding the portal vein, with only mild biliary dilatation (cf. cholangiocarcinoma). Leukaemia can also create a similar appearance.
4. **Extramedullary haematopoiesis**—mimics lymphoma. Look for features of bone marrow failure.

Others

1. **Focal fatty infiltration/sparing**—can occur in periportal region. Geographic appearance, no mass effect.
2. **Peritoneal malignancy**—including direct periportal tumour extension (e.g. from GB, stomach or pancreas), peritoneal metastases, pseudomyxoma peritonei and primary peritoneal tumours, e.g. mesothelioma.

3. **Fluid collections**—following trauma/surgery or tracking from cholecystitis or pancreatitis.
4. **Neurofibroma**—in NF1. Plexiform sheath-like mass encasing but not narrowing the portal vein or obstructing the bile ducts; low attenuation on CT (almost cystic), often extends into mesenteric root or retroperitoneum.
5. **Schwannoma**—well-defined rounded mass ± internal cystic change or calcification.
6. **Sarcomas**—e.g. Kaposi sarcoma (typically causes enhancing periportal nodules + hypervascular nodes), leiomyosarcoma, MPNST.

Further reading

Lee, C.U., Glockner, J.F., 2016. MRI of common and uncommon pathologies involving the periportal space: a pictorial essay. Abdom. Radiol. (N.Y.) 41, 149–161.

Singh, A., Chandrashekhara, S.H., Handa, N., et al., 2016. "Periportal neoplasms" – a CT perspective: review article. Br. J. Radiol. 89 (1060), 20150756.

Tirumani, S.H., Shanbhogue, A.K., Vikram, R., et al., 2014. Imaging of the porta hepatis: spectrum of disease. Radiographics 34 (1), 73–92.

8.16 CYSTIC LIVER LESIONS

Unilocular and thin-walled

Usually anechoic on US, fluid attenuation on CT (0–20 HU), T1 dark and T2 bright on MRI.

1. **Simple cyst**—solitary or multiple, variable size. Usually unilocular with an imperceptible wall. May contain thin nonenhancing septa. Can become haemorrhagic or infected.
2. **Fibropolycystic liver diseases**—these are all caused by congenital ductal plate malformations; end result depends on the size of the ducts involved. The conditions can overlap with each other and with congenital hepatic fibrosis and polycystic kidney disease.
   (a) **Multiple biliary hamartomas**—small ducts. Numerous small cysts (most <1 cm) on CT/MR; can be hypo- or hyperechoic on US ± 'comet-tail' artefact. No communication with biliary tree. Usually nonenhancing, though some may contain enhancing fibrous stromal nodules.
   (b) **Polycystic liver disease**—medium ducts. Multiple cysts of varying size (can be large); no communication with biliary tree. Thin nonenhancing walls, unless complicated by haemorrhage or infection. Some of the cysts may coalesce, mimicking a multilocular cystic lesion, but the presence of cysts elsewhere aids diagnosis.

(c) Caroli disease—large ducts. Multifocal saccular dilatations of intrahepatic bile ducts, often containing a central 'dot' representing portal radicals. May be diffuse or segmental. Intraductal calculi are often seen. Can be associated with medullary sponge kidney.

3. Peribiliary cysts—small (<2 cm) and multiple, seen in cirrhotic or polycystic livers. Located along portal tracts, usually close to the hilum. May mimic biliary dilatation if confluent. No enhancement or communication with the biliary tree.
4. Subcapsular fluid collections—e.g. subcapsular gallbladder rupture, postsurgical seroma or biloma, pancreatic pseudocyst, chronic haematoma; these cause scalloping of the liver margin. An intrahepatic biloma in a posttransplant patient suggests biliary necrosis due to hepatic artery occlusion.
5. Focal bile duct dilatation—e.g. due to a stricture, biliary IPMN or intrahepatic choledochal cyst. See Section 8.3.
6. **Cystic metastases**—can occasionally mimic simple cysts (see later).
7. **Hydatid cyst**—CL and CE1 types (see later).
8. **Ciliated hepatic foregut cyst**—rare; typically a thin-walled unilocular wedge-like cyst located in the periphery of segment 4. May contain mucinous material, increasing attenuation on CT and T1 signal on MRI. Small risk of malignancy—thick septations or solid components are worrying.
9. **Intrahepatic gallbladder**—congenital anomaly. Often small and located close to an empty GB fossa.

8

Multilocular or thick-walled

1. Haemorrhagic or infected simple cyst—common in polycystic livers. T1 hyperintensity suggests haemorrhage; wall thickening and enhancement ± restricted diffusion suggests infection. NB: haemorrhage into a cyst almost excludes hydatid cyst from the differential.
2. Abscess—these typically show internal restricted diffusion on MRI, intense rim enhancement + surrounding oedema ('double-target' sign) ± associated venous thrombosis. Clinical and biochemical signs of infection are typically present.
   (a) Pyogenic—often multilocular or septated ± internal gas (especially with *Klebsiella*). Tend to form clusters when multiple. Klebsiella abscesses may also contain multiple discontinuous T2 hypointense enhancing septa ('turquoise' sign).
   (b) Amoebic—usually large, solitary, round and unilocular, with a thick wall and perilesional oedema. Usually no internal gas. Rupture of an abscess through the diaphragm suggests amoebic abscess.
   (c) Candidiasis—in immunocompromised patients; innumerable microabscesses (most <1 cm), usually involving both liver

and spleen. Mycobacterial and other fungal infections can look identical.

(d) **Melioidosis**—endemic in tropical Australasia. Single or multiple abscesses with a characteristic 'honeycomb' appearance, usually also with splenic involvement.

(e) **Fascioliasis**—parasitic GI tract infection endemic in the tropics. The parasites burrow through the intestinal wall into the peritoneal space, where they migrate to and invade the liver, heading to the bile ducts. This results in a linear array of small subcapsular abscesses along the path of parasite migration through the liver parenchyma towards the hilum. Peripheral eosinophilia is usually present.

(f) **Visceral larva migrans**—parasitic infection (most commonly *Toxocara* from dogs or cats) that can cause clustered or coalescent liver abscesses similar to pyogenic abscesses. The presence of peripheral eosinophilia is suggestive.

(g) **Aseptic abscesses**—most commonly related to IBD (Crohn's > UC); may precede the diagnosis. Usually multiple, variable size. More common in the spleen.

3. **Cystic metastases**—typically multiple. Do not usually exhibit the surrounding rim of oedema ('double-target' sign) or central restricted diffusion seen with abscesses. Three sources:
   (a) **Mucinous tumours**—e.g. from GI tract (intraparenchymal) or ovary (subcapsular). Often have irregular walls and septa.
   (b) **Cystic degeneration of hypervascular metastases**—e.g. NET, melanoma, sarcoma; usually show nodular rim enhancement.
   (c) **Treatment-related cystic change**—especially with GIST metastases; can mimic simple cysts.
4. **Biliary cystadenoma**—typically solitary, large and multilocular with septal vascularity and enhancement ± calcification. Usually in middle-aged women, most often in segment 4. Upstream biliary dilatation is common (rare with simple cysts). Mural or septal nodularity is worrying for malignant transformation to cystadenocarcinoma, although it is often not possible to reliably differentiate the two.
5. **Hydatid cyst**—caused by *Echinococcus granulosus*, usually seen in patients in close contact with sheep. Well-defined rounded margin; may be solitary or multiple ± involvement of other organs (most commonly lung, but can occur anywhere). Characteristic imaging appearance depending on stage of disease (NB: internal septa and solid components never show vascularity or enhancement—cf. other cystic lesions):
   (a) **CL (active)**—simple unilocular cyst, no internal echoes or visible wall. Mimics a simple hepatic cyst; upstream biliary dilatation may help differentiate (very rare with simple cysts).
   (b) **CE1 (active)**—same as CL but with internal echoes (hydatid sand) and a visible thin wall on US.

(c) **CE2 (active)**—multilocular cyst due to filling of 'mother' cyst with several smaller 'daughter' cysts. No solid components.
(d) **CE3a (transitional)**—cyst with detached internal membranes ('water-lily' sign).
(e) **CE3b (transitional)**—similar to CE2 but with solid components between the daughter cysts.
(f) **CE4 (inactive)**—cyst with heterogeneous solid contents ('ball of wool' sign). No daughter cysts.
(g) **CE5 (inactive)**—cyst with solid contents and wall calcification. The entire lesion may become calcified.

6. **Cystic HCC**—rare form of HCC due to marked central necrosis; usually shows mural nodular enhancement + washout. Cystic necrosis within a solid HCC is more commonly seen after RFA/ TACE therapy.
7. **Inflammatory pseudotumour**—can occasionally present as a complex cystic mass with thick enhancing septa.
8. **Multicystic biliary hamartoma**—rare, benign. Tubulocystic honeycomb-like mass with mural and septal enhancement, typically in a peripheral location.
9. **Biliary adenofibroma**—rare benign tumour with some malignant potential; complex multicystic mass + enhancing solid components, indistinguishable from biliary cystadenocarcinoma.
10. **Lymphangioma**—intrahepatic location is rare.
11. **Glomus tumour**—very rare. Complex cystic mass with arterially enhancing mural nodules that persist into the delayed phase.
12. **Mesenchymal hamartoma and embryonal sarcoma**—typically in children; very rare in adults. Both appear as complex multilocular cystic masses.

Further reading

Bächler, P., Baladron, M.J., Menias, C., et al., 2016. Multimodality imaging of liver infections: differential diagnosis and potential pitfalls. Radiographics 36 (4), 1001–1023.

Borhani, A.A., Wiant, A., Heller, M.T., 2014. Cystic hepatic lesions: a review and an algorithmic approach. AJR Am. J. Roentgenol. 203 (6), 1192–1204.

Del Poggio, P., Buonocore, M., 2008. Cystic tumors of the liver: a practical approach. World J. Gastroenterol. 14 (23), 3616–3620.

Qian, L.J., Zhu, J., Zhuang, Z.G., et al., 2013. Spectrum of multilocular cystic hepatic lesions: CT and MR imaging findings with pathologic correlation. Radiographics 33 (5), 1419–1433.

8.17 FAT-CONTAINING LIVER LESIONS

Macroscopic fat

This is fat visible on CT (foci of attenuation less than –20 HU) and showing signal loss on fatsat MRI sequences. Hyperechoic on

US. Beware of normal pericaval fat mimicking a fat-containing liver lesion.

1. Pseudolipoma of Glisson's capsule—small subcapsular fatty nodule, usually located on the liver dome. Represents a detached colonic epiploic appendage that attaches to the liver capsule.
2. Angiomyolipoma—rare; contains fat and enhancing soft tissue, similar to renal AMLs. Can be associated with tuberous sclerosis. Fat content varies; some are fat-poor. The presence of internal vessels is characteristic and aids differentiation from other lesions.
3. HCC/adenoma—can occasionally contain macroscopic fat.
4. **Lipoma**—rare. Purely fatty.
5. **Surgical omentopexy**—flap of omentum is placed on the liver surface, e.g. after hydatid cyst surgery.
6. **Hydatid cyst**—can rarely contain droplets of fat.
7. **Hepatic adrenal rest tumour**—rare; contains a mixture of soft tissue and fat, mimicking AML.
8. **Fatty metastasis**—e.g. from teratoma or liposarcoma; rare. Primary hepatic teratoma or liposarcoma is even rarer.
9. **Lipopeliosis**—rare; can occur in a transplanted liver after an ischaemic insult.
10. **Extramedullary haematopoiesis**—the rare focal intrahepatic form can contain fat.
11. **Langerhans cell histiocytosis***—in children; periportal xanthomatous deposits.

Microscopic fat

This is only visible on MRI, as signal loss on the opposed-phase T1 sequence (relative to the in-phase T1 sequence).

1. Focal fatty infiltration—most common adjacent to the falciform ligament or porta but can occur anywhere; often has a geographic morphology but can appear nodular (focal nodular steatosis). No mass effect, abnormal enhancement or restricted diffusion.
2. HCC—often contains fat. Hypervascular on arterial phase + washout on later phases. Mainly seen in cirrhotic livers.
3. Hepatic adenoma—often contain fat. Hypervascular ± washout. Most common in young women taking oral contraceptives.
4. **Regenerative nodules**—occasionally contain fat; usually multiple. No enhancement (cf. HCC). Seen in cirrhotic livers.
5. **FNH**—uncommonly contains foci of intracellular fat, especially if the background liver is fatty.
6. **Angiomyolipoma**—if fat-poor.

Further reading

Basaran, C., Karcaaltincaba, M., Akata, D., et al., 2005. Fat-containing lesions of the liver: cross-sectional imaging findings with emphasis on MRI. AJR Am. J. Roentgenol. 184 (4), 1103–1110.

Prasad, S.R., Wang, H., Rosas, H., et al., 2005. Fat-containing lesions of the liver: radiologic-pathologic correlation. Radiographics 25 (2), 321–331.

8.18 HYPERVASCULAR LIVER LESIONS

These are lesions that enhance avidly on arterial phase CT/MR and can be characterized by how they behave on subsequent phases (NB: there is some overlap between categories).

Arterial enhancement persisting on the delayed phase

The lesion continues to enhance more than the background liver on the delayed phase.

1. **Haemangioma**—classically shows peripheral nodular (discontinuous) enhancement on arterial phase with progressive centripetal filling on later phases. The enhancement follows the enhancement of the blood pool. Small capillary haemangiomas often 'flash-fill' homogeneously on the arterial phase. Large cavernous haemangiomas may not fill completely even on delayed phases due to central fibrosis. Haemangiomas are typically T2 bright on MRI (almost cyst-like)—most other hypervascular lesions are only mildly-moderately T2 hyperintense. Restricted diffusion may be present.
2. **Vascular malformation/shunt**—has dilated feeding and draining vessels. May be arterioportal, arteriovenous or portosystemic. T2 dark (flow void).
3. **Mass-forming cholangiocarcinoma**—can contain hypervascular areas, especially in the periphery, with central fibrosis that enhances in the delayed phase (± peripheral washout). Also note that mixed HCC-cholangiocarcinoma neoplasms can occur that exhibit imaging features of both tumours.
4. **Treated metastasis**—can show persistent enhancement.
5. **Angiomyolipoma**—typically contains macroscopic fat. Vascular components enhance.
6. **Angiosarcoma**—large aggressive infiltrative mass + satellite nodules; may diffusely infiltrate entire liver. Heterogeneous multifocal arterial enhancement ± partial filling on later phases. Areas of haemorrhage, necrosis and cystic change are common. Often metastatic at presentation. Most common in older men.
7. **Epithelioid haemangioendothelioma**—rare malignant vascular tumour, less aggressive than angiosarcoma. Typically, multifocal subcapsular masses that often coalesce + capsular retraction ± a T2 bright core ('target' sign). Often shows peripheral target-like arterial enhancement ± partial filling on later phases; may mimic haemangioma.

8. **Peliosis hepatis**—single or multiple blood-filled cystic spaces within the liver. Most common in immunocompromised patients (especially AIDS) due to *Bartonella* infection; can also be seen in various chronic illnesses (e.g. diabetes, coeliac disease, vasculitis, TB) and secondary to drugs (e.g. steroids, OCP). Peripheral (ring-like) or central arterial enhancement with centripetal or centrifugal filling on later phases. May rupture into peritoneal cavity. Usually regresses after removing the cause.
9. **Leiomyoma**—rare; usually hypervascular with persistent enhancement in the delayed phase.

Arterial enhancement equilibrating on the delayed phase

The lesion enhances similarly to the background liver on the delayed phase (i.e. almost becomes invisible).

1. Transient hepatic attenuation/intensity difference (THAD/THID)—region of increased arterial enhancement on CT (THAD) or MRI (THID) that equilibrates with the background liver on later phases, usually with no corresponding abnormality on other MRI sequences. Small peripheral wedge-shaped THADs/THIDs are common, especially in cirrhosis, and are of no consequence. Other causes include:
   (a) **Hyperaemia adjacent to inflammation**—e.g. liver abscess, peritonitis (Fitz-Hugh-Curtis syndrome), cholecystitis, duodenitis, colitis. Ill-defined region of arterial hyperenhancement + mild T2 hyperintensity (oedema).
   (b) **Portal vein occlusion**—e.g. due to thrombus or tumour. Causes a wedge of arterial hyperenhancement peripheral to the occluded portal vein.
   (c) **Arterioportal/arteriovenous shunt**—can be congenital (AVM—multiple in HHT) or secondary to cirrhosis, trauma or an underlying hypervascular mass. Focal arterial hyperenhancement around the shunt due to reduced vascular resistance. A dilated feeding artery and draining vein are often seen.
   (d) **Biliary obstruction**—causes arterial hyperenhancement in the surrounding liver due to elevated sinusoidal pressure.
   (e) **SVC/IVC obstruction**—collateral veins entering the liver cause hyperenhancement of the adjacent parenchyma.
2. FNH—focal hyperplastic response around a (central) vascular malformation; usually an incidental finding in young adults (F>M). Typically shows homogeneous arterial enhancement that equilibrates with the background liver on later phases. Often has a T2 hyperintense central scar which enhances in the delayed phase. May be multiple.

3. <u>Hepatic adenoma</u>—clinical and radiological features depend on subtype. Generally, adenomas are mildly T2 hyperintense and hypervascular ± washout ± fat content ± associated haemorrhage. Hepatocyte-specific MR contrast agents (e.g. Primovist) can aid differentiation from FNH (see Section 8.27).
   (a) **Inflammatory**— most common; usually in women on the OCP. Marked arterial enhancement (more than other subtypes) which may persist on the delayed phase. No/minimal fat content. Moderately T2 hyperintense; a peripheral T2 bright rim ('atoll' sign) is characteristic if present. Highest risk of associated haemorrhage.
   (b) **HNF1α-mutated**—almost exclusively in women, usually on the OCP. Diffuse microscopic fat content is characteristic. Often multiple. Least T2 hyperintense and least hypervascular subtype; tends to show washout on later phases.
   (c) **β-catenin-mutated**—more common in men, especially those on anabolic steroids. Also seen in glycogen storage disease (multiple) and FAP. No fat content. May contain a T2 hyperintense scar. Highest risk of malignant transformation.
   (d) **Unclassified**—no specific imaging features.
4. <u>Fibrolamellar HCC</u>—variant of HCC that occurs in noncirrhotic livers, usually in young adults. Mimics FNH on imaging but tends to be larger (>5 cm) with a T2 hypointense central scar and heterogeneous enhancement ± washout. Calcification is common (rare in FNH).
5. **Large regenerative nodules**—seen in chronic Budd-Chiari syndrome; often multiple. Imaging features are identical to FNH.
6. **Intrahepatic splenosis**—post splenectomy. Subcapsular deposits of splenic tissue; heterogeneous arterial enhancement, becoming homogeneous in the portal phase.

8

Arterial enhancement with washout on portal or delayed phase

The lesion enhances less than the background liver on the portal or delayed phase.

1. <u>HCC</u>—usually in cirrhotic livers. Characteristically shows arterial enhancement followed by washout, ± internal fat ± enhancing capsule ± venous invasion (tumour thrombus). May be multiple.
2. <u>Hypervascular metastases</u>—e.g. from NETs, RCC, thyroid, melanoma, breast, sarcoma (including Kaposi), choriocarcinoma. Usually multiple. Often T2 bright + restricted diffusion. Metastases from insulinoma may be surrounded by a halo of fatty infiltration.
3. **Hepatic adenoma**—can show washout (especially the HNF1α-mutated subtype).
4. **Fibrolamellar HCC**—can show washout.

Rare hypervascular tumours with nonspecific appearances

1. **Inflammatory pseudotumour**—variable appearance; may be hypervascular ± washout.
2. **Solitary fibrous tumour**—rare; solitary large well-defined mass with heterogeneous arterial enhancement and areas of both high and low T2 signal.
3. **Primary hepatic NET**—e.g. carcinoid, gastrinoma, paraganglioma; very rare. Often large ± areas of cystic (T2 bright) or haemorrhagic (T1 hyperintense) change. Heterogeneous arterial enhancement that may persist or wash out.
4. **Clear cell myomelanocytic tumour**—rare tumour of perivascular epithelioid cells (PEComa) seen in children and young adults; usually arises from or adjacent to the falciform ligament. Usually large + heterogeneous arterial enhancement and areas of necrosis.
5. **Intrahepatic bile duct adenoma**—very rare; usually small (<2 cm) and subcapsular. Heterogeneous arterial enhancement that may persist or wash out, ± cystic change.
6. **Adenomatoid tumour**—very rare; solid or solid-cystic hypervascular mass.

Further reading

Kamaya, A., Maturen, K.E., Tye, G.A., et al., 2009. Hypervascular liver lesions. Semin. Ultrasound CT MR 30 (5), 387–407.

8.19 LIVER LESIONS WITH GRADUAL DELAYED ENHANCEMENT

Gradual delayed enhancement usually suggests a fibrotic lesion.

1. <u>**Mass-forming cholangiocarcinoma**</u>—classically shows gradual delayed enhancement, especially centrally. Usually causes capsular retraction ± peripheral biliary dilatation ± vascular occlusion ± restricted diffusion.
2. <u>**Confluent hepatic fibrosis**</u>—seen in cirrhosis; see Section 8.25. Can mimic cholangiocarcinoma but tends to be more wedge-like, with no restricted diffusion, biliary dilatation or vascular occlusion.
3. <u>**Haemangioma**</u>—some are late-filling (complete or partial), especially the sclerosing subtype.
4. **Treated metastasis/HCC**—treatment results in fibrosis.
5. **Solid organizing abscess**—this is a partially healed abscess that contains late-enhancing fibrosis/granulation tissue.
6. **Inflammatory pseudotumour**—variable appearance, may show delayed enhancement.
7. **Solitary fibrous tumour**—rare; often contains both hypervascular areas and fibrotic late-enhancing areas.

Further reading

Awaya, H., Ito, K., Honjo, K., et al., 1998. Differential diagnosis of hepatic tumors with delayed enhancement at gadolinium-enhanced MRI: a pictorial essay. Clin. Imaging 22 (3), 180–187.

8.20 HYPOVASCULAR LIVER LESIONS

Excluding cystic lesions (see Section 8.16).

1. Metastases—e.g. from GI tract, pancreas, lung, breast, etc. Most metastases tend to be hypovascular due to central necrosis ± mild peripheral arterial enhancement.
2. Cholangiocarcinoma—may show minimal enhancement.
3. Granulomatous lesions—typically small and numerous.
   (a) Sarcoidosis*—numerous small hypovascular nodules, typically involving both liver and spleen and usually in the presence of nodal and thoracic disease. The nodules are typically T2 hypointense (cf. other granulomatous processes below).
   (b) TB*—numerous small hypovascular nodules, typically involving both liver and spleen. Usually in immunocompromised patients; can mimic fungal infection (e.g. candidiasis) but the presence of necrotic lymph nodes and lung involvement suggests TB. Nodules often calcify after healing.
   (c) **Brucellosis**—can present as a solitary abscess or multiple hypovascular granulomas ± calcification.
   (d) **Cat-scratch disease**—caused by *Bartonella henselae*. Usually involves lymph nodes but hepatic (± splenic) dissemination with multiple hypovascular necrotizing granulomas can occur. May mimic TB or fungal infection, but typically occurs in immunocompetent children or young adults.
4. Nodular steatosis—can mimic malignancy on CT, especially when multifocal. Diagnosis confirmed on in-/opposed-phase MRI. May have a pathognomonic rim of more marked fatty infiltration.
5. Haematoma—due to trauma, coagulopathy or underlying mass lesion. Hyperattenuating on unenhanced CT, no internal enhancement (unless there is active bleeding). Variable MRI signal depending on age.
6. **Sclerosing haemangioma**—may be completely hypovascular with only mild T2 hyperintensity ± capsular retraction, mimicking malignancy. May have calcification or a wedge-like morphology.
7. **Previously treated HCC/metastasis**—e.g. ablation, TACE, chemotherapy.
8. **Lymphoma***—well-defined homogeneous mass, masses or micronodules that may have a periportal distribution. Leukaemia and extraosseous myeloma can have a similar appearance.

9. **Inflammatory pseudotumour**—variable appearance, can be hypovascular.
10. **Hydatid disease***—the two *Echinococcus* species have different imaging features, but neither shows internal enhancement as the contents are derived from the parasite, not the host.
    (a) **Cystic echinococcosis**—*E. granulosus*. Types CE4 and CE5 appear solid, the latter being calcified (see Section 8.16).
    (b) **Alveolar echinococcosis**—*E. multilocularis*. Irregular heterogeneous mass or masses, often with foci of calcification ± peripheral fibrosis showing mild delayed enhancement. No restricted diffusion.
11. **Other rare primary tumours**— e.g. leiomyosarcoma (associated with immunosuppression, may be centrally cystic), other sarcomas (e.g. carcinosarcoma, fibrosarcoma), epithelioid haemangioendothelioma (may be hypovascular), melanoma (may be T1 hyperintense and T2 hypointense), squamous cell carcinoma, GIST, PNET. These are often large nonspecific heterogeneous necrotic masses.
12. **Other rare lesions**—e.g. Langerhans cell histiocytosis, amyloidoma, Rosai-Dorfman disease.

Further reading

Tan, Y., Xiao, E.H., 2013. Rare hepatic malignant tumors: dynamic CT, MRI, and clinicopathological features: with analysis of 54 cases and review of the literature. Abdom. Imaging 38 (3), 511–526.

8.21 LIVER LESIONS WITH A CENTRAL SCAR

Scars often show delayed enhancement, and do not have to be exactly central.

1. **Focal nodular hyperplasia**—the scar is typically T2 hyperintense and noncalcified.
2. **Cavernous haemangioma**—especially if large.
3. **Fibrolamellar HCC**—the scar is typically T2 hypointense and often calcified. Conventional HCCs can also occasionally contain a central scar.
4. **Large regenerative nodules**—seen in chronic Budd-Chiari syndrome. Identical appearance to FNH.
5. **Mass-forming cholangiocarcinoma**—can have a peripheral hypervascular component and a central fibrous component, giving the appearance of a central scar. Look for associated biliary dilatation (rare with benign lesions).
6. **Hepatic adenoma**—occasionally.
7. **Metastases**—can contain a central fibrotic component.
8. **Epithelioid haemangioendothelioma**—rare; peripheral vascular component + central fibrosis often giving a 'target' appearance.

Further reading

Kim, T., Hori, M., Onishi, H., 2009. Liver masses with central or eccentric scar. Semin. Ultrasound CT MR 30 (5), 418–425.

8.22 HEPATIC CAPSULAR RETRACTION

Often a sinister feature.

1. **Metastases**—especially after treatment or with fibrotic/necrotic tumours, e.g. breast, carcinoid, lung, colorectal. Can create a 'pseudocirrhosis' appearance.
2. **Mass-forming cholangiocarcinoma**—classically shows capsular retraction.
3. **Confluent hepatic fibrosis**—seen in cirrhosis; capsular retraction is characteristic (see Section 8.25).
4. **Sclerosing haemangioma**—can cause adjacent capsular retraction.
5. **Post trauma**—including iatrogenic, e.g. biliary drainage, biopsy.
6. **HCC**—following ablation or TACE. Can also be seen with fibrolamellar HCCs.
7. **Epithelioid haemangioendothelioma**—classically shows capsular retraction. See Section 8.18.
8. **Inflammatory pseudotumour**—variable appearance; can mimic cholangiocarcinoma.
9. **Pseudomyxoma peritonei (mimic)**—scalloping of liver surface may resemble capsular retraction.

Further reading

Blachar, A., Federle, M.P., Sosna, J., 2009. Liver lesions with hepatic capsular retraction. Semin. Ultrasound CT MR 30 (5), 426–435.

8.23 T1 HYPERINTENSE LIVER LESIONS

NB: most liver lesions are T1 hypointense.

1. **Fat**—see Section 8.17.
2. **Haemorrhage**—in the subacute stage due to methaemoglobin. Haematomas do not show internal enhancement and can be either traumatic (e.g. post biopsy), spontaneous or related to an underlying mass, e.g. adenoma, HCC. Haemorrhagic cysts are also usually T1 hyperintense, either homogeneously or graduated (slightly higher intensity dependently).
3. **Cirrhotic nodules**—regenerative/dysplastic nodules and HCC can all be T1 hyperintense, even without fat (due to copper content). This can make it difficult to assess arterial enhancement—subtraction images may help.

8

4. Melanoma metastases.
5. **Intrahepatic ductal calculi**—pigment type, seen in PSC, recurrent pyogenic cholangitis and Caroli disease.
6. **Proteinaceous material**—may be seen dependently in abscesses. Can also be seen in the rare ciliated hepatic foregut cyst.
7. **Calcification**—can occasionally be T1 hyperintense.
8. **Chemical**—gadolinium, lipiodol (contains fat).
9. **'Relative'**—i.e. normal-signal liver surrounded by low-signal liver, e.g. iron deposition (haemochromatosis/siderosis), oedema.
10. **Artefact**—pulsation artefact from abdominal aorta can produce a periodic 'ghost' artefact along the phase-encoded direction that can be hypo- or hyperintense depending on the phase.

Further reading

Furlan, A., Marin, D., Bae, K.T., et al., 2009. Focal liver lesions hyperintense on T1-weighted magnetic resonance imaging. Semin. Ultrasound CT MR 30 (5), 436–449.

8.24 T2 HYPOINTENSE LIVER LESIONS

NB: most liver lesions are T2 hyperintense. Diffuse hepatic T2 hypointensity suggests haemochromatosis (± pancreatic and cardiac T2 hypointensity) or secondary haemosiderosis due to chronic blood transfusions/iron therapy (± splenic and bone marrow T2 hypointensity).

1. Siderotic nodules—in cirrhosis, regenerative and low-grade dysplastic nodules containing iron are typically T2 hypointense. Occasionally early HCCs can also appear T2 hypointense due to a combination of iron and copper content.
2. Gas—e.g. pneumobilia or gas within an abscess. Rises to the antidependent surface.
3. Haemorrhage—traumatic, spontaneous, within a cyst or related to a mass, e.g. adenoma, HCC, metastasis, AML, peliosis. T1 and T2 signals vary based on age of blood products.
4. Calcification—see Section 8.7.
5. **Vascular malformation/shunt**—flow voids.
6. **Sarcoidosis***—numerous T2 hypointense nodules in liver and spleen.
7. **Fibrous masses**—often have T2 hypointense areas, e.g. fibrolamellar HCC (especially in central scar), cholangiocarcinoma, some metastases (e.g. from adenocarcinoma or posttreatment), solitary fibrous tumour, solid organizing abscess.
8. **Liver ablation**—e.g. for HCC/metastasis. Causes T2 hypointense coagulative necrosis.
9. **Thick mucin**—e.g. within mucinous metastases.

10. **Leiomyoma**—often T2 hypointense and hypervascular. Rare.
11. **Melanoma metastases**—occasionally T2 hypointense.

Further reading

Curvo-Semedo, L., Brito, J.B., Seco, M.F., et al., 2010. The hypointense liver lesion on T2-weighted MR images and what it means. Radiographics 30 (1), e38.

8.25 LESIONS IN CHRONIC LIVER DISEASE

1. **Regenerative nodules**—typically numerous, small (<2 cm) and T2 iso/hypointense. Variable T1 signal. Variable attenuation on unenhanced CT—siderotic nodules are often dense. No hyperenhancement or restricted diffusion. May contain fat (tend to be multiple—a single fat-containing nodule is worrying).
2. **Dysplastic nodules**—usually small (<2 cm). Tend to be T2 hypointense (low-grade) or mildly T2 hyperintense (high-grade). Variable T1 signal and CT attenuation. No restricted diffusion. High-grade dysplastic nodules may show arterial enhancement, but do not wash out.
3. **HCC**—characteristically shows arterial enhancement followed by washout. NB: the arterial phase must be well-timed to detect the transient arterial enhancement—this may be missed if the phase is too early (no splenic enhancement) or too late (too much portal vein enhancement). Typically mildly T2 hyperintense. Variable T1 signal. May show restricted diffusion. May be well-defined and encapsulated or ill-defined and infiltrative; may also develop within a large dysplastic nodule ('nodule-in-nodule' appearance). Portal vein invasion is diagnostic if present.
4. **Confluent hepatic fibrosis**—peripheral well-defined wedge-like area of volume loss, T2 hyperintensity and capsular retraction which shows gradual delayed enhancement. No restricted diffusion or associated biliary dilatation or vascular occlusion.
5. **Mass-forming cholangiocarcinoma**—especially in PSC. Can mimic confluent hepatic fibrosis but tends to be more mass-like ± associated peripheral biliary dilatation, vascular occlusion and restricted diffusion.
6. **Large regenerative nodules**—seen in chronic Budd-Chiari syndrome. Identical appearance to FNH.

Further reading

Hanna, R.F., Aguirre, D.A., Kased, N., et al., 2008. Cirrhosis-associated hepatocellular nodules: correlation of histopathologic and MR imaging features. Radiographics 28 (3), 747–769.

8.26 FLOWCHART FOR CHARACTERIZING LIVER LESIONS ON MRI

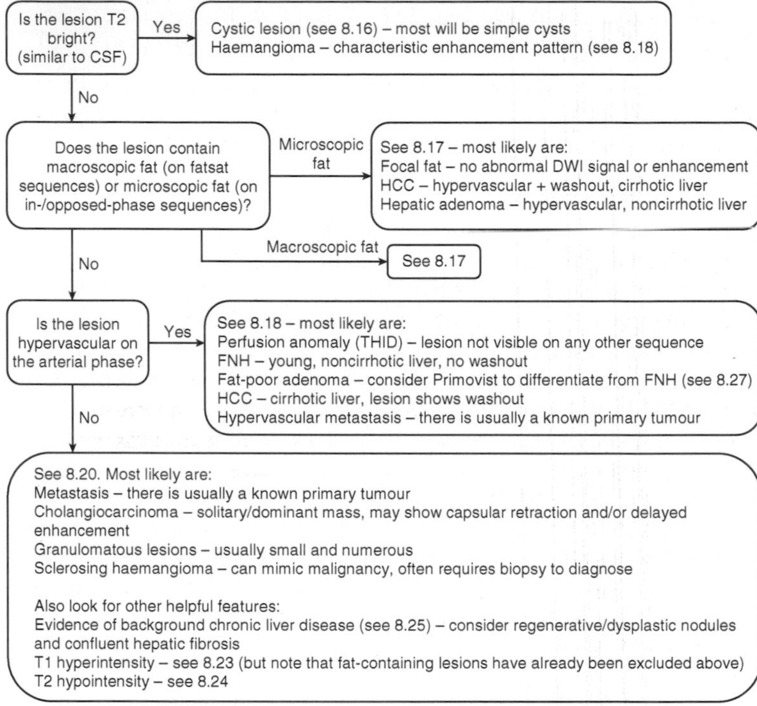

Is the lesion T2 bright? (similar to CSF)
Yes
Cystic lesion (see 8.16) – most will be simple cysts
Haemangioma – characteristic enhancement pattern (see 8.18)
No
Does the lesion contain macroscopic fat (on fatsat sequences) or microscopic fat (on in-/opposed-phase sequences)?
Microscopic fat
See 8.17 – most likely are:
Focal fat – no abnormal DWI signal or enhancement
HCC – hypervascular + washout, cirrhotic liver
Hepatic adenoma – hypervascular, noncirrhotic liver
Macroscopic fat
See 8.17
No
Is the lesion hypervascular on the arterial phase?
Yes
See 8.18 – most likely are:
Perfusion anomaly (THID) – lesion not visible on any other sequence
FNH – young, noncirrhotic liver, no washout
Fat-poor adenoma – consider Primovist to differentiate from FNH (see 8.27)
HCC – cirrhotic liver, lesion shows washout
Hypervascular metastasis – there is usually a known primary tumour
No
See 8.20. Most likely are:
Metastasis – there is usually a known primary tumour
Cholangiocarcinoma – solitary/dominant mass, may show capsular retraction and/or delayed enhancement
Granulomatous lesions – usually small and numerous
Sclerosing haemangioma – can mimic malignancy, often requires biopsy to diagnose
Also look for other helpful features:
Evidence of background chronic liver disease (see 8.25) – consider regenerative/dysplastic nodules and confluent hepatic fibrosis
T1 hyperintensity – see 8.23 (but note that fat-containing lesions have already been excluded above)
T2 hypointensity – see 8.24

NB: DWI and postcontrast sequences are the most sensitive for detecting liver lesions. The lesions can then be characterized using the T2, T1 in-/opposed-phase and postcontrast sequences.

8.27 HEPATOCYTE-SPECIFIC MR CONTRAST AGENTS

These agents (e.g. Primovist) are taken up by hepatocytes and excreted in bile, contrary to extracellular MR contrast agents (e.g. Gadovist), which stay in the extracellular space. This provides the opportunity to obtain an extra 'hepatobiliary' phase post contrast—in the case of Primovist this phase is seen at ~20 min. This can be used as a problem-solving tool in certain circumstances:

1. **Ascertaining the extent of liver metastases**—the hepatobiliary phase has a high sensitivity for detecting even very small liver metastases (which appear hypointense as they do not contain hepatocytes), and aids decision-making when considering liver resection for colorectal liver metastases.

2. FNH vs hepatic adenoma—both lesions are hypervascular, mildly T2 hyperintense and most common in young adult women. In the absence of haemorrhage, washout or internal fat it can be difficult to differentiate the two on conventional imaging—this is important as FNH can be left alone whereas adenomas should be followed up or resected if large (due to risk of haemorrhage). With hepatocyte-specific contrast agents an FNH is characteristically iso- or hyperintense to background liver on the hepatobiliary phase. In contrast, adenomas are typically hypointense to background liver (though inflammatory adenomas may have a rim of hyperintensity).
3. Diagnosing bile leaks—on the hepatobiliary phase contrast should be visible in the biliary tree; in the case of a bile leak contrast extravasation into an adjacent fluid collection can be seen.
4. **Aiding characterization of nodules in a cirrhotic liver**—regenerative and dysplastic nodules are typically iso- or hyperintense on the hepatobiliary phase, whereas HCC is usually hypointense. NB: some well-differentiated HCCs may be iso-/hyperintense, and some high-grade dysplastic nodules may be hypointense, so this is not entirely reliable.
5. **Other biliary applications**—e.g. assessing variant anatomy, bile flow dynamics and obstruction, and differentiating peribiliary cysts from lesions communicating with the biliary tree.

Lesions which take up hepatocyte-specific contrast agents in the hepatobiliary phase include:

1. FNH—uptake > background liver is a characteristic feature. The central scar is often hypointense.
2. Regenerative and dysplastic nodules—in cirrhosis.
3. Lesions communicating with the biliary tree—e.g. choledochal cyst, Caroli disease, biloma (if there is an ongoing bile leak).
4. **Large regenerative nodules**—seen in chronic Budd-Chiari syndrome. Identical imaging features to FNH.
5. **Focal fatty infiltration**—uptake may be less than background liver.
6. **THID**—see Section 8.18.
7. **Hepatic adenoma**—inflammatory subtype can show peripheral uptake.
8. **Well-differentiated HCC**—can show uptake.

Pitfalls of using hepatocyte-specific contrast agents include:

1. **Assessing arterial enhancement**—usually less intense than with extracellular contrast agents, therefore hypervascular lesions (e.g. haemangioma, HCC) may be less appreciable.
2. **Assessing washout on the delayed phase**—by this time hepatocytes have begun to take up the contrast, so lesions that

normally do not wash out (e.g. haemangiomas) often show 'pseudo-washout', appearing less intense than the background liver.

Further reading

Goodwin, M.D., Dobson, J.E., Sirlin, C.B., et al., 2011. Diagnostic challenges and pitfalls in MR imaging with hepatocyte-specific contrast agents. Radiographics 31 (6), 1547–1568.

Seale, M.K., Catalano, O.A., Saini, S., et al., 2009. Hepatobiliary-specific MR contrast agents: role in imaging the liver and biliary tree. Radiographics 29, 1725–1748.

8.28 SPLENOMEGALY

Huge spleen

1. **Chronic myeloid leukaemia.**
2. **Myelofibrosis**—look for bone sclerosis.
3. **Malaria*.**
4. **Gaucher disease***—look for bone infarcts, e.g. in femoral heads.
5. **Lymphoma*.**
6. **Visceral leishmaniasis (kala-azar).**

Moderately large spleen

1. **All of the above.**
2. **Haemolytic anaemias**—including haemoglobinopathies.
3. **Portal hypertension**—e.g. cirrhosis, splenic/portal vein occlusion, right heart failure.
4. **Leukaemias.**
5. **Polycythaemia vera.**
6. **Systemic mastocytosis**—look for bone sclerosis.
7. **Glycogen storage diseases.**

Slightly large spleen

1. **All of the above.**
2. **Infections.**
   (a) **Viral**—infectious hepatitis, infectious mononucleosis, HIV.
   (b) **Bacterial**—septicaemia (e.g. intravenous drug user), brucellosis, typhoid, TB.
   (c) **Rickettsial**—typhus.
   (d) **Fungal**—histoplasmosis.
3. **Sarcoidosis*.**
4. **Rheumatoid arthritis***—Felty's syndrome.
5. **Amyloidosis*.**
6. **Systemic lupus erythematosus (SLE)*.**

8.29 SPLENIC CALCIFICATION

Curvilinear

1. Splenic artery atherosclerosis—especially splenic artery aneurysm.
2. Cyst—any chronic cyst, including hydatid or posttraumatic.

Multiple small nodular/punctate

1. Phleboliths—± small central lucencies. Can be seen in haemangiomas.
2. TB*—usually few in number + calcified intrathoracic nodes and lung granulomas.
3. Histoplasmosis—calcifications are often larger than in TB or other fungal infections, e.g. candidiasis; with calcified intrathoracic nodes and lung granulomas.
4. Gamna-Gandy bodies—siderotic splenic nodules usually due to portal hypertension.
5. **Sickle cell anaemia.**
6. *Pneumocystis jiroveci*—e.g. in AIDS, ± hepatic, renal, adrenal and nodal calcification.
7. **Toxoplasmosis.**
8. **Sarcoidosis*.**
9. **SLE.**
10. **Amyloidosis***—often with hepatic calcification.

8

Diffuse homogeneous

1. Sickle cell anaemia—spleen is shrunken and diffusely calcified.
2. **Previous Thorotrast administration**—with liver and nodal calcification; see Section 8.7.

Solitary >1 cm

1. Healed infarct or haematoma.
2. Healed abscess.
3. Healed granuloma—e.g. TB, histoplasmosis.
4. **Brucellosis**—pathognomonic large 'snowflake' calcification within a chronic brucellar abscess; calcification persists after healing.

8.30 CYSTIC SPLENIC LESIONS

1. Pseudocyst—accounts for most splenic cysts. Usually posttraumatic; can also be seen following infection, infarction or pancreatitis. Can be simple or complex (thick wall, septa, debris, calcification).
2. Epithelial cyst—thin-walled unilocular cyst ± septations, no enhancement.

3. Abscess—pyogenic, TB (may be T2 hypointense), fungal (microabscesses + liver involvement), aseptic (e.g. in IBD, see Section 8.16). Restricted diffusion, ± rim enhancement. A peripheral 'necklace' of small locules suggests melioidosis; a large 'snowflake' calcification suggests brucellosis.
4. Hydatid cyst—usually in the presence of liver involvement; see Section 8.16.
5. **Lymphangioma**—often multilocular with thin enhancing septa, no solid components.
6. **Cystic metastasis**—e.g. from melanoma or mucinous primaries. Rare.

8.31 SOLID SPLENIC LESIONS

Beware of the normal heterogeneous arterial enhancement pattern of the spleen mimicking a lesion. Also note it is often difficult to characterize solid lesions accurately on imaging, although most incidentally detected lesions are benign (especially in the absence of splenomegaly).

Nonneoplastic

1. Infarct—peripheral wedge-shaped area of poor enhancement ± rim of capsular enhancement. Usually embolic (± infarcts elsewhere) or related to a haematological disorder (e.g. sickle cell disease, leukaemia, lymphoma).
2. Haematoma—usually traumatic; can also occur due to coagulopathy or splenomegaly. Hyperattenuating on unenhanced CT, no internal enhancement unless there is active bleeding.
3. Siderotic nodules—also known as Gamna-Gandy bodies, seen in portal hypertension. T1 and T2 dark on MRI; may be calcified. Typically, multiple within an enlarged spleen.
4. Sarcoidosis*—numerous small hypovascular T2 hypointense nodules, usually with hepatic, nodal and thoracic involvement.
5. **Peliosis**—rare; nearly always in the presence of hepatic peliosis and with a similar appearance (see Section 8.18).
6. **Extramedullary haematopoiesis**—usually causes diffuse splenomegaly but can rarely present as a focal hypovascular mass ± internal fat.
7. **Gaucher disease***—marked splenomegaly ± numerous hypovascular nodules. Look for bone infarcts.
8. **Amyloidosis***—usually diffuse, causing strikingly poor arterial enhancement of the spleen and T2 hypointensity on MRI. Focal hypovascular amyloidomas are rare.

Benign neoplasms and hamartomas

1. Haemangioma—most common incidental solid splenic lesion. Usually hyperechoic on US without vascularity on Doppler, ±

calcifications (phleboliths). Hypoattenuating on unenhanced CT. Enhancement varies; may be homogeneous, heterogeneous or similar to hepatic haemangiomas (peripheral and nodular with progressive filling). T2 hyperintense on MRI. May be multiple or diffuse (haemangiomatosis) in Klippel-Trénaunay or Beckwith-Wiedemann syndromes.

2. Hamartoma—solitary well-defined mass with arterial enhancement persisting or equilibrating on the delayed phase, ± calcification ± fat content ± central scar. Usually hyperechoic on US and hypervascular on Doppler. Nearly isoattenuating to background spleen on unenhanced CT, and nearly T1/T2 isointense on MRI (cf. haemangioma). May be multiple in tuberous sclerosis or Wiskott-Aldrich syndrome.
3. **Sclerosing angiomatoid nodular transformation**—fibrosing variant of hamartoma. Solitary well-defined mass with centripetal delayed enhancement due to central fibrosis. Centrally T2 hypointense on MRI ± hypointense bands radiating to the edges.
4. **Littoral cell angioma**—usually numerous ill-defined hypovascular nodules which equilibrate with the background spleen on the delayed phase. Variable T2 signal on MRI depending on haemosiderin content. Splenomegaly is nearly always present.
5. **Other rare lesions**—inflammatory pseudotumour (usually large, variable appearance), lipoma (contains fat only), angiomyolipoma (fat + enhancing soft tissue, usually in tuberous sclerosis), solitary fibrous tumour (well-defined heterogeneous hypervascular mass ± calcification).

8

Malignant neoplasms

1. Lymphoma*—usually with splenomegaly and disease elsewhere. Can present as solitary or multiple homogeneous hypoechoic hypovascular masses, micronodules or diffuse splenomegaly without a discrete lesion. May invade adjacent organs. Leukaemia and extraosseous myeloma can appear similar.
2. Metastases—e.g. from melanoma, lung, breast, GI tract. Nearly always with disseminated metastases elsewhere. Pancreatic tail tumours can also directly invade the spleen.
3. Angiosarcoma—rare overall, but the most common primary nonhaematolymphoid splenic malignancy; usually seen in older adults. Solitary or multiple ill-defined heterogeneously enhancing masses ± calcification ± haemorrhage. Often metastatic at presentation.
4. **Haemangioendothelioma**—rare; usually seen in young adults, less aggressive than angiosarcoma. Large, well-defined, heterogeneous mass ± necrotic, haemorrhagic or calcified areas.
5. **Other rare sarcomas**—e.g. leiomyosarcoma, undifferentiated pleomorphic sarcoma. Large, heterogeneous, nonspecific mass.

Further reading

Ricci, Z.J., Oh, S.K., Chernyak, V., et al., 2016. Improving diagnosis of atraumatic splenic lesions, part I: nonneoplastic lesions. Clin. Imaging 40 (4), 769–779.

Ricci, Z.J., Mazzariol, F.S., Flusberg, M., et al., 2016. Improving diagnosis of atraumatic splenic lesions, part II: benign neoplasms/nonneoplastic mass-like lesions. Clin. Imaging 40 (4), 691–704.

Ricci, Z.J., Kaul, B., Stein, M.W., et al., 2016. Improving diagnosis of atraumatic splenic lesions, part III: malignant lesions. Clin. Imaging 40 (5), 846–855.

8.32 PANCREATIC CALCIFICATION

1. **Chronic pancreatitis**—especially due to alcohol (numerous, various sizes); can also be seen in chronic gallstone pancreatitis (smaller and fewer), hereditary pancreatitis (children and young adults) and tropical calcific pancreatitis (large ductal calculi in young patients in tropical developing countries). Rare in autoimmune pancreatitis. Calcification may be ductal or parenchymal.
2. **Vascular calcification**—e.g. splenic or gastroduodenal artery. Typically linear; may mimic parenchymal calcification.
3. **Pseudocyst**—can rim calcify or contain milk of calcium.
4. **Calcification within a tumour**—e.g. NET (coarse and irregular), serous cystadenoma (in central scar), mucinous cystadenoma (in wall or septa), IPMN, solid pseudopapillary neoplasm (peripheral and punctate), acinar cell carcinoma (variable pattern), haemangioma (phleboliths), pancreatoblastoma (children), mucinous metastasis (e.g. from GI tract). Calcification is almost never seen in primary adenocarcinoma.
5. **Hyperparathyroidism***—due to a combination of metastatic calcification (directly due to hypercalcaemia) and recurrent hypercalcaemia-induced pancreatitis. Most have nephrocalcinosis or urolithiasis, suggesting the diagnosis.
6. **Cystic fibrosis***—typically causes diffuse fatty replacement of the pancreas, but fine granular calcification can occur late in the disease.
7. **Shwachman-Diamond syndrome**—also causes diffuse fatty replacement of the pancreas; calcification is rarer than in CF.
8. **Dystrophic calcification**—e.g. following trauma, infection or infarction.
9. **Other mimics**—distal CBD stone, oral contrast within a duodenal diverticulum.

Further reading

Javadi, S., Menias, C.O., Korivi, B.R., et al., 2017. Pancreatic calcifications and calcified pancreatic masses: pattern recognition approach on CT. AJR Am. J. Roentgenol. 209 (1), 77–87.

8.33 PANCREATIC DUCT DILATATION

NB: the normal PD can measure up to 3.5 mm in the pancreatic head.

1. Pancreatic ductal adenocarcinoma—focal PD dilatation with an abrupt transition point should always be considered suspicious for an underlying adenocarcinoma, as these can be isoattenuating on CT. Look for focal splenic vein/portal confluence narrowing, upstream pancreatic atrophy and CBD dilatation. Endoscopic ultrasound (EUS) may be necessary for further assessment. PD obstruction is much less common with other pancreatic tumours.
2. Obstructing PD calculi—due to chronic pancreatitis.
3. Benign stricture—e.g. due to recurrent/chronic pancreatitis (strictures are often multifocal), trauma or surgery (e.g. pancreaticojejunostomy). Benign strictures tend to be shorter and smoother than malignant strictures.
4. Ampullary tumour/gallstone—CBD dilatation > PD dilatation.
5. Main duct IPMN—markedly dilated PD filled with mucin, usually extending to ampulla (which may bulge into duodenum) with dilated sidebranches ± intraluminal soft tissue. No focal strictures. High risk of malignancy.
6. **Necrotizing pancreatitis**—often results in PD disruption and pancreatic collections, and can cause PD obstruction ± fistula.
7. **Pancreas divisum**—dorsal duct drains into the minor ampulla which may drain poorly, resulting in mild PD dilatation.

8

8.34 CYSTIC PANCREATIC LESIONS

In practice, most indeterminate cystic lesions >2 cm in size will be considered for EUS-FNA if the patient would be fit for surgical resection. A high CEA level within the aspirated fluid suggests a mucinous lesion (i.e. sidebranch IPMN or mucinous cystadenoma), whereas a low CEA suggests either a pseudocyst (high amylase) or serous cystadenoma (low amylase). Mucinous lesions carry a risk of malignancy and are usually resected.

1. Pseudocyst—most common cystic pancreatic lesion. Usually unilocular with a mildly thick fibrous wall, ± internal debris ± fistula with PD. No enhancing solid components. Other signs of chronic pancreatitis are usually present, e.g. atrophy, calcification, PD irregularity, ectatic sidebranches. May become infected.
2. Ectatic PD sidebranch—common and early finding in chronic pancreatitis. Benign stricture at insertion of sidebranch onto the main PD causes focal sidebranch dilatation that can mimic a small (<1 cm) unilocular sidebranch IPMN. Often multiple.

3. Sidebranch IPMN—most common in older men ('grandfather'). Uni-/multilocular cyst communicating with PD (best seen on MRCP). Lower risk of malignancy versus main duct IPMN; enhancing solid components, size >3 cm and extension into the main PD (causing dilatation) are worrying features. Can be multiple.
4. Serous cystadenoma—usually in older women ('grandmother'), most common in the head. Typically multilocular and microcystic with innumerable tiny locules giving a honeycomb or sponge-like appearance. May have a characteristic central scar ± calcification. The cysts may be so small that the lesion appears solid and hypervascular on CT (microcysts are better appreciated on MRI). Occasionally macrocystic, mimicking a mucinous cystadenoma. No communication with PD. No malignant potential. Can be multiple in vHL disease.
5. Mucinous cystadenoma—almost exclusively in women (contains ovarian stroma), usually middle-aged ('mother'). Typically in the body/tail. Typically uni-/multilocular and macrocystic with large locules (>2 cm). No communication with PD. Mural nodularity, septal thickening or calcification are worrying for malignant transformation to mucinous cystadenocarcinoma.
6. Solid pseudopapillary tumour—almost exclusively in young adult women ('daughter'), especially Afro-Caribbeans. Large well-defined encapsulated mixed solid-cystic mass ± calcification, with peripheral irregular soft tissue and central cystic change, haemorrhage and necrosis. Usually benign.
7. **Neuroendocrine tumour**—can occasionally undergo marked cystic change (suggests malignant degeneration). Peripheral irregular/nodular arterial enhancement is usually present, differentiating this from other cystic lesions.
8. **Pancreatic adenocarcinoma**—can rarely be markedly necrotic or mucinous, appearing cystic. Look for associated duct obstruction and vascular occlusion.
9. **Cystic metastases**—e.g. from RCC, melanoma or lung. Rare.
10. **Epithelial (true) cyst**—rare; usually seen in autosomal dominant polycystic kidney disease, vHL disease and cystic fibrosis, where they are usually multiple. Thin-walled, unilocular, no solid components, no communication with PD.
11. **Lymphoepithelial cyst**—rare, benign; usually macrocystic, located in the body/tail. Similar appearance to mucinous cystadenoma except usually seen in men. May contain microscopic fat on in-/opposed-phase MRI ± T2 hypointensity and restricted diffusion due to keratin content.
12. **Acinar cystic transformation**—rare, benign. Solitary or multiple cysts in a clustered, segmental or diffuse distribution ± calcification. No communication with PD (cf. IPMN).

13. **Other rare cystic lesions**—cystic teratoma (+ fat and calcification), lymphangioma (multiloculated and thin-walled), endometrioma (blood products on MRI), hydatid cyst (characteristic appearance; see Section 8.16), pancreatoblastoma (nearly always in children).
14. **Mimics**—a fluid-filled duodenal diverticulum, duplication cyst, cystic dystrophy of the duodenal wall (due to paraduodenal pancreatitis) or CBD diverticulum may mimic a pancreatic cyst.

Further reading

Dewhurst, C.E., Mortele, K.J., 2012. Cystic tumors of the pancreas: imaging and management. Radiol. Clin. North Am. 50 (3), 467–486.

Khan, A., Khosa, F., Eisenberg, R.L., 2011. Cystic lesions of the pancreas. AJR Am. J. Roentgenol. 196 (6), W668–W677.

Sidden, C.R., Mortele, K.J., 2007. Cystic tumors of the pancreas: ultrasound, computed tomography, and magnetic resonance imaging features. Semin. Ultrasound CT MR 28 (5), 339–356.

8.35 SOLID PANCREATIC LESIONS

Best assessed on triple phase CT. Note that on MRI the pancreas is normally homogeneously T1 hyperintense relative to other solid organs, and most pathologies cause a reduction in T1 signal. Beware of tumours arising from adjacent organs mimicking a pancreatic mass, e.g. duodenal carcinoma or carcinoid, gastric GIST, renal and adrenal tumours, peripancreatic adenopathy. Other mimics include a normal duodenum passing through an annular pancreas, and a fatty pancreas with focal fatty sparing (typically in the posterior head/uncinate).

Hypovascular

Often best seen on the arterial phase as an area of reduced enhancement. The portal phase is best for assessing the effect on the portal venous system.

1. <u>Ductal adenocarcinoma</u>—ill-defined infiltrative hypovascular mass, usually causing PD obstruction, upstream atrophy and narrowing/occlusion of the splenic vein, superior mesenteric vein or portal confluence ± encasement of the superior mesenteric artery or coeliac axis. Tumours in the head tend to present earlier due to CBD obstruction and painless jaundice; tumours in the tail tend to present late with metastases. No calcification. The mass may be isoattenuating and very subtle—the secondary signs above may be the only indication of an underlying tumour.
2. <u>Focal pancreatitis</u>—can mimic carcinoma, or both may coexist. Associated nodular fat necrosis can mimic metastatic disease.

Acute inflammation tends to cause more ill-defined fat stranding, usually without CBD/PD dilatation. Portal or splenic vein thrombosis can be seen but narrowing does not usually occur acutely unless compressed by a collection. Other inflammatory mimics of pancreatic cancer include:

(a) **Chronic pancreatitis**—can create a focal fibroinflammatory mass, typically with calcification, most common in the head ± upstream PD dilatation due to obstructing ductal calculi. Mild CBD dilatation and splenic vein occlusion may also be seen. A narrow CBD/PD may be seen to traverse the mass ('duct-penetrating' sign; not seen with carcinoma).

(b) **Paraduodenal pancreatitis**—focal inflammation in the pancreaticoduodenal groove ± ill-defined sheet-like fibrous mass ± mild CBD/PD dilatation ± duodenal stricture. Cystic change is common (not usually seen with carcinoma). Tends to displace the pancreatic head and distal CBD away from the duodenum. Chronic calcific pancreatitis often coexists.

(c) **Autoimmune pancreatitis**—typically causes diffuse 'sausage-like' swelling of the pancreas with a thin discrete halo of fat stranding but can occasionally be focal, mimicking a mass. Common manifestation of IgG4-related disease. An associated stricture of the distal CBD can also be seen ± IgG4-cholangitis upstream. PD dilatation and vascular occlusion are typically absent (useful discriminating feature).

3. **Cholangiocarcinoma of the intrapancreatic CBD**—centered on and obstructs the CBD but does not usually obstruct the PD (cf. pancreatic ductal adenocarcinoma).
4. **Metastasis**—e.g. from lung (especially small-cell carcinoma), breast, melanoma, GI tract. Usually well-defined, often multiple, with disseminated metastases elsewhere. Duct obstruction and venous occlusion are much less common than with primary ductal adenocarcinoma.
5. **Lymphoma***—usually in the presence of nodal disease elsewhere. Homogeneous hypovascular mass which encases vessels without causing narrowing or CBD/PD obstruction.
6. **Solid pseudopapillary tumour**—see Section 8.34; can be completely solid.
7. **Acinar cell carcinoma**—well-defined heterogeneous mass ± necrosis/cystic change ± calcification, usually without CBD/PD dilatation. Can cause ectopic fat necrosis and bone infarcts due to lipase secretion.
8. **Hamartoma**—well-defined solid mass ± fat or cystic change.
9. **TB***—can rarely involve the pancreas creating a hypovascular mass ± cystic change, usually in the presence of TB elsewhere (e.g. necrotic nodes).
10. **Sarcoidosis***—very rare, typically in the presence of disease elsewhere. Single or multiple hypovascular masses.

11. **Other rare tumours**—e.g. granular cell tumour, inflammatory pseudotumour. Nonspecific appearances.

Hypervascular

Best seen on the arterial phase (may be isoattenuating on the portal phase). NB: these do not usually cause CBD/PD dilatation.

1. **Neuroendocrine tumour (NET)**—most are hyperfunctioning, presenting as a small hypervascular mass with a characteristic clinical syndrome. Nonfunctioning tumours are more likely to be malignant and present as a larger heterogeneously enhancing mass ± cystic change ± calcification ± tumour thrombus in the splenic/portal vein. NETs are associated with MEN1 (especially nonfunctioning and gastrinomas, typically multiple), vHL (nonfunctioning, often multiple), NF1 (especially periampullary somatostatinoma) and tuberous sclerosis (especially insulinoma).
   (a) **Insulinoma**—presents with episodes of hypoglycaemia. Usually benign, solitary and <2 cm in diameter. Even distribution throughout the pancreas.
   (b) **Gastrinoma**—presents with multiple peptic ulcers (Zollinger-Ellison syndrome)—look for diffuse gastric fold thickening. The majority are malignant. Typically located in the 'gastrinoma triangle' which includes the pancreatic head and neck. Variable size.
   (c) **Glucagonoma**—presents with 4D syndrome (dermatitis, diabetes, DVT, depression), weight loss and diarrhoea. Most are malignant. Typically >2 cm, usually in the body/tail.
   (d) **VIPoma**—presents with WDHA syndrome (profuse watery diarrhoea, hypokalaemia, achlorhydria)—look for multiple fluid-filled loops of bowel. Most are malignant. Typically >2 cm, most common in the tail.
   (e) **Somatostatinoma**—presents with diabetes, gallstones and steatorrhoea. Most are malignant. Typically >2 cm, most common in the head.
2. **Metastasis**—especially from RCC. May be an isolated finding many years after initial diagnosis, mimicking a NET.
3. **Intrapancreatic splenunculus**—typically small and in the tail. Enhances similarly to spleen (heterogeneous in arterial phase, homogeneous in portal phase). Identical signal characteristics to spleen on MRI.
4. **Vascular anomalies**—e.g. gastroduodenal/splenic artery aneurysms, intrapancreatic venous shunts due to portal venous system thrombosis.
5. **Serous cystadenoma**—can appear solid and hypervascular on CT; MRI better demonstrates microcystic nature (see Section 8.34).
6. **Haemangioma**—peripheral nodular enhancement with centripetal filling ± phleboliths.

8

7. **Schwannoma**—rare; mildly hypervascular ± necrosis/cystic change ± calcification.
8. **Castleman disease**—pancreatic involvement is very rare. Well-defined hypervascular mass ± cystic change ± calcification.
9. **Other rare tumours**—e.g. solitary fibrous tumour, leiomyosarcoma, other sarcomas. These are usually large masses with heterogeneous enhancement ± necrosis/cystic change ± calcification.

Further reading

Al-Hawary, M.M., Kaza, R.K., Asar, S.F., et al., 2013. Mimics of pancreatic ductal adenocarcinoma. Cancer Imaging 13 (3), 342–349.

Barral, M., Faraoun, S.A., Fishman, E.K., et al., 2016. Imaging features of rare pancreatic tumors. Diagn. Interv. Imaging 97 (12), 1259–1273.

De Juan, C., Sanchez, M., Miquel, R., et al., 2008. Uncommon tumors and pseudotumoral lesions of the pancreas. Curr. Probl. Diagn. Radiol. 37 (4), 145–164.

Low, G., Panu, A., Millo, N., Leen, E., 2011. Multimodality imaging of neoplastic and nonneoplastic solid lesions of the pancreas. Radiographics 31 (4), 993–1015.

Adrenals, urinary tract, testes and prostate

Chris J Harvey, Imran Syed, Qaiser Malik

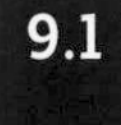 9.1 INCIDENTAL ADRENAL MASS (UNILATERAL)

Common incidental finding on CT. A mass <3 cm in diameter is likely to be benign and a mass >5 cm in diameter is probably malignant. On unenhanced CT, 98% of homogeneous adrenal masses with an attenuation of ≤10 HU will be benign (typically lipid-rich adenomas). Approximately 30% of adenomas will have an attenuation >10 HU (lipid-poor). For indeterminate lesions, i.e. those >10 HU, a contrast-enhanced scan with portal venous and delayed imaging is required to assess degree of enhancement and washout. A relative washout of >40% and an absolute washout of >60% (Table) are highly sensitive and specific for lipid-poor adenomas. Note that lesions with an unenhanced attenuation of >43 HU or a postcontrast attenuation of >120 HU are very unlikely to be adenomas, regardless of washout characteristics. Chemical shift MRI can also characterize lesions by assessing for the presence of microscopic fat (i.e. >20% signal dropout on out-of-phase images). FDG PET/CT can also be used to differentiate benign from malignant tumours, and to detect other metastases/primary tumours. Ultimately, biopsy may be required.

Method for calculating washout on adrenal CT	
Relative percentage washout	$\frac{\text{Enhanced HU} - \text{Delayed HU}}{\text{Enhanced HU}} \times 100$
Absolute percentage washout	$\frac{\text{Enhanced HU} - \text{Delayed HU}}{\text{Enhanced HU} - \text{Unenhanced HU}} \times 100$

Unenhanced HU: unenhanced attenuation (HU) of the lesion measured from a region of interest (ROI) placed on the lesion avoiding foci of calcification, necrosis or haemorrhage and lesion edge.
Enhanced HU: attenuation at 60 seconds following IV contrast (portal phase).
Delayed HU: attenuation at 15 minutes following IV contrast.

Note that collision tumours (a combination of two different neoplasms, most commonly adenoma + myelolipoma or adenoma + metastasis), can occur and will have imaging characteristics of both component tumours.

Functioning tumours

1. Conn's adenoma—accounts for 70% of Conn's syndrome. Usually small, homogeneous, relatively low density due to cholesterol content. 30% of Conn's syndrome is due to bilateral hyperplasia, which can occasionally be nodular and mimic an adenoma. Note that functioning and nonfunctioning adenomas are essentially indistinguishable on imaging, although functioning adenomas tend to be smaller and are more likely to be lipid-rich.
2. Phaeochromocytoma—usually large (>5 cm) with avid contrast enhancement ± central necrosis/haemorrhage (NB: it is safe to administer IV iodinated CT contrast). Often markedly T2 hyperintense on MRI. Rule of tens: 10% malignant, 10% bilateral, 10% ectopic—of these 50% are located around the kidney, particularly the renal hilum (if not seen on CT, MIBG isotope scan may be helpful). 10% show calcification. 10% are multiple and usually part of MEN 2A/B syndrome, NF1, tuberous sclerosis or vHL.
3. Cushing's adenoma—accounts for 10% of Cushing's syndrome. Usually >2 cm. 80% of Cushing's syndrome is due to excess ACTH from a pituitary adenoma (Cushing's disease) or ectopic source (small cell carcinoma, carcinoid, pancreatic NET, phaeochromocytoma, medullary thyroid carcinoma) with resultant adrenal hyperplasia. 10% of Cushing's syndrome is due to adrenal carcinoma. The differentials for an adrenal mass in Cushing's syndrome are:
   (a) Functioning adenoma/carcinoma—atrophy of the contralateral adrenal is suggestive.
   (b) Coincidental nonfunctioning adenoma—both adrenals may be hyperplastic (due to excess ACTH).
   (c) Metastasis from small cell primary.
   (d) Bilateral nodular hyperplasia—see Section 9.2.
4. Adrenal carcinoma—rare, usually large (>5 cm). Functioning tumours (<50%) may present with Cushing's, virilization, feminization or rarely Conn's, and are more common in women.

Malignant tumours

1. Metastases—often bilateral, usually >2 cm, irregular outline with patchy contrast enhancement. Common sources include lung, breast, renal and GI tract. Metastases from melanoma and RCC are usually hypervascular and may mimic phaeochromocytoma. Recent haemorrhage into a vascular metastasis can produce patchy high

attenuation on unenhanced CT. In patients without a known extraadrenal primary tumour, the vast majority of adrenal masses are benign; in the presence of a known primary malignancy 26-36% of adrenal lesions are metastatic.

2. **Carcinoma**—rare, aggressive. Typically a large (>5 cm), irregular, heterogeneously enhancing mass with central necrosis/ haemorrhage ± foci of calcification and nodal, metastatic and/or intravenous spread. May invade the adjacent kidney, making it difficult to distinguish from an advanced RCC. Nonfunctioning tumours (>50%) are more common in men and present at a larger size than functioning tumours.
3. **Lymphoma***—usually secondary in the presence of retroperitoneal nodal disease. Unilateral or bilateral adrenal masses/diffuse enlargement + mild homogeneous enhancement.
4. **Neuroblastoma**—very rare in adults. Usually large (>5 cm), ill-defined and heterogeneous + calcification. Commonly surrounds and displaces vessels (e.g. aorta and IVC) without causing significant narrowing. Metastases are common at presentation.
5. **Sarcoma**—e.g. angiosarcoma, leiomyosarcoma. Very rare. Nonspecific appearances: aggressive, irregular, heterogeneously enhancing mass.

Benign

1. **Nonfunctioning adenoma**—very common. Usually small (50% <2 cm), homogeneous and well-defined. If lipid-rich, will have unenhanced CT attenuation <10 HU and will drop signal on out-of-phase T1-weighted MRI.
2. **Myelolipoma**—benign tumour composed of fat and haemopoietic tissue. Characteristic appearance on CT: discrete mass containing soft tissue and macroscopic fat (<–20 HU) ± calcification. On MRI the fatty component will drop signal on fatsat sequences. If large, may be hard to differentiate from retroperitoneal liposarcoma and exophytic renal AML. Nearly all are found in the adrenal, but extraadrenal tumours (presacral, perirenal, retroperitoneum, mediastinum, liver, stomach, omentum) can occur.
3. **Adrenal haemorrhage**—hyperattenuating mass on unenhanced CT with surrounding fat stranding. Occurs in 25% of severe trauma (usually unilateral, R>L), but can also occur in vascular masses (e.g. phaeochromocytoma, metastases), coagulopathies and severe stress (e.g. surgery, sepsis, burns, pregnancy, hypotension—often bilateral).
4. **Cyst**—round, well-defined, water density, nonenhancing. May contain thin septa ± mural calcification. Pseudocysts due to previous haemorrhage > true cysts. Beware of cystic tumours (e.g. some phaeochromocytomas)—look for nodular wall thickening. If multiloculated, consider lymphangioma and hydatid cyst in the differential.

9

5. Granulomatous disease—e.g. TB, histoplasmosis. More commonly bilateral, see Section 9.2.
6. **Haemangioma**—rare. Often contains phleboliths. Typically demonstrates peripheral nodular enhancement ± partial infilling on delayed phase. Central fibrotic scar usually does not enhance. Peripheral nonfibrotic component is usually markedly T2 hyperintense. May mimic phaeochromocytoma.
7. **Ganglioneuroma**—rare, occurs in children or young adults. Benign counterpart of neuroblastoma, arises from sympathetic ganglia. Well-defined, often shows heterogeneous delayed enhancement. Heterogeneously T2 hyperintense on MRI ± whorled appearance. Calcification is common.
8. **Other very rare lesions**—adrenal lipoma, teratoma and angiomyolipoma can mimic myelolipoma due to macroscopic fat content (a fat–fluid level suggests teratoma). Schwannomas may be cystic ± calcification. Solitary fibrous tumours, leiomyomas, oncocytomas and inflammatory pseudotumours have also been rarely reported in the adrenals
and present as a nonspecific solid heterogeneously enhancing mass.
9. **Pseudolesions**—e.g. exophytic renal/hepatic/pancreatic mass, gastric diverticulum, splenunculus, retroperitoneal varices. These can occasionally mimic an adrenal mass but IV/oral contrast and coronal reconstructions will nearly always clarify the diagnosis.

Further reading

Adam, S.Z., Nikolaidis, P., Horowitz, J.M., et al., 2016. Chemical Shift MR Imaging of the adrenal gland: principles, pitfalls, and applications. Radiographics 36, 414–432.

Blake, M.A., Cronin, C.G., Boland, G.W., 2010. Adrenal imaging. AJR Am. J. Roentgenol. 194, 1450–1460.

Boland, G.W., Blake, M.A., Hahn, P.F., Mayo-Smith, W.W., 2008. Incidental adrenal lesions: principles, techniques, and algorithms for imaging characterization. Radiology 249 (3), 756–775.

Boland, G.W., Dwamena, B.A., Jagtiani Sangwaiya, M., et al., 2011. Characterization of adrenal masses by using FDG PET: a systematic review and meta-analysis of diagnostic test performance. Radiology 259 (1), 117–126.

Johnson, P.T., Horton, K.M., Fishman, E.K., 2009. Adrenal mass imaging with multidetector CT: pathologic conditions, pearls, and pitfalls. Radiographics 29 (5), 1333–1351.

Lattin, G.E., Jr., Sturgill, E.D., Tujo, C.A., et al., 2014. From the radiologic pathology archives: adrenal tumors and tumor-like conditions in the adult: radiologic-pathologic correlation. Radiographics 34, 805–829.

Low, G., Dhliwayo, H., Lomas, D.J., 2012. Adrenal neoplasms. Clin. Radiol. 67, 988–1000.

9.2 BILATERAL ADRENAL MASSES

1. Metastases—bilateral in 15%. Usually do not affect adrenal function; may cause adrenal insufficiency if extensive (replacing >80% of adrenal gland).
2. Phaeochromocytoma—bilateral in 10%. Suggests an underlying hereditary cause, e.g. MEN 2A/B, NF1, tuberous sclerosis or vHL.
3. Adenomas—due to the prevalence of adenomas, they can occasionally be bilateral.
4. Hyperplasia—congenital adrenal hyperplasia results in symmetrically enlarged and thickened adrenal glands in children. In adults, adrenal hyperplasia has several causes:
   (a) ACTH-dependent hyperplasia—more commonly due to ectopic ACTH secretion, but can occur in Cushing's disease. Adrenals are usually mildly and diffusely enlarged but may be nodular in morphology.
   (b) ACTH-independent macronodular adrenocortical hyperplasia (AIMAH)—rare. Multiple bilateral large adrenal adenomas, each typically >1 cm and lipid-rich.
   (c) Primary pigmented nodular adrenocortical disease (PPNAD)—rare, autosomal dominant, typically presents in young females. Multiple bilateral adrenal micronodules, each usually <5 mm. Strongly associated with Carney complex.
5. Adrenal haemorrhage—often bilateral in cases due to severe haemodynamic stress.
6. Granulomatous disease—histoplasmosis/TB. Bilateral adrenal masses/enlargement ± central necrosis ± adrenal insufficiency in the acute setting. Results in adrenal atrophy and calcification in the chronic setting.
7. **Lymphoma***—primary adrenal lymphoma is rare; typically presents with bilateral large homogeneous adrenal masses/diffuse enlargement, often with adrenal insufficiency. Secondary adrenal involvement is more common, usually without adrenal insufficiency.

Further reading

Gupta, P., Bhalla, A., Sharma, R., 2012. Bilateral adrenal lesions. J. Med. Imaging Radiat. Oncol. 56, 636–645.

9.3 ADRENAL CALCIFICATION

1. Previous haemorrhage—unilateral or bilateral depending on aetiology. Old haemorrhage within a mass lesion (e.g. a large adenoma, myelolipoma or hypervascular metastasis) can also lead to calcification.

9

2. **Cystic disease**—curvilinear calcification within the cyst wall/septa. More common in pseudocysts than true cysts. Can also be seen in chronic hydatid cysts.
3. **Chronic TB*/histoplasmosis**—atrophic calcified adrenals (often bilateral).
4. **Calcification within a tumour**—e.g. adrenal carcinoma (irregular punctate calcifications in 30%), phaeochromocytoma (10%), neuroblastoma (up to 90%, coarse/amorphous pattern), ganglioneuroma (fine/speckled pattern), haemangioma (phleboliths), teratoma and certain metastases (e.g. from mucinous adenocarcinoma, osteosarcoma).
5. **Addison's disease**—calcification is rare in primary autoimmune disease, and suggests a secondary cause, e.g. previous haemorrhage, TB or histoplasmosis.
6. **Wolman disease**—rare autosomal recessive lysosomal acid lipase deficiency resulting in accumulation of cholesterol and triglycerides in organs. Presents in early infancy with failure to thrive. Pathognomonic appearance of enlarged densely calcified adrenals on AXR, US or CT. Fatty infiltration and enlargement of the liver, spleen and lymph nodes also occurs.

Further reading

Elsayes, K.M., Emad-Eldin, S., Morani, A.C., Jensen, C.T., 2017. Practical approach to adrenal imaging. Radiol. Clin. North Am. 55 (2), 279–301. Review.

Hindman, N., Israel, G.M., 2005. Adrenal gland and adrenal mass calcification. Eur. Radiol. 15 (6), 1163–1167.

9.4 CONGENITAL RENAL ANOMALIES

These may be anomalies of position, form or number, and are twice as common in men versus women.

Anomalies of position

All malpositioned kidneys are malrotated. Most commonly malrotation occurs around the vertical axis with collecting structures positioned ventrally.

1. **Ectopic kidney**—typically sited caudal to usual site. A pelvic kidney is due to failure of renal ascent. Blood supply is from the iliac artery or aorta. Most ectopic kidneys are asymptomatic, although pelvic kidneys are more susceptible to trauma, reflux, stone formation, PUJ obstruction and infection, and may complicate natural childbirth later in life. Rarely, a kidney may herniate through a Bochdalek hernia during its ascent, giving rise to an intrathoracic kidney.

Anomalies of form

These are associated with an increased risk of reflux, infection, stone formation, PUJ obstruction and other congenital anomalies (e.g. VACTERL association; see Part 2).

1. **Horseshoe kidney**—two kidneys joined by parenchymal/fibrous isthmus, typically at the lower poles. Ascent is arrested by the inferior mesenteric artery. Most common fusion anomaly (1 in 400 births). Both kidneys are malrotated with the renal pelves and ureters situated anteriorly and renal long axis medially oriented. Associated with many congenital syndromes (e.g. Turner) and an increased risk of malignancy (Wilms, TCC, RCC).
2. **Crossed renal ectopia**—kidney is located on opposite side of midline from its ureteral orifice. Usually L→R. The lower kidney is usually ectopic. In 90% there is fusion of both kidneys (crossed fused ectopia).
3. **Pancake/discoid kidney**—bilateral fused pelvic kidneys, usually near the aortic bifurcation.
4. **Renal hypoplasia**—incomplete development results in a smaller kidney (<50% of normal size) with fewer calyces and papillae. Normal function.

Anomalies of number

1. **Unilateral renal agenesis**—1 in 1000 live births. Associated with chromosomal abnormalities, VACTERL anomalies, Müllerian duct anomalies (in women) and Zinner syndrome (in men: renal agenesis + ipsilateral seminal vesicle cyst + ejaculatory duct obstruction). Hyperplastic normal solitary kidney—up to twice the normal size.
2. **Bilateral renal agenesis**—Potter syndrome. 1 in 10,000 live births. Invariably fatal in first few days of life due to pulmonary hypoplasia secondary to the associated oligohydramnios.
3. **Supernumerary kidney**—very rare. Most commonly on left side caudal to normal kidney. May be partially fused with the normal kidney mimicking a duplex kidney, but the two components will have separate arterial and venous supply.

9

Further reading

Cohen, H.L., Kravets, F., Zucconi, W., et al., 2004. Congenital abnormalities of the genitourinary system. Semin. Roentgenol. 39 (2), 282–303.

Servaes, S., Epelman, M., 2013. The current state of imaging pediatric genitourinary anomalies and abnormalities. Curr. Probl. Diagn. Radiol. 42 (1), 1–12.

Surabhi, V.R., Menias, C.O., George, V., et al., 2015. MDCT and MR urogram spectrum of congenital anomalies of the kidney and urinary tract diagnosed in adulthood. AJR Am. J. Roentgenol. 205 (3), W294–W304.

9.5 LOCALIZED BULGE OF THE RENAL OUTLINE ON IVU

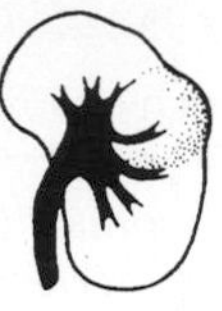

RENAL CYST
US confirms typical echo-free cyst

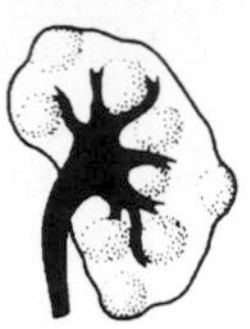

MULTIPLE RENAL CYSTS
e.g. adult type polycystic disease. Spider leg deformity of calyces

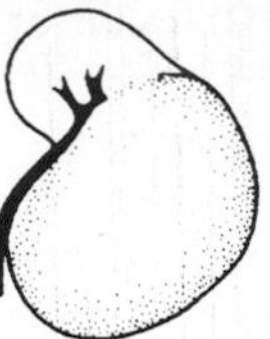

TUMOUR
Replacement of much or all of normal renal tissue

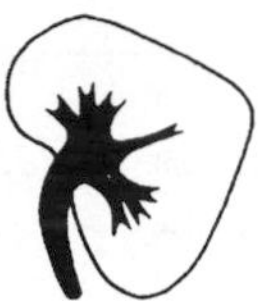

DROMEDARY HUMP
Left-sided variant

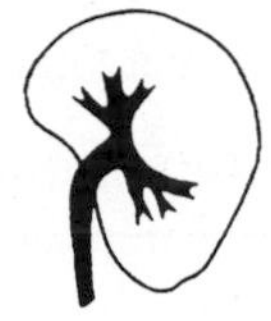

PROMINENT SEPTUM OF BERTIN
Increased activity on Tc-DMSA scanning

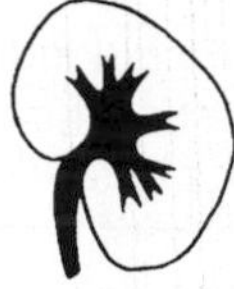

HILAR LIP
Hyperplasia of parenchyma adjacent to the renal hilum. Normal on Tc-DMSA scan

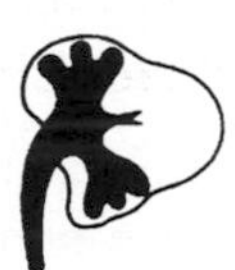

PSEUDOTUMOUR IN REFLUX NEPHROPATHY
Hypertrophy of unscarred renal parenchyma

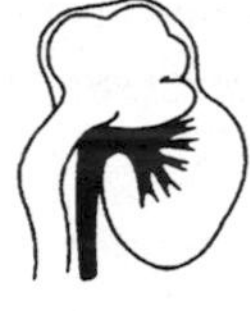

DUPLEX KIDNEY WITH HYDRONEPHROTIC UPPER MOIETY
Drooping flower appearance

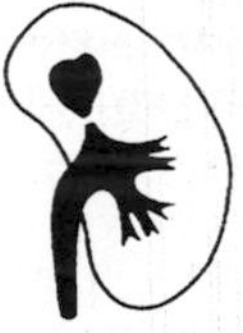

DILATATION OF A SINGLE CALYX
Most commonly due to extrinsic compression by an intrarenal artery (Fraley syndrome)

Redrawn from Taylor C.M. & Chapman S. (1989) *Handbook of Renal Investigations in Children*. London: Wright. By kind permission of the publisher.

1. Cyst—well-defined nephrographic defect with a thin wall on the outer margin. Beak sign. Displacement and distortion of smooth-walled calyces without obliteration.
2. Tumour—mostly RCC in adults and Wilms tumour in children. See Section 9.18.

3. <u>**Fetal lobulation**</u>—the lobule directly overlies a normal calyx. Normal interpapillary line. See Section 9.6.
4. <u>**Dromedary hump**</u>—on the midportion of the lateral border of the left kidney. Due to prolonged pressure by the spleen during fetal development. The arc of the interpapillary line parallels the renal contour.
5. <u>**Splenic impression**</u>—on the left side only, producing an apparent bulge inferiorly.
6. <u>**Enlarged septum of Bertin**</u>—overgrowth of the renal cortex from two adjacent renal lobules. Usually between upper and interpolar portion. Excretory urography shows a pseudomass with calyceal splaying and associated short calyx ± attempted duplication. DMSA accumulates normally or in excess. On US echogenicity is usually similar to the normal renal cortex but may be increased. CT and contrast-enhanced US, enhances similar to the cortex.
7. **Localized compensatory hypertrophy**—e.g. adjacent to an area of pyelonephritic scarring.
8. **Acute focal nephritis (lobar nephronia)**—usually an ill-defined hypoechoic mass on US, but may be hyperechoic. CT shows an ill-defined, low-attenuation, wedge-shaped mass with reduced contrast enhancement.
9. **Abscess**—loss of renal outline and psoas margin on the control film. Scoliosis concave to the involved side. Initially there is no nephrographic defect, but following central necrosis there will be a central defect surrounded by a thick irregular wall. Adjacent calyces are displaced or effaced.
10. **Nonfunctioning moiety of a duplex**—usually a hydronephrotic upper moiety. Delayed films may show contrast medium in the upper moiety calyces. Lower moiety calyces display the 'drooping lily' appearance.

9

Further reading

Bhatt, S., MacLennan, G., Dogra, V., 2007. Renal pseudotumors. AJR Am. J. Roentgenol. 188 (5), 1380–1387.

Israel, G.M., Silverman, S.G., 2011. The incidental renal mass. Radiol. Clin. North Am. 49, 369–383.

O'Connor, S.D., Pickhardt, P.J., Kim, D.H., et al., 2011. Incidental finding of renal masses at unenhanced CT: prevalence and analysis of features for guiding management. AJR Am. J. Roentgenol. 197 (1), 139–145.

Silverman, S.G., Israel, G.M., Herts, B.R., Richie, J.P., 2008. Management of the incidental renal mass. Radiology 249 (1), 16–31.

9.6 UNILATERAL SCARRED KIDNEY

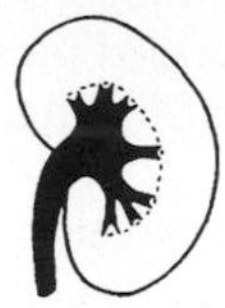

NORMAL
Cortex parallel to interpapillary line

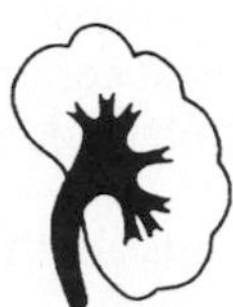

FETAL LOBULATION
Normal size. Cortical depressions between papillae

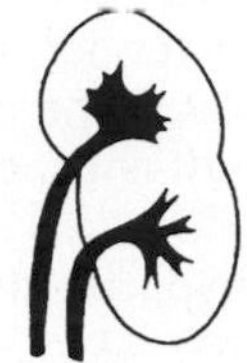

DUPLEX KIDNEY
Renal size usually larger than normal

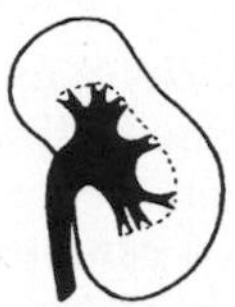

SPLEEN IMPRESSION
Right kidney may show hepatic impression

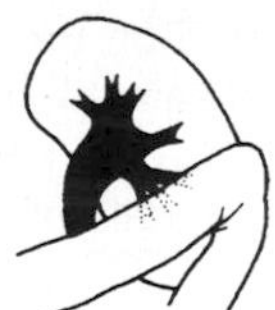

OVERLYING BOWEL
Spurious loss of cortex

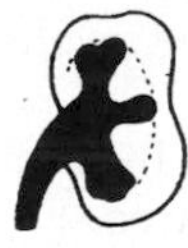

REFLUX NEPHROPATHY
Focal scars over dilated calyces. Most prominent at upper and lower poles. May be bilateral

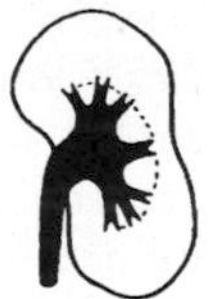

LOBAR INFARCTION
Broad depression over a normal calyx

Redrawn from Taylor C.M. & Chapman S. (1989) *Handbook of Renal Investigations in Children*. London: Wright. By kind permission of the publisher.

1. **Reflux nephropathy**—focal cortical scar over a dilated calyx. Usually multifocal and may be bilateral. Scarring is most prominent at the upper and lower poles.
2. **Tuberculous autonephrectomy** (putty kidney)—calcification differentiates it from the other members of this section.
3. **Lobar infarction**—a broad contour depression over a normal calyx. Normal interpapillary line.
4. **Renal dysplasia**—a forme fruste of multicystic kidney. Dilated calyces. Indistinguishable from chronic pyelonephritis.

Differential diagnosis

1. Persistent fetal lobulation—lobules overlie calyces with interlobular septa between the calyces. Normal size kidney.

9.7 UNILATERAL SMALL SMOOTH KIDNEY

The most common causes are postobstructive, ischaemia and postinflammatory. In all these cases chronic unilateral disease is associated with compensatory contralateral renal hypertrophy.

Prerenal = vascular

Usually with a small volume collecting system. This is a sign of diminished urinary volume and, together with global cortical thinning, delayed opacification of the calyces, increased density of the opacified collecting system and delayed washout following oral fluids or diuretics, indicates ischaemia.

1. Ischaemia due to renal artery stenosis—ureteric notching (due to enlarged collateral vessels) differentiates this from the other causes in this group. See Section 9.25.
2. **Radiation nephritis**—at least 23 Gy over 5 weeks. The collecting system may be normal or small. Depending on the size of the radiation field, both, one or just part of one kidney may be affected.
3. **End result of renal infarction**—due to previous renal artery occlusion or renal vein thrombosis. The collecting system does not usually opacify during excretion urography.

Renal = parenchymal

1. Congenital hypoplasia—<6 calyces. The pelvicalyceal system is otherwise normal.
2. Multicystic dysplastic kidney (adult).
3. Papillary necrosis—late sequela. See Section 9.23.
4. **Postinflammatory**—following acute diffuse nephritis especially in diabetes.
5. **Following partial nephrectomy.**

Postrenal = collecting system

Usually with a dilated collecting system.

1. Postobstructive atrophy—± thinning of the renal cortex and if there is impaired renal function this will be revealed by poor contrast medium density in the collecting system.

9.8 BILATERAL SMALL SMOOTH KIDNEYS

The most common causes are ischaemia due to hypotension, chronic glomerulonephritis, late diabetic nephropathy and chronic pyelonephritis. Most of the unilateral causes can also occur bilaterally.

Prerenal = vascular

1. **Arterial hypotension**—distinguished by the time relationship to the contrast medium injection and its transient nature.
2. **Generalized arteriosclerosis**—normal calyces.

Renal = parenchymal

1. **Chronic glomerulonephritis**—normal calyces. Reduced nephrogram density and poor calyceal opacification.
2. **Hereditary nephropathies**—e.g. Alport's syndrome.

Postrenal = collecting system

1. **Chronic papillary necrosis**—with other signs of necrotic papillae (see Section 9.23).

9.9 UNILATERAL LARGE SMOOTH KIDNEY

The most common causes are duplex kidneys, compensatory hypertrophy and obstruction.

Prerenal = vascular

1. **Acute renal vein thrombosis**—enlarged kidney + surrounding oedema + filling defect in the renal vein (best seen on CT). On US the kidney may be hyper- or hypoechoic ± absent Doppler venous flow ± visible thrombus. Echogenic streaks may be seen radiating from the renal hilum (representing thrombosed veins). Most common causes are nephrotic syndrome (in adults) and dehydration/sepsis (in children). Many other causes including intrinsic renal diseases (pyelonephritis, glomerulonephritis, amyloid), hypercoagulable states (pregnancy, OCP, malignancy, thrombophilia), extrinsic compression (by tumour, nodes or RPF), vasculitis, sickle cell disease, trauma, transplant rejection. Beware of tumour thrombus due to renal vein invasion from RCC—this shows enhancement, whereas bland thrombus is nonenhancing.
2. **Acute arterial infarction**—well-defined wedge-shaped areas of reduced Doppler flow on US and reduced enhancement on CT. Usually embolic, may be bilateral.

Renal = parenchymal

1. **Duplex kidney**—50% are bigger than the contralateral kidney; 40% are the same size; 10% are smaller.
2. **Compensatory hypertrophy**—for an atrophic/absent contralateral kidney.
3. **Crossed fused ectopia**—see Section 9.4.
4. **Acute pyelonephritis**—impaired excretion of contrast medium ± dense nephrogram. Attenuated calyces but may have nonobstructive pelvicalyceal or ureteric dilatation. Completely reversible within a few weeks of clinical recovery.
5. **Diffuse infiltrative tumour**—e.g. lymphoma/leukaemia (usually bilateral).
6. **Malakoplakia**—renal involvement may be diffuse causing enlargement.

Postrenal = collecting system

1. **Obstructed kidney**—dilated calyces and renal pelvis.
2. **Xanthogranulomatous pyelonephritis**—staghorn calculus is typically present with dilated calyces and a contracted renal pelvis (bear's paw appearance) ± distortion of the renal outline and perinephric stranding.
3. **Pyonephrosis**—obstructed kidney + echogenic pus in collecting system + urothelial thickening.

Further reading

Pickhardt, P.J., Lonergan, G.J., Davis, C.J., Jr., et al., 2000. Infiltrative renal lesions: radiologic–pathologic correlation. Radiographics 20, 215–243.

9.10 BILATERAL LARGE SMOOTH KIDNEYS

The most common causes are bilateral duplex kidneys, bilateral hydronephrosis, acute glomerulonephritis and nephrotic syndrome. Most of the unilateral causes can also occur bilaterally.

Developmental

1. **Bilateral duplex kidneys**.
2. **Autosomal recessive polycystic kidney disease***—infantile form. On US, smooth enlarged hyperechoic kidneys with numerous tiny cysts and echobright foci.

Inflammation/oedema

1. **Acute glomerulonephritis**—many different causes including Wegener's granulomatosis, microscopic polyangiitis, Goodpasture's syndrome, SLE, HSP, infections, drugs. Renal cortex may be diffusely hyperechoic on US.

2. Acute tubular necrosis—usually due to hypoperfusion or toxins (e.g. drugs, iodinated contrast, haemolysis, rhabdomyolysis). Hyperechoic (or normal) renal cortex on US. Persistent nephrogram on delayed postcontrast CT.
3. Acute cortical necrosis—>50% of cases are related to pregnancy (placental abruption, infected abortion, preeclampsia). Other causes include shock, sepsis, trauma, hyperacute transplant rejection, HUS, sickle cell disease, NSAIDs. Enhancing medulla and renal capsule with nonenhancing cortex on CT. Hypoechoic renal cortex on US. Cortical calcification is a late finding.
4. **Acute interstitial nephritis**—most commonly an allergic drug reaction. Other causes include autoimmune disease, acute transplant rejection and various infections. Renal cortex may be hyperechoic on US.
5. **Polyarteritis nodosa**—microaneurysms of renal artery branches + small renal infarcts.

Deposition of abnormal proteins

1. Amyloid—secondary > primary amyloid. Kidneys may be enlarged in acute disease ± focal mass lesions. Chronic deposition results in small kidneys ± amorphous calcifications.
2. Multiple myeloma*—kidneys may be enlarged ± focal masses. Usually in the setting of disseminated skeletal disease.

Neoplastic infiltration

Leukaemia and lymphoma*—usually bilateral.

Miscellaneous

1. Bilateral hydronephrosis.
2. Acute renal papillary necrosis (see Section 9.23).
3. Acute uric acid nephropathy/tumour lysis syndrome—massive tumour lysis following chemotherapy results in acute kidney injury due to precipitation of uric acid and calcium phosphate crystals in the renal tubules. Usually occurs in the setting of advanced lymphoma or leukaemia. CT may show enlarged kidneys with acute stone formation and/or milk of calcium in the collecting systems ± obstruction.
4. **Early diabetic nephropathy**—renal echotexture is usually normal.
5. **Sickle cell anaemia***—in early disease. The renal pyramids are often echobright on US ± papillary necrosis. The kidneys atrophy in chronic disease.
6. **HIV-associated nephropathy**—bilateral enlarged hyperechoic kidneys + urothelial thickening ± effacement of renal sinus fat.
7. **Acromegaly* and gigantism**—as part of the generalized visceromegaly. Tall stature, obesity and steroid use can also result in large kidneys with normal echotexture.

Further reading

Davidson, A.J., 1999. Renal parenchymal disease. In: Davidson, A.J., Hartman, D.S., Choyke, P.L., Wagner, B.J. (Eds.), Radiology of the Kidney and Genitourinary Tract, third ed. WB Saunders, Philadelphia, PA, pp. 73–358.

9.11 RENAL CALCIFICATION

Calculi—see Section 9.12.
Nephrocalcinosis—see Section 9.14.

Dystrophic calcification due to localized disease

Usually in one kidney or focally in one kidney.

1. Infections
   (a) **Chronic pyelonephritis**—focal unilateral/asymmetrical cortical calcification with associated parenchymal scarring. Pyogenic abscesses can rarely calcify.
   (b) **Tuberculosis***—variable appearance of nodular, curvilinear or amorphous calcification, usually within dilated calyces or tuberculous abscess → end-stage putty kidney. Typically multifocal with calcification elsewhere in the urinary tract. In the early stage there may be triangular ring-like medullary calcification due to papillary necrosis. The urogenital tract is the second commonest site of involvement after the lungs.
   (c) **Xanthogranulomatous pyelonephritis**—large obstructive calculus in 80% of cases.
   (d) **Hydatid**—the cyst is usually polar and calcification is curvilinear or heterogeneous. 50% of echinococcal cysts calcify.
2. **Tumours**—e.g. RCC, Wilms tumour, TCC, metastasis.
3. **Cysts**—rim/septal calcification, usually related to previous infection or haemorrhage. Common in ADPKD.
4. **Vascular**—e.g. in a chronic perinephric haematoma, or curvilinear calcification in atherosclerotic/aneurysmal renal arteries.

Further reading

Dyer, R.B., Chen, M.Y., Zagoria, R.J., 1998. Abnormal calcifications in the urinary tract. Radiographics 18 (6), 1405–1424.

Dyer, R.B., Chen, M.Y., Zagoria, R.J., 2004. Classical signs in uroradiology. Radiographics 24, S247–S280.

9.12 RENAL CALCULI

Most common cause of renal calcification. Stones <500 HU on CT are likely to be radiolucent on plain film. Stones >1000 HU, homogeneous in density and >10 cm deep to the skin surface are less likely to respond to extracorporeal shock wave lithotripsy.

Ureteric stones <5 mm are likely to pass spontaneously. Obstructing stones cause upstream ureteric and pelvicalyceal dilatation ± perinephric/periureteric stranding. The main differentials for renal stones on unenhanced CT are vascular calcifications (linear, sited within renal sinus fat rather than in the collecting system) and Randall's plaques (<2 mm foci of calcification at the tips of the renal papillae, which act as a nidus for calcium oxalate stone formation). The main differential for a ureteric stone on unenhanced CT is an adjacent phlebolith, particularly in the pelvis. Differentiating features of a phlebolith include round morphology, radiolucent centre, relatively low attenuation (<280 HU) and comet tail sign (streak of soft tissue extending from the calcification, which represents the occluded vein). Small ureteric stones tend to show the 'soft tissue rim' sign which represents the oedematous ureteric wall around the stone.

Calcium-containing

75% are calcium oxalate/phosphate. Usually very dense (up to 1700 HU on CT). Causes include:

1. **With normocalcaemia**—obstruction, UTI, prolonged bed rest, dehydration, congenital renal anomalies (e.g. horseshoe kidney), calyceal/bladder diverticula, Cushing's syndrome, type 1 renal tubular acidosis, medullary sponge kidney, idiopathic hypercalciuria.
2. **With hypercalcaemia**—hyperparathyroidism, milk-alkali syndrome, excess vitamin D, sarcoidosis, idiopathic infantile hypercalcaemia.

Pure calcium oxalate

Due to hyperoxaluria. Can lead to oxalosis (deposition of oxalate in extrarenal organs) if untreated.

1. **Secondary hyperoxaluria**—mainly in patients with Crohn's disease, small bowel resection, high vitamin C intake or chronic renal failure/dialysis.
2. **Primary hyperoxaluria**—rare, autosomal recessive, typically presents in childhood. Radiologically: cortical and medullary nephrocalcinosis (generally diffuse and homogeneous), recurrent renal stones, dense vascular calcification, osteopenia or renal osteodystrophy and abnormal metaphyses (dense/lucent bands).

Struvite

Account for 15% of calculi overall, and 70% of staghorn calculi. Caused by urease-producing bacterial UTI (e.g. *Proteus, Klebsiella, Pseudomonas, Enterobacter*—not *E. coli*); more common in women.

Cystine

Due to inherited cystinuria, presents in younger patients. Stones are usually <550 HU on CT, often large in size (may be staghorn) and homogeneous in density.

Uric acid

Usually <500 HU on CT, typically form in acidic urine. Causes include:

1. **With hyperuricaemia**—gout, myeloproliferative disorders and tumour lysis syndrome.
2. **With normouricaemia**—idiopathic or associated with acidic, concentrated urine, e.g. in hot climates and in chronic diarrhoea (including ileostomy patients).

Xanthine

Rare, due to xanthinuria, which may be primary (hereditary xanthinuria) or secondary (due to allopurinol). Stones are radiolucent on plain film but radiopaque on CT.

Stones radiolucent on CT (soft-tissue attenuation)

Rare. Suspect in patients with ureteric obstruction without a visible cause on unenhanced CT. CT urography will show the stone as a filling defect.

1. **Protease inhibitors, e.g. Indinavir**—used in HIV treatment. Most common medication-induced calculus—other causes include sulphonamides, ciprofloxacin, ephedrine, guaifenesin.
2. **Matrix**—mainly composed of mucoproteins. Tend to occur in patients with a history of UTIs, renal stones or proteinuria on dialysis.

9

Further reading

Blake, S.P., McNicholas, M.M., Raptopoulos, V., 1999. Nonopaque crystal deposition causing ureteric obstruction in patients with HIV undergoing indinavir therapy. AJR Am. J. Roentgenol. 171 (3), 717–720.

Cheng, P.M., Moin, P., Dunn, M.D., et al., 2012. What the radiologist needs to know about urolithiasis: part 1 – pathogenesis, types, assessment, and variant anatomy. AJR 198 (6), W540–W547.

Cheng, P.M., Moin, P., Dunn, M.D., et al., 2012. What the radiologist needs to know about urolithiasis: part 2 – CT findings, reporting, and treatment. AJR 198 (6), W548–W554.

Dyer, R.B., Chen, M.Y., Zagoria, R.J., 1998. Abnormal calcifications in the urinary tract. Radiographics 18 (6), 1405–1424.

Sandhu, C., Anson, K.M., Patel, U., 2003. Urinary tract stones – Part I: role of radiological imaging in diagnosis and treatment planning. Clin. Radiol. 58 (6), 415–421.

Sandhu, C., Anson, K.M., Patel, U., 2003. Urinary tract stones – Part II: current state of treatment. Clin. Radiol. 58 (6), 422–423.

9.13 MIMICS OF RENAL COLIC ON UNENHANCED CT UROGRAPHY

9% to 29% of patients presenting with flank pain may have alternative diagnoses other than renal colic at unenhanced CT. A renal or ureteric stone will be detected on CT in 33%–55% of patients with acute flank pain. If unenhanced CT demonstrates unilateral perinephric stranding or nephromegaly but no stones, the use of IV contrast should be considered.

Nonstone genitourinary

1. **Pyelonephritis**—asymmetric perinephric stranding or mild renal enlargement. Mild disease may have no signs on unenhanced CT. Post IV contrast, pyelonephritis may be seen as a focal region of low attenuation or a more widespread striated enhancement of the kidney. Renal or perinephric abscesses are rare sequelae.
2. **Congenital PUJ obstruction**—hydronephrosis with a sudden transition to normal at the PUJ without a visible cause on CT.
3. **Ureteric obstruction by any other cause**.
4. **Cystitis**.
5. **Renal neoplasm**—e.g. RCC, TCC.
6. **Perinephric/subcapsular haemorrhage**—if no history of trauma or coagulopathy, consider the possibility of an underlying tumour.
7. **Renal infarction or renal vein thrombosis**—difficult to appreciate on unenhanced CT. Perinephric stranding may be the only visible sign. Acute thrombus within the renal vein may appear hyperattenuating compared to flowing blood in the IVC.

Gynaecological

1. **Adnexal masses**—most commonly ovarian cysts (usually haemorrhagic), tuboovarian abscesses, dermoid cysts, endometriomas and ovarian neoplasms.
2. **Cervical cancer**—which may involve the distal ureters.
3. **Degenerating or torted fibroids**.
4. **Ectopic pregnancy**.

Gastrointestinal

1. **Appendicitis**—if pain is right-sided.
2. **Diverticulitis**—usually left-sided. Meckel's diverticulitis may occur on either side.
3. **Abdominal hernias**—particularly inguinal.
4. **Fat necrosis**—e.g. epiploic appendagitis (usually left-sided) or omental infarction (usually right-sided).
5. **Other bowel pathology**—e.g. obstruction, intussusception, ischaemia, IBD or tumour.

Pancreatic and hepatobiliary disorders

1. Gallstones.
2. Pancreatitis and pancreatic tumours.

Vascular

1. Renal artery aneurysm.
2. Ruptured abdominal aortic aneurysm—a crescent-shaped area of high attenuation (> intraluminal blood) in the wall of an AAA on unenhanced CT is a sign of impending rupture. Periaortic stranding or haemorrhage (>60 HU) indicates active bleeding.
3. Aortic dissection—high attenuation in the aortic wall on unenhanced CT indicates intramural haematoma. Displacement of intimal calcification into the aortic lumen and/or renal infarction may be seen.
4. SMA thrombosis, embolism or dissection—pain may radiate to one side. Difficult to appreciate on unenhanced CT, may see vessel enlargement, perivascular stranding, high-attenuation blood clot within the vessel or displacement of intimal calcification (in the case of dissection) + signs of bowel ischaemia.
5. Intraperitoneal and retroperitoneal haemorrhage—e.g. due to trauma, anticoagulants, coagulopathy, vasculitis (PAN), splenic rupture and certain neoplasms.
6. Rectus sheath haematoma—hyperattenuating compared with normal muscle on unenhanced CT. Usually due to anticoagulants/ coagulopathy.

Musculoskeletal

1. Mechanical low back pain.
2. Osteoporotic fracture—usually in the elderly.
3. Bone metastases and myeloma.
4. Psoas haematoma.
5. Discitis—difficult to appreciate on unenhanced CT. May see endplate irregularity and fat stranding adjacent to a disc.

Further reading

Rucker, C.M., Menias, C.O., Bhalla, S., 2004. Mimics of renal colic: alternative diagnoses at unenhanced helical CT. Radiographics 24 (Suppl. 1), S11–S28, discussion S28–33.

9.14 NEPHROCALCINOSIS

Parenchymal calcification associated with a diffuse renal lesion (i.e. dystrophic calcification) or metabolic abnormality, e.g. hypercalcaemia. May be medullary (95%) or cortical (5%).

Medullary (pyramidal)

The first three causes account for 70% of cases.

1. **Medullary sponge kidney**—developmental anomaly causing cystic dilatation of the small collecting ducts in the medullary pyramids; may involve a variable portion of one or both kidneys. The dilated tubules fill with contrast during an IVU, giving a characteristic 'paintbrush' appearance to the pyramids. The tubules may contain small calculi, giving rise to medullary nephrocalcinosis—this usually manifests as focal or asymmetrical clusters of punctate calcification. Kidneys may be enlarged or normal in size. Echobright medullary pyramids on US (even without calcification). MRI may show cystic nature of pyramids on T2 sequences. Associated with Caroli disease of the liver.
2. **Hyperparathyroidism***—usually bilateral and symmetrical, diffuse rather than punctate.
3. **Renal tubular acidosis (type 1)**—most common cause in children, may be associated with osteomalacia or rickets. Calcification tends to be more severe and confluent than in other causes; typically bilateral and symmetrical. Kidneys are usually of normal size.
4. **Renal papillary necrosis**—calcification of necrotic papillae. Usually asymmetrical. See Section 9.23.
5. **Causes of hypercalcaemia or hypercalciuria**—e.g. malignancy (bone metastases, myeloma, paraneoplastic syndromes), sarcoidosis, hypervitaminosis D, milk-alkali syndrome and idiopathic hypercalciuria.
6. **Preterm neonates**—in up to two-thirds. Risk factors include extreme prematurity, severe respiratory disease, gentamicin use, and high urinary oxalate and urate excretion. Echobright medullary pyramids on US, typically bilateral and symmetrical. The majority resolve spontaneously by midchildhood. Main differential in this patient group is papillary necrosis, which also produces echobright medullary pyramids but is usually asymmetrical and results in sloughing of papillae within weeks.
7. **Hyperoxaluria**—typically causes diffuse cortical and medullary nephrocalcinosis as well as nephrolithiasis. Primary form presents in childhood.

Cortical

1. **Acute cortical necrosis**—classically 'tramline' calcification, occurs in the chronic phase.
2. **Chronic glomerulonephritis**—bilateral curvilinear or punctate cortical calcification.
3. **Chronic infection**—multifocal nodular cortical calcification can occur with HIV-related renal infections, e.g. *Pneumocystis jirovecii*, *Mycobacterium avium complex* (MAC) and CMV.

4. **Chronic renal transplant rejection**—due to cortical necrosis.
5. **Hyperoxaluria**—typically causes diffuse cortical and medullary nephrocalcinosis.
6. **Alport syndrome**—rare inherited disorder (most commonly X-linked), presents in adolescence or early adulthood with progressive renal failure and deafness. Renal calcification can look identical to hyperoxaluria.

Further reading

Habbig, S., Beck, B.B., Hoppe, B., 2011. Nephrocalcinosis and urolithiasis in children. Kidney Int. 80 (12), 1278–1291.

Hoppe, B., Kemper, M.J., 2010. Diagnostic examination of the child with urolithiasis or nephrocalcinosis. Pediatr. Nephrol. 25 (3), 403–413.

Narendra, A., White, M.P., Rolton, H.A., et al., 2001. Nephrocalcinosis in preterm babies. Arch. Dis. Child. Fetal Neonatal Ed. 85, F207–F213.

9.15 RENAL CYSTIC DISEASE

Renal dysplasia

1. Multicystic dysplastic kidney—due to ureteric atresia during early fetal life; usually diagnosed antenatally. Multiple cysts replace the kidney with intervening echobright dysplastic tissue (no functioning renal tissue). Typically involutes over time. Associated with contralateral PUJ obstruction (PUJO) and reflux. Typically involves the whole kidney but can rarely be segmental (in the case of a duplex kidney with antenatal atresia of only one ureter), thereby mimicking a multiloculated cystic mass.
2. Localized cystic renal disease—a nonencapsulated cluster of variable-sized cysts replacing part of one kidney. May occasionally involve the entire kidney but is always unilateral.

Polycystic kidney disease*

1. Autosomal recessive polycystic kidney disease*—presents antenatally or in infancy/childhood. Bilateral enlarged echogenic kidneys with multiple microcysts, most of which are too small to resolve individually (often seen as tiny echobright foci). See Part 2 for other features and associations.
2. Autosomal dominant polycystic kidney disease*—usually presents in adulthood (or earlier if undergoing screening). Enlarged kidneys with numerous cysts of varying sizes. See Part 2 for other features and associations.

Cystic tumours

1. Multilocular cystic nephroma—nonhereditary, benign. Usually presents in young children (not neonates) or middle-aged women. Multilocular cystic mass with a fibrous capsule. Linear septal and

9

capsular enhancement is often seen on CT/MRI, but nodular enhancement should not be present. Cannot be reliably differentiated from cystic RCC.

2. Multilocular cystic RCC—5% of RCCs are cystic (variant of clear cell RCC). Nodular components on imaging suggest RCC.
3. **Mixed epithelial and stromal tumour**—rare, typically seen in perimenopausal women particularly those taking OCP/hormone replacement therapy. Complex multiloculated cystic mass on imaging, often with enhancing nodular components ± calcification. Indistinguishable from cystic RCC on imaging.
4. **Angiomyolipoma with epithelial cysts**—rare cystic variant of AML. Indistinguishable from cystic RCC on imaging.
5. **Primary renal sarcoma**—e.g. leiomyosarcoma, angiosarcoma. Rare and aggressive, usually solid but can occasionally be predominantly cystic with enhancing nodular components.
6. **Cystic Wilms tumour**—extremely rare in adults.

Cortical cysts

1. Simple cyst—unilocular, thin-walled, no enhancement. Increase in size and number with age. May become haemorrhagic (>20 HU on unenhanced CT) or infected (thickened enhancing wall ± septations).
2. Syndromes associated with cysts
   (a) von Hippel-Lindau disease*—most patients will have renal cysts. There is also a high risk of RCC, many of which arise from preexisting cysts. Even simple-looking cysts on imaging often contain foci of RCC on histology. Fortunately, RCCs in vHL are slow growing and typically do not metastasize until they are >3 cm, therefore cysts can be followed up to look for malignant transformation.
   (b) Tuberous sclerosis*—cysts are the second most common renal manifestation after angiomyolipomas.
3. End-stage renal disease and haemodialysis—causes interstitial fibrosis and hyperplasia of tubular epithelium leading to cyst formation. On imaging: atrophic kidneys containing multiple cysts (>2 on each side) of varying size ± internal haemorrhage ± rupture. Incidence increases with time on dialysis, but cysts usually involute after a successful renal transplant. Also increased risk of RCC (7%, usually papillary type), increasing with time on dialysis.
4. **Lithium-induced nephrotoxicity**—causes chronic focal interstitial nephritis. Numerous 1–2 mm cortical and medullary cysts in normal-sized kidneys. On US these are often seen as multiple tiny echobright foci (rather than anechoic cysts) due to their small size, and may be mistaken for calcification.
5. **Glomerulocystic kidney disease**—rare, usually presents in children. Multiple bilateral small cysts in a characteristic subcapsular cortical distribution, due to cystic dilatation of

Bowman's capsule. The cysts may be difficult to visualize on US due to their small size and are best seen on T2-weighted MRI.

Medullary cysts

1. Calyceal diverticulum—solitary unilocular cystic space communicating via an isthmus with the fornix of a calyx. Fills with contrast during excretion urography. May contain milk of calcium or dependent calculi—highly suggestive of a diverticulum. Risk of infection, bleeding and rupture.
2. Medullary sponge kidney—bilateral in 60%–80%. Multiple tiny cysts in the medullary pyramids that opacify during excretion urography ('paintbrush' appearance) and often contain tiny calculi. The cysts themselves are usually too small to see on US, and cause a generalized increase in medullary echogenicity.
3. Papillary necrosis—clubbed calyces may mimic cysts on US.
4. **Medullary cystic disease complex**—refers to two clinically similar inherited disorders presenting with polyuria and polydipsia (due to salt-wasting) and progressive renal failure. Adult form (medullary cystic kidney disease) presents at 20–40 years. Juvenile form (juvenile nephronophthisis) presents in children. US shows normal/small echobright kidneys with multiple small cysts in the medulla and corticomedullary junction.

Miscellaneous

1. Infective
   (a) Pyogenic abscess—complex cystic lesion with internal echoes on US and a thick irregular wall on CT ± internal gas. May be within the kidney or perinephric. Renal aspergillosis and actinomycosis can have identical appearances but occur in immunocompromised patients (including diabetics and those on steroid therapy).
   (b) Xanthogranulomatous pyelonephritis—gross cystic dilatation of multiple calyces may mimic a complex cystic mass but the presence of a large renal pelvic calculus aids diagnosis.
   (c) Tuberculosis*—causes papillary necrosis and infundibular stenosis resulting in dilated moth-eaten or clubbed calyces + calcification (late stage). These can be large and mimic a cyst. Tuberculous abscesses can also form if the caseating papillary necrosis does not rupture into the collecting system.
   (d) **Hydatid cyst**—rare. Initially unilocular, later becoming multilocular and thick-walled due to the formation of daughter cysts. The lesion becomes semisolid and calcified after death of the parasite.
   (e) **Candidiasis**—rare, seen in immunocompromised patients. Typically causes multiple microabscesses, also involves the liver and spleen.

2. Traumatic—intrarenal haematoma or urinoma.
3. **Endometriosis***—renal involvement is rare, usually presents with a complex haemorrhagic cystic lesion.

Extraparenchymal renal cysts

1. Parapelvic cyst—essentially just a cortical cyst that extends into the renal sinus fat. Usually single and unilateral but may be multiple. Large cysts may cause haematuria, hypertension or hydronephrosis via local compression.
2. Peripelvic cyst— also known as renal sinus cyst or lymphangioma. Arises from dilated lymphatics in the renal sinus, thus does not involve the renal parenchyma. Usually multiple, small and bilateral; elongated simple cysts that do not communicate with the collecting system. Mimics hydronephrosis but can be differentiated on excretory phase CT. Lymphangiomatosis may also present with bilateral perinephric cystic lesions.

Further reading

Choyke, P.L., 2000. Acquired cystic kidney disease. Eur. Radiol. 10, 1716–1721.

Katabathina, V.S., Kota, G., Dasyam, A.K., et al., 2010. Adult renal cystic disease: a genetic, biological, and developmental primer. Radiographics 30 (6), 1509–1523.

Meister, M., Choyke, P., Anderson, C., Patel, U., 2009. Radiological evaluation, management, and surveillance of renal masses in Von Hippel–Lindau disease. Clin. Radiol. 64 (6), 589–600.

Pedrosa, I., Saiz, A., Arrazola, L., et al., 2000. Hydatid disease: radiologic and pathologic features and complications. Radiographics 20, 795–817.

Saunders, A.J., Denton, E., Stephens, S., et al., 1999. Cystic kidney disease presenting in infancy. Clin. Radiol. 54, 370–376.

Wood, C.G., Stromberg, L.J., Harmath, C.B., et al., 2015. CT and MR imaging for evaluation of cystic renal lesions and diseases. Radiographics 35, 125–141.

9.16 BOSNIAK CLASSIFICATION OF RENAL CYSTS

The Bosniak classification system for CT evaluation of renal cysts is helpful in both assessing malignant risk and determining required follow-up/treatment. Contrast-enhanced CT and MRI are highly accurate in the characterization of Bosniak cysts. Recently contrast-enhanced US has been shown to rival, and in some cases surpass, CT in this respect because of its ability to image the microcirculation and show flow in septa and nodules not seen on CT/MR.

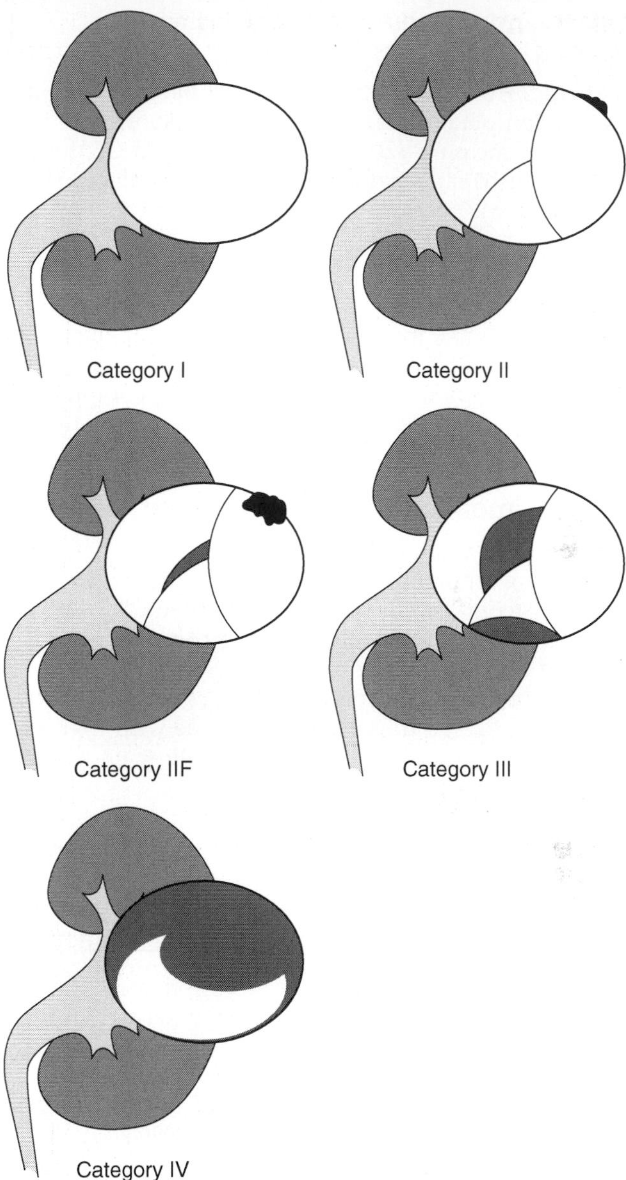

Bosniak I—simple cyst

Water attenuation with no enhancement; imperceptible wall, no septa, calcifications or solid components. No work-up; ~0% malignant.

Bosniak II—minimally complicated

A few thin (<1 mm) septations, fine calcification only, nonenhancing. Homogeneous well-defined partially exophytic high-attenuation renal lesions of <3 cm are also included in this category—these measure >20 HU on unenhanced CT due to proteinaceous or haemorrhagic fluid (>70 HU is diagnostic for a haemorrhagic cyst). No work-up; ~0% malignant.

Bosniak IIF—minimally complicated requiring follow-up

Several thin septations, minimally thickened septa or wall ± thick calcification; no measurable enhancement; includes hyperdense nonenhancing lesions that are >3 cm or almost completely intrarenal (<25% of wall visible). Needs US/CT follow-up; ~5% malignant.

Bosniak III—measurable enhancement/probably malignant

Thick enhancing septations or wall (enhancement = an increase of >15 HU on postcontrast CT versus unenhanced CT). This category includes cystic RCC, multilocular cystic nephroma, mixed epithelial and stromal tumour, renal abscess and complex haemorrhagic or infected cysts. Treatment comprises partial nephrectomy, or RFA in the elderly and those with high surgical risk. If clinical features suggest an abscess, follow-up would be preferable; >30% malignant.

Bosniak IV—clearly malignant

Enhancing nodular component. Treatment comprises partial or total nephrectomy. Nearly all are malignant, although a small few may be benign (e.g. mixed epithelial and stromal tumour).

Further reading

Harvey, C.J., Alsafi, A., Kuzmich, S., et al., 2015. Role of US Contrast agents in the assessment of indeterminate solid and cystic lesions in native and transplant kidneys. Radiographics 35, 1419–1430.

Wood, C.G., Stromberg, L.J., Harmath, C.B., 2015. CT and MR imaging for evaluation of cystic renal lesions and diseases. Radiographics 35, 125–141.

9.17 FAT-CONTAINING RENAL MASS

1. <u>Angiomyolipoma</u>—the vast majority of renal lesions containing macroscopic fat (<–20 HU on unenhanced CT) will be AMLs. Usually solitary, found incidentally on imaging. Typically well-defined and homogeneously hyperechoic on US. Variable amount of fat versus soft tissue. Risk of haemorrhage, particularly if

>4 cm or with intralesional aneurysms >5 mm. May rarely extend into the renal vein ± IVC. AMLs are seen in up to 80% of patients with tuberous sclerosis; usually multiple, bilateral, large and often fat-poor. Can also be seen in LAM, NF1 and vHL.

2. Renal cell carcinoma—microscopic fat is very common (in up to 60%), seen as signal dropout on out-of-phase MRI sequences. Macroscopic fat (i.e. visible on CT) is rare, but the presence of both macroscopic fat and calcification within a renal mass suggests RCC since calcification is very rare in AML.
3. Liposarcoma—arises from perinephric/retroperitoneal fat. Usually large, displaces and compresses the adjacent kidney. Can mimic an exophytic AML, but helpful features favouring AML include a renal cortical defect (representing the site of origin of the AML) and prominent intratumoural vessels extending into the renal cortex.
4. **Lipoma**—rare. Composed entirely of fat, no soft-tissue component. Similar on CT to a fat-rich AML.
5. **Oncocytoma**—can rarely contain a small focus of macroscopic fat.
6. **Xanthogranulomatous pyelonephritis**—xanthomatous material within dilated calyces can be of low attenuation on CT similar to fat density.
7. **Wilms tumour**—very rare in adults.
8. **Teratoma**—very rare, usually found in children or adolescents. Contains varying amounts of soft tissue, fat and calcification. A fat–fluid level is characteristic.
9. **Renal sinus lipomatosis**—expansion of the renal sinus fat without a soft-tissue component, secondary to chronic inflammation.

9

Further reading

Choi, D.J., Wallace, C., Fraire, A.E., et al., 2005. Intrarenal teratoma. Radiographics 25, 481–485.

Helenon, O., Merran, S., Paraf, F., et al., 1997. Unusual fat-containing tumors of the kidney – a diagnostic dilemma. Radiographics 1, 129–144.

Schieda, N., Kielar, A.Z., Al Dandan, O., et al., 2015. Ten uncommon and unusual variants of renal angiomyolipoma (AML): radiologic-pathologic correlation. Clin. Radiol. 70, 206–220.

9.18 SOLID RENAL LESIONS

Well-defined mass

Grows as a discrete rounded mass deforming the renal contour and displacing the normal renal parenchyma and collecting system.

1. Renal cell carcinoma—90% of malignant renal tumours in adults. Multiple or bilateral in 3%–5% (common in polycystic kidneys and vHL). Typically well-defined, may contain

calcification. May be hyperechoic on US, mimicking AML (a hypoechoic rim and heterogeneous echotexture favour RCC, but there is significant overlap). In practice all solid well-defined renal masses are presumed to be RCC due to its frequency and varied appearance. Invades renal vein/IVC in advanced stage. Appearance depends on subtype:

(a) **Clear cell**—most common (80%). Avid heterogeneous arterial enhancement ± washout in the nephrographic phase. Frequently contains cystic, haemorrhagic or necrotic components. Up to 60% contain microscopic fat on in/out of phase MRI, but macroscopic fat (on CT) is rare. Typically T2 hyperintense.

(b) **Papillary**—10%–15% of RCCs, most common form in dialysis patients. Often multiple and bilateral in hereditary papillary RCC syndrome. Typically homogeneous, T2 hypointense and hypovascular with only mild enhancement on CT/MR. Can mimic hyperdense cyst on CT (enhancement in papillary RCC may be very subtle; precontrast T1 hyperintensity on MRI can help confirm haemorrhagic cyst) and fat-poor AML (but microscopic fat on MRI is rare in papillary RCC and common in fat-poor AMLs).

(c) **Chromophobe**—5% of RCCs, best prognosis. Often multiple in Birt-Hogg-Dubé syndrome. Shows moderate enhancement on CT/MR, which may be homogeneous or heterogeneous. Variable T2 signal, may have a T2 hyperintense central fibrous scar which shows delayed enhancement, mimicking oncocytoma—DWI may be helpful (chromophobe RCCs tend to restrict diffusion more than oncocytomas) but not enough to accurately differentiate the two.

2. **Oncocytoma**—most common benign solid nonfatty renal mass, usually solitary and unilateral except in Birt-Hogg-Dubé syndrome, hereditary oncocytosis and some cases of tuberous sclerosis. Typically shows homogeneous early enhancement followed by washout. May have a hypovascular T2 hyperintense central fibrous scar which shows delayed enhancement. Cannot be reliably differentiated from RCC (particularly chromophobe type) therefore is often resected.
3. **Fat-poor angiomyolipoma**—5% of AMLs do not contain macroscopic fat visible on CT (particularly in tuberous sclerosis), although many of these will have microscopic fat on in/out of phase MRI. Usually hyperattenuating on unenhanced CT (>45 HU) with homogeneous enhancement. Typically T2 hypointense on MRI + restricted diffusion. Hard to differentiate from papillary RCC, although the presence of microscopic fat suggests AML (rare in papillary RCC). Epithelioid AML is an aggressive variant that is fat-poor, often bleeds, has malignant potential and is frequently associated with tuberous sclerosis.

4. **Haemangioma**—rare, small, nearly always arises from the renal papillae or pelvis. More common in young adults, including those with Klippel-Trénaunay and Sturge-Weber syndromes. Usually shows avid peripheral enhancement persisting on later phases (no washout). Homogeneously T2 hyperintense on MRI. May contain phleboliths.
5. **Leiomyoma**—rare, usually small and solitary. Most commonly arise from the renal capsule but can arise from the renal pelvis. Typically well-defined, homogeneously hyperattenuating on unenhanced CT with uniform enhancement, but may be heterogeneous if large. T1/T2 hypointense on MRI.
6. **Juxtaglomerular cell tumour**—rare, benign, typically seen in young adults presenting with uncontrolled hypertension, polyuria and polydipsia due to renin secretion. Solitary well-defined hypovascular mass with heterogeneous delayed enhancement.
7. **Metanephric adenoma**—rare benign tumour usually found in middle-aged patients. Polycythaemia is characteristic, but only found in 10% of patients. Well-defined hypovascular mass with heterogeneous enhancement ± haemorrhage, necrosis or calcification.
8. **Medullary fibroma**—benign lesion found in the renal pyramid. Typically <5 mm and hypovascular, thus hard to see on imaging. Can rarely be large, presenting as a heterogeneous mass with low T1 and T2 signal protruding into the renal pelvis.
9. **Papillary adenoma**—common premalignant lesion, particularly in dialysis patients. Typically subcapsular in location, hypovascular and <5 mm by definition, thus hard to see on imaging (usually found incidentally on histology).
10. **Sarcomas**—rare and aggressive, most present as a large well-defined heterogeneous mass ± necrosis, haemorrhage or cystic change. Leiomyosarcoma is most common; other types include osteosarcoma (typically calcified), Ewing sarcoma (usually in children or adolescents), synovial sarcoma, fibrosarcoma, clear cell sarcoma. Note that large RCCs can undergo sarcomatoid transformation—this is more common than primary renal sarcoma.
11. **Other rare lesions not specific to the kidney**—e.g. solitary fibrous tumour (relatively homogeneous enhancement, often has radial bands of low T2 signal on MRI), sarcoidosis (typically multifocal, T2 hypointense on MRI), inflammatory pseudotumour, plasmacytoma, glomus tumour, myopericytoma, schwannoma, paraganglioma, carcinoid. Most of these usually present as nonspecific well-defined heterogeneously enhancing masses indistinguishable from RCC.
12. **Pseudotumours**—e.g. prominent column of Bertin, persistent fetal lobulation, dromedary hump, aneurysms and AVMs. Splenosis on the surface of the left kidney may also mimic a renal

lesion, but the history of splenic trauma/resection and the enhancement pattern is usually diagnostic. Congenital splenorenal fusion (of heterotopic splenic tissue) can have a similar appearance but is very rare. Large adrenal masses inseparable from the kidney may also mimic a renal mass.

Infiltrative lesions

These are ill-defined, hypovascular and do not usually distort the renal contour.

1. **Urothelial carcinoma (aka TCC)**—typically ill-defined and hypovascular, arises from the pelvicalyceal system and may obstruct or obliterate other calyces. May seed further down the urinary tract. Early tumours are seen as a mildly enhancing polypoid or sessile filling defect in the pyelographic phase on IVU, CT or MR.
2. **Squamous cell carcinoma**—usually associated with calculi or chronic UTI, can also occur in XGP. Starts as a plaque or stricture in the pelvicalyceal system but infiltrates the renal parenchyma early on, so there is usually a large parenchymal mass before any sizeable intrapelvic mass. May be very difficult to identify in chronically infected and distorted kidneys, e.g. in XGP.
3. **Infiltrative subtypes of RCC**—medullary carcinoma (nearly always in young patients with sickle cell trait) and collecting duct carcinoma both typically have infiltrative growth patterns and are aggressive, often metastatic at presentation.
4. **Lymphoma***—usually secondary involvement in advanced NHL (primary lymphoma is very rare as there is no renal lymphoid tissue). Usually there are multifocal bilateral infiltrative hypovascular lesions on CT/MR, which are T2 hypointense, but can present as a single ill-defined mass, diffuse renal enlargement, perinephric soft-tissue thickening or direct extension from retroperitoneal lymphadenopathy. Can affect the renal sinus and mimic TCC.
5. **Metastases**—not uncommon, usually in the presence of metastatic disease elsewhere. Ill-defined hypovascular mass or masses. Lung, breast, GI tract, melanoma and the contralateral kidney are the most common sources.
6. **Leukaemia**—typically causes bilateral diffuse renal enlargement but can rarely present with single or multiple masses (chloroma in acute myeloid leukaemia).
7. **Malakoplakia**—uncommon inflammatory condition usually involving the urinary tract, related to recurrent *E. coli* infection. Most commonly involves the urothelium (causing nodules or plaques), but can also involve the renal parenchyma causing focal, multifocal or diffuse infiltrative lesions. May extend into the perinephric fat.

8. **Sarcomas**—rare. Angiosarcoma and rhabdomyosarcoma often have an infiltrative growth pattern.
9. **Other rare lesions**—e.g. plasmacytoma, extramedullary haematopoiesis, inflammatory pseudotumour, Wegener's granulomatosis, Rosai-Dorfman disease, amyloidosis.
10. **Mimics**—focal pyelonephritis often presents as an ill-defined area of hypovascularity or striated enhancement, but the clinical features of sepsis are usually indicative. This is usually T2 hyperintense on MRI and may be hypo- or hyperechoic on US. A renal infarct presents as a peripheral wedge-shaped hypovascular area (± renal capsule enhancement) and may be multifocal. Predisposing factors are usually present. Radiation nephritis (due to spinal or retroperitoneal radiotherapy) presents as a well-defined wedge of hypoenhancement in the medial aspect of one or both kidneys.

Further reading

Baliyan, V., Das, C.J., Sharma, S., Gupta, A.K., 2014. Diffusion-weighted imaging in urinary tract lesions. Clin. Radiol. 69, 773–782.

Heilbrun, M.E., Remer, E.M., Casalino, D.D., et al., 2015. ACR Appropriateness Criteria indeterminate renal mass. J. Am. Coll. Radiol. 12 (4), 333–341.

Jinzaki, M., Silverman, S.G., Akita, H., et al., 2014. Renal angiomyolipoma: a radiological classification and update on recent developments in diagnosis and management. Abdom. Imaging 39 (3), 588–604.

Katabathina, V.S., Vikram, R., Nagar, A.M., et al., 2010. Mesenchymal neoplasms of the kidney in adults: imaging spectrum with radiologic-pathologic correlation. Radiographics 30 (6), 1525–1540.

Mittal, M.K., Sureka, B., 2016. Solid renal masses in adults. Indian J Radiol Imaging 26 (45), 429–442.

Pallwein-Prettner, L., Flöry, D., Rotter, C.R., et al., 2011. Assessment and characterisation of common renal masses with CT and MRI. Insights Imaging 2 (5), 543–556.

Pedrosa, I., Maryellen, R., Sun, M.R., Spencer, M., 2008. MR imaging of renal masses: correlation with findings at surgery and pathologic analysis. Radiographics 28, 985–1003.

Pickhardt, P.J., Lonergan, G.J., Davis, C.J., Jr., et al., 2000. From the archives of the AFIP. Infiltrative renal lesions: radiologic-pathologic correlation. Armed Forces Institute of Pathology. Radiographics 20 (1), 215–243.

Purysko, A.S., Westphalen, A.C., Remer, E.M., et al., 2016. Imaging manifestations of hematologic diseases with renal and perinephric involvement. Radiographics 36, 1038–1054.

Ramamurthy, N.K., Moosavi, B., McInnes, M.D., et al., 2015. Multiparametric MRI of solid renal masses: pearls and pitfalls. Clin. Radiol. 70 (3), 304–316.

Zhang, J., Lefkowitz, R.A., Ishill, N.M., 2007. Solid renal cortical tumors: differentiation with CT. Radiology 244, 494–504.

9.19 RENAL SINUS MASS

Neoplastic

1. **Urothelial carcinoma**—intraluminal filling defect on excretory urography, centred in the renal pelvis which secondarily invades the renal sinus and renal parenchyma. Commonly causes calyceal obstruction.
2. **Squamous cell carcinoma**—strongly associated with renal calculi and chronic UTI.
3. **Metastasis to sinus lymph nodes.**
4. **Lymphoma***—may be limited to the renal sinus, particularly in PTLD. Ill-defined hypovascular mass which characteristically does not cause obstruction.
5. **Mesenchymal tumour**—e.g. lipoma, medullary fibroma, haemangioma, leiomyoma.
6. **Retroperitoneal tumours extending into the renal sinus**—any retroperitoneal tumour but lymphoma most commonly.
7. **Renal parenchymal tumours projecting into the renal sinus.**

Nonneoplastic lesions

1. **Peripelvic cyst**—typically multiple and bilateral, arise from lymphatics within sinus fat. See Section 9.15.
2. **Parapelvic cyst**—single, larger cyst protruding into the sinus, originating from the adjacent parenchyma. See Section 9.15.
3. **Sinus lipomatosis**—echogenic central sinus complex on US. CT and MRI directly reveal fatty nature.
4. **Vascular**—renal artery aneurysm, AVM or renal vein varix can manifest as peripelvic lesions. Colour Doppler or contrast-enhanced CT are diagnostic.
5. **Inflammatory**—soft-tissue thickening in the sinus due to chronic/severe pyelonephritis, XGP or malakoplakia.
6. **Haematoma**—due to anticoagulants or less commonly trauma.
7. **Urinoma**—due to pelvicalyceal rupture, usually associated with ureteral obstruction (e.g. stones), PUJ obstruction or trauma (including surgery).
8. **Rare infiltrative disorders**—any of the following can cause bilateral infiltrative masses in the renal sinus ± hydronephrosis.
   (a) **Rosai-Dorfman disease***—renal involvement is rare but the most common manifestation is bilateral infiltrative renal hilar masses.
   (b) **Retroperitoneal fibrosis**—periaortic soft tissue may extend into the renal sinus.
   (c) **Erdheim-Chester disease***—perinephric soft tissue may extend into the renal sinus.

(d) **Amyloidosis***—can rarely involve the renal sinuses, causing infiltrative soft-tissue masses which may calcify (highly suggestive).
(e) **Extramedullary haematopoiesis**—look for signs of bone marrow failure, e.g. bone sclerosis, splenomegaly. Uptake on sulphur colloid scintigraphy is diagnostic.

Further reading

Purysko, A.S., Westphalen, A.C., Remer, E.M., et al., 2016. Imaging manifestations of hematologic diseases with renal and perinephric involvement. Radiographics 36 (4), 1038–1054.
Rha, S.E., Byun, J.Y., Jung, S.E., et al., 2004. The renal sinus: pathologic spectrum and multimodality imaging approach. Radiographics 24 (Suppl. 1), S117–S131.

9.20 NEOPLASTIC AND PROLIFERATIVE DISORDERS OF THE PERINEPHRIC SPACE

Soft-tissue rind

1. **Lymphoma***—usually due to extension of renal/retroperitoneal lymphoma into perinephric space, but can present as isolated perinephric soft-tissue thickening.
2. **Erdheim-Chester disease***—retroperitoneal involvement is common and produces a characteristic rind of soft tissue around the kidneys and aorta.
3. **Amyloidosis***—may diffusely infiltrate the perinephric and retroperitoneal fat ± foci of calcification (highly suggestive).
4. **Retroperitoneal fibrosis**—periaortic soft tissue may extend into the perinephric space.
5. **Metastases**—most present as focal masses but breast cancer can present as infiltrative retroperitoneal soft tissue, which can involve the perinephric space.
6. **Extramedullary haematopoiesis**—can rarely infiltrate the perinephric fat.
7. **Rosai-Dorfman disease***—can rarely cause subcapsular renal infiltration.
8. **Nephroblastomatosis**—only occurs in infants and children, due to persistent nephrogenic rests. Presents as bilateral confluent subcapsular soft-tissue nodules, which are homogeneous and hypovascular. Risk of malignant transformation to Wilms tumour.

Focal solid lesions

1. **Renal lesions extending into the perinephric space**—e.g. tumours (RCC, TCC), inflammatory lesions (malakoplakia, XGP).

9

2. **Metastases**—common sources include lung and melanoma. Usually in the presence of metastatic disease elsewhere. Lymphoma, leukaemia and myeloma may also rarely present as a focal perinephric mass.
3. **Perinephric haematoma**—may be spontaneous (due to vasculitis, anticoagulation or coagulopathy) or due to an underlying aneurysm or mass lesion, e.g. AML or RCC. Hyperattenuating subcapsular mass that does not enhance post contrast.
4. **Nodular fat necrosis due to severe pancreatitis**—usually presents with numerous small soft-tissue nodules (± central fat) throughout the intraabdominal fat.
5. **Primary sarcoma**—some liposarcomas may present as a solid mass. Other sarcomas can also arise from the perinephric space.
6. **Other rare lesions not specific to the perinephric space**—e.g. haemangioma, solitary fibrous tumour, Castleman disease, desmoid tumour, inflammatory pseudotumour, plasmacytoma.

Fatty lesions

1. **Exophytic angiomyolipoma**—often large, mimics perinephric liposarcoma. Features favouring AML include a focal renal cortical defect (representing the site of origin) and prominent intratumoural vessels extending into the renal parenchyma.
2. **Liposarcoma**—most common primary retroperitoneal malignancy, often arises from perinephric fat. Usually large and unencapsulated, displaces the adjacent kidney. See Section 4.4 for subtypes.
3. **Perinephric lipomatosis**—associated with renal stones and chronic renal infection (including XGP and TB). Expansion of the perinephric and renal sinus fat ± stranding.
4. **Extraadrenal myelolipoma**—can rarely arise from the perinephric space. Mimics liposarcoma due to mix of fatty and soft-tissue components, but typically appears encapsulated. Uptake on sulphur colloid scintigraphy suggests myelolipoma but is also seen in extramedullary haematopoiesis.
5. **Extramedullary haematopoiesis**—may contain foci of macroscopic fat.

Cystic lesions

1. **Exophytic renal cyst or cystic lesions**—including cystic neoplasms and abscesses.
2. **Urinoma**—due to pelvicalyceal rupture, usually associated with ureteral obstruction (e.g. stones), PUJO or trauma/surgery.
3. **Lymphangiomatosis**—rare benign lymphatic malformation resulting in bilateral multiloculated perinephric cysts and usually multiple bilateral peripelvic cysts.

Further reading
Heller, M.T., Haarer, K.A., Thomas, E., Thaete, F.L., 2012. Neoplastic and proliferative disorders of the perinephric space. Clin. Radiol. 67 (11), 31–41.
Purysko, A.S., Westphalen, A.C., Remer, E.M., 2016. Imaging manifestations of hematologic diseases with renal and perinephric involvement. Radiographics 36, 1038–1054.
Surabhi, V.R., Menias, C., Prasad, S.R., et al., 2008. Neoplastic and non-neoplastic proliferative disorders of the perirenal space: cross-sectional imaging findings. Radiographics 28 (4), 1005–1017.

9.21 NEPHROGRAPHIC PATTERNS

Normal kidneys show three phases of contrast enhancement in a symmetrical fashion:

1. Corticomedullary phase—25–80 seconds after contrast injection. Clear corticomedullary differentiation with most of the contrast within the cortex.
2. Nephrographic phase—90–120 seconds after contrast injection. Homogeneous enhancement of both cortex and medulla; best phase for lesion detection.
3. Excretory phase—>3 minutes after contrast injection. Dense contrast fills the collecting system; best phase for detecting urothelial lesions.

Normal transition through these phases depends on normal arterial inflow, normal venous outflow, normal renal tubules and unobstructed urine outflow through the collecting system. There are several patterns of abnormal renal enhancement depending on the cause.

Absent nephrogram

No enhancement of the renal parenchyma.

1. Global—nearly always due to main renal artery occlusion, either due to thrombosis, dissection or traumatic avulsion. Renal vein thrombosis can also give this appearance. A rim of capsular enhancement ('rim nephrogram') may be seen due to patent capsular vessels, usually developing several days after the initial vascular insult.
2. Segmental—due to focal renal infarction (usually embolic or vasculitic), focal pyelonephritis or an infiltrative lesion. A rim of capsular enhancement, if present, indicates infarction.

Unilateral delayed nephrogram

An asymmetrical pattern of renal enhancement is always abnormal, and the delayed side is always the abnormal side. The delayed side may become progressively hyperdense on subsequent phases.

1. **Obstructive uropathy**—e.g. ureteric stone/tumour.
2. **Reduced arterial inflow**—e.g. renal artery stenosis, Page kidney (reduced perfusion due to extrinsic compression by a subcapsular haematoma or collection).
3. **Reduced venous outflow**—e.g. renal vein thrombosis or compression.
4. **Pyelonephritis**—although a striated nephrogram is more common. As opposed to the other differentials, pyelonephritis does not result in a progressively hyperdense nephrogram.

Bilateral persistent nephrogram

Both kidneys are still in the corticomedullary phase >90 seconds or nephrographic phase >3 minutes after contrast injection.

1. **Reduced arterial inflow**—e.g. systemic hypotension/shock, and rarely bilateral renal artery stenosis.
2. **Abnormal renal tubules**—e.g. acute tubular necrosis (including iodinated contrast nephropathy), acute glomerulonephritis, acute papillary necrosis, tumour lysis syndrome or tubular protein deposition (myeloma, rhabdomyolysis, amyloidosis). In acute tubular necrosis the nephrograms may persist for days.
3. **Bilateral obstructive uropathy**—rare.
4. **Reduced venous outflow**—e.g. bilateral renal vein thrombosis. Rare.

Unilateral striated nephrogram

Streaky radial bands of alternating hyper and hypoattenuation, best seen in the excretory phase.

1. **Acute ureteric obstruction**.
2. **Acute pyelonephritis**—may be unilateral or bilateral.
3. **Renal vein thrombosis**.
4. **Traumatic renal contusion**.

Bilateral striated nephrogram

1. **Acute pyelonephritis**—may be asymmetrical.
2. **Abnormal renal tubules**—e.g. acute tubular necrosis, acute interstitial nephritis, tubular protein deposition (rhabdomyolysis, HIV nephropathy).
3. **Hypotension/shock***.

4. Medullary sponge kidney—in the medulla only. Parallel or fan-shaped streaks radiating from the papilla to the corticomedullary junction ('paintbrush' appearance), representing dilated contrast-filled tubules. Nephrocalcinosis often also present.
5. Autosomal recessive polycystic kidney disease*—contrast medium in dilated tubules.

Spotted nephrogram

Multiple segmental areas of nonenhancement. Coarser appearance than a striated nephrogram.

1. Vasculitis—e.g. polyarteritis nodosa, Wegener's granulomatosis, SLE, drug-induced. Causes multiple infarcts of differing ages due to occlusion of small intrarenal arteries.
2. Multiple emboli—usually from a cardiac source.
3. **Pyelonephritis**—less common than a striated nephrogram.

Reverse rim nephrogram

Bilateral nonenhancing renal cortices with enhancement of the medulla and renal capsule. Pathognomonic for acute cortical necrosis, most commonly due to pregnancy-related complications (e.g. placental abruption, infected abortion, preeclampsia). Other causes include shock, sepsis, trauma, hyperacute transplant rejection, HUS, sickle cell disease, NSAIDs.

Further reading

Wolin, E.A., Hartman, D.S., Olson, J.R., 2013. Nephrographic and pyelographic analysis of CT urography: differential diagnosis. AJR 200, 1197–1203.

9

9.22 DIFFUSE LOW SIGNAL IN THE RENAL CORTEX ON MRI

Typically reflects haemosiderin deposition in the renal cortex due to intravascular haemolysis, resulting in low T1 and T2 signal. The renal medulla is spared. The liver, spleen and bone marrow are also normal unless there is coexisting extravascular haemolysis (e.g. sickle cell) or transfusional haemosiderosis.

1. Paroxysmal nocturnal haemoglobinuria—most common cause.
2. **Mechanical haemolysis**—caused by malfunctioning prosthetic heart valves.
3. **Severe sickle cell disease***—although haemolysis is predominantly extravascular (causing haemosiderin deposition in the liver, spleen and bone marrow), intravascular haemolysis can also occur in severe crises.

4. **Renal cortical necrosis**—cortical thinning and low signal due to diffuse calcification.

Further reading

Jeong, J.Y., Kim, S.H., Lee, H.J., Sim, J.S., 2002. Atypical low-signal-intensity renal parenchyma: causes and patterns. Radiographics 22 (4), 833–846.

9.23 RENAL PAPILLARY NECROSIS

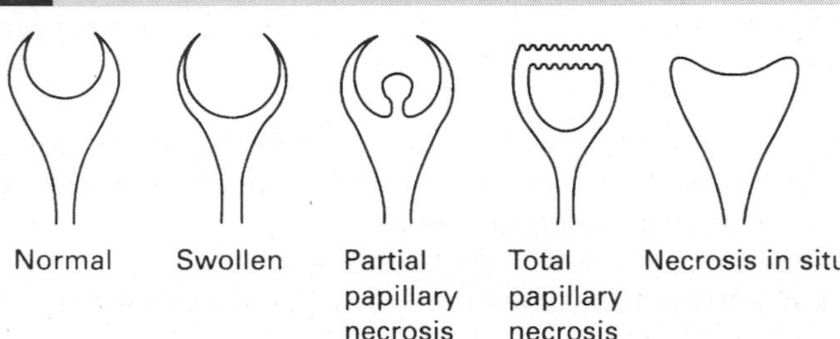

Necrosis of the renal papilla in the medulla due to interstitial nephritis or ischaemia. Involved kidneys are small with smooth outlines in chronic disease, or large in acute fulminant cases.

1. <u>Bilateral</u>—in 85% multiple papillae are affected. Diabetes (50%), analgesics and sickle cell disease are the most important causes; others include trauma, acute tubular necrosis, shock (in infants) and chronic alcoholism.
2. <u>Unilateral</u>—usually due to obstruction, renal vein thrombosis, acute pyelonephritis or TB.
3. <u>Papillae may show:</u>
   (a) Enlargement (early) due to oedema. On CT, early disease presents as ill-defined areas of hypoenhancement in the papillary regions on the nephrographic phase. On US, echogenic rings may be seen in the medulla surrounded by a rim of fluid.
   (b) Partial sloughing—fissuring of the papilla occurs in one of two ways:
      (i) Central (medullary type)—a contrast-filled fissure forms at the tip of the papilla ± a central cavity ('ball-on-tee' or 'egg-in-cup' sign on excretory phase).
      (ii) Forniceal (papillary type)—fissuring occurs at the edges of the papilla causing a 'lobster claw' appearance—if this progresses it leads to total sloughing.
   (c) Total sloughing (signet ring sign)—the sloughed papillary tissue may:
      (i) Fragment and be passed in the urine.
      (ii) Cause ureteric obstruction.
      (iii) Remain free in a calyx as a filling defect (echogenic on US).
      (iv) Remain in the pelvis and form a ball calculus.

   (d) Necrosis in situ—the papilla is shrunken and necrotic but has not separated. This may then become calcified or ossified (particularly in analgesic nephropathy and TB).
4. <u>Calyces</u>—will appear dilated and clubbed following total sloughing of a papilla. On US this presents as a cystic cavity in the medulla contiguous with the calyces.

Further reading

Jung, D.C., Kim, S.H., Jung, S.I., et al., 2006. Renal papillary necrosis: review and comparison of findings at multi-detector row CT and intravenous urography. Radiographics 26 (6), 1827–1836.

Kawamoto, S., Duggan, P., Sheth, S., et al., 2017. Renal papillary and calyceal lesions at ct urography: genitourinary imaging. Radiographics 37, 358–359.

9.24 RENAL CAUSES OF HYPERTENSION

1. <u>**Renal artery stenosis**</u>—see Section 9.25. Note that other arterial abnormalities such as aneurysms and AVMs can also rarely cause renovascular hypertension.
2. **Chronic bilateral parenchymal disease**—e.g. glomerulonephritis, polycystic disease, diabetic glomerulosclerosis, connective tissue diseases (SLE, scleroderma, PAN), analgesic nephropathy.
3. **Chronic reflux nephropathy or obstructive uropathy.**
4. **Tumours producing renin**—characteristic in juxtaglomerular cell tumours (rare, seen in young adults), but can also occur with Wilms tumours and RCC.
5. **Chronic renal infection**—e.g. XGP, TB.
6. **Renal vein thrombosis.**
7. **Radiotherapy.**

9.25 RENAL ARTERY STENOSIS

Diagnosed in up to 5% of hypertensive patients. Conventional angiography is the gold standard but is invasive. CT/MR angiography will directly visualize the stenosis ± other features, e.g. poststenotic dilatation, delayed nephrogram and renal atrophy (these all suggest a haemodynamically significant stenosis). On Doppler US, features include:

1. <u>Direct signs</u>—seen at the site of narrowing.
   (a) Peak systolic velocity (PSV) in main renal artery >200 cm/s. Correlates well with >60% stenosis.
   (b) Renal artery PSV ÷ aortic PSV >3.5 correlates with >60% stenosis.
   (c) Turbulent flow in the poststenotic main renal artery.

(d) Lack of Doppler flow within main renal artery (indicates occlusion).

2. Indirect signs—seen distal to the site of narrowing. Less reliable than direct signs.
   (a) Tardus-parvus intrarenal waveform—blunted and delayed systolic upstroke, demonstrated by loss of the early systolic peak, a systolic upstroke gradient <3 m/s^2 and acceleration time >0.07 s (time from onset of systole to peak systole). High specificity but low sensitivity.
   (b) Intrarenal arterial resistive index >0.8.
   (c) Smooth renal atrophy.

Aetiology

1. Atherosclerosis—in ~75%, most commonly men >50 years. Bilateral in 30%. Stenosis of the proximal 2 cm of the renal artery is typical (± calcification); less frequently the distal artery or early branches at bifurcations.
2. Fibromuscular dysplasia—in ~20%, typically women <50 years. Nonatherosclerotic noninflammatory vasculopathy resulting in mural fibroplasia. Bilateral in 60%. Multiple stenoses ± dilatations, which may give the characteristic 'string of beads' appearance. Most commonly affects the middistal renal artery ± hilar branches, but can also involve carotid, vertebral and mesenteric arteries.
3. **Renal artery dissection**—usually due to extension of aortic dissection into the renal arteries, but can also occur due to trauma, instrumentation or spontaneously related to fibromuscular dysplasia, connective tissue disorders (Marfan and Ehlers-Danlos syndromes), severe atherosclerosis, malignant hypertension and extreme physical exertion. On imaging the dissection flap may be hard to visualize due to the small vessel size. Renal artery occlusion may also occur due to thrombosis or embolism.
4. **Arteritis**—PAN typically causes multiple intrarenal artery microaneurysms ± stenoses ± renal infarcts of different ages. SLE, Wegener's granulomatosis and drug-induced vasculitis can cause a similar appearance. Takayasu arteritis can cause stenosis of the proximal renal artery. Other rare causes include radiation vasculopathy, thromboangiitis obliterans, syphilis and congenital rubella.
5. **Renal artery entrapment**—extrinsic compression of the renal artery by the diaphragmatic crus, due to an anomalous high origin of the renal artery. Usually presents in young patients.
6. **Neurofibromatosis***—can rarely cause long tapered stenoses of the middistal renal arteries, usually seen in patients <50 years.
7. **Midaortic syndrome**—rare, seen in young patients. Causes long smooth narrowing of the suprarenal aorta ± renal artery involvement.

8. **Extrinsic compression**—by tumour, lymph nodes, aneurysm or RPF.

Further reading

Al-Katib, S., Shetty, M., Jafri, S.M., Jafri, S.Z., 2017. Radiologic assessment of native renal vasculature: a multimodality review. Radiographics 37, 136–156.

Hartman, R.P., Kawashima, A., 2009. Radiologic evaluation of suspected renovascular hypertension. Am. Fam. Physician 80 (3), 273–279.

Kawashima, A., Sandler, C.M., Ernst, R.D., et al., 2000. CT evaluation of renovascular disease. Radiographics 20, 1321–1340.

Rankin, S., Saunders, A.J., Cook, G.J., et al., 2000. Renovascular disease. Clin. Radiol. 55, 1–12.

9.26 NONOPACIFICATION OF A CALYX ON CT OR EXCRETORY UROGRAPHY

1. **Technical factors**—incomplete filling during excretory urography.
2. **Tumour**—most commonly RCC (adult) or Wilms tumour (child).
3. **Obstructed infundibulum**—due to tumour, calculus or TB.
4. **Duplex kidney**—with a nonfunctioning upper or lower moiety. Signs suggesting a nonfunctioning upper moiety are:
   (a) Fewer calyces than the contralateral kidney. This sign is only reliable in unilateral duplication. (Calyceal distribution is symmetrical in 80% of normal individuals.)
   (b) A shortened upper calyx that does not reach into the upper pole and may be deformed by a dilated upper pole pelvis.
   (c) The kidney may be displaced downward or laterally by a dilated upper moiety pelvis. The appearances mimic a space-occupying lesion in the upper pole.
   (d) The upper pole may be rotated laterally and downward by a dilated upper moiety pelvis resulting in a 'drooping lily' appearance of the lower pole calyces.
   (e) The lower moiety ureter may be displaced or compressed by the upper pole ureter, resulting in a series of scalloped curves.
   (f) The lower moiety renal pelvis may be displaced laterally and its ureter then takes a direct oblique course to the lumbosacral junction.
5. **Infection**—abscess or TB.
6. **Partial nephrectomy**—± a surgical defect in the twelfth rib.

Further reading

Fernbach, S.K., Feinstein, K.A., Spencer, K., et al., 1997. Ureteral duplication and its complications. Radiographics 17, 109–127.

9.27 FILLING DEFECT IN THE RENAL COLLECTING SYSTEM OR URETER

Beware of technical factors—incomplete filling during excretion.

Extrinsic with a smooth margin

1. Renal sinus masses—especially parapelvic and peripelvic cysts and benign mesenchymal tumours (see Section 9.19). These can indent and distort the pelvicalyceal system.
2. Vascular impression—intrarenal arteries can produce transverse or oblique compression lines, most commonly indenting an upper pole calyx ± calyceal obstruction (Fraley syndrome). Collateral vessels can also cause impressions, e.g. ureteric artery collaterals in RAS (indenting the renal pelvis) and venous collaterals in IVC obstruction or gonadal vein varices (indenting the ureter). Renovascular AVMs can also indent the renal pelvis.
3. Renal sinus lipomatosis—most commonly in older patients with chronic UTI or stones. Fat in the renal hilum produces a relative lucency on IVU and narrows and elongates the major calyces.

Arising from the wall with smooth margins

1. Early urothelial carcinoma—in practice any urothelial mass lesion is considered malignant until proven otherwise, due to the overlap in imaging findings.
2. Papilloma—most common benign ureteric tumour, can be solitary or multiple. Smooth surface, most commonly in distal ureter. Indistinguishable from early TCC and rare benign neoplasms, e.g. nephrogenic adenoma (caused by chronic inflammation), leiomyoma, neurofibroma, haemangioma, solitary fibrous tumour.
3. Pyeloureteritis cystica—due to chronic infection. Multiple 2–4-mm well-defined round submucosal cysts project into the lumen of the renal pelvis and/or ureter (upper > lower).
4. Metastases—rare, usually in the presence of disseminated disease. Lung, breast and GI sources are the most common.
5. **Suburothelial haemorrhage**—usually associated with coagulopathy or anticoagulants. Causes diffuse mural thickening ± filling defects in the renal pelvis and upper ureter. The thickening is hyperattenuating on unenhanced CT and does not usually cause significant obstruction, which can aid differentiation from TCC.
6. **Endometriosis***—stricturing is more common but filling defects can occur, typically in the distal ureter.
7. **Pseudodiverticulosis**—multiple, usually bilateral, small (<5 mm) outpouchings from the upper-mid ureters. Associated with chronic UTI and obstruction, increased risk of malignancy.
8. **Stevens-Johnson syndrome**—can cause multiple small mucosal bullae in both ureters with mucosal sloughing, which may cause

obstruction. On CT there may be diffuse urothelial enhancement. Diagnosis usually already known due to cutaneous features.

Arising from the wall with an irregular margin

1. **Urothelial carcinoma**—most common in the distal ureter, often multifocal. Enhances on CT.
2. **Squamous cell carcinoma**—rare, strongly associated with chronic UTI and stones.
3. **Renal cell carcinoma**—infiltrative subtypes may invade the pelvicalyceal system.
4. **Squamous metaplasia**—associated with chronic infection or calculi. Most common in the bladder and renal pelvis. Premalignant lesion, indistinguishable from tumour.
5. **Tuberculosis***—causes nodular wall thickening and strictures.
6. **Malakoplakia**—granulomatous reaction to chronic *E. coli* infection; causes single or multiple urothelial plaques, nodules or masses indistinguishable from malignancy.
7. **Amyloidosis***—can cause focal urothelial thickening and irregular filling defects ± calcification (highly suggestive).
8. **Sarcoidosis***—can rarely cause a ureteric filling defect (granuloma).

In the lumen

Any of these may be single or multiple.

1. **Calculus**.
2. **Blood clot**—due to trauma, tumour or bleeding diathesis. May be adherent to the wall or free in the lumen. Hyperattenuating on unenhanced CT. Changes in size or shape over several days.
3. **Air bubble**—see Section 9.38.
4. **Sloughed papilla**—due to papillary necrosis. Often triangular, may be rim-calcified. Look for blunted papillae in kidney.
5. **Benign fibroepithelial polyp**—rare, usually in the renal pelvis or ureter in young adults. Elongated, smooth and pedunculated—the stalk may be long, so the polyp can mimic an intraluminal lesion and may protrude into the bladder. Enhances on CT.
6. **Fungus ball**—typically in the renal pelvis, due to aspergillosis or candidiasis in immunocompromised patients.

Further reading

Cowan, N.C., 2012. CT urography for hematuria. Nat. Rev. Urol. 9 (4), 218–226.

9

9.28 SPONTANEOUS URINARY CONTRAST EXTRAVASATION

Seen on CT and excretory urography. Also known as spontaneous pyelorenal backflow. Usually due to forniceal rupture caused by sudden increased pressure in the collecting system, e.g. obstructing stone or iatrogenic (retrograde pyelography). Complications are rare and treatment is conservative. Imaging findings depend on which space the fornix ruptures into. The first two are the most common.

1. **Pyelosinus backflow**—contrast extravasation from fornix rupture into the renal sinus ± perinephric space. Contrast may also track inferiorly alongside ureter.
2. **Pyelotubular backflow**—physiological reflux of contrast from the calyx into the terminal portions of collecting ducts in the renal papilla (not due to forniceal rupture). Fan-like streaks from a calyx into the medullary pyramid.
3. **Pyelointerstitial backflow**—forniceal rupture into the renal interstitium; contrast flows from a calyx into the medullary pyramid ± renal cortex. More amorphous than pyelotubular.
4. **Pyelolymphatic backflow**—forniceal rupture into renal sinus lymphatics; contrast flows into small serpiginous lymphatic channels extending medially towards paraaortic lymphatics.
5. **Pyelovenous backflow**—forniceal rupture into arcuate or interlobar veins, with contrast flowing into the renal vein. Very rare.

Further reading

Cooke, G.M., Batiks, J.P., 1974. Spontaneous extravasation of contrast medium during intravenous urography. Report of fourteen cases and a review of the literature. Clin. Radiol. 25 (1), 87–93.

9.29 COLLECTING SYSTEM DILATATION

Aetiology depends on pattern of dilatation.

Dilated calyx with a narrow infundibulum/renal pelvis

1. Stricture—due to tumour, calculus or TB.
2. Xanthogranulomatous pyelonephritis—typically there is a large calculus in a contracted and thickened renal pelvis, with gross calyceal dilatation and parenchymal atrophy.
3. Infiltrative processes of the renal sinus—these can constrict the renal pelvis and cause calyceal dilatation (see Section 9.19).

4. <u>Extrinsic compression by an artery</u>—most commonly a right upper pole calyx (Fraley syndrome). The renal pelvis is normal.
5. <u>Calyceal diverticulum (mimic)</u>—congenital outpouching that communicates with a calyceal fornix via a thin isthmus. May contain milk of calcium or dependent calculi (highly suggestive of a diverticulum).

Dilated calyx with a wide infundibulum and normal renal pelvis

1. <u>Chronic reflux or obstruction</u>—generally all the calyces are affected + associated parenchymal atrophy. The renal pelvis may be mildly dilated.
2. <u>Papillary necrosis</u>—clubbed calyces due to sloughing of papillae. See Section 9.23.
3. <u>Congenital megacalyces</u>—dilated and clubbed calyces (due to hypoplasia of medullary pyramids) usually with a normal renal pelvis. Number of calyces is often increased (polycalycosis) up to 20–25 (normal 8–12). Normal cortical thickness and good renal function differentiate it from chronic reflux/obstruction.

Dilated renal pelvis with normal calyces

Characteristic of a baggy extrarenal pelvis (normal variant).

Dilated calyces and renal pelvis with a normal ureter

1. <u>Congenital PUJ obstruction</u>—due to abnormal embryogenesis of the PUJ resulting in a variable degree of stenosis. Often presents in childhood (or detected antenatally), but can present in adults. Extrinsic crossing vessels at the PUJ may contribute to obstruction.
2. <u>Acquired PUJ obstruction</u>—due to malignant and benign strictures, calculus (and other filling defects), previous trauma or inflammation.
3. <u>Peripelvic cysts (mimic)</u>—can be hard to differentiate from hydronephrosis on US. Excretory phase CT is diagnostic.

Dilated pelvicalyceal system and ureter

See Section 9.30.

9.30 DILATED URETER

Obstruction

Within the lumen

See Section 9.27.

In the wall

1. **Oedema or stricture due to calculus**—the calculus may have passed.
2. **Primary tumour**—TCC, papilloma and other benign and malignant neoplasms (see Section 9.27).
3. **Metastasis**—can present as a thick-walled stricture. Usually in the presence of disseminated disease. Lung, breast and GI sources are the most common.
4. **Postsurgical**—e.g. a misplaced ligature, following ureteric instrumentation or at a ureteral anastomosis.
5. **Tuberculous stricture**—typically multifocal stricturing causing a beaded or corkscrew ureter ± calcification. A particular hazard during the early weeks of treatment.
6. **Schistosomiasis***—chronic disease causes distal ureteric stricturing ± calcification in the ureter or bladder (pathognomonic).
7. **Ureterocoele**—cystic dilatation of the ureter at the VUJ, projects into bladder. Due to congenital stenosis at ureteric orifice. Commonly associated with ectopic ureteric insertion (e.g. in duplex systems). Beware of a pseudoureterocoele due to an obstructing stone or mass at the VUJ.
8. **Radiation ureteritis.**
9. **Malakoplakia**—causes mural nodules and masses ± obstruction.
10. **Amyloidosis***—can cause a ureteral stricture ± calcification (highly suggestive).
11. **Vasculitis**—e.g. PAN, Wegener's granulomatosis, HSP, Churg-Strauss syndrome. Can rarely cause single or multiple ureteric strictures.
12. **Primary obstructive megaureter**—dilated pelvicalyceal system and ureter (>6 mm) transitioning to a normal calibre aperistaltic distal ureter, without a visible obstructing lesion. Congenital, often diagnosed antenatally but can present at any age.
13. **Congenital midureteric stricture**—short smooth stenosis in the midureter. Presents in infancy or antenatally, but is often mistaken for PUJ obstruction or megaureter.

Outside the wall

1. **Retroperitoneal fibrosis**—tethers and obstructs the midureters + medial deviation. Other infiltrative retroperitoneal processes can also obstruct the ureters but tend not to cause deviation, e.g. amyloidosis, Erdheim-Chester disease and extramedullary haematopoiesis.
2. **Direct invasion of the ureter from pelvic and retroperitoneal malignancies**—e.g. cervix, endometrium, bladder, prostate, rectum, lymphoma.
3. **Stricture due to adjacent inflammation**—e.g. appendicitis, diverticulitis, Crohn's disease, tuboovarian abscess, pelvic actinomycosis, inflammatory AAA.

4. Endometriosis*—typically causes distal ureteric stricturing + other features on MRI.
5. Extrinsic compression from benign pelvic masses—e.g. large uterine fibroids, pelvic lipomatosis.
6. Retrocaval ureter—right side only. Dilated upper ureter with a transition to normal as the ureter courses medially behind IVC.

Vesicoureteric reflux

Dilated pelvicalyceal system and ureter down to the VUJ (as opposed to primary megaureter where the distal ureter is of normal calibre) + demonstrable reflux. The ureter may become very dilated and tortuous. See Section 14.61.

No obstruction or reflux

1. Pregnancy—in the third trimester, R>L side.
2. Residual dilatation following relief of obstruction—most commonly following passage of a ureteric calculus or post prostatectomy.
3. **Polyuria or diuresis**—e.g. medication, diabetes insipidus.
4. **Urinary tract infection**—due to the effect of P-fimbriated *E. coli* on the urothelium.
5. **Primary nonobstructive megaureter**—similar to primary obstructive megaureter except there is usually no hydronephrosis.

Further reading

Mostbeck, G.H., Zontsich, T., Turetschek, K., 2001. Ultrasound of the kidney: obstruction and medical diseases. Eur. Radiol. 11, 1878–1889.

Potenta, S.E., D'Agostino, R., Sternberk, K.M., et al., 2015. CT urography for evaluation of the ureter. Radiographics 35 (3), 709–726.

9.31 DEVIATED URETERS

Medial deviation

1. Normal variant—in 15%, due to large iliopsoas muscles displacing distal ureters medially.
2. Retroperitoneal fibrosis—medially displaced midureters. See Section 9.33.
3. Retrocaval ureter—the right ureter passes behind the IVC at the level of L4. The distal ureter lies medial to the dilated proximal portion.
4. Pelvic lipomatosis—nearly always in men, most common in Afro-Caribbeans. Medial displacement of the distal ureters with elevation and elongation of the bladder ('pear-shaped') and rectum + widened presacral space. Lucent on plain film, CT shows diffuse symmetrical fatty proliferation around bladder and rectum.

May cause ureteric obstruction and cystitis glandularis. Chronic proctitis (e.g. due to UC or radiotherapy) can cause a similar appearance but the fatty proliferation is limited to the mesorectal fat.
5. **Following abdominoperineal resection**—the distal ureters are medially placed.
6. **Pelvic sidewall mass**—e.g. haematoma, lymphadenopathy, iliac artery aneurysm. Medially displaces one or both distal ureters.

Lateral deviation

Much more common than medial deviation.

1. **Hypertrophy of psoas muscles**—can displace upper ureters laterally.
2. **Retroperitoneal mass**—e.g. lymphadenopathy, haematoma, abscess, lymphocoele, sarcoma, neurogenic tumours. Displaces upper ureters.
3. **Pelvic mass**—e.g. fibroids, ovarian tumour. Displaces distal ureters.
4. **Aneurysmal aortic dilatation**—displaces upper ureters.
5. **Postoperative**—e.g. urostomy, ureterolysis.
6. **Prune-belly syndrome**—See Section 14.61.

9.32 RETROPERITONEAL MASS

Note that masses arising from retroperitoneal organs are excluded. Presacral masses are covered in Section 7.29.

Solid

Most solid retroperitoneal masses are malignant. There is significant overlap in imaging findings, but some features can be helpful.

1. **Lymphoma***—most common. Confluent mass or masses of paraaortic/iliac lymph nodes, typically homogeneous and mildly enhancing on CT. Infiltrative, tends to surround vessels without causing significant narrowing. Often lifts the aorta away from the spine ('floating aorta' sign). Necrosis is rare except in very high-grade lymphomas. Calcification is rare except post treatment.
2. **Other causes of retroperitoneal lymphadenopathy**.
   (a) Metastases—common sources include kidneys, cervix, prostate and testes. Central necrosis, if present, aids differentiation from lymphoma. Extranodal retroperitoneal metastases can also rarely be seen, e.g. from lung cancer or melanoma, usually in the presence of metastatic disease elsewhere.

(b) Infection—e.g. TB or MAC. Nodes are typically necrotic. Most common in immunocompromised patients.
(c) Sarcoidosis*—most commonly involves periportal nodes in the abdomen but paraaortic nodes can also be involved. Usually homogeneous, <2 cm and discrete (in contrast to the confluent adenopathy seen in lymphoma).
(d) Castleman disease—benign lymph node hyperplasia. Presents as single or multiple avidly enhancing lymph node masses in the peripancreatic, paraaortic or iliac regions ± intratumoural vessels. Often homogeneous, may be heterogeneous if large ± calcification.
(e) **Rosai-Dorfman disease***—can rarely cause retroperitoneal adenopathy or masses.

3. Nonneoplastic masses and infiltrative disorders
   (a) Vascular malformations—retroperitoneal collateral veins are commonly seen in portal hypertension. IVC anomalies are occasionally seen (e.g. left-sided, double, azygos continuation). Congenital AVMs are rare, usually seen in the pelvis. Haemangiomas are very rare in the retroperitoneum but may show characteristic marked T2 hyperintensity on MRI ± peripheral or progressive enhancement. Phleboliths and peripheral interdigitating fat may also be seen.
   (b) Retroperitoneal fibrosis—see Section 9.33.
   (c) Erdheim-Chester disease*—characteristic rind of soft tissue around the aorta and kidneys. T1/T2 hypointense, minimal enhancement.
   (d) Extramedullary haematopoiesis—well-defined, heterogeneous soft-tissue masses ± fat, in a paravertebral or presacral location. Splenomegaly and diffuse skeletal changes (sclerosis in myelofibrosis, expansion in thalassaemia) are usually also present indicating bone marrow failure.
   (e) Amyloidosis*—infiltrative, poorly enhancing, soft-tissue mass or thickening that may be focal or diffuse throughout the retroperitoneum ± involvement of mesentery and omentum. T2 hypointense on MRI. Often contains characteristic coarse calcification.
   (f) Old rejected renal transplant—located in the right or left iliac fossa. Atrophic and poorly enhancing with areas of calcification, may mimic a tumour. Surgical clips and vascular anastomoses are indicative.
4. Sarcomas—many different types (most common are below). Often large, well-defined ± invasion of adjacent structures. Note that rhabdomyosarcoma is the most common sarcoma in children (very rare in adults).
   (a) Liposarcoma—most are characteristically fatty, but pleomorphic variants contain little or no fat, presenting as a nonspecific heterogeneously enhancing soft-tissue mass.

Myxoid variants appear pseudocystic due to low attenuation on CT and high T2 signal on MRI, but internal reticular enhancement aids differentiation from true cysts.

(b) **Leiomyosarcoma**—often shows extensive necrosis and cystic change. Intravascular extension, e.g. into the IVC, is a characteristic feature if present (although angiosarcoma can also do this). Calcification is rare. F>M.

(c) **Undifferentiated pleomorphic sarcoma**—nonspecific heterogeneously enhancing mass. Calcification is not uncommon, and necrosis is usually less extensive than in leiomyosarcoma. M>F.

5. **Neurogenic tumours**—often occur in younger adults cf. sarcomas. Typically well-defined and usually benign but malignant varieties/transformation can occur.

(a) **Schwannoma**—round/oval encapsulated mass, can be homogeneous (if small) or heterogeneous with areas of cystic degeneration and calcification (if large or 'ancient'). Variable enhancement. Located along peripheral nerves, most commonly paravertebral ± nodular extension along the course of the nerve or towards a neural foramen.

(b) **Neurofibroma**—round or plexiform in shape, located along peripheral nerves. Low attenuation on CT (20–25 HU) with only mild enhancement. On MRI the target sign is characteristic if present: peripheral T2 hyperintensity (myxoid component) + central T2 hypointensity (cellular component). Extension into a spinal neural foramen is also characteristic. Plexiform neurofibromas are diagnostic of NF1 and present as fusiform expansion of peripheral nerves, usually bilateral and symmetrical (most commonly involving the lumbosacral plexus). These are at higher risk of malignant transformation: significant asymmetry, progressive enlargement, irregular infiltrative margins, areas of necrosis or perilesional oedema are worrying features.

(c) **Paraganglioma**—most common extraadrenal location is paraaortic distal to the inferior mesenteric artery origin (organs of Zuckerkandl). Typically shows avid enhancement on CT and MRI ± flow voids. May be homogeneously T2 bright or heterogeneous due to haemorrhage, necrosis and calcification. Uptake on MIBG scintigraphy is diagnostic. Typical clinical features (e.g. hypertension) may be present. Associated with NF1, MEN-2 and vHL. Risk of retroperitoneal haemorrhage. Up to 40% are malignant (large size and irregular margins are worrying features).

(d) **Ganglioneuroma**—benign tumour arising from paravertebral sympathetic ganglia. Well-defined and lobulated, often extending around vessels without causing significant narrowing. May extend into neural foramina.

Homogeneously hypoattenuating on unenhanced CT (myxoid stroma) ± calcification. Heterogeneously T2 hyperintense on MRI ± characteristic whorled appearance. Heterogeneous delayed enhancement. Necrosis is rare. The more malignant ganglion cell tumours (neuroblastoma and ganglioneuroblastoma) nearly always occur in children.

6. <u>Germ cell tumour</u>—nearly always in men. Large lobulated paraaortic mass; homogeneous if seminoma, heterogeneous with haemorrhage and necrosis if nonseminomatous. Calcification and fat suggests teratoma (F>M). Most represent metastatic disease from a testicular primary, but the primary tumour may 'burn out', leaving only a testicular scar and a paraaortic mass—this tends to be ipsilateral to the primary testicular tumour, whereas primary retroperitoneal germ cell tumours tend to be centred on the midline. Elevated serum αFP or ß-HCG can aid differentiation from other heterogeneous tumours.
7. <u>Desmoid tumour</u>—benign but locally aggressive, with a high rate of recurrence. Heterogeneously enhancing infiltrative mass, may be T2 hyperintense (cellular) or hypointense (fibrotic). Often invades the abdominal wall, may encase and narrow vessels. Associated with Gardner variant FAP.
8. <u>Solitary fibrous tumour</u>—well-defined, lobulated, usually benign. Typically shows marked heterogeneous enhancement ± intratumoural vessels—these features are suggestive but can also be seen in paraganglioma (characteristic location ± clinical features), angiosarcoma (usually ill-defined ± intravascular extension) and Castleman disease (often more homogeneous). Cystic change, necrosis or haemorrhage can occur. Calcification is rare.
9. <u>Undescended testis ± tumour</u>—located along the expected course of testicular descent, most commonly close to the deep inguinal ring. Associated gonadal vessels and absence of the testis within the scrotum are pathognomonic. Increased risk of tumour development, usually presents when large.
10. **Leiomyoma**—rare, nearly always in women (often with a history of uterine leiomyomas); usually located in the pelvis. T2 hypointense on MRI ± areas of cystic change (particularly if large) ± intratumoural vessels (angioleiomyoma). May mimic leiomyosarcoma.
11. **Primary sex cord stromal tumour**—very rare, seen only in women (usually peri- or postmenopausal). Usually in the pelvis (broad ligament) but can rarely be higher in the retroperitoneum. Nonspecific, heterogeneous mass ± calcification. An elevated oestrogen level is suggestive.
12. **Perivascular epithelioid cell tumour (PEComa)**—very rare, usually in middle-aged women. Most are benign. Nonspecific, well-defined, heterogeneously enhancing mass.

13. **Extragastrointestinal stromal tumour**—very rare. Nonspecific, well-defined, heterogeneously enhancing mass ± calcification.
14. **Extramedullary plasmacytoma**—very rare, most commonly perinephric in location. Nonspecific, infiltrative mass on imaging.

Cystic

1. **Nonneoplastic cystic lesions**—most common.
   (a) **Pseudocyst**—typically forms after an episode of acute pancreatitis; has a thick, enhancing wall and often heterogeneous contents ± foci of fat. Usually located close to the pancreas. A nonpancreatic pseudocyst can also rarely occur, representing a nonresolving, chronic haematoma.
   (b) **Urinoma**—occurs after rupture of the renal collecting system or bladder. Thin-walled, unilocular, located adjacent to the rupture site. May fill with contrast on delayed postcontrast images if there is an ongoing urine leak.
   (c) **Lymphocoele**—occurs after retroperitoneal lymphadenectomy due to leakage of lymph from cut lymphatics (look for surgical clips). Thin-walled, unilocular, located adjacent to iliac vessels or aorta. Fluid may have negative HU value on CT due to fat content.
   (d) **Haematoma**—most commonly due to coagulopathy; other causes include trauma and bleeding aneurysms or tumours (particularly AML and paraganglioma). Heterogeneous high attenuation on CT ± active contrast extravasation; if fluid–fluid levels are present ('haematocrit' sign) this indicates coagulopathy as the cause.
   (e) **Abscess**—enhancing wall, heterogeneous contents ± gas. Clinical features of sepsis. Common locations include perinephric, within psoas muscle and paravertebral (consider discitis). (a) to (d) can also become infected and resemble an abscess. If the abscess has a well-defined wall with minimal surrounding oedema/fat stranding, consider TB (cold abscess).
2. **Lymphangioma**—congenital malformation; can present at any age, more common in men (cf. items 3-8 below). Often large and elongated, characteristically traversing different compartments. Thin-walled, usually multilocular with no enhancement. May contain fat density/signal due to lymph. Calcification is rare except in lymphangiomatosis (multiple widespread lymphangiomas).
3. **Cystadenoma**—almost exclusively in women, can be mucinous or serous. Thin-walled unilocular cyst, usually in a lateral location. Solid nodules indicate malignant transformation to cystadenocarcinoma.

4. **Epidermoid cyst**—usually in the presacral space in middle-aged women, but can rarely be higher in the retroperitoneal space. Thin-walled, unilocular, typically near the midline.
5. **Müllerian cyst**—only occurs in women, typically obese with menstrual irregularity. Thin-walled, uni- or multilocular, usually in a lateral location.
6. **Cystic mesothelioma**—benign, most common in middle-aged women. Usually arises from the pelvic peritoneum but can rarely be retroperitoneal. Thin-walled, multilocular.
7. **Cystic teratoma**—benign, typically occurs in young girls. Complex cystic mass + characteristic foci of calcification and fat.
8. **Lymphangioleiomyoma**—cystic mass or masses with peripheral enhancement ± chylous ascites. Arises from lymphatics in the paraaortic region or next to iliac vessels. Only occurs in women with lymphangioleiomyomatosis, so look for the characteristic lung cysts.
9. **Bronchogenic cyst**—usually mediastinal, but can rarely be in the subphrenic retroperitoneal space. Thin-walled, unilocular, nonenhancing ± mural calcification. May be hyperattenuating due to proteinaceous contents.
10. **Dilated cisterna chyli**—located to the right of the aorta in the retrocrural space. Tubular, continues cranially as the thoracic duct.
11. **Cystic change in a solid neoplasm**—some solid tumours (such as paragangliomas, schwannomas, leiomyomas, leiomyosarcomas and synovial sarcomas) can show marked cystic change, becoming predominantly cystic with a thick irregular enhancing wall. Note that myxoid tumours appear pseudocystic, but the reticular internal enhancement (best seen on MRI) helps distinguish these from true cystic lesions.
12. **Hydatid cyst**—rare. Encapsulated, multilocular, no internal enhancement.

9

Fat containing

1. Liposarcoma—usually large and unencapsulated, displaces and compresses the adjacent kidney. Contains a mixture of fat and soft tissue ± calcification. Amount of fat is variable: well-differentiated tumours are usually almost entirely fatty + thick fibrous septa; dedifferentiated tumours are fatty with nodular soft-tissue components >1 cm or foci of calcification; myxoid and pleomorphic variants contain little or no fat.
2. Angiomyolipoma—typically arises from the kidney but can be very exophytic or rarely completely extrarenal, mimicking a liposarcoma. Prominent intratumoural vessels or aneurysms and an associated cortical notch in the adjacent kidney indicate AML.

3. Retroperitoneal fat necrosis—usually due to severe acute pancreatitis. Initially presents as ill-defined fat stranding, evolving into multiple fat-containing soft-tissue nodules, which involute over time. Can also involve mesenteric and omental fat. Long-term steroids can also cause fat necrosis but are more localized. Trauma or surgery can cause encapsulated fat necrosis: a thick, enhancing capsule and internal fat–fluid level are characteristic.
4. Perinephric lipomatosis—usually due to chronic infection or stones. Diffuse unencapsulated fatty proliferation with no soft-tissue components. A similar appearance can be seen with antiretroviral-associated lipodystrophy in patients with HIV.
5. **Lipoma**—rare in the retroperitoneum. Even a purely fatty retroperitoneal mass should be treated as suspicious for a well-differentiated liposarcoma.
6. **Teratoma**—rare, typically in young patients. Mature teratomas are encapsulated and contain a mixture of fat, soft tissue and calcification; a fat–fluid level is characteristic. Malignant teratomas usually contain little fat, and in men most represent metastases from a testicular primary (which may have 'burned out').
7. **Hibernoma**—rare, benign tumour of brown fat. Slightly higher attenuation than normal fat on CT (and slightly lower T1 signal on MRI) with internal septa ± enhancement. A prominent feeding vessel is almost pathognomonic. Typically shows high FDG uptake on PET (cf. well-differentiated liposarcomas, which show low grade uptake).
8. **Extraadrenal myelolipoma**—usually presacral, but can rarely arise higher in the retroperitoneum. Encapsulated fatty mass with streaky soft-tissue components. Can mimic liposarcoma but appears more well-defined and shows uptake on sulfur colloid scintigraphy.
9. **Extramedullary haematopoiesis**—haematopoietically inactive areas (yellow marrow) contain fat.
10. **Others**—paragangliomas, ganglioneuromas, haemangiomas and lymphangiomas can rarely contain macroscopic fat. Lipoblastomas appear similar to liposarcomas but occur only in infants and children.

Further reading

Osman, S., Lehnert, B.E., Elojeimy, S., et al., 2013. A comprehensive review of the retroperitoneal anatomy, neoplasms, and pattern of disease spread. Curr. Probl. Diagn. Radiol. 42 (5), 191–208.

Rajiah, P., Sinha, R., Cuevas, C., et al., 2011. Imaging of uncommon retroperitoneal masses. Radiographics 31 (4), 949–976.

Sangster, G.P., Migliaro, M., Heldmann, M.G., et al., 2016. The gamut of primary retroperitoneal masses: multimodality evaluation with pathologic correlation. Abdom Radiol (NY) 41 (7), 1411–1430.

Scali, E.P., Chandler, T.M., Heffernan, E.J., et al., 2015. Primary retroperitoneal masses: what is the differential diagnosis? Abdom. Imaging 40 (6), 1887–1903.

Shaaban, A.M., Rezvani, M., Tubay, M., et al., 2016. Fat-containing retroperitoneal lesions: imaging characteristics, localization, and differential diagnosis. Radiographics 36 (3), 710–734.

Yang, D.M., Jung, D.H., Kim, H., et al., 2004. Retroperitoneal cystic masses: CT, clinical, and pathologic findings and literature review. Radiographics 24 (5), 1353–1365.

9.33 RETROPERITONEAL FIBROSIS

1. Dense retroperitoneal/periaortic fibrotic soft-tissue mass (hypoechoic on US) that typically begins around the aortic bifurcation and extends superiorly to the renal arteries. Can rarely extend into the mesenteric root or into the pelvis. Reactive retroperitoneal lymphadenopathy is not uncommon.
2. Encases the aorta (usually sparing its posterior aspect and not displacing it away from the spine) and IVC, lymphatics and ureters ± obstruction. The ureters are tethered by the fibrosis and deviated medially.
3. In the acute inflammatory phase the mass shows moderate enhancement, T2 hyperintensity on MRI and uptake on PET. In the chronic fibrotic phase the mass shows minimal enhancement, T2 hypointensity and no uptake on PET.

Aetiology

1. <u>Primary ('idiopathic')</u>—>70%. Most cases now found to be autoimmune, due to IgG4-related disease. Similar histologically to chronic periaortitis and inflammatory AAA.
2. <u>Secondary</u>
   (a) **<u>Retroperitoneal malignancy</u>**—lymphoma and some metastases (e.g. from breast, stomach, colon, kidney, bladder, prostate, cervix, carcinoid, sarcomas) can trigger a desmoplastic reaction similar to RPF; lymphadenopathy tends to be more pronounced and metastases may be seen elsewhere. Malignancy often displaces the aorta away from the spine and may invade the psoas muscles or spine. Soft-tissue extension or adenopathy above the renal arteries is also suggestive of malignancy.
   (b) **Retroperitoneal haemorrhage**—e.g. due to ruptured aneurysm, trauma, surgery, coagulopathy. Blood incites a fibrotic reaction similar to RPF.
   (c) **Inflammatory conditions**—e.g. Crohn's, diverticulitis, TB, histoplasmosis, actinomycosis, pyelonephritis and extravasation of urine.

(d) **Connective tissue diseases**—e.g. ankylosing spondylitis, SLE, rheumatoid arthritis, PAN, Wegener's granulomatosis, Churg-Strauss syndrome, sarcoidosis.
(e) **Other infiltrative retroperitoneal processes**—particularly Erdheim-Chester disease, which characteristically causes a soft-tissue rind around the aorta (+ involvement of its posterior margin) and kidneys, usually sparing the ureters. Amyloidosis can also infiltrate the retroperitoneum but appears more diffuse than RPF, and does not usually involve the ureters.
(f) **Drugs**—e.g. ergot derivatives, dopamine agonists, hydralazine, ß-blockers, analgesics.
(g) **Retroperitoneal radiotherapy.**

Further reading

Cronin, C.G., Lohan, D.G., Blake, M.A., et al., 2008. Retroperitoneal fibrosis: a review of clinical features and imaging findings. AJR Am. J. Roentgenol. 191 (2), 423–431.

Runowska, M., Majewski, D., Puszczewicz, M., 2016. Retroperitoneal fibrosis - the state-of-the-art. Reumatologia 54 (5), 256–263.

Zen, Y., Onodera, M., Inoue, D., et al., 2009. Retroperitoneal fibrosis: a clinicopathologic study with respect to immunoglobulin G4. Am. J. Surg. Pathol. 33 (12), 1833–1839.

9.34 FILLING DEFECT OR MASS IN THE BLADDER

Within the lumen

1. Calculus.
2. Foreign body—e.g. catheter, ureteric stent and other self-inserted objects. If chronic these can become encrusted with calcification.
3. Blood clot—hyperattenuating on unenhanced CT, no acoustic shadow on US, no vascularity or enhancement. If serpiginous in appearance, suggests bleed from upper urinary tract.
4. Ureterocoele—cystic dilatation of ureter projecting into the bladder at VUJ or ectopic insertion site, giving a 'cobra-head' appearance on IVU.
5. **Fungus ball**—in immunocompromised patients, due to candidiasis or aspergillosis.

Arising from the wall

1. Malignant neoplasms—much more common than benign neoplasms. In practice all bladder polyps or masses are presumed malignant until proven otherwise, as imaging features overlap widely.
   (a) Urothelial carcinoma—accounts for 90% of bladder tumours in adults. Presents as a polypoid or papillary mass projecting

into the lumen, or as an area of focal wall thickening and/or enhancement. Often multifocal, tends to recur. Invades perivesical fat ± adjacent organs in advanced cases. May have calcification along its surface.

(b) <u>Squamous cell carcinoma</u>—<5% of bladder tumours, but >50% in areas where schistosomiasis is endemic. Other risk factors are chronic UTI and bladder calculi. Usually sessile and locally invasive, but otherwise indistinguishable from TCC.

(c) <u>Adenocarcinoma</u>—<2% of bladder tumours, classically associated with a persistent urachus or bladder exstrophy. Presents as a focal mass/polyp or, in the signet ring variant, as diffuse bladder wall thickening (like linitis plastica).

(d) <u>Metastasis</u>—most commonly from RCC, melanoma, breast or stomach.

(e) <u>Sarcoma</u>—rare in adults, but rhabdomyosarcoma is the most common bladder tumour in children. Leiomyosarcoma is the most common bladder sarcoma in adults, usually large and invasive with areas of necrosis.

(f) **Lymphoma***—rare, secondary > primary. Usually a discrete nonspecific mass.

(g) **Neuroendocrine tumours**—e.g. carcinoid tumour (small, polypoid) and small cell carcinoma (large, highly invasive and aggressive). Rare.

(h) **Melanoma**—rare, may be T1 hyperintense on MRI. Can also arise in urethra.

2. <u>Benign neoplasms</u>.

(a) <u>Papilloma</u>—usually small but essentially indistinguishable from papillary TCC.

(b) **Leiomyoma**—submucosal in location, smooth and well-defined with homogeneous low T2 signal on MRI ± cystic areas. Can be hard to differentiate from well-differentiated leiomyosarcoma on imaging.

(c) **Neurofibroma**—rare. Low attenuation on CT, T2 hyperintense on MRI + central hypointensity. May be focal, or diffuse/plexiform in NF1.

(d) **Paraganglioma**—rare. Avidly enhancing mass ± ring calcification ± characteristic history of micturition-induced hypertension and headache.

(e) **Haemangioma**—rare; small, hypervascular, homogeneously T2 bright.

(f) **Solitary fibrous tumour**—rare; large, well-defined, heterogeneous enhancement.

3. <u>Inflammatory lesions</u>.

(a) <u>Nephrogenic adenoma</u>—metaplastic response to chronic infection, stones, trauma or surgery. Usually solitary, can be polypoid or sessile. Does not invade muscularis or perivesical fat. Not premalignant, but often recurs.

9

(b) Cystitis cystica and glandularis—metaplastic response to chronic infection, obstruction or stones, differentiating into either cystic lesions (cystica) or mucin-secreting glands (glandularis)—both often coexist. Cystitis cystica presents as multiple small submucosal cysts. Cystitis glandularis can present as an enhancing polypoid mass. Does not invade muscularis or perivesical fat.
(c) Malakoplakia—uncommon chronic inflammatory response to *E. coli* infection, most often seen in the bladder. Variable appearances—solitary or multiple, polypoid or plaque-like, small or large, homogeneously or heterogeneously enhancing, intraluminal or invading perivesical fat. Indistinguishable from malignancy.
(d) **Inflammatory pseudotumour**—rare, most often seen in young adults. Single heterogeneously enhancing mass, may invade perivesical fat.
(e) **Eosinophilic cystitis**—rare. May present as diffuse bladder wall thickening or as a focal nonspecific enhancing mass.

4. Infection—TB and schistosomiasis (see Section 9.35).
5. **Amyloidosis***—rare, but the bladder is the most common involved site in the urinary tract. Usually causes focal bladder wall thickening or mass ± characteristic mural calcification.
6. **Ectopic prostate**—rare congenital anomaly. Small intramural nodule usually in the trigone or urethra.

Extrinsic

1. Prostatic enlargement—median lobe often protrudes into the bladder base in benign prostatic hyperplasia (BPH).
2. Pelvic lymphadenopathy, mass or collection—indents bladder outline. Pelvic malignancies (e.g. prostate, cervix, rectum) may also directly invade the bladder.
3. Enlarged uterus—e.g. fibroids, pregnancy. Indents bladder dome.
4. Inflammation adjacent to the bladder—e.g. Crohn's disease, diverticulitis. Causes focal bladder wall thickening adjacent to the inflammatory process. Intravesical gas suggests a fistula.
5. Iliac artery aneurysm—look for curvilinear calcification on XR.
6. **Colonic distension.**
7. **Urachal cyst or mass**—may indent the bladder dome in the midline.
8. **Endometriosis***—most often seen on the serosal surface of the posterior bladder wall in the uterovesical pouch. Deposits can grow through the bladder wall and create filling defects. Typically T1 hyperintense on MRI due to haemorrhage + enhancement + other sites of involvement in the pelvis.

Note that bilateral pelvic lesions (haematomas, collections, lymphadenopathy, lipomatosis, iliac artery aneurysms, iliopsoas hypertrophy or venous collaterals from IVC occlusion) can indent the bladder on both sides and elongate it, giving it a 'pear-shaped' appearance.

Further reading

Wong-You-Cheong, J.J., Woodward, P.J., Manning, M.A., Davis, C.J., 2006. From the archives of the AFIP: inflammatory and nonneoplastic bladder masses: radiologic-pathologic correlation. Radiographics 26 (6), 1847–1868.

Wong-You-Cheong, J.J., Woodward, P.J., Manning, M.A., Sesterhenn, I.A., 2006. From the archives of the AFIP: neoplasms of the urinary bladder: radiologic-pathologic correlation. Radiographics 26 (2), 553–580.

9.35 DIFFUSE BLADDER WALL THICKENING

Normal bladder wall thickness: <5 mm in nondistended bladders, <3 mm in well-distended bladders.

Inflammatory

1. **Any cause of cystitis**—e.g. infection, haemorrhagic cystitis (e.g. due to radiation or chemotherapy—look for intraluminal blood clots), trauma, eosinophilic cystitis, interstitial cystitis.
2. **Tuberculosis***—diffuse bladder wall thickening ± irregular mucosal masses in the acute phase. Contracted thick-walled bladder ± calcification in the chronic phase. Nearly always secondary to renal involvement, so the presence of normal kidneys practically excludes TB.
3. **Schistosomiasis***—diffuse nodular bladder wall thickening in the acute phase, similar to TB except that infection starts in the bladder and progresses up the urinary tract. Diffuse bladder wall calcification ± contraction/fibrosis in the chronic phase.
4. **Malakoplakia**—can involve the bladder circumferentially.

Muscular hypertrophy

Results in a thick-walled and trabeculated bladder.

1. **Chronic bladder outlet obstruction**—e.g. due to BPH, urethral stricture, posterior urethral valves. Bladder is typically distended.
2. **Neurogenic bladder (upper motor neuron damage only)**—characteristic 'pine cone' appearance on cystogram in severe cases due to elongated and trabeculated bladder, which may be distended or small. Note that lower motor neuron damage and sensory neuropathy both lead to a distended, thin-walled bladder.

Neoplastic

Most neoplasms present as masses or focal wall thickening (see Section 9.34), but a few can present as diffuse wall thickening.

1. **Signet-ring adenocarcinoma**—'linitis plastica' appearance.
2. **Metastases**—from gastric cancer or leukaemia.
3. **Lymphoma***—rare; 10% present as diffuse bladder wall thickening.
4. **Plexiform neurofibroma**—can diffusely involve the bladder wall. Low attenuation on CT, T2 hyperintense on MRI + central hypointensity. Rare; diagnostic of NF1.

Further reading

Shebel, H.M., Elsayes, K.M., Abou El Atta, H.M., et al., 2012. Genitourinary schistosomiasis: life cycle and radiologic–pathologic findings. Radiographics 32 (4), 1031–1046.

9.36 BLADDER CALCIFICATION

In the lumen

1. **Calculus**—may have passed through the ureter (typically <5 mm) or grown within the bladder (often large, round, may be laminated or spiculated).
2. **Foreign body**—encrustation of a ureteric stent or catheter balloon.
3. **Tumour**—e.g. TCC, SCC, paraganglioma, inflammatory pseudotumour. Typically surface calcification, so looks intraluminal on unenhanced CT (may be the only sign of an underlying tumour).
4. **Alkaline-encrusted cystitis**—due to *Corynebacterium* infection. Results in encrustation along infected urothelium. Can involve bladder or upper tracts.

In the wall

1. **Schistosomiasis***—infrequent in the Western hemisphere but the most common cause of mural calcification worldwide. Thin curvilinear calcification outlining a bladder of (usually) normal size and shape. Calcification spreads to the distal ureters in 15%.
2. **Tuberculosis***—rare and usually accompanied by calcification elsewhere in the urogenital tract. Contracted fibrotic bladder.
3. **Chronic radiation or chemotherapy-induced cystitis**—e.g. cyclophosphamide and mitomycin C. Contracted thick-walled bladder that can rarely calcify.
4. **Tumour**—mucinous adenocarcinoma may contain fine punctate calcification. Haemangioma may contain phleboliths.
5. **Amyloidosis***—rare. Can cause focal bladder wall calcification.

Further reading

Dyer, R.B., Chen, M.Y., Zagoria, R.J., 1998. Abnormal calcifications in the urinary tract. Radiographics 18 (6), 1405–1424.

Pollack, H.M., Banner, M.P., Martinez, L.O., et al., 1986. Diagnostic considerations in urinary bladder wall calcification. AJR Am. J. Roentgenol. 136, 791–797.

9.37 BLADDER FISTULA

Congenital

1. Bladder exstrophy—extruded bladder communicating with skin surface (surgically corrected in infancy). Markedly widened pubic symphysis on plain film (manta ray sign).
2. Imperforate anus—high type. Rectum can fistulate with bladder or urethra.
3. Patent urachus—bladder communicates with umbilicus.

Inflammatory

1. Diverticular disease—most common cause.
2. Crohn's disease*.
3. Appendix abscess—and other pelvic sepsis.
4. **Tuberculosis***—rare.

Neoplastic

1. Carcinoma of the colon, bladder or reproductive organs.
2. **Radiotherapy**—usually 12–18 months after treatment.

Trauma

1. Accidental.
2. Iatrogenic—particularly in obstetrics and gynaecology (vesicovaginal fistula).

Further reading

Yu, N.C., Raman, S.S., Patel, M., et al., 2004. Fistulas of the genitourinary tract: a radiologic review. Radiographics 24 (5), 1331–1352.

9.38 GAS IN THE URINARY SYSTEM

Gas shadows that conform to the position and shape of the bladder, ureters or pelvicalyceal systems on plain film.

Gas in the bladder lumen

Gas rises and forms an air–fluid level.

1. Following instrumentation—e.g. catheterization or cystoscopy.
2. Vesicointestinal fistula—diverticular disease, Crohn's disease and carcinoma of the colon or rectum.

9

3. <u>Cystitis</u>—due to gas-forming organisms and fermentation, especially in diabetics. Usually *E. coli*. Clostridial infections are rare, and usually secondary to septicaemia.
4. **Penetrating wounds.**

Gas in the bladder wall

String of gas bubbles outlining bladder wall.

1. <u>Emphysematous cystitis</u>—usually in diabetics.

Gas in the ureters and pelvicalyceal systems

1. **<u>Any cause of gas in the bladder</u>**.
2. <u>Ureteric diversion</u>—into the colon or bladder.
3. <u>Fistula</u>—most commonly with colon or duodenum; other sites include stomach, small bowel, skin or vagina. Most commonly iatrogenic (e.g. nephrostomy, nephrolithotomy, hysterectomy); other causes include urinary calculi, XGP, TB, trauma, malignancy, radiotherapy, diverticulitis, Crohn's disease or duodenal ulcer.
4. <u>Emphysematous pyelitis</u>—usually in diabetics. Gas may also be present in the renal parenchyma (emphysematous pyelonephritis) ± retroperitoneum.

Further reading

Grayson, D.E., Abbott, R.M., Levy, A.D., Sherman, P.M., 2002. Emphysematous infections of the abdomen and pelvis: a pictorial review. Radiographics 22 (3), 543–561.

Yu, N.C., Raman, S.S., Patel, M., Barbaric, Z., 2004. Fistulas of the genitourinary tract: a radiologic review. Radiographics 24 (5), 1331–1352.

9.39 URACHAL LESIONS

The urachus is an embryological connection between the anterosuperior bladder dome and the umbilicus, which normally involutes and obliterates completely in utero. It resides in the extraperitoneal space deep to rectus abdominis in the midline.

1. <u>Congenital anomalies</u>—due to incomplete involution. Any of these can be complicated by infection, stone formation or malignant transformation.
   (a) <u>Patent urachus</u>—the entire urachus remains patent, resulting in urine leaking from the umbilicus. Typically presents in neonates.
   (b) <u>Urachal cyst</u>—a focal portion of the urachus remains patent but does not communicate with the umbilicus or bladder, thereby forming a fluid-filled cyst. Unilocular with a thin minimally enhancing wall (unless infected).

(c) Urachal sinus—the umbilical end of the urachus remains patent, resulting in a blind-ending sinus extending inferiorly from the umbilicus ± intermittent discharge.
(d) Vesicourachal diverticulum—the bladder end of the urachus remains patent, resulting in a midline outpouching from the anterosuperior bladder dome.

2. Infection—most common complication of urachal anomalies, most often by *S. aureus* and *E. coli*. Heterogeneous echogenicity on US, mural enhancement + surrounding fat stranding on CT. Can form an abscess ± fistula. May mimic urachal carcinoma if large and complex.
3. Malignancy—usually adenocarcinoma; most are mucinous with areas of calcification. Typically located adjacent to the bladder dome—a midline supravesical mass containing calcification is almost diagnostic of urachal carcinoma. Mucinous components will appear cystic on CT and T2 hyperintense on MRI. Solid components will enhance. Less common malignancies include TCC, SCC and sarcoma.
4. **Benign tumours**—e.g. adenoma, cystadenoma, fibroma, fibroadenoma, fibromyoma, hamartoma. Very rare, indistinguishable from carcinoma.
5. **Mimics of urachal lesions.**
   (a) **At the umbilicus**—an omphalomesenteric duct sinus can mimic an urachal sinus, although the former usually courses to the right (towards the distal ileum) rather than inferiorly in the midline. Other causes of periumbilical inflammation can mimic an infected urachal sinus.
   (b) **Supravesical**—other lesions inseparable from the bladder dome can mimic a urachal tumour or abscess, e.g. endometrioma, ovarian torsion, invasive bladder cancer, malakoplakia, inflammatory pseudotumour, peritoneal metastasis, appendiceal abscess, dropped gallstone.

Further reading

Parada Villavicencio, C., Adam, S.Z., Nikolaidis, P., et al., 2016. Imaging of the urachus: anomalies, complications, and mimics. Radiographics 36 (7), 2049–2063.

9.40 CALCIFICATIONS OF THE MALE GENITAL TRACT

Seminal vesicles and vas deferens

1. Diabetes mellitus—vast majority of cases. Bilateral and symmetrical linear calcification of the vas deferens wall. Ageing and secondary hyperparathyroidism can produce an identical appearance.

9

2. **Chronic infection**—mainly TB but also schistosomiasis, chronic UTI, gonorrhoea and syphilis. Vas deferens calcification is intraluminal and usually unilateral or asymmetrical. Seminal vesicles can show wall calcification in chronic schistosomiasis.
3. **Seminal vesicle/ejaculatory duct calculi**—rare, usually secondary to ejaculatory duct obstruction (e.g. congenital or due to chronic infection).

Prostate

Calcification is common in men >50 years and is nearly always benign.

1. **Benign calcification**—typically located in the periurethral region or at the interface between transitional and peripheral zones. Most commonly due to chronic prostatitis (including TB and schistosomiasis) or BPH, but can also rarely be seen in hyperparathyroidism and may be extensive in alkaptonuria.
2. **Prostate cancer**—calcification within the peripheral zone is suggestive of underlying malignancy.
3. **Impacted calculus in the prostatic urethra**—located in the midline.
4. **Seed brachytherapy**—multiple tiny radioactive seeds implanted for treatment of prostate cancer. Very dense on plain film and CT. Radiation therapy can also cause prostate calcification.

Scrotum

1. **Testicular microlithiasis**—multiple (>4) 1–3mm echogenic nonshadowing intratesticular foci, usually bilateral. Common incidental finding. No follow-up needed in low-risk asymptomatic patients. Note that solitary punctate calcification in an otherwise normal testis usually represents a phlebolith or sperm granuloma.
2. **Scrotal pearl**—represents a previously torted and detached testicular or epididymal appendix. Often mobile, located between the layers of tunica vaginalis. The appendix may also calcify in situ without detaching.
3. **Previous trauma, torsion or infection**—including TB. Calcification may be intratesticular or in the epididymis or tunica albuginea ± a chronic haematocoele or pyocoele. Missed torsion leads to an atrophic testis containing multifocal calcification.
4. **Calcification in a mass lesion**—Sertoli cell tumours and nonseminomatous germ cell tumours often contain calcification, especially those with a teratoma component. A 'burned-out' testicular tumour can regress into an irregular focus of calcification. Calcification can also be seen in the walls of cysts and epidermoids, and within paratesticular fibrous pseudotumours.
5. **Sperm/suture granuloma**—occurs at vasectomy site on vas deferens.

6. **End-stage renal failure**—can produce bilateral epididymal calcification.

Penis

1. **Peyronie's disease**—the fibrous plaques on the tunica albuginea can calcify.
2. **End-stage renal failure**—can cause calcification of vessels or tunica albuginea in the penis.

Further reading

Bushby, L.H., Miller, F.N., Rosairo, S., et al., 2002. Scrotal calcification: ultrasound appearances, distribution and aetiology. Br. J. Radiol. 75 (891), 283–288.

Chen, M.Y., Bechtold, R.E., Bohrer, S.P., et al., 1999. Abnormal calcification on plain radiographs of the abdomen [Review]. Crit. Rev. Diagn. Imaging 40 (2–3), 63–202.

9.41 PROSTATIC LESIONS

Solid

1. **Benign prostatic hyperplasia**—most common prostatic mass. Presents as well-defined nodular enlargement of the transitional zone with heterogeneous T2 signal on MRI. May protrude into the bladder base.
2. **Prostatic adenocarcinoma**—95% of prostate cancers. 70% arise from the peripheral zone (in contrast to BPH). T2 hypointense on MRI + restricted diffusion + early enhancement and washout. Easier to detect in the peripheral zone (which is normally T2 hyperintense) than the transitional zone, where it can be hard to differentiate from BPH nodules—ill-defined margins, lentiform shape, homogeneous T2 hypointensity + restricted diffusion favours carcinoma. Tumours may show extracapsular invasion ± involvement of seminal vesicles, bladder, rectum or pelvic floor/sidewall. Typically metastasizes to lymph nodes and bones (sclerotic deposits), and less commonly to lung and liver.
3. **Benign mimics of prostate cancer**
   (a) **Postbiopsy haemorrhage**—commonly seen in the peripheral zone, usually resolves after 6–8 weeks. Causes T2 hypointensity ± restricted diffusion, but the presence of T1 hyperintensity distinguishes this from cancer.
   (b) **Prostatitis**—acute, chronic and granulomatous (e.g. TB, malakoplakia, sarcoidosis) prostatitis all usually involve the peripheral zone, causing focal or diffuse T2 hypointensity + restricted diffusion indistinguishable from cancer. Granulomatous prostatitis can also extend beyond the prostate. Prostatitis can lead to necrosis and atrophy of the peripheral zone resulting in volume loss, T2 hypointensity and

restricted diffusion. Volume loss and low-level enhancement can help differentiate this from carcinoma.
   (c) Normal structures—the anterior fibromuscular stroma (anterior to transitional zone) and central zone (around ejaculatory ducts) are both homogeneously and symmetrically T2 hypointense and must not be mistaken for carcinoma.
4. Secondary malignancy—usually due to direct prostate invasion from bladder or rectal cancer. Tumours of the prostatic urethra (e.g. carcinoma, melanoma) can also invade the prostate. Metastases (e.g. from lung, melanoma, GI tract) are less common.
5. **Rare prostate neoplasms**—serum prostate specific antigen (PSA) is usually normal. Bone metastases, if present, are usually lytic (in contrast to the sclerotic metastases seen in adenocarcinoma).
   (a) **Other carcinomas**—SCC, TCC and BCC can rarely arise from the prostate. SCC is T2 hypointense, indistinguishable from adenocarcinoma. TCC and BCC may be T2 hyperintense. SCC and TCC have a poor prognosis.
   (b) **Sarcomas**—most common are rhabdomyosarcoma (in children) and leiomyosarcoma (in adults). Usually much larger than adenocarcinoma and more heterogeneous on T2 and postcontrast sequences due to haemorrhage and necrosis. Often invades adjacent structures and metastasizes early.
   (c) **Stromal tumour of uncertain malignant potential (STUMP)**—well-defined heterogeneously enhancing solid-cystic mass, often large. Involves both peripheral and transitional zones (in contrast to BPH, which displaces the peripheral zone). May be adherent to rectum, often recurs after surgery. Can transform into stromal sarcoma.
   (d) **Lymphoma***—homogeneous soft-tissue mass, which can involve the whole prostate. Usually secondary involvement, with disease present elsewhere.
   (e) **Neuroendocrine tumours**—e.g. carcinoid (low grade, heterogeneously T2 hyperintense), small cell carcinoma (high grade, very aggressive), paraganglioma (T2 hyperintense, avid enhancement, characteristic clinical picture of headache, tachycardia and sweating induced by micturition or rectal examination).
6. **Rare benign lesions**—e.g. inflammatory pseudotumour, solitary fibrous tumour, leiomyoma, neurofibroma, haemangioma, dermoid cyst.
7. **Amyloidosis***—rare; T2 hypointense with no restricted diffusion and minimal enhancement.

Cystic

1. Midline—(a)-(c) are located posterior to the prostatic urethra and are unilocular and T2 bright on MRI, with variable T1 signal

depending on protein content. Infection and stone formation can occur.

(a) Utricle cyst—small (8–10 mm), does not extend beyond prostate. Communicates with prostatic urethra. May be associated with other congenital genitourinary anomalies.
(b) Müllerian duct cyst—larger, elongated, usually extends above the prostate. Does not communicate with urethra.
(c) Ejaculatory duct cyst—rare, due to obstruction and dilatation of ejaculatory duct. Usually small and paramedian, may appear in the midline if large. Can communicate with urethra, vas deferens and/or seminal vesicles.
(d) **Cowper's duct cyst (mimic)**—located inferior to the prostatic apex within the urogenital diaphragm or bulb of the corpus spongiosum. Usually unilocular, midline or paramedian. If large, may appear inseparable from the prostate. Usually communicates with the bulbous urethra.
(e) **TURP defect (mimic)**—irregular periurethral urine-filled defect continuous with bladder lumen.

2. **Lateral**
   (a) Cystic degeneration of BPH—most common cystic lesion. Occurs in the transitional zone only. Usually small and multiple, may contain haemorrhage or calculi.
   (b) Retention cyst—also occurs in BPH but can be located in any zone.
   (c) Abscess—clinical features of acute prostatitis are key. Increased risk in diabetic or immunocompromised men. Irregular enhancing walls, heterogeneous contents ± septations + restricted diffusion. May rupture into urethra (creating a urethral pseudodiverticulum) or fistulate with the rectum. A tuberculous abscess may create multiple fistulae to the perineal and scrotal skin ('watering can' perineum).
   (d) **Cavitary prostatitis**—due to chronic prostatitis, resulting in cystic change throughout the gland ('Swiss cheese' appearance).
   (e) **Cystic tumours.**
      (i) **Cystic prostate carcinoma**—some variants of adenocarcinoma (e.g. mucinous or ductal) can show cystic change. Usually located in the peripheral zone (in contrast to cystic BPH).
      (ii) **Multilocular cystadenoma**—benign cystic tumour with multiple enhancing septations, typically very large and extending well above the prostate without invasion of adjacent structures. May contain haemorrhage and small enhancing solid elements. Often appears in the midline due to its large size.
      (iii) **Lymphangioma**—rare. Multiloculated, minimal enhancement.

(f) **Hydatid cyst**—very rare. Encapsulated, multilocular, no internal enhancement.

Further reading

Chang, J.M., Lee, H.J., Lee, S.E., et al., 2008. Pictorial review: unusual tumours involving the prostate: radiological-pathological findings. Br. J. Radiol. 81 (971), 907–915.

Chu, L.C., Ross, H.M., Lotal, T.L., Macura, K.J., 2013. Prostatic stromal neoplasms: differential diagnosis of cystic and solid prostatic and periprostatic masses. AJR 200 (6), W571–W580.

Kitzing, Y.X., Prando, A., Varol, C., et al., 2016. Benign conditions that mimic prostate carcinoma: MR imaging features with histopathologic correlation. Radiographics 36 (1), 162–175.

Li, Y., Mongan, J., Behr, S.C., et al., 2016. Beyond prostate adenocarcinoma: expanding the differential diagnosis in prostate pathologic conditions. Radiographics 36 (4), 1055–1075.

Shebel, H.M., Farg, H.M., Kolokythas, O., El-Diasty, T., 2013. Cysts of the lower male genitourinary tract: embryologic and anatomic considerations and differential diagnosis. Radiographics 33 (4), 1125–1143.

9.42 SEMINAL VESICLE ABNORMALITIES

1. **Congenital**—often associated with other genitourinary tract anomalies.
   (a) **Agenesis/hypoplasia**—bilateral agenesis is associated with cystic fibrosis. Unilateral agenesis is often associated with ipsilateral renal agenesis.
   (b) **Cyst**—bilateral cysts are associated with ADPKD. A unilateral cyst (or cystic dilatation) is often associated with ejaculatory duct obstruction and ipsilateral renal agenesis—the triad of Zinner syndrome. The cyst may contain proteinaceous material (T1 hyperintense). A ureteric remnant is often present and may insert ectopically onto the cystic seminal vesicle or other sites.
2. **Secondary tumour invasion**—most commonly by prostate cancer (stage T3b disease), less commonly by bladder or rectal cancer. The vas deferens may also be involved.
3. **Iatrogenic changes**—prostate biopsy can cause seminal vesicle haemorrhage (intraluminal T1 hyperintensity helps differentiate this from malignant infiltration). Radiotherapy often causes bilateral symmetrical seminal vesicle atrophy with luminal narrowing or obliteration and diffuse mural T2 hypointensity.
4. **Infection**—usually secondary to prostatitis (e.g. bacterial, tuberculous, schistosomiasis). Diffuse mural thickening and enhancement with luminal dilatation in the acute phase. An abscess may form, particularly in diabetics or following instrumentation. In chronic or recurrent infection the seminal vesicles atrophy.

5. **Amyloidosis***—common in the elderly. Bilateral diffuse T2 hypointense mural thickening and luminal narrowing. The lack of restricted diffusion or enhancement helps distinguish this from malignant infiltration.
6. **Primary seminal vesicle tumours**—very rare. Malignant tumours (infiltrative appearance) are more common and include adenocarcinoma, sarcoma and seminoma. Benign tumours (well-defined) include cystadenoma (multiloculated cystic mass), leiomyoma, fibroma, schwannoma, paraganglioma, dermoid cyst.
7. **Hydatid cyst**—very rare. Multiloculated with nonenhancing septa.

Further reading

Kim, B., Kawashima, A., Ryu, J.A., et al., 2009. Imaging of the seminal vesicle and vas deferens. Radiographics 29 (4), 1105–1121.

Mahati, N.R., Verma, S., 2014. Lesions of the seminal vesicles and their MRI characteristics. J Clin Imaging Sci 4, 61.

9.43 ULTRASOUND OF INTRATESTICULAR ABNORMALITIES

Neoplastic

Usually painless. Most are malignant and imaging features overlap, so most solid painless intratesticular masses are presumed malignant until proven otherwise.

1. Germ cell tumours—95% of testicular tumours in young men, nearly always unilateral. Usually hypervascular on US. Risk factors include undescended testes (even if corrected), previous contralateral germ cell tumour or positive family history. The primary tumour may 'burn out', regressing into an irregular focus of calcification, but any metastases will remain.
   (a) Seminoma—~50%. Typically a solid well-defined homogeneously hypoechoic mass contained within the testis. May be multifocal. Necrosis and calcification are rare. 25% have retroperitoneal nodal disease at presentation. αFP and ß-HCG are usually normal.
   (b) Nonseminomatous germ cell tumour—usually contains a mixture of embryonal, teratoma, yolk sac and choriocarcinoma components. More aggressive than seminoma and more heterogeneous due to necrosis, haemorrhage, cystic change and calcification. Often invades tunica albuginea. αFP, ß-HCG and LDH often raised. Pure yolk sac tumour is the most common testicular tumour in children.
   (c) Epidermoid cyst—most common benign testicular tumour. Characteristic 'onion skin' appearance on US: well-defined avascular mass containing concentric echogenic rings of

keratin. Alternatively may be hypoechoic with a central echogenic focus (target appearance). May be rim-calcified.

2. **Sex cord stromal tumours**—usually benign but indistinguishable from malignancy on imaging; usually small, solitary, hypoechoic and hypervascular. Leydig cell tumours are the most common and may secrete testosterone or oestrogen. Sertoli cell tumours can calcify, may secrete oestrogen and are associated with Peutz-Jeghers syndrome and Carney complex. Rarer subtypes include granulosa cell tumour and thecoma-fibroma.
3. Lymphoma*—most common testicular malignancy in men >60 years, usually secondary. Hypoechoic and hypervascular on US, often multifocal and bilateral. May be diffuse. Leukaemia can look identical.
4. **Metastases**—rare, usually in patients >50 years. May be bilateral. Most common sources include prostate, lung, kidney, colon and melanoma.
5. **Cystadenoma of the rete testis**—rare. Multiloculated cystic tumour arising from rete testis. Has mass effect and may extend beyond testis (in contrast to tubular ectasia). Indistinguishable from cystadenocarcinoma therefore needs excision.
6. **Other rare tumours not limited to the testis**—e.g. haemangioma, leiomyoma, lipoma, sarcoma, plasmacytoma, carcinoid tumour, neurofibroma. Apart from lipoma (well-defined and hyperechoic), these do not have specific imaging findings.

Nonneoplastic cysts

Typically painless. Note that cystic tumours usually have complex features, i.e. a perceptible wall, septations ± solid components.

1. Tubular ectasia of the rete testis—geographic cluster of numerous small cysts replacing the mediastinum testis. No mass effect or Doppler flow. Often bilateral, more common in older men.
2. Simple cyst—2–20 mm; unilocular, anechoic with an imperceptible wall. Usually solitary and often located near the mediastinum.
3. Intratesticular varicocoele (mimic)—serpiginous with venous flow on Doppler.

Vascular

Usually painful.

1. Testicular torsion
   (a) Acute—presentation <24 hours. Enlarged isoechoic (early), hypoechoic or heterogeneous (late) testis ± hydrocoele and epididymal enlargement. Colour Doppler: absent testicular flow (complete torsion) or reduced diastolic arterial flow

(partial torsion <360 degrees); normal peritesticular flow. A twist in the spermatic cord may be seen (most specific sign).
   (b) Subacute or missed—presentation at 1–10 days. Hypoechoic heterogeneous testis due to infarction. Colour Doppler: absent testicular flow; increased peritesticular flow. Testis atrophies in the chronic phase.
   (c) Spontaneous detorsion—colour Doppler: normal or increased testicular flow; increased peritesticular flow.
2. Segmental infarction—due to infection, trauma, transient torsion, vasculitis (most commonly PAN), sickle cell disease or hypercoagulable states. Geographic hypoechoic hypovascular area extending to periphery of testis.

Infective

Usually painful. Imaging features can overlap with malignancy but the presence of epididymal enlargement, scrotal thickening and hydrocoele favours infection.

1. Epididymoorchitis—generalized testicular and/or epididymal swelling and hypoechogenicity initially; progresses to patchy focal low reflectivity. Hypoechoic areas are hypervascular. Isolated orchitis is rare except in mumps. Complications occur in 50%—abscess, necrosis, haematoma and testicular atrophy/scarring.
2. Abscess—complicating epididymoorchitis, often in diabetics or those with mumps. Hypoechoic (or mixed) with an irregular ill-defined wall and low level internal echoes. No internal vascularity, but peripheral hyperaemia is often seen.
3. Granulomatous infection—e.g. TB, brucellosis, syphilis, schistosomiasis, leprosy and fungal infections. Presentation is usually subacute, and pain is less marked. US appearances vary, ranging from diffuse epididymoorchitis to a focal abscess or mass mimicking malignancy. In TB and schistosomiasis, other sites of urinary tract involvement are usually present. TB may also create a sinus tract to the scrotal skin. Other infections tend to occur in immunocompromised patients.

Miscellaneous

1. Testicular haematoma—hypoechoic and avascular. History of trauma is indicative.
2. Testicular sarcoidosis—typically presents in Afro-Caribbean men (in whom testicular cancer is rare) with multiple bilateral small painless hypoechoic masses in the testes and epididymides. Usually occurs in the presence of multisystem involvement.
3. Testicular lipomatosis—multiple, usually bilateral, small well-defined hyperechoic lesions. No mass effect or hypervascularity. Pathognomonic for Cowden syndrome.

4. **Testicular adrenal rests**—seen in congenital adrenal hyperplasia. Variable echogenicity; usually multiple, bilateral and located next to mediastinum testis.
5. **Other rare disorders not limited to the testis**—e.g. malakoplakia, amyloidosis, Rosai-Dorfman disease. Nonspecific testicular mass indistinguishable from malignancy.

Further reading

Dogra, V.S., Gottlieb, R.H., Rubens, D.J., et al., 2001. Benign intratesticular cystic lesions: US features. Radiographics 21, S273–S281.

Mirochnik, B., Bhargava, P., Dighe, M.K., Kanth, N., 2012. Ultrasound evaluation of scrotal pathology [Review]. Radiol. Clin. North Am. 50 (2), 317–332.

Moreno, C.C., Small, W.C., Camacho, J.C., et al., 2015. Testicular tumors: what radiologists need to know—differential diagnosis, staging, and management. Radiographics 35 (2), 400–415.

9.44 ULTRASOUND OF EXTRATESTICULAR ABNORMALITIES

Within epididymis

1. **Epididymitis**—acute history of pain. Enlarged, hypoechoic, hypervascular epididymis with a hydrocoele and skin thickening ± involvement of testis (epididymoorchitis). May be complicated by an epididymal abscess: complex cystic lesion with an irregular wall, no internal vascularity with surrounding hyperaemia. Consider granulomatous infection (e.g. TB) if presentation is subacute.
2. **Spermatocoele**—unilocular or multilocular cyst in epididymal head containing low level echoes ('falling snow') representing spermatozoa.
3. **Epididymal cyst**—unilocular simple cyst in any part of epididymis, no internal echoes.
4. **Postvasectomy ectasia**—epididymis enlarges and appears heterogeneous due to obstruction and dilatation of epididymal ducts. A sperm granuloma may also be seen.
5. **Sarcoidosis***—epididymal enlargement or focal hypoechoic nodules. More common than testicular involvement. Usually bilateral, in the presence of disease elsewhere.
6. **Neoplasms**—most are benign.
   (a) **Adenomatoid tumour**—most common, benign. Well-defined, solid, hypovascular, often hyperechoic on US, most common in the tail.
   (b) **Leiomyoma**—well-defined hypoechoic mass ± cystic change, usually in the head.
   (c) **Papillary cystadenoma**—benign. Typically a mixed solid-cystic mass in the head. Associated with vHL (especially if bilateral).

(d) **Lymphoma*/leukaemia**—rare, often bilateral. Testicular involvement is more common and more extensive (in contrast to sarcoidosis and TB).
(e) **Metastasis**—e.g. from prostate, kidney, GI tract, pancreas. Rare.
(f) **Other rare tumours**—e.g. lymphangioma (multiloculated cystic mass), haemangioma, neurofibroma, sarcoma, adenocarcinoma and plasmacytoma.

7. **Epididymal filariasis**—parasites can be seen moving within dilated epididymal lymphatics on US ('filarial dance sign'). Endemic in tropical areas.

Paratesticular

1. **Hydrocoele**—serous fluid collection between layers of tunica vaginalis. Can be congenital (due to patent processus vaginalis) or reactive to scrotal infection, torsion or malignancy. Envelops the testis (cf. large epididymal cysts which displace the testis).
2. **Pyocoele/haematocoele**—due to infection (pyocoele) or trauma/surgery (haematocoele). Complex paratesticular fluid collection with internal echoes and septations, ± gas if pyocoele.
3. **Tunica albuginea cyst**—2–5 mm, unilocular or septated, located on the surface of the testis.
4. **Scrotal pearl**—see Section 9.40.
5. **Fibrous pseudotumour**—benign reactive fibrous proliferation, typically arises from tunica vaginalis. Single or multiple hypoechoic hypovascular masses ± calcification ± hydrocoele.
6. **Other rare benign tumours of the tunica vaginalis**—e.g. adenomatoid tumour, leiomyoma (can also arise from dartos muscle), lipoma, solitary fibrous tumour.
7. **Malignancies of peritoneal origin involving the tunica vaginalis**—rare.
   (a) **Metastasis**—disseminated peritoneal malignancy + a patent processus vaginalis allows spread of tumour (and fluid) into the tunica vaginalis.
   (b) **Mesothelioma**—typically in older men with a history of asbestos exposure. Usually presents as multiple masses or nodules on the tunica vaginalis + hydrocoele. Benign variants can also occur in younger men.
   (c) **Ovarian-type epithelial tumours**—histologically identical to ovarian surface epithelial tumours and primary peritoneal carcinoma. Usually mixed solid-cystic.
8. **Supernumerary testis**—isoechoic to, and smaller than, the adjacent normal testis.
9. **Splenogonadal fusion**—ectopic splenic tissue attached to the testis (nearly always the left; may be undescended). Homogeneously hypoechoic on US, may have a prominent feeding vessel ± a band of splenic/fibrous tissue connecting the testis to the spleen.

Related to spermatic cord

1. Varicocoele—dilated pampiniform plexus of veins >2 mm on US. Seen in 15% of adult men, usually on the left side. Important to exclude a retroperitoneal mass, particularly in the older patient, if bilateral or if the history is short.
2. Inguinoscrotal hernia—protrudes from the inguinal canal into the scrotum, enlarges with Valsalva.
3. Lipoma—most common extratesticular nonepididymal tumour. May mimic a hernia but is separate from the deep inguinal ring and does not enlarge with Valsalva. Well-defined, avascular, usually uniformly hyperechoic.
4. Hydrocoele of the spermatic cord—may be encysted (resembling a simple cyst) or may communicate with peritoneal space via a patent processus vaginalis (funicular type).
5. Sperm granuloma—occurs following vasectomy at the cut ends of the vas deferens. Well-defined hypoechoic mass.
6. Spermatic cord haematoma—most commonly following inguinal hernia repair but can also occur due to trauma, ruptured varicocoele or anticoagulation.
7. **Leiomyoma**—usually in the inguinal part of the spermatic cord (in contrast to leiomyosarcoma, which is usually in the scrotal part).
8. **Sarcoma**—most common spermatic cord malignancy, most often rhabdomyosarcoma (teenagers and children), liposarcoma or leiomyosarcoma (older men). These present as large heterogeneous invasive soft-tissue masses, apart from well-differentiated liposarcomas, which are mostly fatty and well-defined (albeit difficult to characterize on US).
9. **Other rare tumours**—e.g. adenomatoid tumour, aggressive angiomyxoma, cellular angiofibroma, haemangioma, nerve sheath tumours, paraganglioma, rhabdomyoma, dermoid cyst, lymphoma, plasmacytoma.

Further reading

Akbar, S.A., Sayyed, T.A., Jafri, S.Z.H., et al., 2003. Multimodality imaging of paratesticular neoplasms and their rare mimics. Radiographics 23 (6), 1461–1476.

Cassidy, F.H., Ishioka, K.M., McMahon, C.J., et al., 2010. MR imaging of scrotal tumors and pseudotumors. Radiographics 30 (3), 665–683.

Garriga, V., Serrano, A., Marin, A., et al., 2009. US of the tunica vaginalis testis: anatomic relationships and pathologic conditions. Radiographics 29 (7), 2017–2032.

Kim, W., Rosen, M.A., Langer, J.E., et al., 2007. US MR imaging correlation in pathologic conditions of the scrotum. Radiographics 27 (5), 1239–1253.

Woodward, P.J., Schwab, C.M., Sesterhenn, I.A., 2003. From the archives of the AFIP: extratesticular scrotal masses: radiologic-pathologic correlation. Radiographics 23 (1), 215–240.

9.45 MALE URETHRAL STRICTURE

1. **Trauma**—typically short in length, developing weeks or months after the trauma. Straddle injuries cause strictures of the bulbous urethra. High-energy pelvic fractures cause strictures of the membranous urethra. Iatrogenic trauma, e.g. instrumentation and prostatectomy, causes strictures of the bulbomembranous and prostatic urethra respectively.
2. **Infection**—usually due to chronic or recurrent gonococcal urethritis. Strictures are usually long/multiple and irregular, most commonly in the bulbous urethra, and may be complicated by a periurethral abscess ± perineal or scrotal fistula. Small contrast-filled outpouchings (periurethral glands) strongly suggest infection. Urethral TB is rare but causes strictures of the anterior urethra with multiple perineal and scrotal fistulae ('watering can' perineum).
3. **Urethral cancer**—usually SCC (anterior urethra) or TCC (prostatic urethra), but adenocarcinoma and rarely leiomyosarcoma, melanoma and lymphoma can also occur. Most arise from the bulbomembranous urethra and present as a palpable mass ± urinary obstruction or bleeding. An irregular urethral stricture or change in morphology of a previously benign stricture suggests malignancy. MRI shows a T2 hypointense mass and aids local staging.
4. **Secondary urethral malignancy**—rare. Bladder TCC can seed to the urethra. Direct invasion of the urethra can occur from prostatic, rectal and scrotal malignancies. Penile metastases (e.g. from prostate, melanoma, colon) can erode into the urethra.
5. **Balanitis xerotica obliterans**—lichen sclerosus of the penis. Causes meatal stenosis ± strictures of the penile urethra.
6. **Congenital stricture**—rare, usually presents in childhood.
7. **Benign urethral lesions**—very rare, present as a filling defect rather than a stricture. Examples include papilloma, leiomyoma, haemangioma, fibroepithelial polyp (congenital, arises from verumontanum), malakoplakia, amyloidosis and condyloma acuminata (due to HPV infection; multiple papillary filling defects in anterior urethra + cutaneous papillomas on the penis).

Further reading

Kawashima, A., Sandler, C.M., Wasserman, N.F., et al., 2004. Imaging of urethral disease: a pictorial review. Radiographics 24 (Suppl. 1), S195–S216.

9

Gynaecology and obstetrics

Nishat Bharwani, Victoria Stewart

GYNAECOLOGICAL IMAGING

10.1 COMMON INDICATIONS FOR GYNAECOLOGICAL ULTRASOUND

Primary amenorrhoea

1. Constitutional delay.
2. Polycystic ovarian syndrome (PCOS).
3. Congenital genitourinary malformation—broad range of anomalies, see Fig. 10.2.
4. Gartner duct cyst.
5. Complete androgen insensitivity syndrome (CAIS)—Y chromosome present but external genitalia are of female phenotype due to complete insensitivity of cells to androgens.
6. Hyperprolactinaemia secondary to a pituitary tumour.
7. Androgen-secreting ovarian or adrenal tumour.
8. Pregnancy—always consider in a female who is over the expected age of menarche and is not menstruating.

Secondary amenorrhoea

1. Pregnancy.
2. Premature ovarian failure.
3. Prolonged oral contraceptive pill or implant.
4. Significant weight loss or low body mass index.
5. Cervical stenosis/adhesion.
6. Iatrogenic—e.g. Asherman syndrome, surgery, chemotherapy or radiotherapy.
7. PCOS.
8. Androgen-secreting ovarian or adrenal tumour.
9. Other endocrine disorders—e.g. hypothyroidism, pituitary disease, etc.

Postmenopausal bleeding (PMB)

Definition: vaginal bleeding >12 months following menopause.

1. Endometrial/vaginal atrophy.
2. Endometrial cancer, hyperplasia or polyp.
3. Cervical cancer or polyp.
4. Oestrogen-secreting ovarian lesion—e.g. Brenner tumour, granulosa cell tumour.
5. Endometritis.
6. Anticoagulants.

Acute pelvic pain

1. Complicated ovarian cyst—haemorrhage, rupture or torsion. If haemorrhagic rupture, accompanied by high density ascites (>20 HU).
2. Adnexal torsion—enlarged ovary with central oedema, peripherally placed follicles and a twisted pedicle.
3. Acute pelvic inflammatory disease (PID)—e.g. pyosalpinx, tuboovarian abscess.
4. Complicated fibroid—e.g. degeneration, torsion (if pedunculated).
5. Ectopic pregnancy—particularly tubal location or ruptured ectopic.
6. Ovarian hyperstimulation—enlarged multicystic ovaries in a woman undergoing IVF.
7. Nongynaecological causes—e.g. appendicitis, diverticulitis, Crohn's disease, cystitis and urolithiasis.
8. Acute exacerbation of chronic pelvic pain.

Chronic pelvic pain

Definition: cyclical or noncyclical pain in the lower abdomen or pelvis of >6 months duration that limits activities of daily living; may be continuous or intermittent.

1. Adhesions—due to previous pelvic inflammation, surgery or trauma. May be associated with peritoneal inclusion cysts (pelvic fluid collections entrapped by adhesions).
2. Endometriosis and adenomyosis—pre/perimenopausal women.
3. Chronic PID—e.g. hydrosalpinx.
4. Fibroids.
5. Pelvic congestion syndrome—dilated veins in uterus, broad ligament and ovarian plexus.
6. Nongynaecological causes—e.g. musculoskeletal, neurological.

Raised Ca-125 (normal <35 U/mL)

Ca-125 is a nonspecific marker that increases in response to peritoneal irritation.

1. Ovarian malignancy—invasive or borderline; note invasive mucinous tumours are less likely to elevate Ca-125.
2. Other primary malignancies with peritoneal dissemination—e.g. fallopian tube, breast, GI tract and pancreas.
3. Pregnancy.
4. Endometriosis.
5. Pelvic inflammatory disease.
6. Peritoneal inclusion cyst.
7. Nongynaecological—e.g. congestive cardiac failure, cirrhosis, pancreatitis, abdominopelvic tuberculosis, sarcoidosis and peritoneal dialysis patients.

10.2 ABNORMAL UTERINE CONFIGURATION

The normal uterus is generally anteverted but can be retroverted or retroflexed. The degree of bladder filling affects flexion of the uterus. Normal ranges for uterine size (in cm):

		Infantile	Prepubertal	Reproductive[a]	Postmenopausal
Uterus	Length	1.5–2	2–5.4	5–12	3.5–6.5
	Width	0.8–1	1–2.2	4	1.2–1.8
	AP diameter		1	3	1.5–2

[a] *These values all increase, on average by 1.2 cm, following pregnancy.*

Abnormal uterine configuration

Embryology

- The female reproductive organs develop from the Müllerian ducts in the *absence* of testosterone. The caudal portions of the Müllerian ducts fuse to form the uterus, cervix and upper two-thirds of the vagina, whereas the cranial portions remain separate forming the fallopian tubes. The lower third of the vagina develops from the urogenital sinus.
- Abnormal development or fusion of the Müllerian ducts results in a spectrum of anomalies (see Fig. 10.2). These are often accompanied by renal and ureteric anomalies due to a common embryological origin.
- The ovaries develop separately from the primitive yolk sac, so are typically normal in the presence of Müllerian duct anomalies.

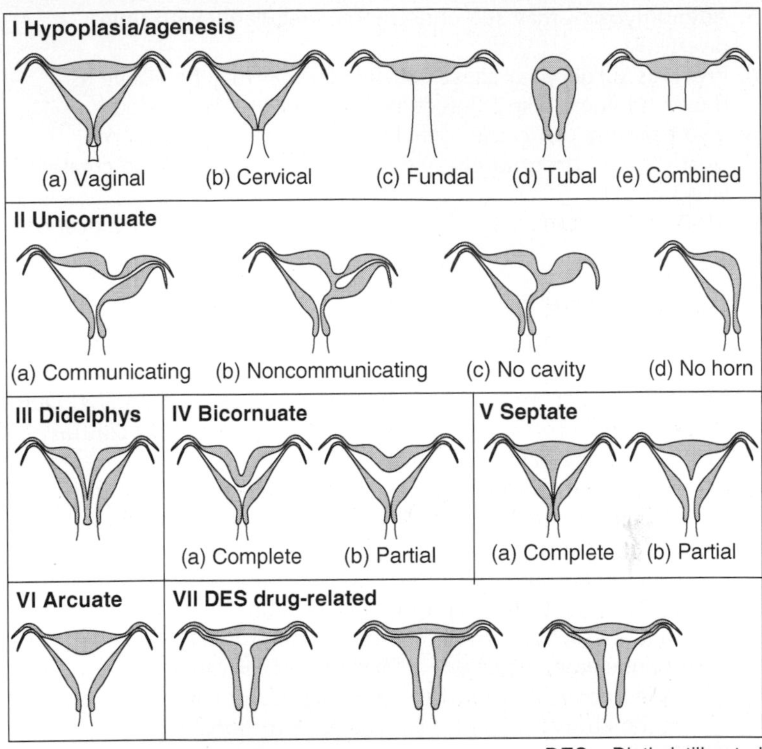

Fig. 10.2. American Fertility Society classification of Müllerian duct anomalies. (Reprinted with permission from Fertil. Steril. 1988, 49, 944–955.)

10.3 HYSTEROSALPINGOGRAPHY (HSG)

Abnormal uterine cavity

Some are better assessed by US, MRI or sonohysterography.

1. <u>Fibroid</u>—submucosal fibroids create a well-defined smooth rounded filling defect. Large intramural fibroids distort the normal contour of the uterine cavity.
2. <u>Endometrial polyp</u>—well-defined filling defect indistinguishable from a submucosal fibroid.
3. <u>Congenital Müllerian duct anomalies</u>—see Section 10.2.
4. <u>Synechiae</u>—intrauterine adhesions, most commonly caused by dilation and curettage procedures. Other causes include previous pregnancy, IUD, radiotherapy or infection (TB, schistosomiasis). Present as linear, angular or stellate filling defects. TB can cause marked distortion of the endometrial cavity. Multiple synechiae + infertility = Asherman syndrome.

5. **Adenomyosis**—may see endometrial irregularity with tiny diverticula.
6. **Previous surgery**—a caesarean-section scar may be visible as a transverse linear filling defect in the lower uterus. Previous myomectomy can cause focal irregularity or a diverticulum.
7. **Unsuspected pregnancy**—very rare. The gestational sac creates a filling defect.
8. **Air bubbles**—can mimic a polyp. Mobile, nondependent location.

Tubal abnormality

HSG is still the best imaging test.

1. Dilated fallopian tube—i.e. hydrosalpinx or haematosalpinx. Due to distal tubal obstruction in the ampullary portion. No contrast spillage into the peritoneal cavity.
   (a) PID—most common cause. Results in hydrosalpinx in the chronic setting (HSG contraindicated in acute infection).
   (b) **Endometriosis***.
   (c) **Tubal malignancy**—primary or secondary.
2. Failure to opacify the whole fallopian tube.
   (a) Tubal occlusion—most commonly due to PID; this can occlude any part of one or both tubes, or cause loculation of spilled contrast around the ampulla. Other causes include endometriosis, TB and fallopian tube malignancy.
   (b) **Tubal spasm**—tube does not fill beyond the cornual portion. Indistinguishable from cornual tubal occlusion. Spasmolytic agents may help.
   (c) **Previous surgery**—tubal ligation results in an abrupt cut-off in the isthmic portion of the fallopian tubes ± mild bulbous dilatation proximally. Hysteroscopically inserted occlusion devices result in total tubal occlusion with a radiopaque linear microinsert visible within the tubes.
3. Tubal irregularity.
   (a) Salpingitis isthmica nodosa (SIN)—idiopathic. Multiple tiny tubal diverticula arising from the isthmic portion. Can affect one or both tubes.
   (b) **Tuberculosis***—usually bilateral. In the acute phase, causes tubal diverticula that tend to be larger and less uniform than in SIN. In the chronic phase, typically causes multiple short tubal constrictions giving a beaded appearance, ± isthmico-ampullary junction obstruction ± peritubal adhesions resulting in a fixed distorted 'corkscrew' tube. Diffuse pipe-stem narrowing can be seen in advanced cases.
   (c) **Tubal polyp**—rare, located in the cornual portion. Smooth, rounded <1 cm filling defect. May be bilateral.

10.4 ENDOMETRIAL ABNORMALITIES

Normal cyclical values of endometrial thickness in premenopausal women:

- During menstruation: <5 mm (echogenic line)
- Proliferative phase (day 6–14): 5–7 mm (echogenic stripe)
- Late proliferative phase (periovulation): up to 11 mm (multilayered appearance)
- Secretory phase (day 15–28): 7–16 mm (homogeneously echogenic)

Normal values in postmenopausal women:

- Without postmenopausal bleeding: <12 mm
- With postmenopausal bleeding: <5 mm

Note that abnormal postmenopausal endometrial thickening usually requires biopsy to exclude malignancy.

Diffusely thickened endometrium

1. **Normal secretory phase**—homogeneously echogenic on US and T2 hyperintense on MRI.
2. **Early pregnancy**—gestation sac can be seen after 5 weeks; if not visible consider ectopic.
3. **Endometrial hyperplasia**—usually homogeneously echogenic ± cystic change, but can be focal or irregular, mimicking malignancy. Due to increased or unopposed oestrogen, e.g. obesity, PCOS, drugs (e.g. Tamoxifen; can cause hyperplasia, polyps, cystic change or, rarely, endometrial cancer), or hormone-secreting ovarian tumour (e.g. fibrothecoma or granulosa cell tumour).
4. **Endometrial carcinoma**—usually heterogeneous and irregular, but can mimic (or coexist with) hyperplasia.
5. **Endometritis**—typically in the postpartum period + clinical signs of sepsis; occasionally due to PID. Intrauterine fluid or gas may also be seen.
6. **Intrauterine fluid**—can mimic endometrial thickening on CT (both hypoattenuating), but not on US (anechoic). Usually related to menstruation or pregnancy in premenopausal women (or infection if clinically septic). In postmenopausal women, usually due to benign cervical stenosis or an obstructing cervical or endometrial tumour/polyp (requires biopsy).

Focal endometrial mass

1. **Endometrial carcinoma**—typically in postmenopausal women with a history of bleeding. Usually heterogeneous and irregular.

On MRI, T2 hypointense relative to normal endometrium, hyperintense relative to junctional zone of myometrium. Enhances less than normal myometrium. Myometrial invasion, if present, is diagnostic.

2. Endometrial polyp—benign, well-defined, homogeneously hyperechoic ± cystic change ± vascular stalk. On MRI, slightly T2 hypointense relative to endometrium.
3. Submucosal fibroid—well-defined, usually hypoechoic on US and T2 hypointense on MRI.
4. Focal endometrial hyperplasia—mimics a sessile polyp or early cancer on imaging.
5. Lesions related to pregnancy.
   (a) Pregnancy or missed miscarriage—visible gestation sac.
   (b) Retained products of conception (RPOC)—heterogeneously echogenic, usually contain Doppler flow; enhance on MRI.
   (c) Intrauterine blood clot—in the postpartum period. Heterogeneous, no internal Doppler flow or enhancement.
   (d) Gestational trophoblastic disease—see Section 10.16.
6. **Endometrial stromal tumours**—rare. Benign forms are nonspecific on imaging, mimicking endometrial polyps. Malignant forms are usually larger than endometrial carcinomas with more avid enhancement, and tend to greatly distend the uterine cavity; high-grade forms are very invasive and aggressive ± metastases.
   (a) **Mixed Müllerian tumours**—contain both epithelial and stromal components; can be benign (adenofibroma), low-grade malignant (adenosarcoma) or high-grade (carcinosarcoma). Adenosarcoma is typically solid-cystic and confined to the uterus, carcinosarcoma is heterogeneous (haemorrhage and necrosis) + restricted diffusion ± extrauterine invasion and metastases. Both may protrude into the endocervical canal.
   (b) **Pure stromal tumours**—can be benign (stromal nodule), low-grade malignant (endometrial stromal sarcoma) or high-grade (undifferentiated endometrial sarcoma). Low-grade sarcoma is heterogeneously T2 hyperintense ± nodular myometrial invasion with characteristic T2 hypointense bands of preserved myometrium. High-grade sarcoma shows more diffuse myometrial invasion. Vascular invasion is common in both malignant forms.
7. **Metastasis to the endometrium**—rare, most commonly from breast or stomach.

Abnormality involving both endometrium and myometrium

1. Adenomyosis—thickening of the junctional zone with irregularity of the endometrial–myometrial interface. May mimic endometrial thickening on US.

2. Submucosal fibroid.
3. Invasive endometrial malignancy.
4. Gestational trophoblastic disease.

10.5 MYOMETRIAL ABNORMALITIES

Diffuse myometrial abnormality

1. Adenomyosis—best seen on MRI. Thickening of the T2 hypointense junctional zone (>12 mm is diagnostic; <8 mm is normal) that may be diffuse, asymmetrical (often posterior) or focal (adenomyoma). T2 hyperintense subendometrial cysts and linear striations are often visible ± myometrial foci of T1 hyperintensity (haemorrhage).
2. Leiomyomatosis—numerous ill-defined T2 hypointense fibroids diffusely replacing the myometrium ± areas of degeneration.
3. Postpartum appearance—after delivery the uterus reduces in size slowly over several weeks. In the first 30 hours the myometrium is heterogeneous with multiple dilated vessels. The junctional zone is usually not visible in the first 6 weeks (or longer after caesarean section).
4. **Oral contraceptives**—can result in diffuse T2 hyperintensity throughout the myometrium ± endometrial atrophy.
5. **Infiltrative malignancy**—rare, mainly lymphoma and leukaemia. Diffuse enlargement and infiltration of the uterus by a homogeneous mildly T2 hyperintense tumour + restricted diffusion. The endometrium is usually spared, but adjacent organs may be involved ± pelvic lymphadenopathy. Aggressive sarcomas can also diffusely replace the uterus but are heterogeneous on imaging.

10

Focal myometrial mass

1. Fibroid (leiomyoma)—very common, particularly in Afro-Caribbeans. Typically hypoechoic on US and T1/T2 hypointense on MRI with homogeneous enhancement and no restricted diffusion. Well-defined, rounded + pseudocapsule. May be intramural, subserosal or submucosal (± pedunculated). Many different variants and forms of degeneration, giving a variety of appearances. Regress after the menopause.
   (a) Degeneration—more common in larger fibroids due to outgrowth of blood supply. Calcification is common after hyaline degeneration and suggests chronicity.
      (i) Hyaline—most common. Heterogeneous T2 hypointensity and enhancement within the fibroid on MRI, may be difficult to see.
      (ii) Cystic—internal well-defined cystic spaces (T2 hyperintense, T1 hypointense, no enhancement).

   (iii) Myxoid—similar in appearance to cystic degeneration but usually appears more complex + internal enhancement.
   (iv) Red—haemorrhagic infarction, usually occurs in pregnancy. Heterogeneous T2 signal with no enhancement and areas of T1 hyperintensity (haemorrhage or thrombosed veins).
   (v) Infection (pyomyoma)—usually postpartum or after instrumentation. Clinical features of sepsis. Fluid and gas within a degenerated fibroid + restricted diffusion + surrounding fat stranding.

(b) Variants.
   (i) Lipoleiomyoma—well-defined, contains a mixture of smooth muscle and fat. May be almost completely fatty. Markedly hyperechoic on US. CT and T1/fatsat MRI are diagnostic. If exophytic, may mimic ovarian teratoma. May rarely transform to liposarcoma.
   (ii) **Cellular leiomyoma**—often larger and more T2 hyperintense than a normal leiomyoma due to minimal collagen. Can show restricted diffusion, mimicking leiomyosarcoma, but usually less heterogeneous and typically well-defined.
   (iii) **Angioleiomyoma**—rare. Usually large with prominent intratumoural vessels ± internal haemorrhage.
   (iv) **Very rare variants**—atypical leiomyoma (mimics cystic degeneration), myxoid leiomyoma (mimics myxoid degeneration), smooth muscle tumour of uncertain malignant potential (STUMP; mimics cellular variant).

(c) Extrauterine manifestations.
   (i) Parasitic leiomyoma—due to torsion and detachment of a pedunculated subserosal leiomyoma, which then attaches onto another site in the peritoneal cavity, usually in the pelvis, e.g. broad ligament. More commonly occurs post myomectomy or hysterectomy due to peritoneal implantation of small leiomyoma fragments.
   (ii) Disseminated peritoneal leiomyomatosis—multiple benign peritoneal leiomyomas, T1/T2 hypointense on MRI with homogeneous enhancement. Rare, occurs in premenopausal women; mimics peritoneal metastases but without ascites and no solid organ involvement apart from uterus and ovaries. No increased uptake on PET.
   (iii) Benign metastasizing leiomyoma—usually seen post hysterectomy performed for fibroids. Typically manifests as multiple discrete lung nodules histologically identical to benign uterine fibroids. Cavitation ± pneumothorax

can occur. Less commonly involves retroperitoneum or lymph nodes.

(iv) **Intravenous leiomyomatosis**—benign uterine fibroids can rarely invade adjacent pelvic veins, and may even extend into the IVC ± right heart. The vascular invasion makes it hard to differentiate from endometrial stromal sarcoma.

2. **Adenomyoma**—focal form of adenomyosis; best seen on MRI. Ill-defined T2 hypointense mass ± small cystic spaces ± foci of T1 hyperintensity. Usually continuous with junctional zone but can be subserosal or submucosal and pedunculated. May rarely appear predominantly cystic with internal haemorrhage, mimicking a fibroid with red degeneration.
3. **Other myometrial tumours**.
   (a) **Leiomyosarcoma**—usually solitary, large and heterogeneous with areas of haemorrhage and necrosis. Mimics a degenerating fibroid, but features suggesting malignancy include irregular or invasive margins, restricted diffusion and rapid growth, particularly in a postmenopausal woman.
   (b) **Metastases**—rare, usually from breast or stomach. Direct invasion from an adjacent tumour (e.g. cervix, colon, bladder) is more common.
   (c) **Lymphoma*/leukaemia**—usually diffuse; can rarely be focal.
   (d) **Other rare tumours**—e.g. melanoma (may be T1 hyperintense), haemangioma (may contain phleboliths), perivascular epithelioid cell tumour (PEComa), inflammatory pseudotumour, nerve sheath tumour, neuroendocrine tumour, plasmacytoma, solitary fibrous tumour.
4. **External invasive endometriosis**—typically in the pouch of Douglas.
5. **Caesarean section haematoma**—in the postpartum period, located at the incision site in the lower anterior wall. In the chronic setting there is focal myometrial thinning or a defect.
6. **Arteriovenous malformation**—usually in young women, often related to previous pregnancy or surgery. US/MRI shows focal ill-defined myometrial thickening with multiple dilated tortuous vessels (high flow and low resistance on Doppler, avid early filling on postcontrast MRI).
7. **Transient physiological myometrial contraction (mimic)**—focal area of T2 hypointense myometrial thickening inseparable from the junctional zone; mimics focal adenomyosis but does not contain cystic spaces and often disappears on subsequent sequences.

10.6 CERVICAL ABNORMALITIES

Generally better assessed on MRI rather than US.

Cystic cervical lesion

1. Nabothian cyst—mucous retention cyst related to chronic cervicitis. Typically unilocular but can be multiple and clustered. Anechoic on US and T2 bright on MRI; mucin content shows variable T1 signal and may create low-level echoes on US. Typically superficial with preservation of the underlying T2 hypointense cervical stroma, but can occasionally extend into the stroma. No vascularity or enhancement (cf. adenoma malignum).
2. **Cervical endometriosis**—can be cystic (T1/T2 hyperintense) or solid (T2 hypointense) in appearance. Other sites of involvement are usually also present.
3. **Postbiopsy haematoma**—T1 hyperintense.
4. **Adenoma malignum**—mucinous adenocarcinoma of the cervix. Presents as a multilocular cystic mass arising from epithelial glands and invading the underlying cervical stroma, with enhancing septa + solid components. Peritoneal metastases are common. Associated with Peutz-Jeghers syndrome.
5. **Ectopic pregnancy**—gestation sac in the endocervical canal, usually with a closed internal os. Can mimic a miscarriage in progress, but in the latter there is no fetal heartbeat and the internal os is usually open. Repeat US should be considered.

Solid cervical lesion

1. Primary cervical carcinoma—most are squamous; less commonly adenocarcinoma or other rarer variants. Arises from epithelium of ectocervix (younger women) or endocervix (older women). Typically homogeneously T2 hyperintense on MRI + restricted diffusion + enhancement; invades and disrupts the underlying T2 hypointense cervical stroma. Can invade the uterus (± obstruction), vagina, parametrium or other adjacent structures.
2. Cervical polyp—well-defined polypoid mass within and expanding the endocervical canal without stromal invasion. Echogenic on US, T2 hypointense on MRI with avid enhancement ± small cystic spaces. Usually pedunculated with a vascular stalk on US; may prolapse into the vagina. Usually benign but may contain foci of noninvasive cancer.
3. Cervical fibroid—usually within the cervical stroma but can rarely be pedunculated and endocervical. Identical imaging features to uterine fibroids.
4. **Endocervical hyperplasia**—diffuse T2 hyperintense thickening of cervical epithelium ± cystic change. Can mimic adenoma malignum, but does not show stromal invasion and is usually hypovascular.

5. **Prolapsed endometrial mass**—e.g. polyp (benign or malignant), fibroid, mixed Müllerian tumour. Distends cervical canal.
6. **Primary endometrial or vaginal tumour invading the cervix**—bladder and rectal tumours may also invade the cervix.
7. **Other rare cervical tumours**—nearly all rare uterine tumours can also arise from the cervix, e.g. lymphoma (homogeneous and diffusely infiltrative, spares cervical epithelium), melanoma (often T1 hyperintense), sarcoma (often large, heterogeneous T2 hyperintensity and enhancement), metastasis (e.g. from breast, stomach), NET (± paraneoplastic syndrome), etc.
8. **Iatrogenic lesions**—e.g. postbiopsy inflammation.

10.7 UTERINE ADNEXA—APPROACH ON US AND MRI

Definition of adnexa: the appendages of the uterus including the ovary, fallopian tube, broad ligament and supporting structures on each side.

Normal ranges for ovarian volume (cm^3)			
Infantile	Prepubertal	Reproductive	Postmenopausal
0.7–3.6	1–6	6–12	<4

Physiological and functional ovarian cysts

Only occur in premenopausal women.

- **Developing follicle**: <1 cm, unilocular, anechoic.
- **Dominant follicle**: 1–3 cm, unilocular, anechoic. There may be one or more smaller cysts around the periphery of the dominant follicle ('cumulus oophorus')—this suggests imminent ovulation and must not be mistaken for a multilocular cystic neoplasm.
- **Corpus luteal cyst**: >3 cm by definition (normal corpus luteum is <3 cm). Typically <5 cm but can reach 8 cm. Thick hypervascular wall ('ring of fire'), crenulated edges, can be haemorrhagic (may appear solid on US).
- **Follicular cyst**: persistent unruptured follicle; >3 cm by definition, usually <5 cm but can be up to 20 cm. Unilocular anechoic cyst. Usually resolves spontaneously within 2–3 months.

Some adnexal masses have characteristic US appearances allowing a definitive diagnosis:

- Unilocular cyst with smooth walls <10 cm in diameter → **simple cyst or cystadenoma**.

10

- Unilocular cyst with ground-glass echogenicity in a premenopausal woman → **endometrioma**.
- Unilocular cystic mass with mixed echogenicity and acoustic shadows in a premenopausal woman → **benign cystic teratoma**.
- Other unilocular cysts with smooth walls → **haemorrhagic cyst** (contains echoes and thin lacy strands) or **hydrosalpinx** (contains incomplete 'septa' representing folds of the fallopian tube).
- Mass with ascites and at least moderate Doppler flow in a postmenopausal woman → **malignant tumour**.

If a lesion does not fit any of these descriptions, the International Ovarian Tumour Analysis (IOTA) Simple Rules can be applied to differentiate benign from malignant lesions (see Table below).

US and MRI features of benign and malignant adnexal masses:

	IOTA Simple Rules (US)[a]	ADNEXMR Scoring System (MRI)[b]
Benign	B features: • Unilocular cyst • Solid components <7 mm in largest diameter • Presence of acoustic shadows • Smooth multilocular cystic mass <10 cm in largest diameter • No blood flow	ADNEXMR Score 2: Benign mass • Purely cystic or fatty or endometriotic • No wall enhancement • ± solid tissue with low signal on DWI and T2 sequences ADNEXMR Score 3: Probably benign • Cystic + wall enhancement but no solid tissue, or • Solid tissue with a type 1 enhancement curve (gradual increase in signal intensity without a well-defined 'shoulder')
Malignant	M features: • Irregular solid tumour • Presence of ascites • >3 papillary structures >3 mm in height • Irregular multilocular cystic-solid tumour ≥10 cm • Very strong blood flow	ADNEXMR Score 5: Probably malignant mass • Peritoneal implants, or • Solid tissue with a type 3 enhancement curve (initial increase in signal intensity steeper than that of myometrium)

US and MRI features of benign and malignant adnexal masses:—cont'd

	IOTA Simple Rules (US)[a]	ADNEXMR Scoring System (MRI)[b]
Comments:	Rule 1: If one or more M features are present in the absence of B features, the mass is classified as *malignant*. Rule 2: If one or more B features are present in the absence of M features, the mass is classified as *benign*. Rule 3: If both M and B features are present, or if no M or B features are present, the result is *inconclusive* and a second stage test is recommended.	NB: ADNEXMR Score 1: No adnexal mass ADNEXMR Score 4: Indeterminate • Solid tissue with a type 2 enhancement curve (moderate initial increase in signal intensity less steep than that of myometrium, followed by a plateau)

[a] *Timmerman, D., Testa, A.C., Bourne, T., et al., 2008. Simple ultrasound-based rules for the diagnosis of ovarian cancer. Ultrasound Obstet. Gynecol. 31, 681–690.*
[b] *Thomassin-Naggara, I., Aubert, E., Rockall, A., et al., 2013. Adnexal masses: Development and preliminary validation of an MR imaging scoring system. Radiology 67, 432 –443.*

10.8 ADNEXAL MASS

10

Unilateral enlarged ovary, no dominant mass

1. **Acute adnexal torsion**—oedematous ovary (hyperechoic on US, T2 hyperintense on MRI) with peripheral follicles and a twisted pedicle + free fluid. The ovary is usually displaced from its normal location, often sited closer to the midline anterior or posterior to the uterus. Haemorrhage may be seen on CT/MRI, suggesting necrosis. Doppler flow may be normal, or absent in advanced cases. Most cases occur in the presence of a mass, e.g. large cyst or dermoid; torsion of a normal ovary most commonly occurs in children due to developmental hypermobility.
2. **Massive ovarian oedema**—due to chronic intermittent partial torsion; clinical presentation is usually subacute with intermittent pelvic pain (in contrast to acute severe pain in acute torsion). Imaging appearance is similar to torsion, except Doppler flow is typically present and ascites is less common. In some chronic cases, areas of T2 hypointensity may be seen, representing ovarian

fibromatosis—this may be peripheral and ring-like ('black garland' appearance).

Bilateral enlarged ovaries, no dominant mass

1. <u>Polycystic ovarian morphology (PCOM)</u>—ovaries ≥10 cm^3 in volume with ≥25 subcapsular follicles, typically measuring 2–9 mm. Hormonal and clinical correlation is required for diagnosis of PCOS.
2. <u>Ovarian hyperstimulation syndrome</u>—complication of exogenous hormonal stimulation for IVF. Grossly enlarged ovaries with multiple peripheral follicles of varying size (typically >1 cm) creating a 'spoke-wheel' appearance. This may mimic a multilocular cystic mass but the bilaterality and clinical context are indicative. Ascites and pleural ± pericardial effusions may be present and suggest increasing severity.
3. **Hyperreactio luteinalis (theca lutein cysts)**—due to high levels of endogenous human chorionic gonadotropin (hCG), typically caused by gestational trophoblastic disease, but occasionally seen in multifetal pregnancy. Similar on imaging to ovarian hyperstimulation syndrome, but free fluid is usually absent.
4. **Stromal hyperplasia/hyperthecosis**—clinical features similar to PCOS but typically occurs in postmenopausal women. Ovaries may be enlarged with hyperechoic stromal expansion and T2 hypointensity; the number of follicles is not increased.

Simple cystic adnexal lesion

Unilocular, anechoic and thin-walled.

1. <u>Follicular cyst</u>—premenopausal women only; >3 cm by definition, usually <5 cm. May show smooth wall enhancement on MRI. Resolves spontaneously, usually within 2–3 months.
2. <u>Paraovarian cyst</u>—separate from ovary, within broad ligament. Usually <5 cm.
3. <u>Ovarian inclusion cyst</u>—in postmenopausal women. Benign, typically ≤1 cm.
4. <u>Serous cystadenoma</u>—usually >5 cm, unilocular and anechoic ± smooth wall enhancement. Occasionally bilateral. Does not resolve spontaneously. Cystadenofibromas and mucinous cystadenomas can also rarely be unilocular.
5. <u>Hydrosalpinx</u>—tubular with partial 'septa' representing folding of the fallopian tube.
6. **Peritoneal inclusion cyst**—premenopausal women only, typically with a history of pelvic surgery or inflammation. Caused by peritoneal adhesions that entrap fluid released by physiological rupture of ovarian follicles, resulting in loculated peritoneal fluid adjacent to or surrounding the ovary; often has an unusual shape, following the contours of adjacent structures without much mass

effect. Can be large ± bilateral, may contain thin septa that are mobile ('flapping sail' sign).

7. **Dermoid cyst**—can rarely appear anechoic if filled with sebum and fluid.

Unilocular cyst with internal echoes on US or T1 hyperintensity on MRI

1. **Haemorrhagic functional cyst**—typically solitary and unilocular. On US, contains low-level echoes and thin lacy fibrin strands ('cobweb' appearance) ± fluid–fluid level or echogenic retracting clot. Hypervascularity of the wall is common but internal flow is absent. May occasionally appear solid on US, but posterior acoustic enhancement and absent internal vascularity help exclude a solid mass. On unenhanced CT, the cyst is typically hyperattenuating. MRI often shows T1 hyperintensity (best seen on T1 fatsat) and T2 hyperintensity ± restricted diffusion but no signal voids on SWI. Retracting clots, if present, show lower T1/T2 signal but do not enhance. Typically resolves within 2–3 months; if persistent, consider endometrioma or haemorrhagic cystic neoplasm.
2. **Endometrioma**—usually in premenopausal women. Often multiple, may be septated, do not usually resolve over time. On US, typically contain diffuse low-level echoes giving a ground-glass appearance ± echogenic avascular foci adherent to the cyst wall. The wall is usually hypovascular ± calcification. On MRI, contents typically show uniform T1 hyperintensity and reduced T2 signal (T2 shading—may be uniform or layered) ± restricted diffusion + signal voids in the wall on SWI. A characteristic nonenhancing T2 dark spot adherent to the wall may be seen. A mural nodule which is not T2 hypointense and shows enhancement or Doppler flow is suspicious for malignant change, or if pregnant, a decidualized endometrioma (in which case the nodule should be isointense to the placenta on all sequences and regress postpartum).
3. **Corpus luteal cyst**—develops after ovulation; >3 cm, thick hypervascular wall ('ring of fire' on Doppler), crenulated edges. Can be haemorrhagic and may appear solid on US.
4. **Dermoid cyst**—typically found in young patients. Variable appearance on US depending on contents. Usually a unilocular cyst containing multiple linear echoes (hair) and a characteristic very echogenic, densely shadowing, mural nodule (dermoid plug). Densely packed hair can create a 'dermoid mesh' appearance. The acoustic shadowing created by a large dermoid plug may obscure the rest of the lesion ('tip of the iceberg' sign). Fluid–fluid levels, floating balls of fat/keratin and foci of calcification may also be seen. No internal vascularity. Pathognomonic appearance on CT/MRI: well-defined adnexal mass containing fat, fluid, soft tissue and calcification (often tooth-like). Restricted diffusion may be present. Usually does not enhance except in rare cases, e.g. if

thyroid or carcinoid tissue is present. Can be complicated by torsion, rupture (free intraperitoneal fat) and malignant transformation (foci of avid enhancement or extramural invasion are suggestive).

5. **Haematosalpinx/pyosalpinx**—due to haemorrhage or infection respectively. Tubular cystic structure with internal echoes on US. T1 hyperintensity is more common in haematosalpinx. With a pyosalpinx there is hypervascularity and wall thickening (>5 mm, often has a 'cogwheel' appearance on US in cross-section) + restricted diffusion on MRI.
6. **Haemorrhage within a cystic neoplasm**—e.g. cystadenoma.

Multilocular cystic lesion

Without solid or papillary components.

1. **Mucinous ovarian tumours**—typically unilateral, large and multilocular + low-level echoes ± 'stained-glass' appearance on MRI due to differing amounts of proteinaceous material in different locules. Smooth enhancement of the wall and septa. Difficult to differentiate benign from borderline and malignant varieties on imaging, but bilaterality or high locularity makes malignancy more likely. Serous cystadenomas can also occasionally be multilocular.
2. **Tuboovarian abscess**—complication of PID; pain and clinical features of infection are indicative. Complex cystic mass containing debris and septations ± gas, with a thick hypervascular wall. On MRI, contents are heterogeneous and usually show restricted diffusion. May be bilateral, and may be associated with perihepatitis (Fitz-Hugh-Curtis syndrome). If there is diffuse peritoneal thickening, consider TB.
3. **Ovarian cystadenofibroma**—solid components may be absent in some cases. Septa are characteristically T2 hypointense.
4. **Benign cystic mesothelioma**—separate from ovary, arises from pelvic peritoneum.
5. **Ovarian lymphangioma**—very rare, more commonly arises from retroperitoneum. Multilocular, no or minimal vascularity.
6. **Hydatid cyst**—very rare.

Solid-cystic lesion

With vascular solid components (i.e. excluding blood clots and dermoids).

1. **Epithelial ovarian tumours**—including serous borderline tumours, serous and mucinous cystadenocarcinomas and endometrioid and clear cell carcinomas—the imaging features of these overlap. Typically presents in peri- or postmenopausal women as a multilocular cystic mass with papillary projections or solid components showing vascularity and restricted diffusion.

Bilaterality or calcification, if present, suggests a serous tumour. Small papillary projections can rarely be seen in serous cystadenomas, but are larger and more numerous in borderline and malignant serous tumours. Endometrioid and clear cell carcinomas can arise within endometriomas (rapid growth or enhancing nodules are suspicious). Endometrioid carcinomas may be accompanied by uterine endometrial hyperplasia or synchronous carcinoma.

2. **Ovarian metastasis**—usually from a signet-ring adenocarcinoma of the GI tract (Krukenberg metastasis). Typically bilateral. Solid components enhance and may be T2 hypointense. Usually occurs in the presence of disease elsewhere, especially the peritoneum.
3. **Ovarian cystadenofibroma**—cystic mass with fibrous septa and mural nodules that cause acoustic shadowing on US and are very T2 hypointense on MRI + enhancement + internal cystic change (characteristic 'black sponge' appearance). Typically no restricted diffusion (in contrast to ovarian carcinoma).
4. **Granulosa cell tumour**—malignant stromal tumour, usually seen in peri- or postmenopausal women but a rare juvenile form also exists. Variable appearance, usually large; can be solid ± numerous small cystic spaces ('Swiss cheese' appearance) or can be cystic with a rind of soft tissue. Secretes oestrogen, causing endometrial hyperplasia, polyps or carcinoma.
5. **Primary fallopian tube carcinoma**—rare. May present as a hydrosalpinx containing nodular enhancing components, or as a predominantly solid sausage-shaped mass. Often mimics ovarian carcinoma. There may be a suggestive history of colicky pelvic pain and an intermittent serosanguinous vaginal discharge that relieves the pain.
6. **Struma ovarii**—rare subtype of mature teratoma composed mostly of thyroid tissue; usually found in premenopausal women, may present with hyperthyroidism. Multilocular cystic-solid mass + hypervascular nodules on imaging; nonenhancing areas of very high attenuation (>90 HU on unenhanced CT) and very low T2 signal on MRI are suggestive, representing colloid.

Purely/mainly solid lesion, T2 hypointense

With fibrous elements.

1. **Fibrothecoma spectrum**—composition ranges from purely fibrous (fibroma) to purely theca cells (thecoma). Apart from pure thecomas, these are typically solid and hypoechoic ± acoustic shadowing on US, and T2 hypointense on MRI with minimal enhancement. Cystic change and calcification may be seen. Fibromas can be associated with ascites and pleural effusions (Meigs syndrome), and are common in women with Gorlin-Goltz syndrome (usually bilateral).

2. Brenner tumour—benign transitional cell tumour. Typically <2 cm (smaller than fibrothecomas) + characteristic amorphous calcification. T2 hypointense on MRI + mild-moderate enhancement. May coexist with a cystadenoma. Malignant form (TCC) is rare and indistinguishable from other malignant epithelial tumours.
3. Uterine fibroid—separate from the ovary; either pedunculated and projecting into the adnexa (± vessels extending to the uterus) or parasitic (attached to broad ligament). T2 hypointense on MRI, enhances more than ovarian fibroma.
4. **Ovarian adenofibroma**—solid form of cystadenofibroma. T2 hypointense + enhancement.
5. **Ovarian fibromatosis (mimic)**—peripherally located follicles are indicative.
6. **Lithopaedion**—rare; also known as 'stone baby'. Results from an abdominal ectopic pregnancy where the dead fetus is too large to be broken down and absorbed by the mother's body, so it becomes heavily calcified instead. Characteristic appearance on plain film and CT.

Purely/mainly solid lesion, not T2 hypointense

1. Ovarian metastasis—e.g. from breast, stomach or uterus. Typically bilateral and usually in the presence of disease elsewhere.
2. **Ovarian stromal tumours.**
   (a) **Pure thecoma**—rare, usually seen in postmenopausal women. Well-defined, intermediate T2 signal + moderate enhancement. May show microscopic fat on in/out of phase sequences. Secretes oestrogen so can cause endometrial thickening.
   (b) **Sertoli-Leydig cell tumour**—usually presents in young women with virilization. Typically a heterogeneous hypervascular mass ± foci of T2 hypointensity and/or cystic change.
   (c) **Sclerosing stromal tumour**—rare, benign, typically seen in young women with menstrual irregularity. Heterogeneously T2 hyperintense solid mass ± small cysts. Characteristic avid peripheral enhancement with centripetal filling.
3. **Malignant ovarian germ cell tumours**—typically in children or young adults. Usually solid but cystic change can occur due to haemorrhage and necrosis. Note that there may be a mixture of cell types.
   (a) **Dysgerminoma**—solid, intermediate T2 signal with avidly enhancing T2 hypointense fibrovascular septa ± calcification.
   (b) **Immature teratoma**—usually contains small foci of fat and calcification.
   (c) **Yolk sac tumour**—large hypervascular mass + prominent intratumoural vessels. Often appears solid-cystic due to haemorrhage and necrosis. Raised serum αFP.

(d) **Choriocarcinoma**—aggressive, rare (more commonly metastatic from an intrauterine primary). Large hypervascular mass + central necrosis/haemorrhage. Raised serum ß-hCG.

(e) **Embryonal carcinoma**—very rare in pure form. Nonspecific large solid mass with areas of necrosis and haemorrhage. Raised serum ß-hCG.

4. **Primary ovarian carcinomas**—can occasionally be mainly solid.
5. **Pelvic actinomycosis**—subacute presentation, associated with a longstanding IUD. Bilateral predominantly solid tuboovarian abscesses + ill-defined infiltrative soft tissue invading adjacent structures—this can be extensive ± fistulae with bowel or skin.
6. **Lymphoma***—usually secondary, often bilateral. Homogeneous ovarian masses without ascites. Disease elsewhere is usually present.
7. **Polypoid endometriosis**—rare form, histologically similar to an endometrial polyp. T2 hyperintense enhancing mass with a T2 hypointense rim.
8. **Carcinosarcoma**—rare, aggressive, usually metastatic at presentation. Heterogeneous enhancing solid mass ± cystic change/necrosis ± invasion of adjacent structures.
9. **Carcinoid tumour**—rare, usually in peri- or postmenopausal women. Solid hypervascular mass; may arise within a mature cystic teratoma. Carcinoid syndrome is common.
10. **Massive ovarian oedema (mimic)**—peripherally located follicles are indicative.

Bilateral adnexal masses

1. <u>PID</u>—bilateral hydrosalpinx or tuboovarian abscesses.
2. <u>Endometriosis</u>*—bilateral endometriomas ± haematosalpinx. The ovaries are often pulled towards the midline by adhesions and may touch ('kissing' ovaries).
3. <u>Invasive/borderline ovarian malignancy</u>—particularly serous tumours. Stage 1b if bilateral. Benign serous cystadenomas can also be bilateral.
4. <u>Metastases</u>—including lymphoma. Typically bilateral.
5. **Germ cell tumours**—dermoid cysts and dysgerminomas are bilateral in 10%–20%.
6. **Ovarian hyperstimulation syndrome/theca lutein cysts**—clinical context is indicative.
7. **Ovarian hyperthecosis**—mildly enlarged T2 hypointense ovaries.
8. **Sarcoidosis***—very rare.

Typical imaging appearances of common adnexal masses by histological subtype.

	Serous adenocarcinoma	Borderline serous tumour	Mucinous adenocarcinoma	Borderline mucinous tumour	Cystadenoma	Cystadenofibroma	Fibrothecoma	Dermoid	Malignant germ cell tumour	Endometrioma	Metastasis
Cystic	√	√	√	√	√	√	x	√	√	√	√[e]
Thin septations	x	√	x	√	√	√	x	√	x	x	x
Irregular/thick septations	√	x	√	x	x	√	x	x	√	x	√
Papillary projections	√	√	x	x	x	√	x	x	x	x	x
Predominantly solid	x	x	x	x	x	x	√	x	√	x	√[e]
Contains fat	x	x	x	x	x	x	x	√	(√)[d]	x	x
Contains low T2 signal	x	x	x	x	x	√	√	√	x	√	x
Contains high T1 signal	x	x	√	√	(√)[b]	(√)[b]	x	√	(√)[d]	√	x
Enhances avidly	√	x	√	x	x	x	x	x[c]	√	x	√
Restricted diffusion	√	√	√	x	x	x	x	√	√	√	√
Bilateral	x[a]	x	x	x	x	x	x	x[c]	x	√	√

[a]*Note: higher stage invasive ovarian cancer can involve both ovaries.*
[b]*If mucinous.*
[c]*Dermoids can have components that enhance avidly with IV contrast; bilateral in 10%.*
[d]*If an immature teratoma.*
[e]*Metastases can be cystic or solid.*

10.9 GYNAECOLOGICAL FISTULAE

1. GI inflammation—e.g. Crohn's disease (enterovaginal), diverticulitis (colovaginal), anal fistula (anovaginal).
2. Iatrogenic—e.g. hysterectomy (ureterovaginal), obstetric trauma (vesicovaginal).
3. Malignancy—of gynaecological tract or other pelvic organs.
4. **Infective**—e.g. actinomycosis, TB.
5. **Post radiotherapy.**
6. **Endometriosis*.**
7. **Congenital**—e.g. high imperforate anus + rectovaginal fistula. Seen in neonates.

10.10 NONGYNAECOLOGICAL PELVIC MASS LESION

Ovaries and uterus can be clearly defined separately.

1. Bowel origin—e.g. diverticular/Crohn's abscess, colorectal cancer, appendix mass, GIST.
2. Bladder origin—e.g. tumour, malakoplakia.
3. Nodal mass—e.g. lymphoma.
4. Peritoneal origin—e.g. inclusion cyst, cystic mesothelioma, metastases, desmoid tumour.
5. **Retroperitoneal origin**—e.g. lymphocele, haematoma, lymphangioma, liposarcoma, neurogenic tumour, solitary fibrous tumour.
6. **Presacral**—e.g. chordoma, epidermoid cyst, tailgut cyst, myelolipoma, extramedullary haematopoiesis.

10.11 VAGINAL AND VULVAL LESIONS

Cystic vaginal/vulval mass

NB: 1–5 can be T1 hyperintense if high protein content.

1. Gartner duct cyst/Müllerian cyst—indistinguishable on imaging, both typically located in the anterolateral wall of the upper vagina, above the lower margin of the symphysis pubis. Gartner duct cysts arise from Wolffian ducts, so can be associated with renal anomalies.
2. Epidermal inclusion cyst—due to previous trauma or surgery. Usually in the posterolateral wall of the lower vagina or vulva.
3. Bartholin cyst—in the posterolateral wall of the lower vagina/ introitus, medial to the labia minora.
4. Skene duct cyst—lateral to the urethral meatus.

5. **Urethral diverticulum**—periurethral cystic lesion, usually at the level of the midurethra. Often has a horseshoe configuration ± stones. Due to Skene gland infection and abscess formation that then ruptures into the urethra, forming a diverticulum.
6. **Hydrocele of the canal of Nuck**—due to a patent processus vaginalis resulting in encysted fluid within the inguinal canal that can extend into the labia majora.
7. **Vulvar abscess**—higher risk in diabetics and pregnancy. Clinical features of infection. Complex cystic lesion + wall enhancement and surrounding fat stranding. Note that the other cysts in this list can also become infected and form an abscess.
8. **Vascular lesions of the vulva**—varicosities of the labia or round ligament can develop in pregnancy. Vascular malformations, including lymphangiomas, can involve the vulva.
9. **Haematocolpos**—distended vagina filled with menstrual blood. Due to either an imperforate hymen, vaginal atresia, a transverse vaginal septum or a longitudinal vaginal septum + obstructed hemivagina. Presents in adolescence after menarche.
10. **Ectopic ureterocoele**—can insert onto the urethra.
11. **Periurethral collagen injection**—treatment for stress incontinence. Can mimic a urethral diverticulum. Other periurethral bulking agents can mimic a mass or calcification.
12. **Endometrioma**—rare; can be superficial (related to surgery, e.g. episiotomy) or deep (usually in the posterior fornix, related to pelvic endometriosis).

Solid vaginal/vulval mass

Excluding foreign bodies (e.g. tampon/pessary).

1. **Secondary vaginal malignancy**—more common than primary tumours; usually via contiguous spread. Common sources include ovaries, cervix, endometrium and anorectum.
2. **Primary vaginal malignancy**—usually SCC; enhancing infiltrative mass with intermediate T2 signal, most commonly arising from the upper vaginal wall in postmenopausal women. Less commonly adenocarcinoma (young women, T2 hyperintense), melanoma (usually postmenopausal, lower vagina, may be T1 hyperintense), leiomyosarcoma (discrete heterogeneous submucosal mass + haemorrhage and necrosis), rhabdomyosarcoma (in children), yolk sac tumour (<3 years old), lymphoma (homogeneous mass; more commonly secondary).
3. **Leiomyoma**—can arise from submucosa of vagina (usually anterior wall) or urethra. Well-defined, low or intermediate T2 signal, homogeneous enhancement.
4. **Aggressive angiomyxoma**—arises from vulval/perineal soft tissues; usually large and extends cranially through the pelvic floor between the pelvic viscera without invading them.

Heterogeneously T2 hyperintense with a characteristic swirled appearance + avid enhancement. Benign but high rate of local recurrence. Similar but less invasive variants (cellular angiofibroma, angiomyofibroblastoma) can also occur—these are usually smaller (<5 cm), limited to the vulva/perineum, and tend to appear more homogeneous on MRI but can also have a swirled appearance.

5. **Fibroepithelial polyp**—usually small and polypoid, arising from the lateral wall of the lower vagina.
6. **Condyloma acuminatum**—due to HPV infection. Large irregular superficial carpet-like mass involving the anus and vulva ± vagina. Can be invasive and transform to SCC.
7. **Endometriosis***—can appear solid and T2 hypointense.
8. **Labial haematoma**—e.g. due to surgery or straddle injuries.
9. **Lichen sclerosus**—diffuse T2 hypointensity in the perineum and labia + mild enhancement.
10. **Urethral caruncle**—benign ectropion of urethra. Cuff of T2 hyperintense tissue surrounding urethral meatus.
11. **Other rare tumours not specific to the vagina/vulva**—e.g. lipoma, haemangioma, solitary fibrous tumour, nodular fasciitis, nerve sheath tumour, paraganglioma, hidradenoma, Merkel cell tumour.

OBSTETRIC IMAGING

Obstetric imaging is no longer part of the Radiology core curriculum in the UK and so will only be covered briefly. It is important to be aware of current practice in obstetric scanning and of potential early pregnancy complications that may present to the radiology department.

10

10.12 ULTRASOUND FEATURES OF A NORMAL INTRAUTERINE PREGNANCY

- 4.5 weeks: visible gestational sac (2–5 mm).
- 5.5 weeks: visible yolk sac (should be seen when gestational sac is 12 mm).
- 6 weeks: embryonic pole is visible and heart rate may be seen
- 6.5 weeks: normal sac growth 1.2 mm per day (on transvaginal scanning). Embryo 4–10 mm with a heartbeat. If not seen, missed miscarriage highly likely.
- 7 weeks: crown–rump length (CRL) 11–16 mm. Cephalad and caudal poles distinguished.
- 8 weeks: CRL 17–23 mm. Forebrain, midbrain, hindbrain and limb buds visible.

10.13 FEATURES OF MISCARRIAGE ON ULTRASOUND

1st trimester pregnancy failure is common and affects 15%–20% of conceptions. Typically presents with vaginal bleeding and pelvic pain.

- **Threatened miscarriage**—live fetus visible; pregnancy will be subsequently lost in 15%.
- **Missed miscarriage**—retention of gestational sac following fetal death. Typically asymptomatic. Most reliable US features to confirm fetal death are:
  - Gestational sac: mean sac diameter ≥25 mm without a yolk sac or fetal pole.
  - Fetal pole: CRL ≥7 mm without detectable cardiac activity.
  - Other signs include deformity or abnormally low position of the gestational sac.
- **Incomplete miscarriage**—pregnancy has incompletely discharged. RPOC have variable appearances and vascularity on US, and can be hard to differentiate from blood clots. Clinical and biochemical correlation essential to exclude ectopic pregnancy.
- **Complete miscarriage**—no residual uterine pregnancy. Empty uterus with normal endometrial thickness (may be subtly irregular). Difficult to diagnose, as an empty uterus can also be seen in ectopic pregnancy and very early intrauterine pregnancy.

10.14 ECTOPIC PREGNANCY

Classic presentation of pain, vaginal bleeding and pelvic mass is neither common nor specific, and not all women have missed a period. US (preferably transvaginal) and serum ß-hCG are therefore vital to early diagnosis. Risk factors include previous ectopic pregnancy, tubal surgery or PID (particularly chlamydia), having an IUD in situ, and undergoing IVF.

US findings of ectopic pregnancy

1. No evidence of an intrauterine pregnancy—highly suggestive if ß-hCG >1800 IU/L.
2. Endometrial thickening—pseudogestational sac may be seen in 10%–29%; this is a small amount of intrauterine fluid that can mimic a gestational sac (but tends to have an irregular shape).
3. Fluid in pelvis—often slightly echogenic as it is usually blood.
4. Adnexal mass—often complex and vascular.
5. Live fetus/fetal cardiac activity outside uterus occurs in about 10%.
6. No ultrasound abnormality does not exclude ectopic gestation.

7. Live intrauterine gestation normally excludes the diagnosis of ectopic pregnancy but beware the coincidental ectopic twin gestation (~1 : 30,000 in unstimulated population).
8. Location of ectopic pregnancy can vary:
   (a) Tubal—most common (>90%), usually in the ampullary portion. Implantation in the isthmic or interstitial portions has a higher risk of rupture.
   (b) Abdominal—usually implants on the pelvic ligaments or pouch of Douglas, but can be found anywhere in the peritoneal cavity (may need CT/MRI to locate). Can obtain blood supply from abdominal organs. Higher risk of mortality.
   (c) Ovarian—can mimic a corpus luteal cyst in the early stages.
   (d) Cervical—can mimic a miscarriage in progress. Features favouring miscarriage include absent fetal heartbeat, an irregular sac and an open cervical os. Repeat US may be required.
   (e) Caesarean scar—gestational sac located anteriorly in the lower uterus; may look similar to cervical ectopic. High risk of uterine rupture.

10.15 PLACENTAL ABNORMALITIES

1. Placental abruption—premature separation of a normally sited placenta, resulting in antepartum haemorrhage. Associated with maternal hypertension, smoking, drug abuse, trauma, fibroids and other risk factors. Haematoma may be hyperechoic (acute), isoechoic or hypoechoic (subacute) relative to placenta, and is usually located at the placental margin; less commonly retroplacental or preplacental. If isoechoic, mimics placental thickening; if hypoechoic, can mimic focal myometrial contraction (transient), uterine fibroid, venous lake or chorioangioma. Haematoma is avascular on Doppler, aiding differentiation from mimics. Note that in many cases a haematoma is not seen—this does not exclude the diagnosis.
2. Placenta praevia—a portion of the placenta covers the internal cervical os; high risk of maternal and fetal haemorrhage during labour. US diagnosis at the 18–20 week scan is far greater than incidence at term due to differential growth of the lower uterine segment. 'Low-lying placenta' and 'touching the os' are terms no longer advised on the 18–20 week scan. The placenta must cross the internal os to initiate a follow-up scan (NICE).
3. Vasa praevia—abnormal fetal vessels coursing through the membranes over the internal cervical os; high risk of fetal haemorrhage during labour. Usually associated with velamentous insertion of the umbilical cord (i.e. inserting directly onto the membranes), but can also occur in placentas with >1 lobe where vessels traverse the membranes to connect the lobes.

4. **Morbidly adherent placenta**—abnormal myometrial adherence or invasion by placental chorionic villi. Caused by a focal decidual defect typically related to previous caesarean section(s) or other uterine interventions; often occurs in the presence of placenta praevia. High risk of catastrophic maternal haemorrhage during labour. Depth of invasion determines subtype, but this is often difficult to classify on imaging—general features on US include multiple turbulent linear vascular channels (lacunae) extending from placenta into myometrium, loss of the retroplacental hypoechoic clear space and myometrial thickness <1 mm. On MRI, the placenta may contain heterogeneous T2 signal with hypointense bands of fibrosis, and there may be focal bulging or interruption of the myometrium.
   (a) **Placenta accreta**—placenta is attached to myometrium (rather than decidua) without direct invasion. Commonest form, least severe.
   (b) **Placenta increta**—placenta partially invades myometrium.
   (c) **Placenta percreta**—placenta invades full thickness of myometrium ± adjacent structures, e.g. bladder. Suggestive imaging features include loss of the fat plane between uterus and bladder, increased vascularity in the bladder wall or direct extension of placental tissue beyond the uterus. Least common form, most severe—high risk of uterine rupture.
5. **Placental masses**—excluding abruption (avascular haematoma, see above).
   (a) **Placental lake**—well-defined hypoechoic vascular space containing slow nonturbulent blood flow (cf. lacunae). May thrombose (intervillous thrombus).
   (b) **Placental cyst**—well-defined, anechoic, avascular. Usually asymptomatic unless large (>4.5 cm) or multiple.
   (c) **Chorioangioma**—benign hamartoma, most common placental tumour. Well-defined, hypoechoic and hypervascular; usually located on the fetal side of placenta close to the umbilical cord. Fetal complications can occur if >5 cm or diffuse in nature (chorioangiomatosis).
   (d) **Gestational trophoblastic disease**—see Section 10.16.
   (e) **Placental mesenchymal dysplasia**—large thick placenta containing multiple cysts. Can cause fetal growth restriction, death or preterm delivery. Associated with Beckwith-Wiedemann syndrome. Mimics partial molar pregnancy, but multiple fetal anomalies and markedly elevated ß-hCG levels are usually seen in a partial mole.
   (f) **Placental metastases**—rare, most commonly from maternal melanoma, lymphoma, breast or lung cancer, or fetal neuroblastoma.
   (g) **Placental teratoma**—very rare; usually on the fetal side of placenta. Well-defined heterogeneous mass + calcification with

minimal internal flow on Doppler. Can mimic an acardiac twin—absence of organized fetal structures or umbilical vessels aids differentiation.

10.16 GESTATIONAL TROPHOBLASTIC DISEASE

Uncommon neoplastic proliferation of trophoblastic tissue. Usually presents with hyperemesis and markedly elevated ß-hCG. Ovarian theca lutein cysts may be seen. Subtypes include:

1. <u>Complete hydatidiform mole</u>—most common, due to fertilization of an empty ovum. Large complex echogenic hypervascular multicystic mass with no identifiable fetal tissue. May mimic placental hydropic degeneration after a failed pregnancy, but is usually more vascular with higher ß-hCG levels. Rarely, a complete mole may coexist with a normal twin, thereby mimicking a partial mole or placental mesenchymal dysplasia—but the presence of a second normal placenta helps exclude these.
2. <u>Partial hydatidiform mole</u>—due to fertilization of a normal ovum by two sperm. Similar appearance to a complete mole except fetal tissue is present, albeit growth-restricted with multiple anomalies.
3. <u>Invasive mole</u>—most commonly develops after evacuation of a hydatidiform mole. Heterogeneous echogenic hypervascular mass + small cysts or foci of haemorrhage and necrosis. Locally invades the myometrium ± adjacent structures, but does not typically metastasize.
4. <u>Gestational choriocarcinoma</u>—similar appearance to an invasive mole but often metastasizes (most commonly to lungs). The primary tumour may be very small. 50% develop after a molar pregnancy, the rest after abortion, miscarriage or normal pregnancy (usually within 1 year, but can be longer).
5. **Placental site trophoblastic tumour**—rare. Similar appearance to choriocarcinoma but produces little ß-hCG and is chemoresistant, requiring surgery.
6. **Epithelioid trophoblastic tumour**—very rare, produces little ß-hCG. Can occur many years after pregnancy.

10.17 MATERNAL COMPLICATIONS DURING PREGNANCY

1. <u>Nongynaecological</u>—e.g. appendicitis, urinary tract infection or obstruction, biliary obstruction or infection. CT is best avoided, US ± MRI are preferable. In the case of suspected pulmonary embolus, low-dose perfusion-only scintigraphy is recommended unless the CXR is abnormal, in which case low-dose CTPA is preferable.

2. **Red degeneration of a uterine fibroid**—not uncommon, particularly in large fibroids. Contains cystic spaces on US with internal echoes and absent internal Doppler flow. Contains T1 hyperintensity on MRI.
3. **Adnexal torsion**—usually occurs at 12–14 weeks gestation.
4. **HELLP syndrome**—complication of preeclampsia characterized by **H**aemolysis, **E**levated **L**FTs and **L**ow **P**latelets, which can result in hepatic subcapsular haemorrhage, rupture or infarction.
5. **Hyperreactio luteinalis**—see Section 10.8.
6. **Ovarian luteoma**—rare benign ovarian tumour that occurs in pregnancy and can cause maternal virilization. Solid, hypoechoic and vascular on US. Regresses after delivery.
7. **Ectopic deciduosis**—this can occur in two settings (both regress after delivery):
   - **(a)** Within preexisting endometriomas, creating enhancing mural nodules that are isointense to the placenta on all sequences on MRI.
   - **(b)** In the peritoneum, due to progesterone-induced metaplasia of mesenchymal cells, creating peritoneal nodules (mainly in the pelvis) that can mimic metastatic disease. If peritoneal deciduosis occurs on the serosal surface of the appendix, it can mimic appendicitis.

10.18 POSTPARTUM COMPLICATIONS

1. **Haemorrhage**—causes include uterine atony, RPOC, morbidly adherent placenta and uterine rupture or dehiscence. Intrauterine blood clots may be seen on imaging.
2. **Endometritis**—pelvic pain and clinical features of sepsis; more common after caesarean section. Can be related to RPOC or intrauterine blood clots. Imaging features are nonspecific and overlap with normal postpartum state, so mainly a clinical diagnosis. Intrauterine fluid, gas, debris and RPOC ± increased vascularity may be seen.
3. **RPOC**—can occur postpartum or after miscarriage or abortion. Heterogeneous echogenic material within endometrial cavity that usually demonstrates vascularity on US/MRI (cf. intrauterine blood clots which are avascular and usually more hypoechoic). May contain calcification. Note that a normal postpartum uterus may contain fluid and echogenic foci.
4. **Uterine rupture/dehiscence**—rupture usually occurs during labour at a previous caesarean-section site, but can be delayed and occur postpartum. A myometrial defect ± haematoma ± haemoperitoneum may be seen on imaging. Dehiscence of a recent caesarean-section incision is often due to infection and can be associated with a bladder flap haematoma (situated between the bladder and uterus).

5. **Adnexal torsion**—can occur as the uterus returns to the pelvis.
6. **Ovarian vein thrombosis**—R>L, usually due to endometritis leading to ascending septic pelvic thrombophlebitis. High attenuation thrombus within a distended ovarian vein on unenhanced CT ± surrounding fat stranding. Hypoattenuating on postcontrast CT, may be mistaken for a dilated ureter.

Further reading

Chudleigh, T., Thilaganathan, B., 2004. Obstetric Ultrasound: How, Why and When, third ed. Churchill Livingstone. Trish Chudleigh PhD DMU; Basky Thilaganathan, ed.

Santos, P., Cunha, T.M., 2015. Uterine sarcomas: clinical presentation and MRI features. Diagn. Interv. Radiol. 21 (1), 4–9.

Shah, S.H., Jagannathan, J.P., Krajewski, K., et al., 2012. Uterine sarcomas: then and now. AJR Am. J. Roentgenol. 199 (1), 213–223.

Nalaboff, K.M., Pellerito, J.S., Ben-Levi, E., 2001. Imaging the endometrium: disease and normal variants. Radiographics 21 (6), 1409–1424.

Sudderuddin, S., Helbren, E., Telesca, M., et al., 2014. MRI appearances of benign uterine disease. Clin. Radiol. 69 (11), 1095–1104.

Arleo, E.K., Schwartz, P.E., Hui, P., McCarthy, S., 2015. Review of leiomyoma variants. AJR Am. J. Roentgenol. 205 (4), 912–921.

Okamoto, Y., Tanaka, Y.O., Nishida, M., et al., 2003. MR imaging of the uterine cervix: imaging-pathologic correlation. Radiographics 23 (2), 425–445.

Wildenberg, J.C., Yam, B.L., Langer, J.E., Jones, L.P., 2016. US of the nongravid cervix with multimodality imaging correlation: normal appearance, pathologic conditions, and diagnostic pitfalls. Radiographics 36 (2), 596–617.

Jung, S.E., Lee, J.M., Rha, S.E., et al., 2002. CT and MR imaging of ovarian tumors with emphasis on differential diagnosis. Radiographics 22 (6), 1305–1325.

Foti, P.V., Attina, G., Spadola, S., et al., 2016. MR imaging of ovarian masses: classification and differential diagnosis. Insights Imaging 7 (1), 21–41.

Levine, D., Brown, D.L., Andreotti, R.F., et al., 2010. Management of asymptomatic ovarian and other adnexal cysts imaged at US: Society of Radiologists in Ultrasound consensus conference statement. Radiology 256 (3), 943–954.

Thomassin-Naggara, I., Aubert, E., Rockall, A., et al., 2013. Adnexal masses: development and preliminary validation of an MR imaging scoring system. Radiology 267 (2), 432–443.

Timmerman, D., Testa, A.C., Bourne, T., et al., 2008. Simple ultrasound-based rules for the diagnosis of ovarian cancer. Ultrasound Obstet. Gynecol. 31 (6), 681–690.

Hosseinzadeh, K., Heller, M.T., Houshmand, G., 2012. Imaging of the female perineum in adults. Radiographics 32 (4), E129–E168.

Agarwa, M.D., Resnick, E.L., Mhuircheartaigh, J.N., Mortele, K.J., 2017. MR imaging of the female perineum. Magn. Reson. Imaging Clin. N. Am. 25 (3), 435–455.

Parikh, J.H., Barton, D.P., Ind, T.E., Sohaib, S.A., 2008. MR imaging features of vaginal malignancies. Radiographics 28 (1), 49–63.

10

Walker, D.K., Salibian, R.A., Salibian, A.D., et al., 2011. Overlooked diseases of the vagina: a direct anatomic-pathologic approach for imaging assessment. Radiographics 31 (6), 1583–1598.

Jha, P., Paroder, V., Mar, W., et al., 2016. Multimodality imaging of placental masses: a pictorial review. Abdom. Radiol. (NY) 41 (12), 2435–2444.

Elsayes, K.M., Trout, A.T., Friedkin, A.M., et al., 2009. Imaging of the placenta: a multimodality pictorial review. Radiographics 29 (5), 1371–1391.

Shaaban, A.M., Rezvani, M., Haroun, R.R., et al., 2017. Gestational trophoblastic disease: clinical and imaging features. Radiographics 37 (2), 681–700.

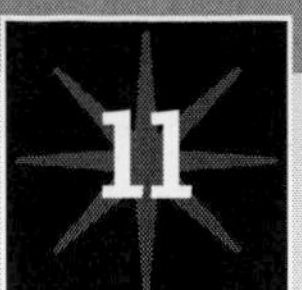

Breast disease and mammography

Neil Upadhyay, Arne Juette, Erika Denton

In UK practice, breast abnormalities are evaluated as part of a 'triple assessment' process: clinical examination, imaging and subsequent image-guided tissue diagnosis. All breast-imaging tests are assigned a numerical score from 1 to 5 with a prefix for each score: P for clinical examination findings, M for mammography, U for ultrasound and MRI for findings on MRI studies. Subsequent histology/cytology results are similarly described.

The UK classification system for imaging is:

1 = normal
2 = benign findings, no further evaluation required
3 = indeterminate/probably benign findings, small risk of malignancy, requires further evaluation
4 = suspicious findings with a moderate risk of malignancy, requires further evaluation
5 = highly suspicious findings with a high risk of malignancy, requires further evaluation

Further evaluation typically means image-guided core biopsy, and increasingly vacuum biopsy for microcalcification (FNA is not recommended as first line).

These UK categories broadly align with the widely used American College of Radiology breast imaging data and reporting system (BIRADS) classification.

11.1 MAMMOGRAPHIC, SONOGRAPHIC AND MRI FEATURES OF BREAST ABNORMALITIES

This table describes the classical appearances of benign and malignant abnormalities on mammography, US and MRI, but note that there is significant overlap between the categories. Breast cancers may be occult on imaging, and sensitivity decreases as mammographic breast density increases.

Lesion characteristics	Typically benign	Typically malignant
Mass	Smooth margin, up to three gentle lobulations	Indistinct, spiculated or microlobulated margins
	Low density on mammogram	High density on mammogram
	Wider than tall on US	Taller than wide on US
Echogenicity on US	Variable depending on lesion	Markedly hypoechoic, often with echogenic halo
Enhancement characteristics on MRI	Slow and prolonged moderate enhancement[a]	Rapid marked enhancement with early washout
Calcification	See Section 11.2	
Surrounding parenchyma	Normal[b]	Disrupted/distorted[c]
Nipple/areola	Normal	Retracted
Skin	Normal	Thickened[d]
Ducts	See Section 11.11	
Subcutaneous/ retromammary space on mammogram	Normal	Obliterated

[a] *Lobular carcinoma can also have these characteristics.*
[b] *Except in infection where the surrounding breast can be oedematous.*
[c] *This may also be seen due to postsurgical/radiotherapy change.*
[d] *This may also be seen due to postsurgical/radiotherapy change, inflammation, heart failure or lymphoedema.*

11.2 CALCIFICATION

Microcalcification is defined as individual calcific densities measuring <0.5 mm in diameter. Microcalcification is not specific to carcinoma, whereas coarse calcification may also be found in carcinoma. This table describes the classical mammographic features. Please note that skin/subcutaneous calcification is covered in Chapter 4.

Definitely benign (see figure)	Probably benign	Suspicious of malignancy
Arterial: tortuous, tramline (1) Widely separated, radiolucent centre (2) Plasma cell mastitis: linear, thick, rod-like ± radiolucent centre (3) Egg-shell or curvilinear margin of cyst/fat necrosis (4) Popcorn within fibroadenoma (5) Large individual >2 mm (6) Floating or layering on lateral mammogram: 'milk of calcium' in microcysts (7) Coarse irregular dystrophic calcification after radiotherapy or trauma Suture calcification (curvilinear, looped, calcified knots)	Widespread in both breasts or symmetrical Macrocalcification of uniform size Superficial distribution (i.e. within skin)	Linear (ductal) or segmental distribution[a] Pleomorphic, linear branching shape[a] Increasing on serial mammography

[a] *See figure.*

11

Examples of definitely benign calcification.

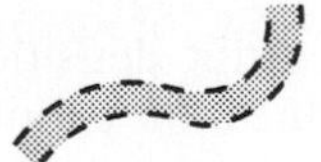

1. Arterial

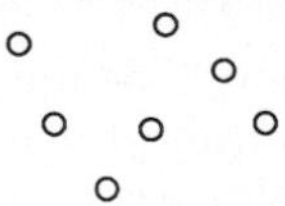

2. Smooth ± lucent centre widely separated

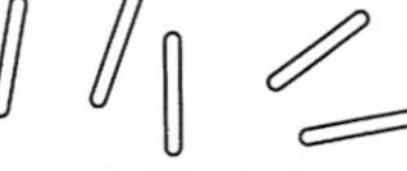

3. Linear, thick, rod-like ± lucent centres

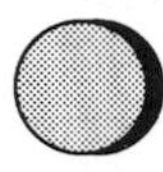

4 'Egg-shell'

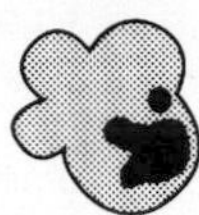

5. 'Pop-corn'

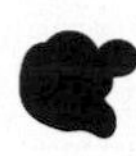

6. Large calcific opacity

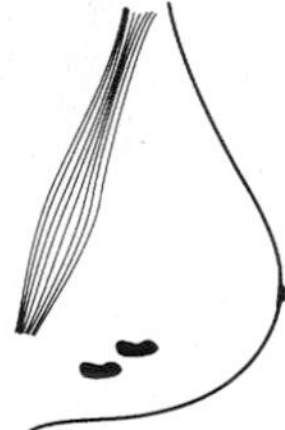

7. Floating calcification

*Suspicious microcalcification; mixture of sizes, shapes, cluster, haphazard arrangement, linear branching patterns

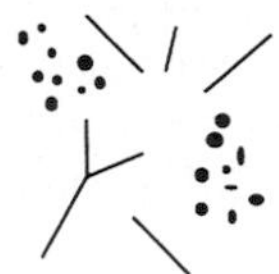

11.3 BENIGN LESIONS WITH TYPICAL IMAGING APPEARANCES

1. Fibroadenoma—involuting fibroadenomas may contain typical 'popcorn' calcification on mammography, which precludes the need for further imaging or biopsy. In the UK national guidance recommends that biopsy in women <25 years is not necessary for confirmation if typical features of a fibroadenoma are present (well-defined, ovoid/round, up to three gentle lobulations). Other countries follow BIRADS recommendations, which advocate US follow-up.
2. Intramammary lymph node—most often in the upper outer quadrant. A fatty hilum is a characteristic feature, typically seen in normal and reactive lymph nodes, but may also be present in pathological nodes—this is seen as a focal radiolucency within the node on mammography (may be difficult to appreciate), fat signal on MRI or hyperechoic on US. Normal or reactive nodes often have 'suspicious' enhancement characteristics on MRI.
3. Lipoma—well-defined, rounded, exclusively fat-containing.
4. Oil cyst—well-defined, lucent on mammography ± 'egg-shell' peripheral calcification. The presence of multiple subcutaneous oil cysts is characteristic for steatocystoma multiplex (many other subcutaneous oil cysts will also be present on the trunk).
5. Hamartoma—'breast tissue within breast tissue' or 'salami-slice' appearance on imaging due to variable mix of fatty and glandular tissue.

11.4 SINGLE WELL-DEFINED MAMMOGRAPHIC SOFT-TISSUE OPACITY

As a general guide any well-defined opacity >1.0 cm in diameter is usually subjected to US and, if solid, biopsy is performed.

Benign

1. Cyst—round/oval, low-density mass. In the case of an oil cyst: rounded, fat density mass ± peripheral calcification.
2. Fibroadenoma—round/oval mass, similar density to glandular breast parenchyma. Cysts and fibroadenomas can have similar appearances on mammography.
3. Intramammary lymph node—common in normal breasts. Pathological causes are the same as those in Section 11.12.
4. Skin lesion—e.g. irregular 'warty' skin papillomas. The air/soft-tissue interface creates a characteristic hypodense halo around skin lesions. Skin markers may be used to confirm.

5. Nipple not in profile—may resemble a soft-tissue opacity on the mediolateral oblique (MLO) view.
6. Hamartoma—variable appearance depending on composition—if mostly glandular tissue it can present as a well-defined mass with density identical to surrounding glandular parenchyma. If mostly fatty, it can present as a well-defined lucent mass.
7. Galactocoele—round/oval mass in a lactating woman. Appearance depends on proportion of fat, water and milk content. May mimic lipoma (if high fat content), hamartoma (if mixed viscous contents) or cyst. May contain characteristic fat-fluid level if contains fresh liquid milk. Can become infected.
8. **Sebaceous cyst**—opacity related to the dermis.
9. **Lactating adenoma**—occurs during lactation or in the third trimester of pregnancy. Imaging features are similar to fibroadenoma. Regresses spontaneously after cessation of breast feeding.
10. **Pseudoangiomatous stromal hyperplasia (PASH)**—the rare tumoural form presents as a well-defined, noncalcified mass in a premenopausal woman. Can mimic fibroadenoma on US.
11. **Myofibroblastoma**—rare benign spindle cell tumour usually found in postmenopausal women and older men. Well-defined, round/oval, noncalcified mass, hypoechoic on US, mimicking fibroadenoma (patient age can be a useful discriminator).
12. **Other rare soft-tissue masses not specific to the breast**—e.g. haemangioma (± phleboliths), leiomyoma (often near areola), schwannoma, neurofibroma, solitary fibrous tumour. These are typically well-defined and hypoechoic on US (mimicking fibroadenoma), although haemangiomas may be microlobulated and have variable echogenicity.

Malignant

1. Carcinoma—a small number of carcinomas can look 'benign' on mammography: high-grade invasive ductal carcinoma, mucinous carcinoma (often mixed solid-cystic), medullary carcinoma, papillary carcinoma (often within a cyst or dilated duct) and adenoid cystic carcinoma.
2. Phyllodes tumour—indistinguishable from a fibroadenoma on mammography, but characterized by its rapid growth and often large by time of presentation. Usually present in an older age group than fibroadenomas. Most are benign, but borderline and malignant varieties exist. Calcification is rare. Malignant lesions metastasize to lung and bone, and may invade the chest wall.
3. **Metastasis to the breast**—can be solitary, see Section 11.5.
4. **Lymphoma***—can appear as a single, well-defined, noncalcified mass. Spiculations and architectural distortion are usually absent. May be primary (rare) or secondary.

11.5 MULTIPLE WELL-DEFINED MAMMOGRAPHIC SOFT-TISSUE OPACITIES

1. Cysts—most common cause.
2. Fibroadenomas—10-20% are multiple.
3. Skin lesions—e.g. cutaneous papillomas, neurofibromas (NF1).
4. Intramammary lymph nodes.
5. **Metastases**—lymphoma, leukaemia (especially acute myeloid leukaemia), melanoma, lung and ovaries are the most common sources. Often involve the subcutaneous fat. Calcification is rare (except in ovarian cancer). Metastases elsewhere are usually also present.
6. **Silicone or paraffin injections**—usually very dense and widely distributed in the breast, accompanied by dense striated appearing fibrosis (sclerosing lipogranulomatosis) ± dense calcification.
7. **Cowden syndrome**—may present with multiple fibroadenomas, fatty hamartomas and/or tubular adenomas. Increased risk of breast cancer.

11.6 LARGE (>5 CM) WELL-DEFINED MAMMOGRAPHIC ABNORMALITY

1. Giant cyst—radiopaque, usually low density.
2. Giant fibroadenoma—radiopaque.
3. Lipoma—radiolucent.
4. Phyllodes tumour—radiopaque, indistinguishable from fibroadenoma.
5. Hamartoma—mixed density, depending on composition of fatty and glandular tissue.
6. **PASH**—see Section 11.4.

11

11.7 BENIGN CONDITIONS THAT MIMIC MALIGNANCY

1. Microcalcification
   (a) **Sclerosing adenosis**—calcification can have suspicious appearances (e.g. clustered/pleomorphic) resembling ductal carcinoma in situ (DCIS).
   (b) **Amyloidosis***—can produce suspicious microcalcification.
   (c) **Pseudoxanthoma elasticum**—can produce microcalcifications in the breast, vessels and skin (especially in the axilla)—if all three are present this is highly suggestive of the diagnosis.
   (d) **Other causes of skin calcification**—e.g. chronic renal failure.

2. Suspicious soft-tissue opacity
   (a) Summation of normal tissues—giving the impression of a suspicious abnormality on mammography. A common reason for recall after screening mammography. Small paddle compression or tomosynthesis can help separate the individual components.
   (b) Fibroadenoma/cyst—when one margin appears ill-defined.
   (c) Fat necrosis—typically seen after surgery, radiotherapy or trauma. Usually superficial. Ill-defined in the early stages ± a radiolucent centre. Often hyperechoic on US (a helpful feature as malignancy is usually hypoechoic). Often contains 'malignant-appearing' dystrophic calcification peripherally, which progresses with time. In later stages it usually becomes well-defined, resulting in an oil cyst, but if it heals with prominent fibrosis it can mimic a spiculated mass.
   (d) Postbiopsy scar.
   (e) Radial scar (<1 cm)/complex sclerosing lesion (>1 cm)—presents as a distortion on mammography or a spiculate lesion with a low density centre—'black star' appearance (malignancy tends to have a higher density centre). As there is a risk of associated carcinoma, these lesions are usually widely sampled with image-guided vacuum excision—there is currently a move away from surgical excision.
   (f) **Haematoma**—varied appearance. Usually a history of trauma, but not always. Resolves over time, but may evolve into fat necrosis or a seroma.
   (g) **Irregular skin lesion**—e.g. wart. Look for the tell-tale hypodense halo.
   (h) **PASH**—may have indistinct borders.
   (i) **Lymphocytic mastitis**—ill-defined mass or masses with marked posterior acoustic shadowing on US (often more than would be expected with malignancy). Usually associated with diabetes (aka diabetic mastopathy) or autoimmune diseases such as Hashimoto thyroiditis, SLE or Sjögren's syndrome.
   (j) **Wegener's granulomatosis*, sarcoidosis* and amyloidosis***—any of these can rarely produce an irregular breast mass or masses, usually in the context of widespread disease elsewhere, therefore the diagnosis may already be suspected (although biopsy is still required to exclude malignancy).
   (k) **Eosinophilic mastitis**—very rare. Usually accompanied by peripheral eosinophilia. Can present as an ill-defined mass or an oedematous/inflamed breast.
   (l) **Other rare soft-tissue masses not specific to the breast**—e.g. desmoid tumour (usually close to pectoral muscles), nodular fasciitis (usually located on the subcutaneous fascia), granular cell tumour (may be well- or ill-defined,

usually upper inner quadrant in supraclavicular nerve territory), inflammatory pseudotumour, Rosai-Dorfman disease. All of these appear as nonspecific, ill-defined masses indistinguishable from malignancy.

11.8 OEDEMATOUS BREAST

Signs on mammography: diffuse increased density with skin thickening and thickening of Cooper's ligaments producing a coarse reticular pattern.

Causes without erythema/inflammation

1. **Previous surgery/radiotherapy**—common, particularly after axillary clearance (obstructing lymphatic drainage). Oedema is most pronounced 6–12 months after treatment, and gradually resolves, usually within 1–3 years. Malignant axillary nodes may also obstruct lymphatic drainage.
2. **Venous obstruction**—e.g. subclavian vein occlusion.
3. **Heart failure/nephrotic syndrome**—more commonly bilateral but can be unilateral, e.g. if patient always lies on one side in bed.
4. **Angioedema**—rare.

Causes with erythema/inflammation

1. **Mastitis**
   (a) **Acute infectious mastitis**—clinical signs of infection. Most common in lactating women. Increased echogenicity in inflamed fat lobules, hypoechoic areas in glandular tissue ± duct ectasia. May be associated with an abscess, presenting as an irregular mass on mammogram and US.
   (b) **Zuska's disease**—usually in nonlactating smokers. Caused by epithelial squamous metaplasia obstructing the lactiferous ducts in the nipple–areola complex, resulting in duct ectasia, recurrent infection, subareolar abscess formation and a lactiferous fistula. Surgical excision of the abscess, fistula and involved lactiferous duct is required for definitive treatment.
   (c) **Granulomatous mastitis**
      (i) **Idiopathic granulomatous lobular mastitis**—usually in young women <5 years after childbirth. Ill-defined mass with inflammatory change ± fistulation with skin ± axillary adenopathy. The mass is usually wider than tall and may have tubular components on US. Other causes of granulomatous inflammation (e.g. sarcoidosis, Wegener's, TB, fungal infection) must be excluded.
      (ii) **TB***—three patterns: nodular (ill-defined mass ± cutaneous fistulation), diffuse (breast oedema + skin

11

thickening) and sclerosing (fibrosis + architectural distortion + reduced breast size). Axillary adenopathy is common and if nodal calcification is present this suggests TB. Breast macrocalcification may be present but microcalcification is rare.

(iii) **Actinomycosis**—may be primary (inoculation via the nipple) or secondary (direct extension from intrathoracic disease). Primary disease presents as an ill-defined retroareolar mass ± cutaneous fistulation ± breast oedema, without calcification or adenopathy. Secondary syphilis (very rare) and TB can have similar appearances.

2. **Inflammatory carcinoma**—can mimic mastitis. Usually a short (<3 months) history of symptoms. Trabecular thickening and skin thickening on mammography. Altered echogenicity ± mass on US with skin thickening. Microcalcifications and axillary adenopathy may also be present. The inflammation is caused by the tumour obstructing the subcutaneous lymphatics.
3. **Localized scleroderma of the breast (morphea)**—can mimic inflammatory carcinoma. More common in younger patients.

11.9 ARCHITECTURAL DISTORTION ON MAMMOGRAPHY WITHOUT A VISIBLE MASS

1. **Radial scar/complex sclerosing lesion**—see Section 11.7.
2. **Invasive breast cancer**—the presence of a correlative abnormality on US significantly increases the probability of malignancy.
3. **DCIS**—suspicious microcalcification is usually also present.
4. **Sclerosing adenosis**—microcalcification may also be present.
5. **Scarring or fat necrosis post biopsy/surgery/infection/trauma**—clinical history is key. Dystrophic calcification may be present.

11.10 SHRUNKEN BREAST

NB: this refers to progressive shrinking of the breast rather than longstanding stable breast asymmetry, which is nearly always a normal variant or rarely due to Poland syndrome.

1. **Following radiotherapy/trauma/burns**—clinical history important. Dystrophic calcification is common. Thoracic radiotherapy in childhood can result in longstanding breast asymmetry due to stunted breast development.
2. **Breast cancer**—especially invasive lobular carcinoma, where a discrete mass may not be visible on mammography.
3. **TB***—particularly the sclerosing form.

11.11 DUCT DILATATION

Benign

1. **Duct ectasia**—Dilated subareolar ducts ± debris on US, due to chronic inflammation/fibrosis leading to duct blockage. On a spectrum alongside plasma cell mastitis, periductal mastitis and Zuska's disease.
2. **Physiological changes during lactation.**
3. **Blocked ducts**—during lactation due to sedimented secretions. Echogenic material in dilated ducts on US.
4. **Papilloma**—well-defined intraductal mass with associated duct dilatation. Usually solitary in a central duct, but may be multiple in distal ducts (papillomatosis). Highly vascular ± a vascular stalk on colour Doppler. May contain calcification.
5. **Apocrine metaplasia**—associated with fibrocystic disease. Consists of dilated ducts and adjacent septated cysts ± inspissated/calcified secretions. Often seen in patients with extensive cystic disease.

Malignant

1. **Ductal carcinoma in situ**—can present as an intraductal mass with duct dilatation (seen on US as a soft-tissue mass filling a duct).
2. **Intraductal papillary carcinoma**—indistinguishable from a benign papilloma on imaging.
3. **Invasive ductal carcinoma**—an irregular mass extending into a duct (and therefore widening the duct) is a highly specific sign of malignancy, but is not commonly seen in isolation.

11.12 AXILLARY LYMPHADENOPATHY

1. Nonspecific reactive hyperplasia—enlarged nodes with preserved fatty hila and normal node morphology. Idiopathic.
2. Malignancy—usually from breast cancer. Other common sources include lymphoma, leukaemia, melanoma. Involved nodes often lose their fatty hilum and elongated shape, becoming more rounded. Other features include eccentric cortical thickening and capsular irregularity. Involved nodes in lymphoma may be markedly hypoechoic, almost cystic in appearance on US. Nodes involved by metastatic thyroid or ovarian cancer may contain peripheral amorphous calcification. Nodal microcalcification can rarely be seen in breast cancer.
3. Infection—e.g. mastitis, soft-tissue infection in the arm, cat-scratch disease, infectious mononucleosis, TB and HIV. Coarse nodal calcification suggests TB (or sarcoidosis).
4. Silicone lymphadenopathy—in patients with silicone breast implants that have ruptured/leaked or following silicone injections

into the breast. Silicone deposits in axillary nodes are very dense on mammography and cause a 'snowstorm' appearance on US.

5. **Connective tissue disease**—e.g. rheumatoid arthritis, SLE, psoriatic arthritis, dermatomyositis, scleroderma. Patients with a history of gold salt therapy for rheumatoid arthritis may have punctate high-density gold deposits within axillary nodes (similar heavy metal nodal deposits can be seen in patients with large tattoos on the arms).
6. **Granulomatous disease**—e.g. sarcoidosis, Wegener's granulomatosis.

11.13 MALE BREAST DISEASE

Common benign conditions in women such as fibrocystic change and fibroadenomas do not typically occur in men. Lobular carcinoma and phyllodes tumours are also very rare in men. In practice, any lesion that is not typical for gynaecomastia will usually be biopsied.

1. **<u>Gynaecomastia</u>**—most common condition. Proliferation of glandular tissue that is typically subareolar, central and fan-shaped. Usually bilateral and asymmetrical. On US gynaecomastia can have spiculated margins, resembling breast carcinoma. In patients on hormonal therapy for gender reassignment or prostate cancer, the gynaecomastia is marked and may look similar to female breasts.
2. **<u>Pseudogynaecomastia</u>**—proliferation of fatty tissue only (no glandular proliferation).
3. **<u>Male breast cancer</u>**—typically eccentric in location. Invasive ductal carcinoma is the most common histological subtype. Imaging features are similar to female breast cancer although microcalcification is less common. Lesions looking like simple cysts should be evaluated carefully as simple cysts do not typically occur in men. Complex cysts should be biopsied—a solid component within a cyst may represent papillary carcinoma (or a benign intraductal papilloma).
4. **Abscess**—commonly subareolar in location, with ill-defined margins ± surrounding trabecular thickening. Clinical signs of infection are typically present.
5. **Haematoma/fat necrosis**—e.g. due to trauma.
6. **Metastases**—rare. In men, prostate is the most common source.
7. **PASH**—similar appearance to that seen in women.
8. **Diabetic mastopathy**—similar appearance to that seen in women.

9. **Myofibroblastoma**—rare, usually found in older men. Imaging features similar to fibroadenoma (but fibroadenoma is exceptionally rare in men). See Section 11.4.
10. **Granulomatous mastitis**—including TB and sarcoidosis. Very rare.
11. **Other soft-tissue masses not specific to the breast**—e.g. sebaceous cyst, lipoma and others (see Sections 11.4 and 11.7).

11.14 MRI IN BREAST DISEASE

Indications

1. **Evaluate local extent of cancer**—when tumour size is uncertain on conventional imaging (typically young women with dense background breast tissue on mammography). Can also potentially assess chest wall invasion.
2. **Lobular carcinoma**—may be mammographically occult and can be multifocal/bilateral.
3. **Metastatic axillary adenopathy of unknown primary**—to identify occult breast cancer.
4. **High-risk screening**—those with a history of mantle radiotherapy or genetic mutation.
5. **Evaluation of implant integrity.**
6. **Monitor response to neoadjuvant chemotherapy.**

Enhancement patterns

1. **Mass-like enhancement**—see Section 11.1 for characteristics of benign and malignant masses. Enhancement curves are important for assessing mass lesions: a progressive enhancement pattern is usually benign, a plateau pattern is indeterminate and a washout pattern is associated with an increased risk of malignancy. Fibroadenomas and phyllodes tumours may contain nonenhancing septa (a helpful feature).
2. **Non-mass enhancement**—ill-defined areas of enhancement that do not form a discrete mass. Linear, segmental, clumped and clustered ring patterns of enhancement are suspicious for DCIS or early invasive carcinoma, but can also be seen in fibrocystic change or PASH. Small foci of enhancement <5 mm in size are usually benign unless the kinetics are suspicious.

11.15 BREAST AUGMENTATION

Types of breast augmentation

1. Silicone implants.
2. Saline implants—less dense than silicone implants on mammography. These first two implants represent the most common types.
3. **Double or triple-lumen implants with silicone and saline compartments.**
4. **Free silicone/polyacrylamide gel injections (historic practice).**
5. **Autologous fat transplantation.**

Normal imaging appearances of breast implants

Implants may be placed superficial or deep to pectoralis major. Saline and silicone both demonstrate high T2 and low T1 signal on MRI, but silicone-specific sequences can differentiate the two. A fibrous capsule normally forms around the elastomer shell of a breast implant, appearing as parallel echogenic lines on US. Radial folds of the elastomer shell are commonly seen and may trap a little fluid between the shell and the fibrous capsule, mimicking implant rupture on MRI (silicone-specific sequences will help differentiate).

Complications of breast implants

1. Rupture—saline implants tend to collapse/deflate when rupture occurs (the leaked saline is then absorbed by the body), whereas silicone implants tend to maintain their shape so rupture may be clinically occult. Two types of rupture (see also table below):
   (a) Intracapsular—rupture of the elastomer shell with an intact surrounding fibrous capsule. Gel bleed (diffusion of silicone through an intact shell) may mimic intracapsular rupture.
   (b) Extracapsular—rupture of both the elastomer shell and fibrous capsule, with leakage of silicone into the surrounding tissues.
2. **Capsular contracture**—contraction of the fibrous capsule distorting the shape of the implant, becoming more rounded. The capsule may be thickened on US and radial folds may be increased in size and number.
3. **Herniation through fibrous capsule**—contour bulge on mammography.
4. **Haematoma**—usually occurs soon after implantation, but chronic expanding haematomas have been reported due to intermittent bleeding from capsular vessels.
5. **Infection**—most common in the early postoperative period. Intact implant shell with surrounding fluid which does not contain free silicone on silicone-specific MRI sequences.

6. **Seroma**—periprosthetic fluid collection. May be early or late (>1 year after implantation).
7. **Breast implant associated anaplastic large cell lymphoma**—very rare. Can occur many years after implantation. Usually confined within the capsule and most commonly presents as an enlarging intracapsular effusion around the implant shell, often without a discrete mass on imaging. FNA is required to confirm the diagnosis and should be performed in any patient with an enlarging periimplant effusion occurring >1 year after implantation.

Intracapsular versus extracapsular rupture		
Modality	**Intracapsular**	**Extracapsular**
Mammography	Usually occult. Contour bulge is a nonspecific sign (may represent implant herniation)	Densely radiopaque silicone in breast parenchyma and/or lymph nodes
Ultrasound	Stepladder sign—multiple parallel linear echoes within implant (US counterpart of MRI linguine sign)	Snowstorm sign—free silicone seen as an echogenic nodule with incoherent posterior shadowing. This may be seen in the breast parenchyma or lymph nodes
MRI	Linguine sign—collapsed elastomer shell within implant Noose sign—small amount of leaked silicone trapped in a radial fold Subcapsular line sign—small amount of silicone outside elastomer shell but within fibrous capsule	Free silicone away from breast implant: best seen on silicone-specific sequences

Further reading

Cao, M.M., Hoyt, A.C., Bassett, L.W., 2011. Mammographic signs of systemic disease. Radiographics 31 (4), 1085–1100.

Dall, B.J., Vinnicombe, S., Gilbert, F.J., 2011. Reporting and management of breast lesions detected using MRI. Clin. Radiol. 66 (12), 1120–1128.

Ferris-James, D.M., Iuanow, E., Mehta, T.S., et al., 2012. Imaging approaches to diagnosis and management of common ductal abnormalities. Radiographics 32 (4), 1009–1030.

Harvey, J.A., 2007. Unusual breast cancers: useful clues to expanding the differential diagnosis. Radiology 242 (3), 683–694.

Lattin, G.E., Jr., Jesinger, R.A., Mattu, R., Glassman, L.M., 2013. From the radiologic pathology archives: diseases of the male breast: radiologic-pathologic correlation. Radiographics 33 (2), 461–489.

Maxwell, A.J., Ridley, N.T., Rubin, G., et al., 2009. The Royal College of Radiologists Breast Group breast imaging classification. Clin. Radiol. 64 (6), 624–627.

NHS Breast Screening Programme. Clinical guidance for breast cancer screening assessment. NHSBSP publication no 49. 4th ed; 2016.

Trop, I., Dugas, A., David, J., et al., 2011. Breast abscesses: evidence-based algorithms for diagnosis, management, and follow-up. Radiographics 31 (6), 1683–1699.

Wilkinson, L., Thomas, V., Sharma, N., 2016. Microcalcification on mammography: approaches to interpretation and biopsy. Br. J. Radiol. 90 (1069), 20160594.

Willet, A.M., Michell, M.J., Lee, M.J.R. (Eds.). Best Practice Diagnostic Guidelines for Patients Presenting with Breast Symptoms. DoH: 2010.

Head and neck

Sami Khan, Elena Boyd, Simon Morley

12.1 PARAPHARYNGEAL SPACE LESIONS

The parapharyngeal space (PPS) contains primarily fat, small vessels and small nerves. It lies between the parotid, masticator, carotid and pharyngeal mucosal spaces. Primary pathology in the PPS is rare (e.g. schwannoma, branchial cleft cyst, venolymphatic malformations and tumours arising from ectopic salivary tissue). More commonly lesions from other spaces bulge into or invade the PPS. The key to identifying the site of origin is assessing the pattern of displacement of the parapharyngeal fat.

1. **Deep lobe parotid neoplasm**—widens stylomandibular notch and displaces parapharyngeal fat medially. See Section 12.5.
2. **Masticator space pathology**—displaces parapharyngeal fat posteriorly. See Section 12.4.
3. **Carotid space mass**—displaces parapharyngeal fat anteriorly. See Section 12.7.
4. **Pharyngeal mucosal space mass**—tumours of the nasopharynx or oropharynx can infiltrate the parapharyngeal fat or displace it laterally. See Sections 12.2 and 12.3.

12.2 PHARYNGEAL MUCOSAL SPACE LESIONS: NASOPHARYNX

1. **Nasopharyngeal carcinoma**—SCC or undifferentiated. Infiltrative intermediate T2 signal mass enhancing less than normal mucosa, centred on fossa of Rosenmüller. Produces middle ear effusion via eustachian tube dysfunction. Can invade nasal cavity, prevertebral muscle, pterygopalatine fossa, skull base and intracranial space (via foramen lacerum and perineural spread along CN V3). Nodal disease commonly retropharyngeal, posterior triangle and posterior deep cervical chain. Distant metastatic disease in 20% (lung, bone, liver) means PET-CT mandatory as part of work-up.

2. <u>**Lymphoma**</u>*—NHL. Bulky homogeneous intermediate T2 signal mass, variable enhancement. May extend into PPS, retropharyngeal space or skull base.
3. <u>**Lymphoid hyperplasia**</u> —normal finding in teens and 20s. May relate to viral infection including HIV. Symmetrical, shows vertical 'tiger stripe' enhancement, often with small mucous retention cysts at the bases. No extension beyond nasopharynx.
4. <u>**Tornwaldt cyst**</u>—thin-walled midline submucosal cyst with variable T1/T2 signal depending on protein content. No internal enhancement.
5. <u>**Juvenile angiofibroma**</u>—benign locally invasive vascular tumour seen almost exclusively in adolescent or young adult males. Avidly enhancing mass centred on the nasopharynx and sphenopalatine foramen, often extending into the pterygopalatine fossa, nasal cavity, paranasal sinuses, masticator space, inferior orbital fissure and middle cranial fossa (via vidian canal or foramen rotundum). Bone remodelling > destruction.
6. **Minor salivary gland malignancy**—infiltrative enhancing mass with propensity for perineural and perivascular spread.

12.3 PHARYNGEAL MUCOSAL SPACE LESIONS: OROPHARYNX

Clinical findings direct the most likely cause. An ulcerating oropharyngeal soft-tissue mass suggests malignancy. An enlarged tonsil with fever and odynophagia suggests infection or abscess.

1. <u>**Tonsil SCC**</u>—lingual (tongue base) or faucial (palatine). Associated with smoking and HPV. Mucosal ulceration or mass evident on inspection. On MRI, the mass is isointense on T1 and iso/↑ to muscle on T2, + enhancement. Level II and III adenopathy is common at presentation. HPV–ve tumours tend to be more ill-defined and invasive (e.g. into adjacent muscle); enhancement helps delineate extent. HPV+ve tumours (p16+ve on histology) tend to be more well-defined, exophytic and enhancing, with cystic nodal metastases.
2. <u>**Palatine tonsil inflammation/abscess**</u>—enlarged poorly enhancing tonsil. Nonenhancing central low attenuation ± gas indicates abscess, which may extend beyond constrictor into PPS.
3. <u>**Lymphoma**</u>*—extranodal NHL involving lingual or palatine tissue (Waldeyer's ring). Cervical adenopathy also seen in most. Imaging: bulky homogeneous nonnecrotic mass, isoattenuating to muscle, intermediate T2 signal.
4. **Minor salivary gland malignancy**—variable appearance depending on histology.

5. **Crohn's disease***—can rarely involve the oropharynx, causing diffuse mucosal thickening and oedema.

12.4 MASTICATOR SPACE LESIONS

1. Abscess—secondary to dental infection/manipulation → osteomyelitis of posterior body of mandible → cortical dehiscence → extension of pus into masticator space. Clinical: trismus, tenderness and fever. CT: cortical destruction ± periosteal reaction at posterior body/ramus. 'Empty socket' if following dental extraction. 'Dirty' fat planes. CT/MRI: swollen and enhancing muscles (myositis) + rim enhancing fluid attenuation abscess ± enhancing phlegmon. T1↓ in marrow, STIR↑ in marrow and soft tissue. May extend into supra-zygomatic masticator space ± associated epidural/subdural empyema.
2. Bony lesions of mandible—see Sections 12.21 and 12.22.
3. **Incidental benign conditions.**
   (a) **Masticator muscle hypertrophy**—smooth, diffuse enlargement of masticator muscle due to bruxism, habitual gum chewing or temporomandibular joint dysfunction. Often bilateral, usually asymmetrical. Clinical: nontender lateral facial mass which enlarges with jaw clenching. CT/MRI: enlarged (>1.5 cm depth) masseter muscle isoattenuating and isointense to normal skeletal muscles on pre- and postcontrast sequences.
   (b) **Masticator space pseudolesions**—incidental small masticator muscle → pseudohypertrophy of contralateral side. Clinical: no facial mass on jaw clenching.
   (c) **Pterygoid venous plexus asymmetry**—unilateral prominence of deep facial venous plexus from cavernous sinus and orbit. CT and MRI: prominent asymmetrical serpiginous vessels in masticator space, enhancing like other veins.
4. **Motor denervation cranial nerve (CN) VIII**—cause: benign or malignant tumours, surgical trauma. Phases:
   (a) **Acute (≤1 month)**—enlarged muscle with STIR↑ (oedema) and ↑enhancement.
   (b) **Subacute (≤12–20 months)**—↓oedema, partial atrophy. STIR normal or mildly ↑. T1↑ due to fatty change. No or mild enhancement.
   (c) **Chronic (>12–20 months)**—fatty atrophy of muscle. T1↑↑. No oedema or enhancement.
5. **Sarcoma**—rhabdomyosarcoma, leiomyosarcoma, liposarcoma, Ewing sarcoma, osteosarcoma, chondrosarcoma or synovial sarcoma. Mean age: 35 years. Can be associated with Gardner syndrome. CT/MRI: aggressive, ill-defined mass ± bone destruction.

12

6. **Perineural tumour extension**—enhancement of CN V3 in masticator space → foramen ovale → Meckel's cave. Can be seen with SCC, melanoma, sarcoma, NHL and adenoid cystic carcinoma (of parotid gland).
7. **Schwannoma of CN V3**—age: third to fourth decade (younger in NF2). CT: smooth enlargement of foramen ovale. MRI: variable T1/T2 signal depending on cystic change or haemorrhage. Homogeneous or heterogeneous enhancement. Well-defined, ovoid or fusiform/tubular shape ± signs of motor denervation.

12.5 FOCAL PAROTID SPACE LESIONS

Overlapping features make imaging diagnosis difficult, FNA or core biopsy often needed for diagnosis; imaging guides surgery. Larger masses with ill-defined margins—consider malignancy.

1. **Pleomorphic adenoma**—80% of parotid tumours. Well-defined lobulated mass, homogeneous when small, heterogeneous when large. Hypoechoic on US ± posterior acoustic enhancement. CT/MRI: prominent homogeneous enhancement when small (less so when large) ± calcification. T1↓, T2↑↑ (especially myxoid type), often with a T2↓ rim (fibrous capsule).
2. **Warthin tumour**—second most common parotid tumour, often in the tail (may be mistaken for lymph node if exophytic). Bilateral or multifocal in 20%; most common cause of multiple solid parotid masses. Peak in sixth decade; the vast majority are smokers. Well-defined and heterogeneous. Greater tendency for cystic change than other salivary gland tumours. Often hypervascular on US with multiple small irregular sponge-like anechoic areas. Large tumours (>5 cm) are more cystic. CT: no calcification; cyst + mural nodule strongly suggestive. MRI: heterogeneous T1/T2 signal. Minimal enhancement on CT/MR.
3. **Nodal metastases or lymphoma***—metastases usually from scalp, external auditory canal (EAC), cheek skin SCC or melanoma. Ill-defined irregular lymph nodes (LNs), often with other abnormal periparotid, occipital or level II/V nodes. Lymphoma may be adenopathy from generalized disease or MALT lymphoma in Sjögren's syndrome.
4. **Salivary gland carcinomas**—mucoepidermoid, adenoid cystic, malignant mixed tumour, acinic cell, adenocarcinoma, ductal carcinoma, SCC. When small or low grade, indistinguishable from pleomorphic adenoma or LNs. Ill-defined margins are clue to diagnosis. T2↓ in a solid mass suggests malignancy. Look for perineural spread to temporal bone along CN VII.

5. **First branchial cleft cyst**—either preauricular/intraparotid (± sinus tract to middle ear or medial EAC) or posterior/inferior to angle of mandible (± sinus tract to lateral EAC).

12.6 DIFFUSE PAROTID ENLARGEMENT

If unilateral, think acute infection or malignancy. In acute infections, look for ductal calculi and drainable abscess.

1. **Parotitis**—acute (viral/bacterial) or acute-on-chronic (due to obstructing calculus). Unilateral enlargement of hyperattenuating parotid + subcutaneous stranding. Chronic: small heterogeneous gland ± calculi in dilated ducts. NB: mumps parotitis is usually bilateral.
2. **Sjögren's syndrome***—multiple bilateral cysts and hypoechoic nodules, ± submandibular/lacrimal gland involvement.
   Look carefully for solid lesions as increased risk of MALT lymphoma.
3. **Benign lymphoepithelial lesions of HIV**—mimics Sjögren's, but other glands are spared. Look for adenoidal hypertrophy and reactive adenopathy of HIV.
4. **Sarcoidosis***—mimics Sjögren's; no increase in NHL risk. Cervical and mediastinal adenopathy is suggestive.
5. **Lymphoma***—usually part of systemic NHL with uni/bilateral solid nodules. Primary NHL is much less common.

12.7 CAROTID SPACE LESIONS

1. **Carotid body paraganglioma**—most common paraganglioma of head and neck; located at carotid bifurcation + characteristic splaying of internal carotid artery (ICA) and external carotid artery (ECA) ('lyre' sign). Rarely associated with MEN 2A/B, Carney triad, tuberous sclerosis, NF1 or vHL—often multicentric when syndromic. Dense vascularity, avid contrast enhancement on CT/MR. MRI: T1↓ usually with 'salt and pepper' appearance due to punctate haemorrhages/slow flow (salt) and flow voids (pepper). T2↑ with multiple flow voids. Angiography: lyre sign with an intense blush in tumour ± 'early vein' due to arteriovenous shunting. Usually supplied by ascending pharyngeal artery. Scintigraphy: not specific, but MIBG and octreotide uptake can be useful for multiple lesions.
2. **Vagal schwannoma**—fusiform, lies along the course of the vagus nerve; tends to displace both ICA and ECA anteriorly ± medially together, rather than splaying them. Imaging: T2↑, intense enhancement ± intramural cysts.

3. **Jugular vein thrombosis**—expansion and lack of contrast/flow void in internal jugular vein (IJV). Causes: IV drug abuse, indwelling IJV catheter or deep neck space infection (Lemierre's syndrome).
4. **Glomus vagale paraganglioma**—identical appearance on CT/MR to carotid body paraganglioma, but located higher below the skull base. Displaces ICA and ECA anteriorly (without splaying) and IJV posteriorly. Vocal cord paralysis is common. Does not widen the jugular foramen.
5. **Pseudoaneurysm**—post trauma or carotid dissection. Imaging: focal dilatation of carotid artery + mural thrombus or calcification. Flow void changes on MRI, complex wall sign; CTA or MRA correlation required.
6. **Neurofibroma**—solitary tumours are fusiform, well-defined and usually sporadic. CT: ↓ attenuation. Plexiform tumours are seen in NF1; see Section 12.8.

12.8 PERIVERTEBRAL SPACE LESIONS

This space has two components: prevertebral (vertebral body, prevertebral and scalene muscles, brachial plexus) and paraspinal (paraspinal muscles, posterior spinal elements; deep layer of deep cervical fascia surrounds and contains lesions).

1. **Vertebral body metastasis**—MRI: replacement of normal marrow signal. CT: lytic or sclerotic vertebral body lesions with perivertebral soft-tissue extension.
2. **Infection**—clinical: local pain, raised inflammatory markers. Discitis or vertebral body osteomyelitis + contiguous inflammatory mass. Epidural extension may cause cord compression or radicular symptoms. CT: peripherally enhancing fluid collection/abscess.
3. **Schwannoma**—may appear embedded in scalene muscles. CT: may extend into spinal canal + smoothly enlarged neural foramen. MRI: T2↑, heterogeneous enhancement and cyst formation when large.
4. **Chordoma**—rare in cervical vertebral body; destructive enhancing mass + perivertebral extension. MRI: characteristic T2↑↑.
5. **Plexiform neurofibroma**—seen in NF1, involves multiple nerve roots. CT: isoattenuating to cord and nerve roots, may follow path of brachial plexus. MRI: isointense to nerve roots or cord, variable enhancement. Characteristic 'target' sign: T2↑ in periphery, T2↓ in centre.

12.9 POSTERIOR CERVICAL SPACE LESIONS

Posterior cervical triangle contains fat, level V LNs, CN XI and distal brachial plexus.

1. **Lymphadenopathy**—e.g. metastatic SCC, thyroid malignancies, lymphoma, suppurative LNs, granulomatous disorders (including TB, sarcoidosis and cat-scratch disease) and Rosai-Dorfman disease.
2. **Third branchial cleft cyst**—congenital cyst posterolateral to carotid space.
3. **Nerve sheath tumour**—e.g. schwannoma, neurofibroma.
4. **Nodular fasciitis**—rapidly growing painful soft-tissue mass, usually related to the subcutaneous or muscular fascia. Variable enhancement and T1/T2 signal (see Section 4.4).
5. **Thoracic duct cyst**—in left supraclavicular fossa. Fluid attenuation and signal.
6. **Venous diverticulum**—arises from the confluence of IJV and subclavian vein. Can mimic a supraclavicular node on CT, as it may not fill well with contrast. Diagnosis confirmed on US (may need Valsalva to visualize).

12.10 RETROPHARYNGEAL SPACE LESIONS: FOCAL

Retropharyngeal space (RPS) lesions lie posterior to the pharynx and anterior to prevertebral muscles. Focal masses are usually high in RPS, medial to carotid arteries. In an adult with an oval T2↑ RPS lesion, consider schwannoma versus lymph node.

1. **Reactive lymph node**—common in children.
2. **Metastatic lymph node**—SCC of naso/oro/hypopharynx. If large but not necrotic, more likely nasopharyngeal carcinoma. Also may be from sinonasal or thyroid malignancies.
3. **Lymphoma***—often with Waldeyer's ring involvement; solid and homogeneous even when large.
4. **Multinodular goitre**—extends from enlarged thyroid, often with cysts and calcifications. Look for tracheal displacement/narrowing.
5. **Ectopic parathyroid adenoma**—4D CT or SPECT aids differentiation from LN.
6. **Sympathetic schwannoma**—slow-growing; fusiform enhancing mass medial to ICA.

12.11 RETROPHARYNGEAL SPACE LESIONS: DIFFUSE

1. **Abscess**—crucial to avoid delay in diagnosis, as this may cause airway compromise or extend into danger space. Usually from pharyngitis or tonsillitis, in children, elderly or the immunocompromised. Rim-enhancing fluid collection; mass effect on surrounding structures helps differentiate from effusion.
2. **Effusion**—fluid from impaired lymphatic drainage, often due to IJV thrombosis, radiotherapy or pharyngitis. Nonenhancing fluid collection with only mild mass effect.
3. **Suppurative adenopathy**—hypoechoic/hypoattenuating enlarged LNs.
4. **Longus colli tendonitis**—neck pain and stiffness. Acute inflammatory process with nonenhancing reactive RPS effusion and pathognomonic calcific deposits in longus colli insertion at C1–C2 levels.
5. **Hypopharyngeal SCC**—posterior wall or pyriform sinus SCC can extend posteriorly into and distend the RPS. Look for prevertebral involvement and RPS nodes.

12.12 ORAL CAVITY: ORAL MUCOSAL SPACE LESIONS

The oral cavity lies above the hyoid bone, anterior to the oropharynx and lingual tonsils and inferior to the sinuses and nose. Four distinct areas: oral mucosal space (OMS), sublingual space (SLS), submandibular space (SMS) and root of tongue (ROT). Each area offers anatomy-based differential diagnoses (see also Sections 12.13–12.15).

OMS lesions are usually evident on examination. Imaging helps stage involvement and nodal disease (levels I and II).

1. **SCC of different OMS subsites**.
2. **Minor salivary gland carcinoma**—second most common submucosal mass, most often in the hard palate. Look for perineural spread along CN V2 branch.
3. **Radiation mucositis**—acute/subacute phase. Diffuse mucosal enhancement.

12.13 ORAL CAVITY: SUBLINGUAL SPACE LESIONS

1. **Simple ranula**—postinflammatory unilateral sublingual mucous retention cyst. Imaging similar to lymphatic malformation, epidermoid and sialocoele.
2. **Abscess**—caused by tooth abscess or submandibular duct stone. Rim-enhancing fluid collection with duct stone or tooth abscess.
3. **Sublingual gland sialadenitis**—enlarged, enhancing sublingual glands.
4. **Sublingual gland carcinoma**—90% of sublingual gland masses are malignant. Most commonly adenoid cystic, mucoepidermoid, or acinic cell. CT/MR: heterogeneous invasive mass, variable enhancement. Tends to recur late (5–10 years).
5. **Sialocoele**—cystic lesion due to trauma, surgery, stone or stenosis of submandibular duct. True sialocoele: distended duct. False: ruptured duct + pseudocyst due to extravasated saliva. May enhance peripherally after 2 weeks.
6. **Dermoid**—from ecto- and mesodermal remnants. Mixed density, may contain fat (T1↑) or calcifications (T1↓).
7. **Epidermoid**—ectoderm only. Homogeneous fluid density; T1↓, T2↑, restricted diffusion.

12.14 ORAL CAVITY: SUBMANDIBULAR SPACE LESIONS

1. **Submandibular gland (SMG) sialadenitis**—swollen, painful SMG ± calculus and dilated duct if acute; atrophic SMG if chronic.
2. **Diving ranula**—simple ranula of SLS ruptures into SMS through mylohyoid defect, forming a thin-walled, comet-shaped pseudocyst.
3. **Pleomorphic adenoma of SMG**—50% of SMG tumours. Heterogeneous, well-defined, T1↓, T2↑, variable enhancement, ± calcifications, haemorrhage or necrosis. Hypoechoic on US.
4. **SMG carcinoma**—usually adenoid cystic or mucoepidermoid. Invasive mass arising from SMG. Look for perineural spread in adenoid cystic carcinoma.
5. **Sjögren's syndrome***—parotids, SMGs and lacrimal glands are usually involved. See Section 12.6.
6. **Benign lymphoepithelial lesions of HIV**—more common in parotid glands. See Section 12.6.
7. **Accessory salivary tissue**—similar attenuation/signal as adjacent SMG, extends into anterior SMS through mylohyoid defect.
8. **Second branchial cleft cyst**—cystic mass in posterior SMS in a child or young adult. Usually thin-walled unless infected.

12

9. **Küttner pseudotumour**—chronic sclerosing sialadenitis, seen as part of IgG4-related disease. Produces firm swelling and pain, or asymptomatic. MRI: T1↓, T2/STIR↑. US: hypoechoic, usually well-defined.

12.15 ORAL CAVITY: ROOT OF TONGUE LESIONS

Contains genioglossus and geniohyoid muscles and lingual septum.

1. **Abscess**—no LNs in root of tongue (ROT), so abscess results from haematogenous spread, foreign body or dental disease. Rim-enhancing mass splitting genioglossus muscles.
2. **SCC invasion**—infiltrative mass arising from floor of mouth or oral tongue.
3. **Thyroglossal duct cyst**—unilocular midline ROT cyst. T2↑, T1↓ (or ↑ if proteinaceous contents). Thin rim of enhancement.
4. **Dermoid and epidermoid**—see Section 12.13.
5. **Ectopic thyroid tissue**—well-defined ROT mass with signal/density similar to thyroid gland: hyperattenuating on CT, T1/T2↑ relative to tongue muscles on MRI. Homogeneous enhancement. NB: this may be the patient's only functioning thyroid tissue. Can undergo goitrous, nodular or malignant change.
6. **Foregut duplication cyst**—congenital cystic lesion between genioglossus muscles, lined with alimentary tract epithelium. Well-defined thick-walled cyst, variable contents, may mimic epidermoid due to protein content. US: visible bowel wall layers.

12.16 TRANSSPATIAL NECK LESIONS

These are lesions that readily cross fascial planes in the neck. Two groups: (1) congenital lesions, which develop before the fascias form; (2) aggressive processes that break through the fascia.

1. **Venous malformation**—congenital slow-flow vascular mass. Lobulated, infiltrative margins, phleboliths on CT, T2↑ on MRI, moderate enhancement.
2. **Venolymphatic malformation**—congenital; lymphatic and venous components. Lymphatic components show fluid characteristics ± blood-fluid levels. Venous components show solid enhancement and phleboliths.

3. <u>Infection</u>—often odontogenic, may spread from superficial to deep, and from deep spaces into mediastinum. Heterogeneous rim-enhancing mass. Check airway and vascular patency.
4. <u>SCC</u>—most common head and neck neoplasm. Deep spread = T4 stage. Nodal conglomerates may involve multiple spaces.
5. **Lymphatic malformation**—congenital uni/multilocular cystic mass. Well-defined, thin-walled, fluid attenuation on CT, blood-fluid levels on MRI. No enhancement.
6. **Plexiform neurofibroma**—seen in NF1. See Section 12.8.

12.17 VISCERAL SPACE LESIONS

This cylindrical space is contained by the middle layer of the deep cervical fascia and is the infrahyoid counterpart of the pharyngeal mucosal space down to the thoracic inlet. Contains thyroid (see Section 12.18), parathyroid glands, level VI lymph nodes, larynx, cervical trachea (see Section 5.1) and oesophagus (see Sections 7.3–7.7). Malignancies may present with recurrent laryngeal nerve palsies. NB: lesions of the thyroid, trachea and oesophagus (including pharyngeal pouches) are covered in other sections.

Laryngeal lesions

Some diagnoses are indicated by the clinical setting, e.g. recent trauma (haematoma, fracture) or radiotherapy (diffuse oedema).

1. <u>SCC</u>—classified as supraglottic, glottic, subglottic or transglottic (>1 site). Linked to smoking and alcohol. Irregular, enhancing, exophytic or infiltrative soft-tissue mass. Look for effacement of paralaryngeal fat and cartilage invasion. Nodal disease is common.
2. <u>Vocal cord paralysis</u>—usually unilateral, L>R due to longer recurrent laryngeal nerve on L side. May be life-threatening if bilateral. Caused by damage to recurrent laryngeal or vagus nerve, either due to tumour infiltration, trauma (e.g. postthyroidectomy), carotid dissection or dilated cardiovascular structures (e.g. aortic aneurysm). The involved cord is medialized with anteromedial deviation of the ipsilateral arytenoid cartilage and aryepiglottic fold.
3. <u>Laryngocoele</u>—air- or fluid-filled cystic dilatation of laryngeal ventricle. May be contained within larynx (internal) or herniate through thyrohyoid membrane beyond confines of larynx (external). Usually due to increased intralaryngeal pressure, e.g. due to chronic cough, occupation (glass blowers, wind instruments) or an obstructing laryngeal tumour.
4. **Laryngeal reflux**—of stomach acid, causing diffuse oedema and mucosal enhancement of larynx and hypopharynx.

5. **Other tumours**—e.g. chondrosarcoma (T2↑, chondroid calcification, minimal enhancement), paraganglioma (discrete hypervascular mass), papilloma (polypoid, seen in papillomatosis related to HPV infection; biopsy required to exclude carcinoma), melanoma (primary or metastatic), inflammatory pseudotumour (nonspecific mass).
6. **Wegener's granulomatosis***—classically causes subglottic stenosis ± inflammatory mass. Look for associated bony erosions in the paranasal sinuses.
7. **Rheumatoid arthritis***—can affect the cricoarytenoid and cricothyroid joints, resulting in sclerosis, fixation ± ankylosis. A poorly enhancing inflammatory mass ± cartilage erosion may also be seen, mimicking malignancy.
8. **Amyloidosis***—submucosal soft-tissue mass or diffuse infiltration + homogeneous enhancement ± calcification. Usually T2 isointense (cf. chondrosarcoma). Most commonly supraglottic. No cartilage destruction.

Other lesions

1. **Thyroglossal duct cyst**—most common congenital neck cyst. May be suprahyoid (in tongue base), level with hyoid or infrahyoid (most common); usually paramedian and intimately related to strap muscles. US: anechoic and thin-walled (unless infected), no internal vascularity. In adults, may contain debris. CT: thin-walled, smooth, well-defined, fluid attenuation. MRI: T2↑, may be T1↑ if haemorrhagic, infected or proteinaceous. No enhancement if uncomplicated, otherwise thin rim enhancement.
2. **Lymphadenopathy**—e.g. lymphoma (homogeneous; when in level VI, often also in mediastinum) or nodal involvement by differentiated thyroid cancer (heterogeneous; may be calcified in papillary and medullary cancer, or cystic in medullary cancer). See Section 12.20 for US assessment of lymph nodes.
3. **Parathyroid adenoma**—benign, most common cause of primary hyperparathyroidism. Majority are solitary, located posterior or inferior to thyroid. May rarely be ectopic, e.g. in mediastinum, carotid sheath, retropharyngeal, or intrathyroid. US: ovoid, homogeneous, hypoechoic to thyroid. Doppler US: characteristic feeding vessel from the poles with vascular rim. NM: ↑ Sestamibi uptake. SPECT may improve anatomical localization. 4DCT is more sensitive than US or scintigraphy for localization; low attenuation precontrast, avid arterial enhancement with washout on delayed phase.
4. **Fourth branchial cleft cyst**—cystic neck mass adjacent to or within thyroid, ± fistula to skin ± recurrent suppurative thyroiditis (intrathyroid abscess). L>R. Imaging: CT best, consider with oral barium (may show connection from cyst to pyriform sinus).

5. **Thymic remnant**—ectopic thymic tissue seen along the path of descent (thymopharyngeal duct).

12.18 THYROID ENLARGEMENT

1. **Multinodular goitre**—diffuse nodular enlargement with benign change, fibrosis, haemorrhage, cysts and calcifications. Patients are usually euthyroid. Look for retrosternal extension and tracheal compression.
2. **Thyroiditis**—may be the following:
   (a) **Autoimmune**—related to thyroid antibodies:
      (i) **Hashimoto's thyroiditis**—lymphocytic thyroiditis. Typically in middle-aged women, usually hypothyroid + goitre, but can be hyperthyroid in ~5%. First gradual painless enlargement, then atrophy and fibrosis. US: depends on phase and severity. Enlarged heterogeneous gland + hypoechoic nodular texture with reactive LNs especially in level VI. Doppler vascularity is usually normal/low. Increased risk of papillary thyroid cancer and NHL.
      (ii) **Graves' disease**—most common cause of thyrotoxicosis, usually in middle-aged women. US: enlarged and patchy hypoechoic thyroid ± marked hypervascularity on Doppler ('thyroid inferno'). NM: enlarged gland with homogeneous ↑ uptake on ^{123}I and ^{99m}Tc-pertechnetate scintigraphy.
      (iii) **Riedel's thyroiditis**—rare, part of IgG4-related disease. Painless, may grow rapidly + dysphagia/stridor, hard fixed 'woody' thyroid. Parenchyma replaced by fibrosis, which extends into surrounding tissues; can mimic anaplastic thyroid carcinoma. US: homogeneously hypoechoic thyroid with ill-defined margins. CT: enlarged hypoattenuating gland + compression of local structures. MRI: ↓ on T1 and T2, variable enhancement.
      (iv) **Postpartum thyroiditis**—seen in 5%–9% of women in the first year after childbirth or abortion; usually transient, lasting several weeks to months. Clinical: hyper- or hypothyroid. US: variable, often hypoechoic thyroid.
   (b) **De Quervain's subacute granulomatous thyroiditis**—self-limiting thyroiditis, often after a viral URTI. US: usually nonenlarged gland, ill-defined geographic hypoechoic and hypovascular areas interspersed with normal parenchyma. The key to diagnosis is that the thyroid is tender and painful.
   (c) **Suppurative thyroiditis**—rare, as the thyroid is normally resistant to infection. Can occur in an abnormal thyroid gland (e.g. Hashimoto's) or due to infection of a fourth branchial

cleft cyst (see Section 12.17). A rim-enhancing abscess may be seen.

3. **Primary thyroid carcinoma**—90% of thyroid malignancies. Risk factors: prior irradiation (especially for papillary type), family history of thyroid cancer. NB: incidental FDG-avid thyroid nodules on PET/CT have ~40% risk being a primary thyroid malignancy. Four main types:
   (a) **Papillary**—most common (60%–80%). F>M, peak in third to fourth decades. US: solitary hypoechoic ill-defined mass + microcalcification. 50% have local adenopathy at presentation, usually ipsilateral levels III and IV, tend to become cystic ± microcalcification. NM: usually concentrates radioiodine but not pertechnetate. Prognosis is excellent even with metastatic disease.
   (b) **Follicular**—10%–20%. F>M, peak in fifth to sixth decades. US: hypoechoic solid tumour. Nodal spread occurs late, haematogenous metastases are more common. NM: typically concentrates pertechnetate but not radioiodine. FNA cannot differentiate between follicular adenoma and carcinoma; surgical resection is required.
   (c) **Medullary**—5%. Most are sporadic, seen in third to fourth decades. When familial (e.g. part of MEN 2A/B syndromes), tend to be multiple and in younger patients. US: hypoechoic mass with punctate (coarse) calcification in primary and involved LNs (cf. fine calcification in papillary type), and in distant metastatic sites on CT. Calcitonin levels are invariably high and can be used for follow-up.
   (d) **Anaplastic**—1%–2%. Highly aggressive, worst prognosis, 5-year survival ~5%. Typically elderly (sixth to seventh decades), F>M, ± previous multinodular goitre. Infiltrative mass ± microcalcification. Nodal ± distant metastases common at presentation.
4. **Thyroid adenoma**—benign, often incidental finding. Well-defined mass, may be heterogeneous ± cystic degeneration.
5. **Thyroid lymphoma***—NHL, ~2.5% of thyroid malignancies. Primary or secondary, peaks at 50–70 years, F>M. Hashimoto's thyroiditis is a major risk factor, but still rare in this group. Clinical: rapidly enlarging goitre, compressive symptoms and cervical lymphadenopathy. B-symptoms rare, ~50% euthyroid. US: may be a hypoechoic nodular mass, diffuse heterogeneous infiltration or both. Calcification rare. CT: goitre, hypoattenuating to adjacent muscle, heterogeneous enhancement. More compressive than invasive. MRI: T1/T2 iso- to ↑, ± pseudocapsule.

6. **Thyroid metastasis**—rare. Most often from breast, kidney, colon or lung. Nonspecific on imaging. Often detected on FDG PET/CT.
7. **Paraganglioma**—can rarely occur within the thyroid. Well-defined, hypervascular + intratumoural vessels (rare with other thyroid masses).
8. **Fourth branchial cleft cyst**—see Section 12.17.
9. **Parathyroid adenoma (mimic)**—at posterior aspect of thyroid, or rarely within the thyroid.

12.19 BRITISH THYROID ASSOCIATION ULTRASOUND GRADING

Thyroid nodules are common incidental findings. The British Thyroid Association (BTA) issued guidelines in 2014 on management of thyroid cancer to enable stratification of thyroid nodules and appropriate selection for FNA (recommended for grades U3–U5).

Features associated with benign nodules

1. Spongiform/honeycomb appearance comprising >50% of the nodule.
2. Purely cystic, or solid-cystic with colloid (ring-down/comet-tail artefact).
3. Eggshell calcification.
4. Iso- or mildly hyperechoic with a hypoechoic halo.
5. Peripheral vascularity on colour flow/Doppler.

Features associated with malignant nodules

1. Solid hypoechoic nodule ± hyperechoic foci (microcalcification).
2. Irregular margin, intranodular vascularity and absent halo.
3. Taller than wide (i.e. anteroposterior > transverse diameter).
4. Interrupted eggshell calcification with hypoechoic soft-tissue extension beyond it.

Features associated with follicular lesions

NB: these are classified as U3, since it is not possible to reliably differentiate follicular adenoma from carcinoma on imaging or FNA—surgical resection is required.

1. Markedly hyperechoic and homogeneous with a hypoechoic halo.
2. Hypoechogenicity or loss of the halo is associated with follicular carcinoma.

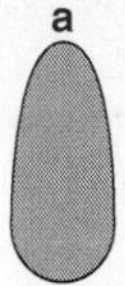

U1. Normal

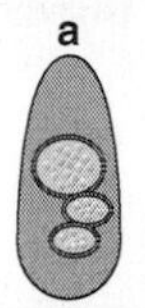

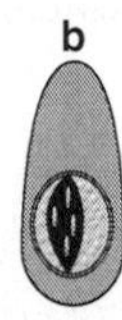

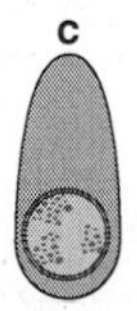

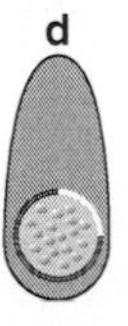

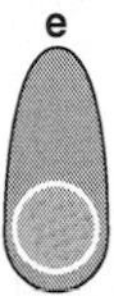

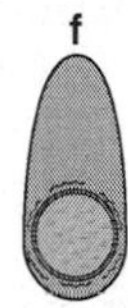

U2. Benign:
(a) halo, iso-echoic/mildly hyperechoic
(b) cystic change +/– ring down sign (colloid)
(c) microcystic/spongiform
(d & e) peripheral egg shell calcification
(f) peripheral vascularity

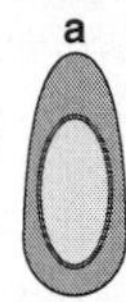

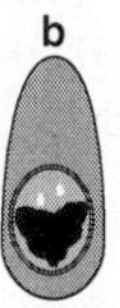

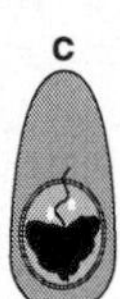

U3. Indeterminate/equivocal:
(a) homogenous, hyperechoic (markedly), solid, halo (follicular lesion)
(b) ? hypoechoic, equivocal echogenic foci, cystic change
(c) mixed/central vascularity

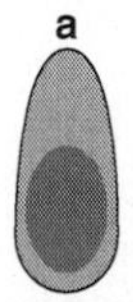

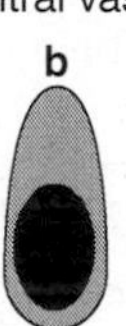

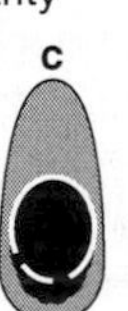

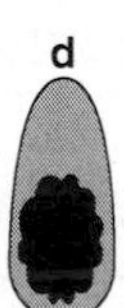

U4. Suspicious:
(a) solid, hypoechoic (cf. thyroid)
(b) solid, very hypoechoic (cf. strap muscle)
(c) disrupted peripheral calcification, hypoechoic
(d) lobulated outline

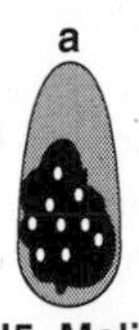

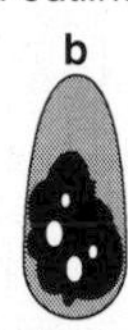

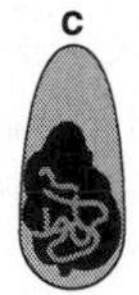

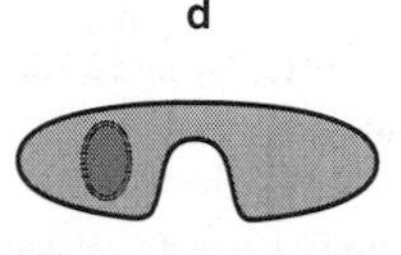

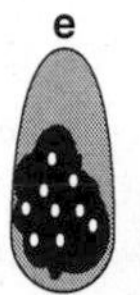

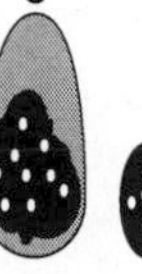

U5. Malignant:
(a) solid, hypoechoic, lobulated/irregular outline, microcalcification (? papillary carcinoma)
(b) solid, hypoechoic, lobulated/irregular outline, globular calcification (? medullary carcinoma)
(c) intranodular vascularity
(d) shape taller than wide (AP>TR)
(e) characteristic associated lymphadenopathy

(Reproduced with permission from Steve Colley in *Clinical Endocrinology*, 2014, 81, 1–122, John Wiley and Sons Ltd.)

12.20 SONOGRAPHIC FEATURES OF NORMAL VERSUS ABNORMAL LYMPH NODES

US is useful to evaluate LNs and select LNs for FNA. US + FNA is more accurate than CT, MRI or US alone for assessment of neck node metastases. Certain US features are associated with normal or abnormal LNs. NB: the context is important—in a patient with known malignancy differing criteria may be appropriate.

1. **Size**—short axis is measured. Poor predictor for malignancy when used alone. Higher size cut-off yields higher specificity but lower sensitivity. Upper neck nodes are larger than lower neck nodes. Cut-off of 7 mm for level I and 8 mm for all other cervical nodes is recommended for 70% accuracy.
2. **Shape**—metastatic, lymphomatous (Hodgkin/NHL) and tuberculous nodes are rounded. Normal or reactive nodes are usually oval or flat. Short/long axis ratio can be measured: <0.5 = oval; ≥ 0.5 = round. However, normal submandibular and parotid nodes are usually round.
3. **Echogenic hilum**—normal feature. May be absent in metastatic, lymphomatous and tuberculous nodes, but not always.
4. **Nodal border**—in proven malignant nodes, irregular ill-defined borders and hypoechoic change around LNs indicate extranodal extension (ENE). Clinical and histological evidence of ENE is now part of AJCC 8th edition; however, radiological appearances suggesting ENE may aid treatment planning at an earlier stage.
5. **Echogenicity**—metastatic nodes are usually hypoechoic. Papillary cancer metastases are hyperechoic (thyroglobulin deposition). Tuberculous nodes are hypoechoic. Lymphomatous nodes are hypoechoic (often markedly) with posterior acoustic enhancement ± intranodal reticulation/micronodular pattern.
6. **Calcification**—common in metastases from papillary (fine and peripheral) and medullary (coarse) thyroid carcinomas. Calcification may be seen in other metastatic LNs after radiotherapy or rarely after chemotherapy.
7. **Intranodal necrosis**—late event in tumour invasion, may appear cystic or echogenic (coagulative necrosis). Cystic necrosis is common in SCC metastases (especially p16+ve), papillary thyroid carcinoma and TB. Coagulative necrosis is uncommon and may be seen in malignant or inflammatory nodes.
8. **Vascular pattern**—normal and reactive nodes tend to show hilar vascularity or appear avascular. Metastatic nodes tend to have peripheral vascularity. Mixed vascularity is also common in lymphomatous nodes.

9. **Ancillary features**—matting (common in TB) and adjacent soft-tissue oedema (may be seen around metastatic, suppurative or tuberculous nodes).

12.21 BONY LESIONS OF MANDIBLE/ MAXILLA: CYSTIC

NB: most of these are odontogenic in origin.

1. **Periapical (radicular) cyst**—well-defined ovoid ≤1 cm cyst at the apex of a dead (nonvital) tooth, due to inflammation and necrosis from dental caries (often visible as erosion of the crown enamel). Most common odontogenic cyst.
2. **Nasopalatine duct cyst**—asymptomatic incidental developmental cyst arising from nasopalatine duct. Well-defined ≥1 cm midline cyst in the anterior maxilla (incisive canal).
3. **Dentigerous cyst**—developmental cyst associated with the crown of an unerupted or impacted tooth. Most in mandible, especially at third molar. Variable size, usually unilocular with a thin sclerotic border. Maxillary cysts expand into maxillary sinus. No enhancement or solid component on CT/MR.
4. **Odontogenic keratocyst**—benign cystic lesion with aggressive behaviour and high recurrence rate. 75% in posterior mandible, near third molar. In maxilla, most often near canine. May be multiple in Gorlin-Goltz syndrome. OPG/CT: solitary expansile unilocular cyst + sclerotic rim, may be near an unerupted tooth but not related to crown; ± displacement of developing tooth or resorption of roots. CT/MR: no solid nodule or mass, ± thin enhancing rim. Due to the keratin content, these usually have soft-tissue attenuation on CT and variable T1/T2 signal. May contain internal foci of calcification (calcifying odontogenic cyst).
5. **Ameloblastoma**—benign, locally aggressive neoplasm arising from tooth-bearing area of jaws. Age: 30–50 years. Most in mandible, especially near third molar and ramus. In maxilla, most often near premolar and first molar. OPG/CT: usually multilocular ('bubbly') and expansile with cortical scalloping and resorption of adjacent teeth. Possible associated unerupted molar tooth. No internal calcification. CT/MR: enhancing mural nodule and septa. Malignant transformation in 1% (ameloblastic carcinoma).
6. **Residual cyst**—at site of dental extraction, abutting alveolar crest. Absent overlying tooth.
7. **Simple bone cyst**—age: 10–30 years. 50% have history of trauma. Mandible >> maxilla. OPG/CT: nonexpansile unilocular cyst with marginal sclerosis, no internal septation and no association with teeth. MRI: T2↑ with fluid-fluid levels, mild rim enhancement.

8. **Aneurysmal bone cyst**—age: <20 years. Can occur spontaneously or related to trauma or other lesions, e.g. giant cell tumour (secondary ABC). Most at mandibular ramus. OPG/CT: uni- or multilocular, expansile + cortical thinning ± dehiscence. Sharp margins, even with cortical destruction, ± shallow reactive bone. Partially cystic meshwork divided by coarse septa. MRI: T2↑ with fluid-fluid levels and 'bubbly' appearance. 'Honeycomb' pattern of enhancement, no mural nodules (cf. ameloblastoma).
9. **Primordial cyst**—a dental follicle without a developing tooth.
10. **Stafne cyst (mimic)**—a medial cortical defect (containing fat or salivary gland tissue) in the posterior mandible measuring <2 cm, unrelated to the teeth. May mimic a cyst on OPG, diagnosis can be confirmed on CT/MR.

12.22 BONY LESIONS OF MANDIBLE/ MAXILLA: SOLID

Lytic

These may mimic cystic lesions on OPG, but their solid nature is revealed on CT/MR.

1. **Malignant infiltration by adjacent tumour**—SCC most common. CT/MRI: destructive bony lesion with adjacent soft-tissue mass.
2. **Myeloma**—most common in posterior mandible. Lytic punched-out lesion without sclerosis or bone expansion.
3. **Metastasis**—e.g. from breast or lung, often multiple. Mandible (especially molar region) > maxilla. MRI: marrow replacement with T1↓, STIR↑ + enhancement.
4. **Lymphoma***—primary or systemic NHL. Infiltrative or destructive lesion + soft-tissue mass ± adenopathy. The degree of bone destruction is often less than with other malignant processes.
5. **Leukaemia**—common in acute leukaemia. Loss of definition of lamina dura, lytic bony destruction or diffuse osteopenia.
6. **Eosinophilic granuloma**—in children. Well- or ill-defined, ± soft-tissue mass ± surrounding reactive sclerosis and periosteal reaction.
7. **Ewing sarcoma**—age 5–25 years. Mandible > maxilla. Ill-defined bony destruction ± periosteal reaction (may be sunburst). Large soft-tissue mass.
8. **Other malignant tumours**—e.g. odontogenic carcinoma, ameloblastic carcinoma, various sarcomas. Ill-defined destructive mass. Rare.
9. **Giant cell granuloma**—benign, mean ~25 years. Mandible (especially midline) > maxilla. CT: expansile lytic mass with coarse

or thin wavy septations, often at right angle to cortex ± cortical scalloping and dehiscence ± tooth root resorption. MRI: T2↓ or isointense ± fluid-fluid levels (intralesional ABC), heterogeneous enhancement.

10. **Ameloblastic fibroma**—benign well-defined lucent lesion. May be multilocular, mimicking ameloblastoma, or unilocular and associated with the crown of an unerupted tooth, mimicking dentigerous cyst.
11. **Odontogenic myxoma**—benign well-defined multilocular lucent lesion indistinguishable from ameloblastoma.
12. **Nerve sheath tumour**—e.g. schwannoma, neurofibroma. May widen inferior alveolar nerve canal.
13. **Intraosseous arteriovenous malformation**—multilocular lucent lesion on OPG. Vascular nature revealed on CT/MR.

Sclerotic, calcified or ossified

Unrelated to the teeth

1. **Osteoma**—small well-defined homogeneously sclerotic lesion unrelated to the teeth, may be exophytic. No hypodense halo. If multiple, consider Gardner syndrome.
2. **Metastasis**—e.g. from prostate or breast. Usually multiple + bone metastases elsewhere.
3. **Exostosis**—also known as torus. Similar to exostoses in other bones. Can arise from mandible or maxilla, grows inwards into the oral cavity.

Related to the teeth

1. **Condensing osteitis**—reactive ill-defined nonexpansile periapical sclerosis around a diseased tooth.
2. **Odontoma**—benign hamartoma. May be simple (supernumerary tooth), compound (a cluster of small tooth-like denticles) or complex (dense amorphous mass of enamel and dentin). Well-defined with a hypodense halo. Often associated with an impacted tooth.
3. **Cementoblastoma**—in children and young adults. Well-defined round sclerotic lesion fused to the apical portion of a tooth, with a radiolucent halo.

Ground-glass, mixed or variable density

Unrelated to the teeth

NB: these may appear related to the teeth if large.

1. **Fibrous dysplasia (FD)**—face and calvarium involvement in 25% of monostotic FD and >50% of polyostotic FD (e.g. McCune-Albright and Mazabraud syndromes). Maxilla > mandible > rest of skull. OPG/CT: typically an ill-defined expansile

ground-glass density lesion, but may also be cystic (lucent + sclerotic border, active disease) or pagetoid (mixed lucent and sclerotic). MRI: variable appearances. Ossified and fibrous areas are T1/T2↓; cystic areas are T2↑. Fibrous areas may enhance. Bone scan and PET-CT: nonspecific ↑ uptake depending on activity. Malignant transformation (e.g. osteosarcoma) is rare. May be associated with ABC. Pagetoid FD mimics Paget's disease; however, Paget's occurs in the elderly and involves skull vault and base, usually sparing the facial bones.

2. **Osteonecrosis**—can occur after local radiotherapy (peaks at 6–12 months, can persist for years) or in patients on bisphosphonates (especially after tooth extraction). Mandible > maxilla. CT: ill-defined bone destruction with mixed lysis and sclerosis ± sequestra ± gas bubbles. MRI: T1↓ and STIR↑ + marrow enhancement and surrounding soft-tissue thickening.
3. **Renal osteodystrophy***—mixed bone sclerosis and resorption with loss of definition of lamina dura ('floating teeth') ± lytic brown tumour.
4. **Osteosarcoma**—mean ~35 years. Mandible > maxilla. Ill-defined destructive lesion with osteoid matrix and periosteal reaction. May be related to previous radiotherapy.
5. **Paget's disease***—may rarely involve maxilla > mandible, usually with skull involvement. Most commonly symmetrical. OPG/CT: trabecular thickening with ground-glass and sclerotic islands. Hypercementosis around tooth roots.
6. **Ossifying fibroma**—benign fibroosseous lesion. Typically a well-defined, solitary, expansile ground-glass density mass ± a sclerotic margin. May also appear lucent (early) or ossified (cementoossifying subtype). May mimic FD but appears more well-defined, tends to displace or erode teeth and peaks at an older age (20–40 years). Mandible > maxilla > other bones. MRI: variable T1/T2 signal ± fluid-fluid levels + enhancement of fibrous component. If multiple, consider hyperparathyroidism-jaw tumour syndrome.
7. **Osteoblastoma/osteoid osteoma**—mixed lucent and sclerotic lesion ± lucent nidus, usually in patients <20 years. Typically painful, unlike most other fibroosseous lesions.
8. **Intraosseous haemangioma**—rare; usually lucent with multiple coarse trabeculations ± phleboliths.

Related to the teeth

1. **Osteomyelitis**—see Section 12.4. Mandible >> maxilla. May be destructive or sclerotic (Garré's sclerosing osteomyelitis) ± sequestra, gas bubbles, fistula, abscess and periostitis.
2. **Cementoosseous dysplasia**—benign hamartomatous lesion mostly seen in middle-aged Afro-Caribbean or East Asian women. May be lytic (early), sclerotic (late) or mixed, ± radiolucent halo. Periapical

location; may be focal or florid (involving ≥2 jaw quadrants). Mandible > maxilla.

3. **Pindborg tumour**—rare; well-defined and lucent + variable scattered or trabecular calcifications (may have a 'driven snow' appearance). May be associated with an unerupted tooth.
4. **Adenomatoid odontogenic tumour**—rare; well-defined lucent lesion related to the crown of an unerupted tooth. Maxilla > mandible. Can mimic dentigerous cyst, but usually contains flakes of calcification.
5. **Ameloblastic fibroodontoma**—rare; well-defined lucent lesion containing a dense mass of enamel and dentin (a hybrid of ameloblastic fibroma and complex odontoma).

12.23 NASAL SEPTAL PERFORATION

1. <u>Trauma</u>—external, self-inflicted (e.g. nose picking) or iatrogenic (e.g. septoplasty, nasal packing, cauterization for epistaxis, nasotracheal intubation). Laceration or septal haematoma → elevation of mucoperichondrium from the septal cartilage → ischemia, necrosis and perforation.
2. <u>Cocaine necrosis</u>—vasoconstriction → ischemic necrosis.
3. <u>Wegener's granulomatosis</u>*—most patients will have involvement of nose (septum > turbinates) and sinuses ± orbit, nasopharynx, larynx, oral cavity, temporal bone and salivary glands. CT/MRI: enhancing nodular soft-tissue masses in nasal cavity ± chronic sinusitis. Commonly causes nasal septal perforation ± destruction of turbinates, lateral nasal wall and hard palate (sinonasal–oral fistula). Sclerotic bone thickening of the sinus walls. MRI: nodular masses are T2↓ relative to inflamed T2↑ mucosa.
4. **Rhinitis medicamentosa**—vasoconstrictive and steroid nasal sprays → ischemic necrosis and perforation.
5. **Invasive fungal sinusitis**—see Section 12.25.
6. **Sarcoidosis***—sinonasal disease is uncommon. Generalized mucosal thickening often centred on the anterior nasal cavity and nasal septum + bone erosion.
7. **Sinonasal SCC**—see Section 12.25. May destroy nasal septum.
8. **Lymphoma***—usually natural killer cell NHL. Age 60–80 years. Nasal cavity > sinuses, ± involvement of nasopharynx, oropharynx and LNs. Infiltrative mass ± bone destruction or remodelling. CT: may be high attenuation. MRI: T2↓ or intermediate due to high cellularity. Variable enhancement.
9. **Melanoma**—arises from melanocytes in sinonasal mucosa. Typically in Caucasians aged 50–90 years. Nasal cavity > sinuses. Infiltrative, avidly enhancing mass with bony destruction ± remodelling. Classically T1↑ (if melanotic) and T2↓. Blooming on

T2* due to haemorrhage. Amelanotic melanoma has variable T1/T2 signal.

10. **Nasal septal abscess**—due to acute rhinosinusitis. Can cause septal perforation.

12.24 PARANASAL SINUS LESION WITHOUT BONE DESTRUCTION

Inflammatory

1. **Chronic rhinosinusitis**—sinonasal inflammation for ≥12 consecutive weeks. Ethmoid > maxillary > frontal and sphenoid. CT: mucosal thickening + bony sclerosis and thickening without destruction or sinus expansion. Sinus secretions may be hyperdense if high protein or fungal content, ± occasional calcification. MRI: variable T1 signal (↑ if proteinaceous). Mucosa is T2↑, secretions vary depending on water content. Smooth mucosal enhancement. Complications: osteomyelitis, subgaleal abscess (Pott's puffy tumour), subperiosteal abscess, myositis of extraocular muscles, pre- or postseptal cellulitis or abscess, optic neuritis, meningitis, epidural or subdural abscess, cerebritis, brain abscess, cavernous sinus thrombosis.
2. **Acute rhinosinusitis**—sinonasal inflammation ≤4 weeks, most commonly ethmoid and maxillary. CT: air-fluid level ± bubbly or strand-like secretions in sinus with mucosal thickening and obstruction of ostiomeatal complex. Enhancement of inflamed mucosa, nonenhancing central secretions. MRI: mucosa and secretions T2↑ and T1↓. If secretions are proteinaceous, T1↑ and T2↓. Same potential complications as above.
3. **Retention cyst**—well-defined rounded cyst, usually in the maxillary sinus. Fluid attenuation on CT and fluid signal on MRI (may be proteinaceous). The rest of the involved sinus is typically aerated (cf. mucocoele). May be associated with sinusitis.
4. **Mucocoele**—completely opacified and expanded sinus with smooth remodelling of walls due to obstruction of sinus ostium. Frontal > ethmoid (may extend into orbit) > maxillary > sphenoid (may extend into cranial cavity). Cause: polyps, sinusitis, trauma, surgery or tumour. CT: fluid or soft-tissue attenuation (if desiccated secretions or fungal colonization). Sinus wall may be normal, thin or focally absent. MRI: fluid signal (may be proteinaceous). Minimal peripheral enhancement only. Thick peripheral mucosal enhancement suggests superadded infection (mucopyocoele). Nodular enhancement suggests an underlying tumour.
5. **Sinonasal polyposis**—inflammatory swelling of sinonasal mucosa that buckles to form 'polyps'. Usually multiple and bilateral, involving both nasal cavity and sinuses. Often obstructs sinus drainage pathways in the superior nasal cavity, resulting in sinusitis.

CT: soft-tissue attenuation, may be hyperattenuating if ↑ protein or colonization with fungus; ± bony remodelling or erosion. MRI: usually T1↓ and T2↑ of mucosa and associated secretions; T1↑ if secretions are proteinaceous. Peripheral mucosal enhancement with central nonenhancing secretions.

6. **Solitary sinonasal polyp**—inflammatory polyp arising from sinus, herniating through major or accessory ostium into nasal cavity ± prolapse into nasopharynx. Antrochoanal polyp is the most common, arising from the maxillary sinus. Sphenochoanal and ethmochoanal polyps are rare. Most common in adolescents and young adults. CT: dumbbell-shaped low attenuation mass arising from maxillary antrum, extending through widened ostium or accessory ostium into ipsilateral nasal cavity + bone remodelling. Can be ↑ density if fungal colonization. MRI: variable T1 signal (↑ if proteinaceous), T2↑. Thin peripheral enhancement.
7. **Allergic fungal sinusitis**—chronic noninvasive fungal sinusitis in an immunocompetent nondiabetic young adult with a long history of chronic rhinosinusitis, allergy ± polyposis. Multiple sinuses involved, may be unilateral or bilateral. Ethmoid > maxillary > frontal > sphenoid, ± sinus expansion with bony remodelling or erosion. CT: ↑ attenuation in opacified sinus with hypoattenuating rim of mucosa. MRI: variable T1 signal depending on protein, water and fungal content. T2↓↓ centrally due to dense fungal concretions and heavy metals. Peripheral enhancement of inflamed mucosa.
8. **Mycetoma**—chronic noninvasive form of fungal sinusitis where material in the sinonasal cavity is colonized by fungus. Indolent clinical course. More common in the elderly. Usually affects a single sinus; maxillary > sphenoid > frontal > ethmoid. CT: thick mucosa with central high attenuation ± calcification ± thick sclerotic sinus wall. MRI: T2↓↓, can be mistaken for air.
9. **Silent sinus syndrome**—chronic occlusion of the maxillary sinus ostium → resorption of sinus gas → retraction of maxillary sinus walls and reduced sinus volume (atelectasis). Symptoms of sinusitis are characteristically absent. CT/MRI: small volume and opacified maxillary sinus with retraction of walls including the orbital floor, resulting in enophthalmos.

Neoplastic

1. <u>**Osteoma**</u>—benign bone-forming tumour that typically arises from the sinus wall and protrudes into the lumen. Almost exclusive to the craniofacial skeleton; frontal and ethmoid >> maxillary and sphenoid sinuses. Usually incidental and asymptomatic; can rarely obstruct sinus drainage, causing sinusitis or a mucocoele. CT: well-defined and uniformly sclerotic, may be ground-glass. Multiple in Gardner syndrome. See Sections 12.21 and 12.22 for other lesions arising from bone, e.g. fibrous dysplasia and ossifying fibroma.

2. Inverted papilloma—benign epithelial tumour of sinonasal mucosa with histology showing epithelial proliferation into underlying stroma. 10% either degenerate or coexist with SCC. Age 40–70 years. Usually arises from lateral nasal wall in middle meatus ± extension into maxillary antrum ± bone remodelling and obstructive sinusitis. Uncommonly arises from sinuses. Often has entrapped bone/tumourous calcification ± focal hyperostosis of adjacent bone at site of origin. CT/MRI: convoluted 'cerebriform' pattern of enhancement. Secretions and areas of necrosis do not enhance. High rate of local recurrence after surgical resection.
3. Juvenile angiofibroma—see Section 12.2.
4. **Pleomorphic adenoma**—can rarely arise from minor salivary gland tissue in the nasal cavity, extending into paranasal sinuses. Nonspecific soft-tissue mass + bone remodelling.
5. **Nerve sheath tumour**—e.g. schwannoma or neurofibroma. Well-defined, expansile, variably enhancing mass centred on the nasoethmoid region + adjacent bone remodelling.

12.25 PARANASAL SINUS LESION WITH BONE DESTRUCTION

1. Sinonasal SCC—most common sinonasal malignancy; sinuses (especially maxillary) > nasal cavity. Age 50–70 years. Infiltrative mass with destruction of sinus wall. The mass shows intermediate T2 signal and heterogeneous nodular enhancement (cf. benign mucosal thickening which is T2↑ with smooth uniform enhancement).
2. Invasive fungal sinusitis—different clinical presentations and course:
   (a) **Acute invasive fungal sinusitis**—immunocompromised patient, rapidly progressive or fatal within days to weeks, ± orbital and intracranial extension.
   (b) **Granulomatous invasive fungal sinusitis**—immunocompetent patient. Slowly progressive over >12 weeks. Enlarging cheek, orbit or sinonasal mass. Primarily seen in the Middle East and on the Indian subcontinent.
   (c) **Chronic invasive fungal sinusitis**—slowly progressive over >12 weeks, usually in patients with AIDS, diabetes or on steroids. CT: soft-tissue opacification and mucosal thickening of sinuses. High attenuation secretions ± septal/sinus wall erosion ± narrowing or occlusion of adjacent arteries or veins ± intraorbital or meningeal extension. MRI: variable T1 signal depending on protein/water content. Fungal elements are T2↓↓ with surrounding soft tissue T2↑ and enhancement.
3. Olfactory neuroblastoma—rare, slow-growing, malignant tumour arising from olfactory neuroepithelium in the roof of the nasal cavity. Dumbbell-shaped enhancing tumour with upper portion in

the anterior cranial fossa, waist at level of cribriform plate and lower portion in upper nasal cavity, + bone destruction (especially cribriform plate) and remodelling ± areas of haemorrhage and necrosis. A peritumoural cyst at the margin of the intracranial component is characteristic. Two peaks: in young adults and middle age. Tends to recur after treatment (may be years later).

4. **Wegener's granulomatosis***—see Section 12.23.
5. **Lymphoma***—see Section 12.23.
6. **Other carcinomas**—e.g. undifferentiated, adenoid cystic, adenocarcinoma. Aggressive ill-defined mass with bony destruction ± perineural spread. Age 40–80 years.
7. **Sarcoidosis***—see Section 12.23.
8. **Osteosarcoma**—age 30–50 years (older than osteosarcoma of long bones). Mandible > maxilla. CT/MRI: aggressive mass with calcified osteoid matrix and periosteal reaction ± soft-tissue component.
9. **Chondrosarcoma**—age 50–80 years. Arises from the nasal septum. CT: well-defined mass with a nonsclerotic margin ± chondroid matrix calcification. Most show bony destruction. MRI: T1↓ or intermediate, T2↑ ± foci of T2↓ (calcification). Heterogeneous enhancement.

12.26 ORBIT: LESIONS INVOLVING THE GLOBE

1. **Haemorrhage**—due to trauma or surgery. Usually vitreal or suprachoroidal, rarely retinal. CT: patchy or lenticular hyperattenuation in vitreous or suprachoroidal space ± evidence of trauma, e.g. globe rupture, dislocated lens or bone fracture. MRI: acute haematoma T1/T2↓; subacute haematoma T1↑.
2. **Retinal or choroidal detachment**—accumulation of fluid or haemorrhage within detached layers of retina or in suprachoroidal space. Retinal: leaves of retina converge at optic disc, forming a 'V' shape. Anterior end extends towards (but not anterior to) ciliary body. Choroidal: does not converge at the optic disc, forming two separate lenticular shapes. Anterior end can extend beyond ciliary body. CT/MR: attenuation and intensity depends on content (fluid, protein or blood). Usually ↑ density on CT and T1↑ on MRI.
3. **Orbital pseudotumour**—various patterns; can involve the globe causing irregular scleral thickening and enhancement, usually extending posteriorly to involve the optic nerve sheath. See also Section 12.29.
4. **Melanoma**—most common primary intraocular tumour in adults. Usually arises from choroid. CT/MRI: dome or mushroom shaped enhancing mass with broad choroidal base ± choroidal or retinal detachment. No calcification (unless following therapy). T1↑ (unless amelanotic), T2↓.

5. **Endophthalmitis**—purulent inflammation of intraocular fluid due to contiguous spread of infection, usually from pre- or postseptal cellulitis, trauma or surgery. More common in children and young adults. CT/MRI: thickening and enhancement of uvea/sclera ± restricted diffusion ± features of panophthalmitis (intraconal fat stranding, oedema and enhancement of extraocular muscles, subperiosteal or intraorbital abscess, septal thickening). Complications: cavernous sinus thrombosis, intracranial spread of infection.
6. **Ocular calcification**—e.g. drusen (at optic disc), choroidal osteoma (close to optic disc), phthisis bulbi (shrunken 'end-stage' eye).
7. **Surgical inserts**—e.g. scleral buckle (dense ring around sclera) or vitreous silicone oil (rounded uniformly dense material within vitreous cavity, T1↑ on MRI). Both are treatments for retinal detachment.
8. **Staphyloma/coloboma**—both are focal posterior outpouchings of the globe, usually bilateral; staphyloma is due to acquired scleral thinning related to severe myopia; coloboma is due to a congenital scleral defect.
9. **Choroidal haemangioma**—benign hamartoma. Avidly enhancing ± calcification; may be circumscribed and lentiform (middle-aged patients, sporadic) or diffuse mild choroidal thickening (younger patients, associated with Sturge-Weber syndrome).
10. **Lymphoproliferative lesions**—see Section 12.30. Can rarely involve the globe.
11. **Ocular metastases**—e.g. from lung or breast. Rare; may be multiple and bilateral.
12. **Sarcoidosis***—see Section 12.30. Can involve iris, ciliary body and/or choroid.
13. **Retinoblastoma**—extremely rare in adults.

12.27 ORBIT: LESIONS OF THE OPTIC NERVE OR SHEATH

1. Optic nerve sheath meningioma—age: fourth to fifth decade (~10 years in NF2). Usually tubular but may be pedunculated or fusiform. Linear or punctate calcification is common (cf. glioma). Homogeneous 'tram-track' enhancement is typical but not pathognomonic. Typically spares distal-most segment of the optic nerve sheath—CSF may become trapped here, creating a perioptic cyst.
2. Optic pathway glioma—age varies (occurs in children when associated with NF1). If bilateral, highly suggestive of NF1. CT/MRI: diffuse sausage-shaped or fusiform enlargement of optic nerve (often kinked) ± chiasm, with variable enhancement ± cystic

spaces. May extend to hypothalamus, optic tracts and radiations. Calcification very rare. Look for cerebral features of NF1.

3. <u>**Optic neuritis**</u>—age 15–50 years. Autoimmune optic nerve inflammation; 50%–60% will develop multiple sclerosis. Focal or segmental T2 hyperintensity of optic nerve ± enhancement ± mild nerve swelling. Look for cerebral features of MS.
4. **Orbital pseudotumour**—various patterns; can involve the optic nerve sheath causing irregular thickening and enhancement (may be 'tram-track') ± involvement of retrobulbar fat.
5. **Lymphoproliferative lesions**—see Section 12.30. May cause 'tram-track' enhancement.
6. **Sarcoidosis***—see Section 12.30. May cause 'tram-track' enhancement.

12.28 ORBIT: LESIONS ARISING WITHIN INTRACONAL FAT

1. <u>**Orbital pseudotumour**</u>—various patterns; can present as an ill-defined infiltrative enhancing intraconal mass ± involvement of other parts of orbit. Does not distort globe or erode bone. MRI: T1↓, T2 signal usually less than other orbital lesions due to cellular infiltrates and fibrosis. See also Section 12.29.
2. <u>**Cavernous haemangioma**</u>—encapsulated vascular malformation, usually an incidental finding on CT/MR. Most common in intraconal fat. CT: iso- or hyperattenuating (due to microcalcification). No phleboliths, unlike venous varix. Avid enhancement. MRI: T1 isointense or ↑. T2↑ ± internal septations. Dynamic post contrast: early patchy enhancement → homogeneous filling on delayed sequences.
3. <u>**Venous varix**</u>—slow-flow venous malformation, distends with Valsalva. Tubular or tortuous retrobulbar lesion with intense enhancement ± phleboliths.
4. **Lymphoproliferative lesions**—see Section 12.30.
5. **Sarcoidosis***—see Section 12.30.
6. **Erdheim-Chester disease***—orbital involvement is common, usually manifesting as bilateral infiltrative enhancing intraconal masses, which are T1/T2↓ on MRI. The pattern of disease elsewhere aids differentiation from orbital pseudotumour.
7. **Nerve sheath tumour**—e.g. schwannoma, neurofibroma. Well-defined intraconal mass.

12.29 ORBIT: CONAL LESIONS

1. <u>**Thyroid ophthalmopathy**</u>—most common orbital disorder and cause of proptosis. Autoimmune process associated with Graves' disease involving extraocular muscles, fat and connective tissue ±

lacrimal glands. Typically bilateral and symmetrical. Muscle involvement: inferior > medial > superior > lateral > obliques (I'M SLO). Muscle belly thickness ≥5 mm is abnormal. Tendons are typically spared (cf. orbital pseudotumour). Acute phase: T2↑ in muscles (oedema, best seen on T2 fatsat). Chronic phase: T2↓ due to fibrosis. Increased orbital fat → stretching of optic nerve.

2. **Orbital pseudotumour**—most common painful orbital mass in adults, usually unilateral. Various patterns; extraocular muscle involvement is the most common, especially superior and medial rectus, superior oblique and levator palpebrae. Shaggy thickening and enhancement of involved muscles + tendinous insertions. Associated with IgG4-related disease.
3. **Lymphoproliferative lesions**—see Section 12.30.
4. **Sarcoidosis***—see Section 12.30.
5. **Metastasis**—most commonly from breast, lung, melanoma. Nonspecific mass, usually in the presence of metastases elsewhere.
6. **Extraocular myositis**—usually due to sinusitis + orbital cellulitis (see Section 12.24). Muscle and fat infiltration + enhancement ± subperiosteal abscess. Most commonly medial rectus secondary to ethmoid sinusitis.
7. **Rhabdomyosarcoma**—usually <15 years. Infiltrative mass ± extension into eyelid and paranasal sinuses.

12.30 ORBIT: EXTRACONAL LESIONS

Lesions arising within the orbital cavity

1. **Lymphoproliferative lesions**—second most common orbital disorder. Spectrum of benign lymphoid hyperplasia to malignant lymphoma (± systemic disease). Age >60 years. Can involve any part of orbit, most commonly anterior extraconal space and lacrimal gland. Mostly unilateral. CT: slightly hyperattenuating due to high cellularity + homogeneous enhancement. MRI: mildly T1/T2↑ relative to muscle. Bone destruction if aggressive histology.
2. **Orbital pseudotumour**—lacrimal gland involvement is the second most common pattern: diffuse enlargement + ill-defined margins + enhancement. Orbital apex involvement can also occur ± intracranial extension through fissures into cavernous sinus (Tolosa-Hunt syndrome). See also Section 12.29.
3. **Pleomorphic adenoma**—most common epithelial tumour of lacrimal gland. Age: second to fifth decades. CT/MRI: well-defined enhancing mass ± cystic change ± calcification ± scalloping of adjacent bone. Risk of malignant transformation.
4. **Malignant lacrimal gland tumour**—e.g. adenoid cystic carcinoma (most common), malignant mixed tumour, adenocarcinoma, SCC. Ill-defined enhancing mass, often with bony destruction.

5. Sarcoidosis*—can involve any part of orbit, most commonly the lacrimal gland. Diffuse nonspecific lacrimal gland enlargement or ill-defined orbital masses with homogeneous enhancement. Lacrimal gland involvement may be isolated without systemic disease.
6. **Sjögren's syndrome***—chronic systemic autoimmune exocrinopathy; usually involves salivary glands, but can also involve lacrimal glands, which become enlarged and heterogeneous.
7. **Dacryocystocoele**—cystic mass at medial canthus + enlarged nasolacrimal duct. Rim enhancement suggests infection (dacryocystitis).

Lesions arising from the orbital wall

1. Subperiosteal abscess—due to orbital cellulitis or adjacent sinusitis (most commonly ethmoidal); see Section 12.24. In this setting any soft-tissue thickening adjacent to the orbital wall must be considered suspicious for an abscess, even in the absence of rim enhancement.
2. Sinonasal mucocoele—see Section 12.24. May bulge into orbit.
3. Sinonasal SCC—see Section 12.25. May invade the orbit.
4. Metastasis to orbital wall—see Section 12.34.
5. Dermoid and epidermoid—developmental ectodermal inclusion cyst, most common in children. Slowly progressive nontender mass → inflammation if ruptures. Located adjacent to sutures, especially frontozygomatic suture ± adjacent bone remodelling. Dermoid contains macroscopic fat ± calcification ± fluid-fluid levels. Epidermoid appears cystic + restricted diffusion.
6. Sphenoid wing dysplasia—seen in NF1, ± other features, e.g. optic nerve glioma, plexiform neurofibroma, buphthalmos and cerebral T2 hyperintensities. X-ray: absent innominate line due to absent greater wing of sphenoid. CT/MRI: hypoplastic or absent sphenoid wing ± herniation of middle cranial fossa contents into the orbit ± associated arachnoid cyst.
7. **Fibrous dysplasia**—see Section 12.22.
8. **Paget's disease***—see Section 12.34.
9. **Intraosseous meningioma**—e.g. in sphenoid wing; either primary or secondary intraosseous extension. CT: bony thickening and permeative sclerosis + enhancing dural mass or thickening.

12.31 EXTERNAL AUDITORY CANAL LESIONS

1. Earwax plug—very common especially in elderly, often bilateral. Low attenuation on CT, usually with a rim of gas.
2. Cholesteatoma—nonenhancing EAC mass with bone erosion ± bone fragments within lesion.

3. <u>Carcinoma</u>—usually SCC but minor salivary gland tumours, e.g. adenoid cystic carcinoma can occur. Infiltrative enhancing mass ± bone destruction ± parotid space nodes. Usually extends inwards from pinna.
4. <u>Necrotizing otitis externa</u>—painful, severe, invasive infection of EAC in elderly diabetics and immunocompromised patients due to *Pseudomonas aeruginosa*. Soft-tissue thickening in the EAC extending to the outer soft tissues (especially below skull base) + fat stranding ± abscess ± erosion or osteomyelitis of the mastoid bone ± skull base. Infection can spread into the intracranial cavity causing venous sinus thrombosis, subdural empyema or brain abscess.
5. **Congenital ear malformations**—variable severity. External ear: EAC stenosis or atresia ± malformed pinna. Middle ear: small cavity ± calcified tympanic membrane ± malformed or fused ossicles. Inner ear usually normal.
6. **Osteoma**—solitary pedunculated bony outgrowth, located laterally in EAC at junction of bony and cartilaginous portions.
7. **Exostosis**—benign lobulated bony overgrowth circumferentially narrowing the EAC bilaterally, due to chronic cold water exposure (surfer's ear).
8. **Medial canal fibrosis**—crescent of fibrous soft tissue in the medial EAC overlying the tympanic membrane. No middle ear involvement or bony changes. Bilateral in 50%.
9. **Keratosis obturans**— abnormal accumulation of desquamated keratin causing partial or complete filling of EAC ± mild expansion. No bony erosion (cf. cholesteatoma). Bilateral in 50%.

12.32 MIDDLE EAR LESIONS

1. <u>Chronic otitis media</u>—either erosive, tympanosclerotic, or both. Erosions and/or sclerosis of ossicles (especially erosion of the distal long process of incus), ± calcification elsewhere in middle ear cavity. Tympanic membrane retraction ± calcification. Under pneumatization of mastoid.
2. <u>Acquired cholesteatoma</u>—focal accumulation of exfoliated keratin within stratified squamous epithelium. Two types based on site of origin (see below). CT: nondependent soft-tissue mass + local bone erosion. MRI: T1↓ (cf. cholesterol granuloma), T2↑ and marked restricted diffusion. No enhancement, though surrounding granulation tissue may enhance. Complications: dural extension, meningitis, subperiosteal or intracranial abscess, labyrinthitis and venous sinus thrombosis. In postsurgical patients it is hard to differentiate recurrent cholesteatoma from granulation tissue, fluid and fibrosis on CT; on nonEPI DWI MRI, only recurrent cholesteatoma will show significant restricted diffusion.

(a) **Pars flaccida**—80%. Arises in Prussak's space (between scutum and malleus) + erosion of scutum and ossicles; if large, can cause dehiscence of lateral semicircular canal, tegmen tympani, tegmen mastoideum and facial nerve canal.

(b) **Pars tensa**—20%. Arises medial to ossicles ± extension into sinus tympani, facial recess, aditus ad antrum ± mastoid air cells. Erosion of adjacent ossicles, mastoid antrum and anterior tegmen mastoideum.

3. **Cholesterol granuloma**—mass of granulation tissue associated with recurrent haemorrhage and cholesterol deposition in patients with chronic otitis media. CT: expansile mass in middle ear ± mastoid air cells. Large lesions cause ossicular displacement ± erosion. MRI: characteristically T1↑ (methaemoglobin); T2↑ centrally (granulation tissue) with a T2↓ rim (haemosiderin). No enhancement (beware of inherent T1↑ signal).
4. **Glomus tympanicum**—benign paraganglioma arising from glomus body situated on cochlear promontory. Most common tumour of middle ear; age 40–60 years. May be associated with paragangliomas elsewhere. Clinical: pulsatile tinnitus, red anteroinferior mass on otoscopy. CT/MRI: avidly enhancing 2–20 mm mass with a flat base on the cochlear promontory. Floor of middle ear cavity intact.
5. **Glomus jugulare**—paraganglioma centred on jugular foramen. Typically large, can extend into middle ear cavity (glomus jugulotympanicum). May be multiple and familial (e.g. MEN 1, NF1). Clinical: pulsatile tinnitus ± cranial nerve palsies (especially CN IX), retrotympanic mass on otoscopy. CT/MRI: avidly enhancing mass in jugular foramen + bone destruction and dehiscence of jugular bulb ± extension of mass into middle ear. Tumours >2 cm show a 'salt and pepper' appearance due to foci of T1↑ (haemorrhage or slow flow) and T1↓ (flow voids).
6. **Acute otomastoiditis with abscess**—clinical: otalgia, otorrhoea, fever and hearing loss. CT: opacified mastoid air cells + cortical and trabecular erosion ± subperiosteal, epidural or brain abscess ± venous sinus thrombosis.
7. **Dehiscent jugular bulb**—normal variant with superolateral protrusion of jugular bulb into middle ear cavity through dehiscent sigmoid plate. No bone destruction. Important incidental finding for surgical planning. Usually asymptomatic.
8. **Aberrant ICA**—normal variant with posterolateral displacement of the petrous portion of the ICA, which protrudes into the middle ear cavity. Important to recognize for surgical planning. Mostly asymptomatic.
9. **Intraosseous meningioma**—see Section 12.30. Temporal bone is a common site. Soft tissue may extend into middle ear cavity.

10. **Middle ear schwannoma**—primary schwannoma arises from tympanic segment of CN VII, Jacobson nerve or chorda tympani. Secondary schwannoma arises from outside middle ear, e.g. jugular foramen schwannoma or acoustic schwannoma (CN VIII). Enhancing mass contiguous with long axis of parent nerve.
11. **Perineural tumour spread along CN VII**—most commonly seen with adenoid cystic carcinoma of parotid. Ill-defined enhancing tubular lesion extending from parotid tumour through stylomastoid foramen → mastoid segment of CN VII ± extension proximally to internal auditory meatus. Best seen on MRI (fatsat T1+C).
12. **Endolymphatic sac tumour**—sporadic or associated with vHL. May be bilateral. CT: permeative destructive mass centred posterior to labyrinth + central spiculated calcification. Thin calcified rim along posterior margin. MRI: T1↑ foci due to haemorrhage. Heterogeneous enhancement.

12.33 PETROUS APEX LESIONS

Normal variants

These are all asymptomatic and incidental.

1. **Asymmetrical marrow**—degree of petrous apex pneumatization is variable and can be asymmetrical; nonpneumatized marrow space may simulate a mass. No bony expansion. MRI: T1↑ due to normal fatty marrow, with signal loss on fatsat sequences (cf. cholesterol granuloma).
2. **Trapped fluid**—sterile residual fluid in pneumatized petrous apex due to previous otomastoiditis. T2↑, variable T1 signal depending on protein content. No bony expansion or erosion. No concurrent middle ear or mastoid inflammation.
3. **Petrous apex cephalocoele**—herniation of posterolateral wall of Meckel's cave into petrous apex. Fluid attenuation and signal on CT/MRI.

12

Well-defined and expansile + bone remodelling

1. **Cholesterol granuloma**—most common petrous apex lesion. T1/T2↑ on MRI (see Section 12.32).
2. **Epidermoid cyst**—also known as congenital cholesteatoma. T1↓ (cf. cholesterol granuloma), T2↑ + restricted diffusion. No enhancement.
3. **Petrous apex mucocoele**—T2↑, variable T1 signal depending on protein content (though not as T1↑ as cholesterol granuloma). No restricted diffusion (cf. epidermoid cyst) or enhancement.

4. **Trigeminal nerve schwannoma**—CT: smooth expansile remodelling of foramen ovale. MRI: enhancing tubular lesion in continuity with the trigeminal nerve in Meckel's cave.
5. **Petrous ICA aneurysm**—see Section 12.35.

Destructive

1. **Metastasis**—e.g. from breast, lung, prostate, RCC. The petrous apex is the most common site of metastasis in the temporal bone.
2. **Petrous apicitis**—suppurative infection of pneumatized petrous apex due to extension of mastoiditis. Age: children and adolescents. Clinical: otorrhea, deep facial/ear pain, fever ± Gradenigo syndrome (retroorbital pain + lateral rectus palsy + otitis media) ± cranial neuropathy (CN V–VIII). CT/MRI: fluid in petrous apex + bony erosion ± enhancing soft-tissue phlegmon or abscess. Complications: dural involvement, cavernous sinus thrombosis, fistula with bony labyrinth.
3. **Chondrosarcoma**—see Section 12.35.
4. **Plasmacytoma***—lytic lesion with nonsclerotic margin. MRI: T1↓ and T2↑ or intermediate; heterogeneous enhancement.
5. **Langerhans cell histiocytosis***—see Section 12.34.

Other

1. **Meningioma**—see Section 12.35.
2. **Paget's disease***—see Section 12.34.
3. **Fibrous dysplasia**—see Section 12.22.

12.34 DIFFUSE OR MULTIFOCAL SKULL BASE LESIONS

1. **Metastasis**—most commonly from breast, lung, prostate. Can be solitary, multifocal or diffuse. Most common where bone marrow is abundant, i.e. clivus, nonpneumatized petrous apex and greater wing of sphenoid. CT: lytic, sclerotic or mixed. MRI: T1↓ lesion replacing high signal marrow; enhances post contrast.
2. **Paget's disease***—calvarium > skull base > temporal bone. Diffuse bone thickening with lysis (early), sclerosis (late) or mixed density (may have a 'cotton wool' appearance). May rarely undergo malignant transformation to osteosarcoma.
3. **Fibrous dysplasia**—see Section 12.22.
4. **Myeloma**—CT: punched-out lytic lesions of calvarium, facial bones and skull base with no marginal sclerosis. MRI: T1↓ and T2↑ or intermediate, + enhancement and restricted diffusion. Bone scan: cold lesion.
5. **Osteomyelitis**—acute or chronic, may relate to necrotizing otitis externa or previous radiotherapy. CT: bone destruction ± sequestra,

can be lytic or sclerotic (if chronic). MRI: T1↓ and T2↑ in marrow + enhancement ± adjacent dural enhancement.

6. **Langerhans cell histiocytosis***—usually in children or young adults. CT: punched-out lytic lesions with bevelled margins ± surrounding sclerosis ± button sequestrum. Heterogeneous enhancement with soft-tissue mass and dural involvement ± thickening of pituitary infundibulum.
7. **Intracranial inflammatory pseudotumour**—see Section 12.30. Extends from orbit to central and anterior skull base ± cavernous sinus, Meckel's cave, falx, tentorium, pterygopalatine fossa, nose and nasopharynx.
8. **Lymphoma***—can cause diffuse or multifocal skull base involvement ± cervicofacial or systemic disease. Most commonly originates from nasal cavity or paranasal sinuses. Permeative bone destruction, sclerosis or both, with a homogeneous soft-tissue mass.

12.35 UNIFOCAL SKULL BASE LESION

See Section 12.36 for clivus lesions.

1. <u>Any multifocal skull base lesion</u>—see Section 12.34. Any of these can be unifocal.
2. <u>Meningioma</u>—avidly enhancing dural based mass + dural tail + bony hyperostosis and sclerosis ± invasion. May extend below skull base through neural and vascular foramina.
3. <u>Chondrosarcoma</u>—arises from skull base synchondroses (petroclival, sphenopetrosal, petrooccipital or sphenooccipital). Lytic mass + chondroid calcification on CT, T2↑ on MRI + variable enhancement. Tumours are often indolent/low grade.
4. <u>ICA aneurysm</u>—if large and involves cavernous portion, causes bony remodelling of adjacent sella, clivus and petrous apex. Continuity with ICA confirmed on CTA/MRA. Variable T1/T2 signal due to turbulent flow voids ± mural thrombus.
5. **Ossifying fibroma**—see Section 12.22.
6. **Haemangiopericytoma**—rare locally aggressive tumour of meninges. Avidly enhancing mass invading and eroding the skull ± dural tail ± internal flow voids. Can mimic meningioma but tends not to calcify or cause bony hyperostosis. Peak age 30–40 years, can also occur in children (cf. meningioma peak age >50 years).
7. **Giant cell tumour**—extremely rare. Age: third to fourth decade. Sphenoid bone most common. CT: expansile lytic lesion with cortical thinning + soft-tissue component ± 'soap bubble' appearance. MRI: T2↓ (haemosiderin), heterogeneous enhancement.

12.36 CLIVUS LESIONS

1. **Skull base lesions not specific to the clivus**—e.g. fibrous dysplasia, Paget's disease, metastasis, lymphoma, myeloma, meningioma. See Sections 12.34 and 12.35.
2. **Nasopharyngeal carcinoma**—see Section 12.2. May invade and destroy clivus ± intracranial extension.
3. **Pituitary macroadenoma**—if large, can invade the clivus and sphenoid sinus. The mass is centred on an enlarged sella.
4. **Chordoma**—peak age 30–50 years. Arises in the midline near sphenooccipital synchondrosis. CT/MRI: expansile lytic clival mass + soft-tissue component + bony sequestra floating within the mass ± intralesional haemorrhage. Classically T2↑↑ with heterogeneous or 'honeycomb' enhancement.
5. **Chondrosarcoma**—see Section 12.35. Tends to be paramidline (cf. chordoma).
6. **Ecchordosis physaliphora**—asymptomatic incidental finding on CT/MR. Benign notochord remnant, either within the clivus (well-defined and lytic on CT) or attached to it by an osseous stalk (characteristic appearance on CT). T2↑↑ on MRI with no or minimal enhancement (cf. chordoma). Histologically very similar to chordoma.

12.37 JUGULAR FORAMEN LESIONS

1. **Glomus jugulare**—see Section 12.32.
2. **Schwannoma**—can arise from CN IX, X or XI. Mean age 45 years. Large tubular or dumbbell-shaped tumour with jugular foramen enlargement and bony remodelling. Uniformly enhancing unless there is cystic change. May extend to adjacent carotid space.
3. **Necrotizing otitis externa**—infection can spread to the jugular foramen either via the bones or soft tissues, ± IJV thrombosis.
4. **Skull base lesions not specific to the jugular foramen**—e.g. meningioma, metastasis, myeloma, chondrosarcoma. See Sections 12.34 and 12.35.

Further reading

1. Koch, B.L., Hamilton, B.E., Hudgins, P.A., Harnsberger, H.R., 2016. Diagnostic Imaging: Head and Neck, third ed. Elsevier.
2. Harnsberger, H.R., Koch, B.L., Phillips, C.D., et al., 2009. Expert DDX: Head and Neck, first ed. Amirsys.
3. Shin, J.H., Lee, H.K., Kim, S.Y., et al., 2001. Imaging of parapharyngeal space lesions: focus on the prestyloid compartment. AJR 177 (6), 1465–1470.
4. Amin, M.B., Greene, F.L., Edge, S.B., et al. (Eds.), 2017. AJCC Cancer Staging Manual, eighth ed. Springer.
5. Cantrell, S.C., Peck, B.W., Li, G., et al., 2013. Differences in imaging characteristics of HPV-positive and HPV-negative oropharyngeal cancers: a

blinded matched-pair analysis. AJNR Am. J. Neuroradiol. 34 (10), 2005–2009.
6. Howlett, D.C., Kesse, K.W., Hughes, D.V., Sallomi, D.F., 2002. The role of imaging in the evaluation of parotid disease. Clin. Radiol. 57 (8), 692–701.
7. Gadodia, A., Bhalla, A.S., Sharma, R., et al., 2011. Bilateral parotid swelling: a radiological review. Dentomaxillofac Radiol. 40 (7), 403–414.
8. Kuwada, C., Mannion, K., Aulino, J.M., Kanekar, S.G., 2012. Imaging of the carotid space. Otolaryngol. Clin. North Am. 45 (6), 1273–1292.
9. Mills, M.K., Shah, L.M., 2015. Imaging of the perivertebral space. Radiol. Clin. North Am. 53 (1), 163–180.
10. Parker, G.D., Harnsberger, H.R., 1991. Radiologic evaluation of the normal and diseased posterior cervical space. AJR 157 (1), 161–165.
11. Hang, J.K., Branstetter, B.F., Eastwood, J.D., Glastonbury, C.M., 2011. Multiplanar CT and MRI of collections in the retropharyngeal space: is it an abscess? AJR 196 (4), W426–W432.
12. Davis, W.L., Harnsberger, H.R., Smoker, W.R., Watanabe, A.S., 1990. Retropharyngeal space: evaluation of normal anatomy and diseases with CT and MR imaging. Radiology 174 (1), 59–64.
13. Law, C.P., Chandra, R.V., Hoang, J.K., Phal, P.M., 2011. Imaging the oral cavity: key concepts for the radiologist. Br. J. Radiol. 84 (1006), 944–957.
14. La'porte, S.J., Juttla, J.K., Lingam, R.K., 2011. Imaging the floor of the mouth and the sublingual space. Radiographics 31 (5), 1215–1230.
15. Agarwal, A.K., Kanekar, S.G., 2012. Submandibular and sublingual spaces: diagnostic imaging and evaluation. Otolaryngol. Clin. North Am. 45 (6), 1311–1323.
16. Fang, W.S., Wiggins, R.H., Illner, A., 2011. Primary lesions of the root of the tongue. Radiographics 31 (7), 1907–1922.
17. Castellote, A., Vázquez, E., Vera, J., 1999. Cervicothoracic lesions in infants and children. Radiographics 19 (3), 583–600.
18. Pameijer, F., Beek, E., Joosten, F., Smithuis, R., Infrahyoid neck; Normal anatomy and pathology [online]. Radiology department of the University Medical Centre of Utrecht, the Rijnstate Hospital in Arnhem and the Rijnland Hospital in Leiderdorp, the Netherlands. Radiology Assistant 2009.
19. Yuen, H.Y., Wong, K.T., Ahuja, A.T., 2016. Sonography of diffuse thyroid disease. AJUM 19 (1), 13–29.
20. Perros, P., Boelaert, K., Colley, S., et al., 2014. British Thyroid Association guidelines for the management of thyroid cancer. Clin. Endocrinol. (Oxf) 81 (s1), 1–122.
21. Van den Brekel, M.W., Castelijns, J.A., Stel, H.V., et al., 1993. Modern imaging techniques and ultrasound-guided aspiration cytology for the assessment of neck node metastases: a prospective comparative study. Eur. Arch. Otorhinolaryngol. 250 (1), 11–17.
22. Ying, M., Ahuja, A., 2003. Sonography of neck lymph nodes. Part I: normal lymph nodes. Clin. Radiol. 58 (5), 351–358.
23. Ahuja, A., Ying, M., 2003. Sonography of neck lymph nodes. Part II: abnormal lymph nodes. Clin. Radiol. 58 (5), 359–366.
24. Van den Brekel, M.W., Castelijns, J.A., Stel, H.V., et al., 1991. Occult metastatic neck disease: detection with US and US-guided fine-needle aspiration cytology. Radiology 180 (2), 457–461.
25. Fernandes, T., Lobo, J.C., Castro, R., et al., 2013. Anatomy and pathology of the masticator space. Insights Imaging 4 (5), 605–616.

26. Dunfee, B.L., Sakai, O., Pistey, R., Gohel, A., 2006. Radiologic and pathologic characteristics of benign and malignant lesions of the mandible. Radiographics 26 (6), 1751–1768.
27. Scholl, R.J., Kellett, H.M., Neumann, D.P., Lurie, A.G., 1999. Cysts and cystic lesions of the mandible: clinical and radiologic-histopathologic review. Radiographics 19 (5), 1107–1124.
28. Cure, J.K., Vattoth, S., Shah, R., 2012. Radiopaque jaw lesions: an approach to the differential diagnosis. Radiographics 32 (7), 1909–1925.
29. Asaumi, J., Konouchi, H., Hisatomi, M., et al., 2003. MR features of aneurysmal bone cyst of the mandible and characteristics distinguishing it from other lesions. Eur. J. Radiol. 45 (2), 108–112.
30. Momeni, A.K., Roberts, C.C., Chew, F.S., 2007. Imaging of chronic and exotic sinonasal disease: review. AJR 189 (6), S35–S45.
31. Eggesbo, H.B., 2012. Imaging of sinonasal tumours. Cancer Imaging 12, 136–152.
32. Kirsten, A.M., Watz, H., Kirsten, D., 2013. Sarcoidosis with involvement of the paranasal sinuses – a retrospective analysis of 12 biopsy-proven cases. BMC Pulm. Med. 13, 59.
33. Tailor, T.D., Gupta, D., Dalley, R.W., et al., 2013. Orbital neoplasms in adults: clinical, radiologic, and pathologic review. Radiographics 33 (6), 1739–1758.
34. Smoker, W.R., Gentry, L.R., Yee, N.K., et al., 2008. Vascular lesions of the orbit: more than meets the eye. Radiographics 28 (1), 185–204.
35. Radhakrishnan, R., Cornelius, R., Cunnane, M.B., et al., 2016. MR imaging findings of endophthalmitis. Neuroradiol J 29 (2), 122–129.
36. Singh, S.K., Das, D., Bhattacharjee, H., et al., 2011. A rare case of adult onset retinoblastoma. Oman J Ophthalmol 4 (1), 25–27.
37. Izumi, M., Eguchi, K., Uetani, M., et al., 1998. MR features of the lacrimal gland in Sjogren's syndrome. AJR 170 (6), 1661–1666.
38. Karcioglu, Z.A., Hadjistilianou, D., Rozans, M., DeFrancesco, S., 2004. Orbital rhabdomyosarcoma. Cancer Control 11 (5), 328–333.
39. Juliano, A.F., Ginat, D.T., Moonis, G., 2013. Imaging review of the temporal bone: part I. Anatomy and inflammatory and neoplastic processes. Radiology 269 (1), 17–33.
40. Juliano, A.F., Ginat, D.T., Moonis, G., 2015. Imaging review of the temporal bone: part II. Traumatic, postoperative, and noninflammatory nonneoplastic conditions. Radiology 276 (3), 655–672.
41. Razek, A.A., Huang, B.Y., 2012. Lesions of the petrous apex: classification and findings at CT and MR imaging. Radiographics 32 (1), 151–173.
42. Policeni, B.A., Smoker, W.R., 2015. Imaging of the skull base. Radiol. Clin. North Am. 53 (1), 1–14.
43. Smith, A.B., Horkanyne-Szakaly, I., Schroeder, J.W., Rushing, E.J., 2014. From the radiologic pathology archives: mass lesions of the dura: beyond meningioma – radiologic-pathologic correlation. Radiographics 34 (2), 295–312.
44. Lee, J.A., Bank, W.O., Gonzalez-Melendez, M., et al., 1998. Giant cell tumor of the skull. Radiographics 18 (5), 1295–1302.

Skull and brain

Luke Dixon, Joseph Lansley,
Chandrashekar Hoskote, Janak Saada

13.1 SOLITARY ACUTE INTRACRANIAL HAEMORRHAGE

1. **Intracerebral**.
   (a) **Hypertension**—basal ganglia, pons, cerebellum.
   (b) **Cerebral amyloid angiopathy**—lobar location, peripheral microhaemorrhages (often multifocal).
   (c) **Haemorrhagic lesions**—e.g. metastases, primary tumours, infarcts.
   (d) **Traumatic**—more commonly multifocal (see Section 13.3).
2. **Subarachnoid**—see Section 13.2. Extends into sulci ± basal cisterns.
3. **Subdural**—most common in elderly post trauma (which may be minor); also associated with intracranial hypotension or dural arteriovenous fistula (AVF). Crescentic shape, does not cross falx.
4. **Extradural**—traumatic; usually arterial bleed, rarely venous. Lentiform shape, does not cross cranial sutures.
5. **Intraventricular**—usually due to extension from subarachnoid or intracerebral bleed; isolated intraventricular haemorrhage is rare and due to subependymal vein rupture.

13.2 SUBARACHNOID HAEMORRHAGE (SAH)

Unless there is a clear history of trauma (with typical SAH distribution) most cases will require angiography to look for the underlying cause. If the blood load is centred on the posterior fossa or foramen magnum (FM), consider a posterior inferior cerebellar artery aneurysm or spinal AVM, which may require imaging of the spine. Beware of 'pseudosubarachnoid' sign in hypoxic brain injury (look for loss of grey–white matter [WM] differentiation). Polycythaemia may also cause hyperdensity mimicking SAH on plain CT.

1. Trauma—often localized to coup and contrecoup injuries, i.e. superficial.
2. Intracranial aneurysm—haemorrhage typically centred on the aneurysm (e.g. sylvian fissure = MCA aneurysm; interhemispheric fissure = anterior communicating artery aneurysm). Blood usually within basal cisterns, whereas nonaneurysmal causes are more often sulcal in location. An aneurysm may be seen as a filling defect within the acute haemorrhage.
3. Arteriovenous shunt—AVM (indirect shunt with nidus of vessels) or AVF (direct shunt between artery and vein). Prominent draining veins, may be partially calcified.
4. Vasculopathy—cerebral amyloid angiopathy, reversible cerebral vasoconstriction syndrome (RCVS; reversible arterial stenosis often associated with certain drugs) and vasculitis (multifocal arterial stenoses). Haemorrhage may be multifocal.
5. Venous thrombosis—look for venous hyperdensity/expansion.
6. Perimesencephalic—typically limited to the basal cisterns around the midbrain ± pons, especially interpeduncular cistern. Spontaneous, has a benign course. No cause is found on angiography; thought to be due to a venous bleed.
7. **Iatrogenic**—following lumbar puncture or surgery.

13.3 MULTIFOCAL ACUTE INTRACEREBRAL HAEMORRHAGE

1. Trauma—contusions (common, typically seen in the anteroinferior frontal lobes and temporal poles at sites of impact with the skull); haemorrhagic shear injury (i.e. diffuse axonal injury, located at grey-WM junction [GWMJ], corpus callosum and brainstem).
2. Septic embolism.
3. Haemorrhagic neoplastic lesions—metastasis, leukemia.
4. Coagulopathy—horizontal blood-blood levels are suggestive.
5. Venous sinus thrombosis.
6. Vasculopathy—drugs, cerebral amyloid angiopathy, vasculitis, posterior reversible encephalopathy syndrome (PRES) and RCVS.
7. **Multiple cavernomas**—rare, syndromic, young males.

13.4 MICROHAEMORRHAGES ON MRI

Definition: <5 mm foci of signal loss on blood sensitive MRI sequences (susceptibility-weighted imaging [SWI]/T2*) not due to calcifications or flow voids.

1. Acute trauma—haemorrhagic shear injury (see Section 13.3). MRI is more sensitive than CT.
2. Hypertensive vasculopathy—central pattern involving the basal ganglia, thalami, brainstem and cerebellum.

3. Cerebral amyloid angiopathy—typically peripheral cortical/subcortical, usually spares the basal ganglia. Associated with lobar and subarachnoid haemorrhages.
4. Cavernomas—including familial syndromes.
5. **Venous thrombosis/congestion.**
6. **Radiotherapy**—radiation-induced capillary telangiectasia within the radiation field.
7. **Cerebral vasculitis**—usually at GWMJ.
8. **Septic emboli**—e.g. from infective endocarditis.
9. **Haemorrhagic metastases**—especially melanoma, RCC and intravascular lymphoma.
10. **Sickle cell anaemia and beta thalassaemia***—associated with cerebral fat embolism from bone marrow infarcts. Seen in cerebral and cerebellar WM and corpus callosum.
11. **CADASIL**—symmetrical multifocal WM hyperintensity in frontal and anterior temporal lobes and external capsule, with noncharacteristic distribution of microhaemorrhages.
12. **PRES**—parietooccipital and superior frontal gyral predominance of microhaemorrhages.
13. **Fat/air embolism**—microbleeds may be associated with foci of restricted diffusion.
14. **Critical illness-associated cerebral microbleeds**—may be related to hypoxaemia, high altitude or disseminated intravascular coagulation.
15. **Drugs**—cocaine abuse.

Further reading

Noorbakhsh-Sabet, N., Pulakanti, V.C., Zand, R., 2017. Uncommon causes of cerebral microbleeds. J. Stroke Cerebrovasc. Dis. 26 (10), 2043–2049.

Chiang, F., Tedesqui, G., Mauricio Varon, D., et al., 2016. Imaging spectrum of brain microhemorrhages on SWI. Neurographics 6 (3), 174–186.

13.5 SUPERFICIAL SIDEROSIS

Best seen on SWI/T2* as curvilinear low signal coating the leptomeninges. Two different patterns:

Classical

Involves the infratentorial regions and spinal cord. Clinical triad of sensorineural hearing loss, ataxia and pyramidal weakness, related to toxic effects of iron on neurons. Due to chronic recurrent low-volume SAH, which is clinically silent. Causes include:

1. Dural defect—either intracranial or spinal. Usually due to previous trauma or surgery. May see extraarachnoid CSF collection or

pseudomeningocoele on MRI. Dural defect may be visible on CT myelography.
2. **Dural ectasia**—e.g. in Marfan.
3. **CNS tumours.**
4. **Vascular malformations.**

Cortical

Involves the supratentorial compartment (especially cerebral convexities) but may also extend to the infratentorial region. Causes include:

1. **Previous SAH**—of any cause (see Section 13.2), including subarachnoid extension of intracerebral haemorrhage and bleeding neoplasms.
2. **Cerebral amyloid angiopathy**—in older patients (>60 years). Intracerebral microhaemorrhages may also be seen.
3. **RCVS**—in younger adults (<60 years), associated with pregnancy and certain drugs.
4. **Cerebral vasculitis.**
5. **Hyperperfusion syndrome**—after revascularization, e.g. carotid stenting or endarterectomy.
6. **Infective endocarditis.**

Mimics of superficial siderosis

1. **Acute SAH**—hyperattenuating on CT, increased signal in subarachnoid space on FLAIR/T1.
2. **Sequelae of cerebral infarction**—petechial haemorrhages and laminar cortical necrosis both cause susceptibility effects but are centred on the cortex rather than the subarachnoid space.
3. **Cortical vein thrombosis**—susceptibility effect follows the cortical veins.
4. **Cortical calcification**—e.g. in Sturge-Weber syndrome. Very dense on CT.

Further reading

Charidimou, A., Linn, J., Vernooij, M.W., et al., 2015. Cortical superficial siderosis: detection and clinical significance in cerebral amyloid angiopathy and related conditions. Brain 138 (8), 2126–2139.

Wilson, D., Chatterjee, F., Farmer, S.F., et al., 2017. Infratentorial superficial siderosis: classification, diagnostic criteria, and rational investigation pathway. Ann. Neurol. 81 (3), 333–343.

13.6 HYDROCEPHALUS

Large ventricles do not always equate to hydrocephalus: cerebral atrophy can lead to relative enlargement of ventricles. Hydrocephalus is more likely if:

- Commensurate enlargement of temporal horns.
- Ventricles disproportionately enlarged compared to sulci.
- Blunted third ventricular recesses.
- Evidence of periventricular CSF transudation.

Hydrocephalus can be caused by increased CSF production, reduced CSF absorption through arachnoid granulations (communicating) or obstruction to CSF flow (obstructive). A 'compensated' hydrocephalus cannot be readily determined on imaging from a single time point but is likely if the appearances are static and asymptomatic.

CSF overproduction

1. **Choroid plexus tumours**—i.e. papilloma, carcinoma; see Section 13.33.

Communicating

1. **Posthaemorrhagic**—especially SAH.
2. **Bacterial meningitis**—small cortical infarcts may be present as a complicating feature.
3. **Leptomeningeal carcinomatosis**—look for leptomeningeal enhancement.
4. **Idiopathic normal pressure hydrocephalus**—dilated ventricles with a narrowed callosal angle, crowding of gyri at the vertex and widened sylvian fissures. Classic clinical triad of dementia, urinary incontinence and gait apraxia.
5. **Increased venous pressure**—venous obstruction, vein of Galen malformation.
6. **Vestibular schwannoma**—rare, thought to be due to increased CSF protein impairing CSF absorption.

Obstructive

Pattern of ventricular enlargement depends on level of obstruction:

Any level

1. **Haemorrhage**.
2. **Intraventricular tumours**—see Section 13.33.
3. **Ventriculitis**—complication of meningitis, surgery or haemorrhage. Look for subtle ependymal enhancement and dependent sediment in lateral ventricles (restricts on DWI).
4. **Neurocysticercosis**—can cause obstruction either due to location of cyst or by causing ventriculitis. Cysts are best seen on steady-state gradient echo sequences such as CISS/FIESTA-C.

Foramen of Monro

Dilated lateral ventricle(s), normal third and fourth ventricles.

1. Any cause of significant midline shift—compresses the ipsilateral lateral ventricle and obstructs the contralateral lateral ventricle.
2. Colloid cyst—characteristically located in the anterior roof of the third ventricle. Well-defined, nonenhancing, hyperdense on CT due to protein content.
3. Subependymal giant cell astrocytoma—in young patients with tuberous sclerosis. Typically within a lateral ventricle near foramen of Monro, avidly enhancing, often calcified.

Cerebral aqueduct

Dilated lateral and third ventricles, normal fourth ventricle.

1. Aqueduct stenosis—congenital, presents in childhood, 'beak–like' appearance of aqueduct, no obstructing mass lesion.
2. Tectal plate glioma—typically in children or adolescents. Diffuse enlargement and T2 hyperintensity of tectal plate, usually with no enhancement due to low grade nature of tumour.
3. Pineal region tumour—see Section 13.32.

Fourth ventricle

1. Any posterior fossa mass—e.g. in fourth ventricle (ependymoma, medulloblastoma), within cerebellum or brainstem or extraaxial tumours obstructing the foramina of Luschka and Magendie.
2. Chiari 1 malformation.

13.7 INTRACRANIAL CALCIFICATION

Physiological

Choroid plexus, basal ganglia, pineal, dural (e.g. falx).

Deep grey matter

1. Primary—also known as Fahr disease. Familial, usually autosomal dominant, typically presents in middle age. Symmetrical involvement of basal ganglia > thalami > cerebellar dentate nuclei > WM. Other causes (following) must be excluded first.
2. Endocrine—hyper- and hypoparathyroidism, pseudo- and pseudopseudohypoparathyroidism. Appearance identical to Fahr disease.
3. **Inherited**—Down's, mitochondrial disorders; rarely in Cockayne and Aicardi-Goutieres syndromes. Seen in children.
4. **SLE**—thought to be related to microangiopathy. Background of cerebral volume loss and WM lesions (see Section 13.20).
5. **Toxins**—lead, carbon monoxide.
6. **Posttherapeutic**—mineralizing microangiopathy following chemoradiotherapy in childhood.

Ependymal/periventricular

1. Tuberous sclerosis*—calcified subependymal nodules (hamartomas); associated with cortical tubers (hallmark of the disease, often calcify) and transmantle WM dysplasia. If large or growing + intense enhancement, suggests subependymal giant cell astrocytoma.
2. **Perinatal TORCH infections**—toxoplasma, rubella, CMV (most common) and herpes simplex virus.

Gyriform

1. **Sturge-Weber syndrome***—usually unilateral with associated cerebral atrophy. Look for retinal enhancement and ipsilateral choroid plexus enlargement.
2. **Post infarction**—due to cortical laminar necrosis.
3. **CEC syndrome**—rare disorder characterized by occipital calcifications in a patient with seizures and coeliac disease.

Focal lesions with calcification

1. Tumours.
   (a) **Meningioma**—may be partly or completely calcified.
   (b) **Oligodendroglioma**—most contain calcification. Other low-grade gliomas can also calcify.
   (c) Craniopharyngioma—suprasellar location. Calcification is common (in contrast to pituitary adenomas).
   (d) **Dermoid**—also contains fat.
   (e) **Ependymoma**—located in fourth ventricle.
   (f) **Central neurocytoma**—arises from septum pellucidum.
   (g) **Pineal region tumours**—either engulf or 'explode' the normal pineal calcification.
   (h) **Metastasis**—e.g. from breast, mucinous GI tumours, lung, osteosarcoma.
2. **Infections**.
   (a) **Neurocysticercosis**—multiple small calcifications in brain parenchyma and CSF spaces; reflects end-stage quiescent disease.
   (b) **Tuberculosis***—foci of calcification are usually larger and fewer in number versus cysticercosis.
   (c) **Perinatal TORCH infections**.
3. Vascular.
   (a) **Atherosclerosis**.
   (b) **AVM**.
   (c) **Aneurysm**—rim calcification.
   (d) **Cavernoma**.

13

Further reading

Kıroğlu, Y., Callı, C., Karabulut, N., Oncel, C., 2010. Intracranial calcifications on CT. Diagn. Interv. Radiol. 16, 263–269.

13.8 SOLITARY INTRACEREBRAL MASS

Infiltrative, ill–defined

1. Primary tumour—diffuse glioma, or gliomatosis cerebri if ≥3 lobes involved. Ill-defined T2 hyperintensity with no or minimal mass effect, enhancement or restricted diffusion. Extensive despite minimal symptoms. Look for scalloping of overlying calvarium (suggests longstanding slow-growing mass).
2. Cerebritis/encephalitis—acute clinical presentation (cf. diffuse glioma).
3. Infarction—in both arterial and venous infarction vascular occlusion suggested by hyperdense thrombus (CT), absent flow voids and focal increased intravascular susceptibility on SWI (MRI). Pattern of infarction is different:
   (a) Arterial—follows vascular territory, typically shows restricted diffusion.
   (b) Venous—near to occluded vein, greater oedema and risk of parenchymal haemorrhage (typically has a fragmented appearance). DWI signal variable.
4. **Demyelination**—Neuromyelitis optica (NMO) spectrum disorders, Behçet's.
5. **Contusion**—in the context of trauma.

Discrete, well-defined

1. Haematoma—hypertensive haemorrhage classically ganglionic; cf. amyloid angiopathy where sulcal siderosis and peripheral microhaemorrhages are commonly seen.
2. Metastasis—e.g. from lung, breast, colorectal, melanoma, renal. Appearance varies depending on primary; often considerable oedema in surrounding WM (usually more than primary tumours). Typically located at GWMJ, may be solitary (20%) or multiple (80%).
3. Primary tumour—high-grade gliomas tend to have discrete enhancement with central necrosis (glioblastoma). Typically centred on WM (cf. metastasis). May infiltrate or cross corpus callosum—this can also be seen in lymphoma, but lymphoma typically shows homogeneous enhancement with no central necrosis (unless immunocompromised).
4. Abscess—central restricted diffusion and usually considerable associated oedema. Thin enhancing rim, thicker superficially and thinner at ventricular surface, may 'point' towards ventricle (more likely to rupture into the ventricles, causing ventriculitis and hydrocephalus). 'Dual rim' sign on SWI (cf. primary or metastatic tumour).
5. Cavernoma—characterized on MRI by complete haemosiderin rim and central mixed 'popcorn' components.

6. Tumefactive demyelination—incomplete rim enhancement is characteristic. More likely in younger age group (20–40s) versus metastases.

Further reading

Essig, M., Anzalone, N., Combs, S.E., et al., 2012. MR imaging of neoplastic central nervous system lesions: review and recommendations for current practice. AJNR Am. J. Neuroradiol. 33, 803–817.
Omuro, A.M., Leite, C.C., Mokhtari, K., Delattre, J.Y., 2006. Pitfalls in the diagnosis of brain tumours. Lancet Neurol. 5 (11), 937–948.

13.9 SOLITARY HYPERDENSE INTRACRANIAL LESION ON UNENHANCED CT

Hypercellular mass

1. Lymphoma*—avid homogeneous enhancement and periventricular location are characteristic features.
2. Metastasis—e.g. from small-cell lung cancer.
3. Medulloblastoma—typically in children, located in the cerebellum.
4. Germinoma—young patients, located in the pineal or suprasellar region.

Lesion containing blood/protein

1. Acute haematoma—higher attenuation than adjacent brain parenchyma for up to 7–10 days.
2. Haemorrhagic tumours—especially metastases (e.g. from melanoma); less commonly glioblastoma, or pituitary adenoma with apoplexy.
3. Colloid cyst—homogeneously hyperdense due to protein content, nonenhancing, located in anterior roof of third ventricle.
4. Cavernoma—can mimic intracerebral haematoma on CT. On MRI, characteristically has complete haemosiderin rim with central mixed signal.
5. AVM.

Lesion containing calcification

See Section 13.7.

Further reading

Ishikura, R., Ando, K., Tominaga, S., et al., 1999. CT diagnosis of hyperdense intracranial neoplasms: review of the literature. Nihon Igaku Hoshasen Gakkai Zasshi 59 (4), 105–112.

13.10 INTRINSIC CORTICAL MASS

1. Acute cortical infarction—results in cortical swelling/oedema with localized mass effect. Intense restricted diffusion on DWI.

2. Acute cerebritis/encephalitis—can show restricted diffusion, but less intense and more patchy versus acute infarction.
3. Metastasis—centred on GWMJ (see Section 13.8).
4. Neuronal-glial and glial tumours—apart from (a), these typically present in children or young adults with intractable seizures.
   (a) Oligodendroglioma—middle-aged patients. Cortical/subcortical mass, well- or ill-defined, often calcified. Heterogeneous T2 signal and enhancement. No restricted diffusion.
   (b) Dysembryoplastic neuroepithelial tumour (DNET)—benign, slow-growing, may scallop overlying skull. Well-defined T2 bright cortical mass ('bubbly'), partial FLAIR suppression and characteristic hyperintense rim. No oedema. Variable calcification/microhaemorrhage. No restricted diffusion/enhancement. Associated with focal cortical dysplasia.
   (c) Ganglioglioma—classically cystic mass with an enhancing mural nodule, but can be purely solid. No surrounding oedema. Calcification is common.
   (d) **Pleomorphic xanthoastrocytoma (PXA)**—similar appearance to ganglioglioma, but calcification is rare. Often associated with reactive dural thickening mimicking a dural tail.
5. Focal cortical dysplasia (FCD)—focal cortical thickening with blurring of the GWMJ + T2 hyperintensity of the involved cortex and subcortical WM. Can mimic (or be associated with) a tumour. Potential epileptogenic lesion.
6. Cortical tubers—FLAIR and T2 bright cortical/juxtacortical lesions, found in tuberous sclerosis, <10% enhance.
7. **Cavernoma**—look for blood degradation products.
8. **Haematoma**—usually post trauma.

13.11 POSTERIOR FOSSA MASS (ADULT)

1. Metastasis—most common infratentorial lesion (see Section 13.8).
2. Haemangioblastoma—typically cerebellar hemisphere cystic tumour, avidly enhancing solid mural nodule abutting the pia mater with a nonenhancing cyst wall. Associated with vHL.
3. Astrocytoma.
   (a) Pilocytic—children and young adults, cyst with mural nodule and enhancing cyst wall (cf. haemangioblastoma).
   (b) **Glioblastoma**—older adults, heterogeneous ill-defined mass with irregular intrinsic enhancement.
4. Ependymoma—children and young adults, floor of fourth ventricle with 'plastic-like' extension through ventricular

foramina. Heterogeneous, calcified and cystic. Associated with NF2.

5. **Subependymoma**—older adults, usually small, fourth > lateral ventricle. No enhancement.
6. **Epidermoid**—on CT, T1 and T2 indistinguishable from CSF but hyperintense on DWI and usually incomplete suppression of signal on FLAIR.
7. **Dermoid**—well-defined midline mass with fat and calcification. No enhancement.
8. **Abscess**—intrinsic restricted diffusion (see Section 13.8).
9. **Haematoma/cavernoma**—susceptibility effects from blood can cause variable DWI signal. Cavernoma often associated with nearby developmental venous anomaly.
10. **Diffuse midline glioma**—children and young adults, most commonly pontine, but can occur anywhere in the midline of the CNS.
11. **Hamartoma**—also known as Lhermitte-Duclos disease; characteristic thickened and striated appearance of usually one cerebellar hemisphere with T2 hyperintensity. No enhancement. Associated with Cowden syndrome.
12. **Rosette-forming glioneuronal tumour**—young adults, typically in the midline at the posterior aspect of the fourth ventricle + local parenchymal invasion; mixed solid-cystic.
13. **Any cerebellopontine angle (CPA) mass**—see Section 13.34.

Further reading

Shih, R.Y., Smirniotopoulos, J.G., 2016. Posterior fossa tumors in adult patients. Neuroimaging Clin. N. Am. 26 (4), 493–510.

13.12 SOLITARY RING-ENHANCING LESION

Infection

1. **Pyogenic abscess**—thin regular enhancing capsule; see Section 13.8.
2. **Tuberculoma**—uniformly round with adjacent leptomeningeal enhancement and characteristic central low T2 signal. Look for associated basal leptomeningitis and hydrocephalus.
3. **Toxoplasmosis**—usually multiple; see Section 13.13.
4. **Neurocysticercosis**—usually multiple; see Section 13.13.

Neoplastic

1. **Metastasis**—central necrosis with thick, irregular, nodular rim enhancement, no intrinsic restricted diffusion; see Section 13.8.
2. **Glioblastoma**—centred on WM but often indistinguishable from a single metastasis; see Section 13.8.

3. **Ganglioglioma/cytoma**—children and young adults. Temporal lobe, calcified, slow growing ± bony remodelling, no perilesional oedema (cf. glioblastoma, metastases).

Inflammatory

1. **Demyelination**—incomplete rim enhancement, typical locations; see Section 13.13.
2. **Radiation necrosis**—months to years after radiotherapy. Heterogeneous (linear, nodular and cortical) pattern of contrast enhancement in radiation field. May mimic tumour recurrence but does not show elevated cerebral blood volume (CBV) on perfusion and may regress over follow-up.
3. **Sarcoidosis***—isolated granuloma very rare, often coexistent dural or cranial nerve disease.
4. **PML-IRIS**—see Section 13.20.

Vascular/trauma

1. **Subacute haematoma**—variable signal and diffusion dependent on age; signal drop out on SWI/T2*.
2. **Subacute infarct**—conforms to vascular territory, rim or gyriform pattern of enhancement.
3. **Thrombosed or inflammatory aneurysm**—arises from intracranial artery, appearance dependent on degree of thrombosis/flow and local inflammation.
4. **Contusion**—see Section 13.3.

13.13 MULTIPLE RING-ENHANCING LESIONS

Knowledge of the patient's immune status is essential. Conditions associated with immunocompromised state (HIV, immunosuppression etc.) are labelled with †.

Neoplastic

1. **Metastases**—at GWMJ, rarely involve corpus callosum (cf. glioma, lymphoma); see Section 13.8.
2. **Multifocal glioma**—often lesions are connected by abnormal T2 signal (nonenhancing tumour) and conform to path of WM tracts (e.g. along genu of corpus callosum); see Section 13.8.
3. **Lymphoma†***—typically solid enhancement but in the immunocompromised (or after steroid treatment) may show atypical ring enhancement. Important to differentiate from toxoplasmosis (see following); lymphoma tends to be fewer in number with a subependymal distribution.

Infection

1. **Abscesses†**—may be localized due to direct spread from adjacent structures, e.g. sinusitis/mastoiditis; if haematogenous in origin

then can be scattered across all vascular territories; see Section 13.8 and septic emboli, below.

2. **Septic emboli**†—multiple microabscesses and associated infarcts; check for arteritis (arterial irregularity and stenoses) and mycotic aneurysms. Risk factors: infective endocarditis, IV drug abuse, arteriovenous shunts and indwelling vascular lines.
3. **Tuberculoma**†—see Section 13.12.
4. **Toxoplasmosis**†—basal ganglia and GWMJ, concentric alternating low and high T2 signal, eccentric 'target sign' enhancement.
5. **Neurocysticercosis**—endemic in South America, Asia and Africa. Cysts in subarachnoid space or parenchyma; appearance depends on stage (see Part 2).

Inflammatory

1. **Demyelination**—acute demyelinating plaques may enhance, usually with an 'open ring' pattern incomplete to the gyral surface. Characteristic locations: periventricular, juxtacortical, infratentorial and spinal cord; see Section 13.20.
2. **Radiation necrosis**—see Section 13.12.
3. **PML-IRIS**†—see Section 13.20.

Vascular/trauma

Contusion/haematoma—orbitofrontal and anterior temporal regions; see Section 13.3.

Further reading

Garg, R.K., Sinha, M.K., 2012. Multiple ring-enhancing lesions of the brain. AJNR Am. J. Neuroradiol. 33 (8), 1534–1538.

13.14 INTRACRANIAL CYST WITH MURAL NODULE

Neoplastic

1. **Haemangioblastoma**—nonenhancing cyst wall, posterior fossa; see Section 13.11.
2. **Pilocytic astrocytoma**—enhancing cyst wall, posterior fossa; see Section 13.11.
3. **Cystic metastasis**—adenocarcinoma, SCC. Thick irregular wall ± haemorrhage.
4. **Pleomorphic xanthoastrocytoma**—young adults, temporal lobe; see Section 13.10.
5. **Craniopharyngioma**—multilocular cystic lesion, often in suprasellar region with variable calcification and high T1 signal; see Section 13.28.
6. **Ganglioglioma**—see Section 13.10.

7. **Rosette-forming glioneuronal tumour**—see Section 13.11.
8. **Pineocytoma**—see Section 13.32.

Infection

1. Neurocysticercosis—vesicular and colloidal vesicular stages, central dot from scolex; see Part 2.

13.15 ENHANCING LESIONS IN PERIVASCULAR SPACES

Normal vascular enhancement is regular and linear. Pathological enhancement is more prominent and can be ill-defined/irregular.

1. **Chronic lymphocytic inflammation with pontine perivascular enhancement responsive to steroids (CLIPPERS)**—characteristic punctate and linear enhancement in pons with minimal oedema/mass effect; normal intracranial arteries.
2. **Neurosarcoid**—associated with abnormal thickening and enhancement of dura, cranial nerves and pituitary stalk.
3. **Vasculitis**—evidence of arteritis with stenoses, beading and infarcts.
4. **Lymphoma***—elderly, fluctuating areas of T2 and diffusion abnormality, surrounding mass-like enhancement.
5. **Lymphomatoid granulomatosis**—in the immunocompromised. Multifocal periventricular linear T2 hyperintensities + enhancement.
6. **Behçet's***—young adults, orogenital ulcers. Brainstem and deep ganglionic structures, oedema and mass effect (cf. CLIPPERS).
7. **Langerhans cell histiocytosis***—children and young adults, commonly presents with diabetes insipidus; see Section 13.28.

Further reading

Tsitouridis, I., Papaioannou, S., Arvaniti, M., et al., 2009. Enhancement of Virchow-Robin spaces: an MRI evaluation. Neuroradiol. J. 21 (6), 773–779.

13.16 MENINGEAL ENHANCEMENT

Some degree of dural enhancement is normally seen at the falx, tentorium and cavernous sinus. Hints to pathological enhancement/meningeal disease include:

- Dural enhancement seen on contiguous coronal slices.
- Rim enhancement anteriorly capping the brainstem.
- Abnormal cranial nerve enhancement or thickening.
- Presence of coexistent FLAIR sulcal hyperintensity (see Section 13.36).

Pachymeningeal (dura–arachnoid)

1. Postoperative—greatest at site of craniotomy, usually unilateral, smooth and thin dural enhancement.
2. Intracranial hypotension—due to a drop in CSF volume. Orthostatic headaches, brainstem 'slumping', subdural effusions and convex dural venous sinuses and bulky pituitary from pull of negative pressure. Bilateral smooth and thin dural enhancement.
   (a) **Following lumbar puncture**—mild and transient.
   (b) **Overshunting**—slit-like ventricles.
   (c) **Skull base leak**—following surgery/trauma, presents with CSF rhinorrhoea or otorrhoea. Diagnosed with skull base CT looking for a fracture or defect.
   (d) **Spinal leak**—e.g. meningocoele, posttraumatic. Often subtle, may need a myelogram to localize.
3. Infection—localized to adjacent osteomyelitis or sinusitis. Irregular, thick enhancement.
4. Neoplastic.
   (a) Meningioma—reactive tapered dural thickening around lesion ('dural tail').
   (b) Metastasis—e.g. breast, prostate; smooth or nodular enhancement.
   (c) **Secondary CNS lymphoma***—meningeal > parenchymal involvement.
   (d) **Solitary fibrous tumour of the dura**—similar appearance to meningioma, but tends to be of lower T2 signal, with internal flow voids and a higher propensity for skull invasion. No calcification or associated hyperostosis.
5. Granulomatous disease—TB, sarcoid, Wegener's, rheumatoid, Sjögren's, Behçet's, Erdheim-Chester, syphilis, fungal disease. Multifocal nodular and thick enhancement. Basal distribution in TB meningitis.
6. **Extramedullary haematopoiesis**—dural involvement rare, seen in thalassemia and myelofibrosis. Widened diploic space in skull.
7. **Idiopathic hypertrophic cranial pachymeningitis**—mass-like thickening of the dura, often with cranial nerve involvement. Some cases are due to IgG4-related disease.

Leptomeningeal (pia–arachnoid)

Look for subtle cranial nerve enhancement indicating leptomeningeal pathology.

1. Carcinomatosis—typically nodular. Metastatic (breast, lung), lymphoma, ependymoma, germinoma, medulloblastoma, glioblastoma, pineoblastoma. Image whole neuraxis to assess extent of disease.

2. <u>Meningoencephalitis</u>—bacterial, viral, fungal, Lyme disease. Cerebral swelling.
3. <u>Granulomatous disease</u>—TB, sarcoid, Wegener's, rheumatoid nodules, fungal disease.
4. <u>Vascular</u>—collateral flow (ischaemia) or increased flow, e.g. dural fistula, pial angioma of Sturge-Weber (see Section 13.19).

Further reading

Smirniotopoulos, J.G., Murphy, F.M., Rushing, E.J., et al., 2007. Patterns of contrast enhancement in the brain and meninges. Radiographics 27, 525–551.

13.17 EPENDYMAL ENHANCEMENT

Look specifically for hydrocephalus and radiological contraindications to lumbar puncture.

1. <u>Infection</u>—ventriculitis.
   (a) <u>Bacterial</u>—intraventricular pus restricts diffusion, and may be related to an adjacent cerebral abscess. Ependymal enhancement is an early sign of ventriculitis and warrants escalation of therapy and consideration of shunting for hydrocephalus.
   (b) **Viral**—CMV, VZV; immunocompromised patients.
2. <u>Neoplastic</u>—abutting ventricular surface or intraventricular.
   (a) **Nodular/linear**—lymphoma, glioblastoma, ependymoma, germ cell tumour, metastases.
   (b) **Mass-like**—ependymoma, giant cell astrocytoma.
3. <u>Granulomatous</u>—TB (basal meningitis), sarcoidosis (cranial nerves and dura).
4. <u>Intraventricular haemorrhage</u>—hyperdense blood within the ventricles.
5. **Subependymal venous congestion**—can mimic ependymal enhancement.
   (a) **Deep cerebral vein thrombosis**—hyperdense vein, oedema.
   (b) **AVM or AVF**—dilated abnormal vessels.
   (c) **Sturge-Weber***—cortical calcification, cerebral atrophy and enlarged ipsilateral choroid plexus.

13.18 CRANIAL NERVE (CN) ENHANCEMENT

Rules:

- Enhancement of cisternal and cavernous sinus CN segments always abnormal.

- CN VII enhancement—abnormal in the cisternal, meatal and extracranial segments. Venous plexus causes normal enhancement of the labyrinthine, tympanic and mastoid segments.
- Multiple nerves—metastases, leukaemia, lymphoma, NF2, Lyme disease, chronic inflammatory demyelinating polyneuropathy.
- Optic nerve (CN II)—different pathologies as not a true nerve but CNS WM tract: demyelination, gliomas.

Neoplastic

1. **Primary.**
   (a) **Schwannoma**—CN VIII; sporadic or NF2 (diagnostic if bilateral).
   (b) **Meningioma**—'tram-track' enhancement, CN II.
   (c) **Neurofibroma**—rarer to involve CN, T2 hyperintense rim with central low signal (target sign). NF1: plexiform neurofibromas of CN III and CN V.
   (d) **Optic nerve glioma**—pilocytic astrocytomas, associated with NF1 (see Section 13.31).
2. **Secondary.**
   (a) **Leptomeningeal dissemination**—nodular involvement, seeding from primary CNS (ependymoma, medulloblastoma, germinoma, lymphoma) or secondary metastatic (breast, lung, melanoma).
   (b) **Perineural spread**—from head and neck tumours, e.g. mucosal SCC and salivary gland adenoid cystic carcinoma (CN VII), lymphoma, melanoma.

Infection

1. **Meningitis.**
   (a) **Viral infections**—HSV type 1, CMV, and VZV (Ramsay Hunt Syndrome—vesicular eruptions). CN VII.
   (b) **TB***—cisternal segments of CN, surrounding exudate.
   (c) ***Cryptococcus neoformans***—infiltration of meninges around optic tracts, nerves and chiasm.
2. **Lyme disease**—may involve CN III to VII.
3. **Fungal**—aspergillosis, mucormycosis, actinomycosis. Perineural spread from sinus disease. Elderly diabetic patients are most at risk.

Inflammatory

1. **Bell's palsy**—uniform linear enhancement of CN VII.
2. **Miller-Fisher syndrome**—variant of Guillain-Barré, multiple CN, linear enhancement.
3. **Chronic inflammatory demyelinating polyneuropathy**—'onion bulb' thickening of multiple peripheral and cranial nerves, with diffuse enhancement.
4. **Demyelinating**—multiple sclerosis (MS) and NMO. CN II (optic neuritis).

Granulomatous

1. Sarcoidosis*—any CN with thickening, most commonly CN II centred around chiasm and pituitary stalk.
2. **Wegener's granulomatosis***—spread from sinuses, associated with dural thickening, vasculitis with infarcts.
3. **Tolosa-Hunt**—idiopathic inflammation of cavernous sinus and orbital apex. Painful ophthalmoplegia, enlarged cavernous sinus with internal carotid artery (ICA) narrowing and enhancement of CNs that pass through.

Other

1. **Post radiation neuritis**—limited to radiation field.
2. **Ischaemic**—diabetics, vasculopaths; transient enhancement followed by gradual atrophy. CN II, III and VI.

Further reading

Saremi, F., Helmy, M., Farzin, S., et al., 2005. MRI of cranial nerve enhancement. AJR Am. J. Roentgenol. 185 (6), 1487–1497.

13.19 ENLARGED LEPTOMENINGEAL PERFORATORS

1. **Collateralization due to proximal progressive steno-occlusive disease.**
   (a) Moyamoya disease—idiopathic, progressive occlusion of the proximal intracranial arteries. 'Puff of smoke'—angiographic appearance of small abnormal net-like collateral vessels. 'Ivy sign'—pial collaterals have serpentine sulcal FLAIR hyperintensity and enhancement.
   (b) **Moyamoya-like syndromes**—other proximal intracranial artery steno-occlusive diseases that mimic Moyamoya disease, e.g. post radiation, NF1, Down's syndrome, SCD and atherosclerosis.
2. **Secondary to a distal 'sump' effect.**
   (a) AVM—tangle of abnormal vessels with feeding arteries and draining veins. Often multiple dilated vessels, no stenoses (cf. Moyamoya).
   (b) **Tumour**—vascular tumours recruit increased arterial flow to both tumour and surrounding parenchyma/leptomeninges.
3. **Sturge-Weber***—phakomatosis; facial cutaneous and leptomeningeal haemangiomas. Steal phenomenon causes atrophy of subjacent cortex and WM + 'tram-track' calcification.

13.20 WM LESIONS WITH LITTLE MASS EFFECT

WM lesions are common, of varied aetiologies and frequently an incidental finding, which creates management and follow-up challenges. They may be classified based on pattern into punctate, confluent and diffuse lesions.

Punctate lesions

1. Nonspecific and age-related—small peripheral lesions in nontypical locations for an inflammatory cause (see following). Greater number reported in patients with migraine. Spare subcortical U-fibres (SCUF). Some authors arbitrarily say one lesion per decade is within normal limits.
2. Vascular.
   (a) Small-vessel disease (SVD)—periventricular WM lesions (>3 mm from surface, cf. MS) and deep WM lesions; tends to spare corpus callosum (cf. MS). Varies from punctate to confluent. Spares SCUF due to end-arterial distribution.
   (b) Hypertensive encephalopathy—ganglionic lacunar infarcts and microhaemorrhages. Interrelated with SVD.
   (c) Multi-infarct encephalopathy—SVD + additional embolic cortical and pontine infarcts.
   (d) Cerebral amyloid angiopathy—see Section 13.4.
3. Inflammatory.
   (a) Multiple sclerosis (MS)—perivenous distribution, periventricular (contacting surface, cf. SVD), infratentorial, cortical/juxtacortical with involvement of SCUF (cf. vascular aetiologies). Involves corpus callosum at callososeptal interface. Incomplete ring enhancement (cf. infection). Short segment spinal cord lesions.
   (b) Neuromyelitis optica (NMO)—often indistinct/fluffy lesions, classic locations: periaqueductal grey matter and area postrema (posterior medulla abutting fourth ventricle) + optic neuritis. Long segment spinal cord lesions (cf. MS).
   (c) Vasculitis—wide spectrum of vasculitides defined by size of vessel involvement and whether confined to CNS arteries or systemic. Multiple infarctions, usually bilateral in different vascular territories. Angiography demonstrates multifocal stenoses and occlusions. Black-blood contrast MRI may show enhancing inflammatory tissue cuffing arteries.
   (d) **Sarcoidosis***—see Section 13.15.
   (e) **Connective tissue disease (CTD)**—can be indistinguishable from MS, e.g. SLE (associated with infarcts), Sjögren's. Other signs of CTD.
4. Miliary metastases—e.g. lung, melanoma, breast. Often at GWMJ. Greater mass effect and perilesional oedema. Callosal involvement very rare (cf. MS).
5. Infection—granuloma, septic emboli; ± punctate restricted diffusion, microhaemorrhages, complete ring enhancement (see Section 13.13).

13

6. Diffuse axonal injury (DAI)—shear-related injuries often with microhaemorrhage; common locations GWMJ, splenium and middle cerebellar peduncles.

Confluent WM lesions (up to 20 mm in size)

1. Neoplastic—e.g. glioma, lymphoma, metastases. Generally have more mass versus other differentials (see Section 13.8).
2. Vascular—same as above due to coalescence of multiple vascular insults.
3. Hypotensive cerebral infarction—deep and superficial watershed territories, typical signs of infarction if acute.
4. Infection.
   - (a) Encephalitis—HSV predilection for medial temporal lobes; other non-herpes encephalitides can involve basal ganglia (BG), thalamus, brainstem and cerebellum. Ill-defined, variable enhancement and restricted diffusion. Acute presentation with fevers, seizures, reduced Glasgow Coma Scale (GCS) and nonspecific neurology.
   - (b) Progressive multifocal leukoencephalopathy (PML)—JC polyomavirus opportunistic infection causing demyelination in immunocompromised patients (HIV, patients on immunotherapy). Multifocal periventricular and subcortical lesions involving SCUF. No contrast enhancement. Late cavitation/cystic change.
   - (c) **PML-immune reconstitution inflammatory syndrome (PML-IRIS)**—paradoxical deterioration in PML due to exaggerated inflammatory reaction after reconstitution of immune system. Classically seen in HIV patients on therapy, but also recognized with MS immunotherapies. Associated with mass effect and irregular enhancement (cf. PML).
   - (d) **Lyme disease**—resembles MS but greater abnormalities in BG and brainstem ± CN enhancement.
5. Inflammatory.
   - (a) MS, NMO, vasculitis, sarcoidosis*—see earlier.
   - (b) Tumefactive demyelination—large demyelinating lesion with relatively little mass effect or oedema, often unifocal. Open-ring enhancement, low CBV on perfusion (cf. tumour). Like MS often perivenous in distribution.
   - (c) Acute disseminated encephalomyelitis (ADEM)—monophasic demyelination following infection/vaccination, usually in children or adolescents. Bilateral asymmetrical subcortical lesions, spare callososeptal interface (cf. MS).
6. Osmotic myelinolysis—acute demyelination from rapid change in serum osmolality (classically rapid correction of hyponatraemia). Typically a round or trident-shaped lesion in central pons, but can be extrapontine, e.g. symmetrical in BG and/or WM.
7. **Radiation necrosis**—see Section 13.12.

Diffuse WM lesions (spanning ≥2 cerebral lobes)

1. Vascular—see earlier.
2. Neoplastic—diffuse glioma (see Section 13.8).
3. Inflammatory.
   (a) MS, NMO, vasculitis, sarcoidosis*—see earlier.
   (b) **Rasmussen encephalitis**—children and young adults with intractable seizures; chronic encephalitis of one hemisphere with ipsilateral patchy WM lesions and volume loss.
4. **Leukoencephalopathies**—all tend to cause symmetric, multifocal lesions. Most present in childhood.
   (a) **Inherited**—early adult onset.
      (i) **CADASIL**—recurrent lacunar and subcortical infarcts, especially in anterior temporal and frontal lobes (see Section 13.4).
      (ii) **COL4A1**—small-vessel disease, dilated perivascular spaces, microhaemorrhages and intracerebral haemorrhages. SCUF spared.
      (iii) **X-linked adrenoleukodystrophy**—adult-onset phenotype, frontal lobe and genu of corpus callosum involvement predominates (cf. child onset, which has a predilection for occipitoparietal regions).
      (iv) **Krabbe disease**—adult-onset phenotype, slower progression. CT: hyperdense thalami, cerebellum and caudate nuclei. Periventricular abnormal WM signal.
   (b) **Toxic–metabolic**—dependent on cause, typically symmetrical and often involve splenium + corresponding restricted diffusion.
   (c) **HIV encephalopathy**—symmetric periventricular and deep WM lesions + volume loss.
5. **Degenerative**—e.g. frontotemporal lobar degeneration and corticobasal degeneration; associated volume loss (see Section 13.42).
6. **Radiation leukoencephalopathy**—diffuse confluent lesions with volume loss and evidence of indications for radiotherapy, e.g. intracranial or head and neck tumour.

Further reading

Geraldes, R., Ciccarelli, O., Barkhof, F., et al., 2018. The current role of MRI in differentiating multiple sclerosis from its imaging mimics. Nat. Rev. Neurol. 14 (4), 199–213.

Kim, K.W., MacFall, J.R., Payne, M.E., 2008. Classification of white matter lesions on magnetic resonance imaging in elderly persons. Biol. Psychiatry 64 (4), 273–280.

13.21 CORPUS CALLOSUM (CC) LESIONS

Atrophic/dysplastic callosum

1. Agenesis/dysgenesis—CC develops from anterior to posterior; early embryonic insult = CC agenesis, late embryonic insult = CC dysgenesis limited to rostrum or splenium. Complete agenesis = parallel ('racing car') lateral ventricles, WM tracts paralleling the interhemispheric fissure (Probst bundles), high-riding third ventricle. Associated with pericallosal lipoma, dermoid and interhemispheric arachnoid cysts.
2. Atrophy—small-vessel ischaemia, radiation therapy, leukodystrophy. Extensive abnormal WM signal and volume loss beyond CC.

Multifocal lesions

1. **Demyelination**—MS, NMO. Lower border of CC at callososeptal interface (see Section 13.20).
2. **Vascular**—e.g. embolic infarcts, Susac syndrome. Asymmetric, adjacent to the midline. Callosal lesions are characteristic in Susac syndrome and typically spare the callososeptal interface, ± restricted diffusion and enhancement if acute; patients are typically young adult females presenting with a clinical triad of encephalopathy, bilateral sensorineural hearing loss and branch retinal artery occlusions.
3. DAI—asymmetric involving both midline and borders of CC + microhaemorrhage on SWI (see Section 13.20).
4. **Marchiafava-Bignami syndrome**—chronic alcoholics with vitamin B deficiency. Body of CC > genu/splenium. Large lesions in the central layer of CC (cf. demyelination).

Neoplasms

1. **Butterfly glioma**—high grade glioma, symmetric midline-crossing lesion most common in frontal lobes crossing and expanding genu, heterogeneous enhancement + central necrosis.
2. **Lymphoma***—hypercellular (dense on CT), homogeneous restricted diffusion and solid enhancement (cf. butterfly glioma).

Transient lesions

1. Cytotoxic lesions of the corpus callosum—transient cytotoxic oedema of the splenium; well-defined, oval, in the midline. T2 hyperintense + restricted diffusion but no enhancement. Many causes: seizures, metabolic (hypoglycaemia, sodium imbalance), infections, drugs and toxins.

Hydrocephalus-related

1. **Corpus callosum impingement syndrome**—impingement of CC against falx due to severe chronic hydrocephalus; abnormal signal + atrophy in rostral CC.
2. **Post shunt decompression**—typically diffuse oedema in CC occurring after shunt insertion for chronic severe hydrocephalus.

13.22 DEEP GREY MATTER ABNORMALITIES

Deep grey matter (DGM) = basal ganglia and thalamus
Basal ganglia = caudate + globus pallidus (GP) + putamen
Corpus striatum = caudate + putamen
Lentiform nucleus = putamen + GP

Physiological

1. **Age-related**—incidence of GP calcification increases with age. Increased iron deposition causes reduced T2 signal in GP and putamen (see Section 13.24).
2. **Perivascular spaces (PVS)**—CSF signal on all sequences.

Vascular

1. **Lacunar infarct**—well-defined CSF density/intensity lesions + surrounding high signal rim evident on FLAIR.
2. **Hypertensive haemorrhage**—background of DGM lacunes, enlarged PVS and microhaemorrhages.
3. **Global hypoxic ischaemic injury**—bilateral infarcts in regions of high metabolic demand: GP, posterior putamen, ventrolateral thalami, perirolandic regions, occipital cortex and hippocampal formations.
4. **Venous infarction**—due to internal cerebral vein thrombosis; bithalamic involvement (see Section 13.25). Marked swelling from venous congestion.
5. **Central variant PRES**—can involve brainstem.

Neurodegenerative

1. **Parkinson's**—^{18}F-DOPA PET scan: loss of normal comma-shaped tracer uptake in the corpus striatum with full stop-shaped uptake only seen in the caudate head.
2. **Multiple system atrophy-Parkinson's type (MSA-P)**—reduced putamen volume with reduced T2 signal relative to globus pallidus. High T2 rim surrounding putamen ('putaminal rim' sign).
3. **Huntington's disease**—atrophy of caudate heads, 'boxcar' frontal horns.

Toxins

1. **Chronic bilirubin encephalopathy (kernicterus)**—increased T1 and T2 signal in GP.
2. **Hypermanganesaemia**—e.g. total parenteral nutrition, haemodialysis, liver failure. High T1 signal in BG.
3. **Exogenous toxins.**
   (a) **Carbon monoxide**—GP.
   (b) **Methanol**—putamen.
   (c) **Cyanide**—corpus striatum and perirolandic cortex.

Acquired metabolic disease

1. <u>Uraemic encephalopathy</u>—bilateral basal ganglia, thalamus and midbrain. 'Lentiform fork' sign—T2 hyperintense internal and external capsule.
2. <u>Hyperammonaemic/hepatic encephalopathy</u>—acute liver failure. Symmetric insular, thalamic and posterior limb of internal capsule (PLIC) T2 hyperintensity.
3. **Hypoglycaemia**—symmetric high T2 and restricted diffusion in basal ganglia, PLIC, splenium and parietooccipital cortex.

Inherited metabolic disease

1. **Wilson's disease**—copper deposition disease. High T2 and volume loss in striatum and ventrolateral thalamus. 'Face of giant panda' sign in midbrain and 'miniature panda' sign in pons—'double panda' sign if both are present.
2. **Mitochondrial cytopathies.**
   (a) **Kearns-Sayre syndrome**—GP and cortical calcification.
   (b) **Leigh syndrome**—putamen, thalamus and periaqueductal grey matter.
3. **Lipid storage disorders**—Krabbe disease (see Section 13.20).
4. **Amino acid disorders**—e.g. methylmalonic acidaemia; selective necrosis of GP.
5. **Neurodegeneration with brain iron accumulation (NBIA)**—see Section 13.24.
6. **Fahr disease**—symmetrical calcification of basal ganglia, dentate nuclei and subcortical WM (see Section 13.7).

Infectious

1. **Variant CJD (vCJD)**—'hockey stick' sign: T2 hyperintensity in pulvinar and dorsomedial thalamus (cf. sporadic CJD which spares thalamus).

Further reading

Hegde, A.N., Mohan, S., Lath, N., Lim, C,C., 2011. Differential diagnosis for bilateral abnormalities of the basal ganglia and thalamus. Radiographics 31 (1), 5–30.

13.23 BASAL GANGLIA: BRIGHT ON T1

Correlate with CT (to determine if the high signal is due to calcium), clinicoradiological features of cirrhotic liver disease and liver function tests (LFTs).

Paramagnetic substances

1. **Methaemoglobin**—hypertensive haemorrhage, haemorrhagic infarction. Includes haemorrhagic necrosis, e.g. in carbon monoxide (GP) or methanol (putamina) poisoning.
2. **Copper**—Wilson's disease.
3. **Manganese**—parenteral nutrition, haemodialysis, liver failure.
4. **Calcification**—some crystalline forms of calcium cause T1 shortening (e.g. Fahr, hypoparathyroidism).
5. **Chronic bilirubin encephalopathy (kernicterus)**—increased T1 and T2 signal in GP.
6. **Prior administration of linear gadolinium chelates.**

Unknown cause

1. **Diabetic striatopathy**—non-calcific hyperdensity is a characteristic feature; typically manifests with hemiballism-hemichorea caused by nonketotic hyperglycaemia.
2. **Fabry disease**—typically pulvinar T1 hyperintensity (cf. vCJD with T2 hyperintensity). Associated with posterior circulation infarcts.
3. **NF1**—focal areas of signal intensity (FASI), high on T1 and T2, in the basal ganglia; most common neuroimaging feature of NF1.

Further reading

Lai, P.H., Chen, C., Liang, H.L., Pan, H.B., 1999. Hyperintense basal ganglia on T1 weighted MR imaging. AJR Am. J. Roentgenol. 172 (4), 1109–1115.

13.24 SYMMETRICAL BASAL GANGLIA SUSCEPTIBILITY CHANGES

Most commonly related to calcification (diamagnetic) or iron deposition (paramagnetic). Differentiation of calcification versus iron is easiest via correlation with CT: calcification is hyperdense, whereas iron is not overtly appreciable on CT. Normal physiological mineralization occurs as follows. (NB: this does not normally involve the caudate nuclei.)

1. 10–20 years—iron deposition starts in GP.
2. 20–40 years—iron deposition increases in GP + mildly visible in putamina.
3. >40 years—iron deposition increases in GP and putamina to a lesser extent. Calcification of the GP is also variably present.

Calcium

See Section 13.7 (DGM).

Iron

1. **Neurodegeneration with brain iron accumulation (NBIA)**—group of progressive neurological disorders that feature prominent extrapyramidal symptoms and iron deposition. Reduced signal in GP on T2/T2*/SWI sequences with central high signal: 'eye of the tiger' sign. Most common is pantothenate kinase-associated neurodegeneration (PKAN), which has abnormalities restricted to the GP and substantia nigra. Presence of pigmentary retinopathy is strongly suggestive of PKAN and is not seen in other forms of NBIA.
2. **Huntington's disease**—atrophy of caudate heads.

Further reading

Kruer, M.C., Boddaert, N., 2012. Neurodegeneration with brain iron accumulation: a diagnostic algorithm. Semin. Pediatr. Neurol. 19 (2), 67–74.

13.25 BILATERAL THALAMIC LESIONS

Vascular

1. **Artery of percheron infarct**—variant solitary arterial trunk that arises from one of the posterior cerebral arteries supplying both paramedian thalami and rostral midbrain.
2. **Basilar tip thrombosis**—hyperdense thrombus/loss of flow void in the basilar tip.
3. **Internal cerebral venous infarct**—look for deep cerebral vein thrombus on CT (hyperdense) and MRI (loss of T2 flow void). Greater local swelling than arterial infarcts. SWI may show serpiginous thrombosed deep medullary veins and associated microhaemorrhage.
4. **Hypertensive haemorrhage.**
5. **Hypoxic ischaemic encephalopathy.**

Infection

1. **Encephalitis**—caused by arboviruses transmitted by mosquito or tick bites, e.g. Japanese encephalitis (Asia), West Nile encephalitis (Middle East), Murray Valley encephalitis (Australasia), St Louis encephalitis (USA). Bilateral thalamic involvement is typical ± extension into brainstem or basal ganglia; usually haemorrhagic. Fevers and fulminant course.
2. **Variant CJD**—see Section 13.22.

3. **Acute necrotizing encephalitis**—haemorrhagic parainfectious syndrome in young children. Thought to be an immune overreaction to a mild antecedent viral infection.

Metabolic

1. **Carbon monoxide poisoning**—bilateral GP and thalamus.
2. **Wernicke's encephalopathy**—triad of mental status, gait and oculomotor dysfunction. Due to thiamine deficiency. Symmetric abnormal signal in thalami, mammillary bodies, tectal plate and periaqueductal areas.
3. **Mitochondrial cytopathies**—Leigh, Kearns-Sayre (see Section 13.22).
4. **Fabry disease**—see Section 13.23.
5. **Wilson's disease**—see Section 13.22.

Neoplastic

1. **Bithalamic glioma**—low-grade astrocytoma in children and young adults; expansile and often nonenhancing tumour ± obstructive hydrocephalus.

13.26 BILATERAL MIDDLE CEREBELLAR PEDUNCLE (MCP) LESIONS

Degenerative (~40%)

1. **MSA-cerebellar type (MSA-C)**—symmetrical high T2 signal and volume loss in MCPs, 'hot cross bun' sign in pons: cross of abnormal signal due to selective degeneration of pontocerebellar tracts.
2. **Fragile X**—lesions in MCPs and splenium.

Metabolic/toxic (~20%)

See Section 13.22.

1. **Wilson's disease**.
2. **Cirrhotic liver disease.**
3. **Adrenoleukodystrophy**—see Section 13.20.
4. **Hypoglycemia.**
5. **Solvent abuse.**
6. **Heroin inhalation**—symmetrical involvement of PLIC and cerebellar WM.

Cerebrovascular (~15%)

1. **PRES (central variant)**—typically precipitated by drugs or hypertension.

13

2. Anterior inferior cerebellar artery (AICA) infarction—look for restricted diffusion and signs of vertebral artery occlusion or dissection.

Infection/Inflammatory (~15%)

See Section 13.20.

1. MS.
2. Behçet's*—may involve bilateral basal ganglia, brainstem and thalamus.
3. ADEM.
4. HIV.
5. **Japanese encephalitis**—bilateral thalamic involvement.
6. **PML and PML-IRIS.**

Neoplastic (~10%)

1. **Lymphoma*.**
2. **Brain stem glioma.**
3. **Meningeal carcinomatosis**—leptomeningeal enhancement and FLAIR sulcal hyperintensity.

Further reading

Okamoto, K., Tokiguchi, S., Furusawa, T., et al., 2003. MR Features of diseases involving bilateral middle cerebellar peduncles. AJNR Am. J. Neuroradiol. 24 (10), 1946–1954.

13.27 INTRASELLAR MASS

Approach to sellar lesions

1. Lesion intrinsic or extrinsic to pituitary gland? Sometimes difficult, see if pituitary is displaced or surrounding the lesion.
2. Arising from sella or extending inferiorly from suprasellar? Diaphragma sellae displaced superiorly or inferiorly, respectively.
3. Slow or fast growing? Slow growth implied by bony remodelling and expansion of the sella.
4. Check for cavernous sinus involvement, optic nerve/chiasm compression or infiltration and obstructive hydrocephalus from compression of the third ventricle.
5. Correlate with pituitary function.

Intrinsic to the gland

1. Pituitary adenoma—mildly T2 hyperintense and T1 hypointense relative to normal gland.
   (a) Microadenoma—<10 mm, shows slightly delayed (60 secs) enhancement relative to normal gland.

   (b) Macroadenoma—>10 mm, often demonstrates suprasellar and/or cavernous sinus extension, ± cystic degeneration and high T1 signal from internal haemorrhage or proteinaceous material. Sellar expansion from gradual remodelling.
2. Pituitary hyperplasia—enlarged normal signal gland.
   (a) Physiological—pregnancy, postpartum, lactation and postpubertal females.
   (b) Pathological—end-organ failure, e.g. hypothyroidism.
3. Pituitary haemorrhage/infarction—associated with macroadenoma. Blood-fluid levels, dense intrasellar mass on CT and variable signal and diffusion on MRI. 'Apoplexy' when haemorrhage/infarction is associated with acute clinical symptoms—headache, sudden vision loss and oculomotor palsy.
4. Intracranial hypotension—slightly swollen convex pituitary often extending just above sella, due to negative intracranial pressure (see Section 13.16).
5. Inflammatory hypophysitis—these can involve anterior and/or posterior pituitary and/or infundibulum, typically causing enlargement and avid homogeneous enhancement, but without sellar remodelling (cf. adenoma). Pituitary dysfunction is common. If the posterior pituitary is involved the normal T1 'bright spot' is absent.
   (a) Lymphocytic hypophysitis—typically in late pregnancy or postpartum.
   (b) Granulomatous hypophysitis—e.g. sarcoid, TB, Wegener's.
   (c) IgG4-related hypophysitis—as part of systemic IgG4-related disease.
6. **Metastasis**—rare, males = lung, females = breast. Pituitary or infundibulum. Normal fossa size, bony destruction, dural thickening and irregular margins (cf. adenoma).
7. **Pituitary abscess**—rare, cystic lesion + peripheral enhancement, likely associated meningitis. Fever, meningism.

Extrinsic to the gland

1. Meningioma—sphenoid, diaphragma sellae or cavernous sinus. Typically projects into sella displacing diaphragma sellae inferiorly + enhancing dural tail ± skull hyperostosis (cf. macroadenoma).
2. Rathke's cleft cyst—also known as pars intermedia cyst, typically lies between anterior and posterior pituitary. Usually <1 cm but can be large. 50% have intracystic nodule. 'Claw sign' of normal displaced pituitary.
3. **Craniopharyngioma**—purely intrasellar rare, usually suprasellar and sellar.

Further reading

Go, J.L., Rajamohan, A.G., 2017. Imaging of the sella and parasellar region. Radiol. Clin. North Am. 55 (1), 83–101.

13

13.28 PITUITARY INFUNDIBULAR LESION

Normal pituitary stalk diameter: 2 mm just above gland, 4 mm at level of optic chiasm. Infundibular lesions are often associated with diabetes insipidus and panhypopituitarism.

Neoplastic

1. **Metastases**—e.g. from lung or breast; see Section 13.27.
2. **Lymphoma***—may present as isolated stalk thickening or periventricular enhancing masses. Seen in primary and secondary CNS involvement.
3. **Leukaemia**—acute/chronic myeloid leukemia. Diagnosis usually known prior to infundibular involvement. Look for dural and optic nerve sheath deposits.
4. **Germ cell tumours**—children/young adults. Germinoma most common, other types: embryonal carcinoma, yolk sac tumour, choriocarcinoma, teratoma and mixed. Hyperdense on CT, homogeneous solid enhancement and restricted diffusion.
5. **Craniopharyngioma**.
   (a) **Adamantinomatous** (90%)—children > adults, 90% cystic, 90% calcified and 90% enhance. Multilocular, large with high T1 (oily) contents.
   (b) **Papillary** (10%)—adults, typically a solid enhancing mass. Small water-signal cysts, minimal enhancement. Calcification is rare.
6. **Langerhans cell histiocytosis (LCH)***—children/young adults, stalk thickening and enhancement ± meningeal and choroid plexus involvement. Posterior pituitary bright spot absent. Look for lung, bone and skin disease.
7. **Pituicytoma**—benign, men in 40–50s. Enhances homogeneously. No sellar enlargement.
8. **Other primary tumours**—gliomas, choristomas and tanycytomas (encase circle of Willis).
9. **Pituitary adenoma**—may occasionally arise in the infundibular region (pars tuberalis).

Nonneoplastic

1. **Neurosarcoid**—enhancing stalk granuloma, which often involves adjacent optic pathways and floor of third ventricle. Check for dural, leptomeningeal and CN involvement. Consider systemic involvement.
2. **Lymphocytic infundibuloneurohypophysitis (LINH)**—variant of lymphocytic hypophysitis that predominantly affects infundibulum; see Section 13.27.
3. **Other granulomatous hypophysitis**—TB, Wegener's, Erdheim-Chester, Whipple's disease. In isolation generally

indistinguishable from sarcoidosis. TB associated with basal meningitis. Wegener's associated with sinonasal disease (see Section 13.30).
4. **Ectopic posterior pituitary**—T1 bright spot located on median eminence of hypothalamus ± pituitary stalk/gland hypoplasia. Look for other midline abnormalities, e.g. deficient septum pellucidum.
5. **Infundibular cysts**—pars intermedia cysts may rarely be confined to the stalk.

Further reading

Hamilton, B.E., Salzman, K.L., Osborn, A.G., 2007. Anatomic and pathologic spectrum of pituitary infundibulum lesions. AJR Am. J. Roentgenol. 188 (3), W223–W232.

13.29 SUPRASELLAR MASS

Considerable overlap with infundibular lesions (see Section 13.28) and pituitary lesions with suprasellar extension (see Section 13.27).

Meningeal

1. **Meningioma**—see Section 13.27.
2. **Granulomatous**—TB, sarcoid, LCH. Enhancing granulomas may be T2 hypointense.

Vascular

1. **Saccular aneurysm**—giant aneurysms (>25 mm) may erode bone in the supra or parasellar region, appearances may be complicated by thrombus and flow void. Look for pulsation artefact in phase encoding direction. Angiographic imaging essential.

Parenchymal

1. **Pituitary lesions**—with suprasellar extension.
2. **Infundibular masses**—especially craniopharyngioma (often large, making it difficult to verify infundibular origin).
3. **Hypothalamic hamartoma**—arises from tuber cinereum; T2 iso/hyperintense to cerebral cortex, no enhancement. Gelastic seizures, precocious puberty and developmental delay.
4. **Germ cell tumours**.
5. **Metastases/lymphoma***.

Optic chiasm

1. **Hypothalamic chiasmatic glioma**—pilocytic astrocytoma typically arising from optic nerve/chiasm with variable involvement of hypothalamus. Variable enhancement. Associated with NF1.
2. **Chiasmal optic neuritis**—NMO, MS. High T2 signal and swelling. Signs of demyelinating disease elsewhere.

Cisternal

1. Epidermoid—paramidline cystic lesion, CSF density (CT) and T1/T2 signal (MRI). Incomplete signal suppression on FLAIR and characteristic restricted diffusion enable differentiation from arachnoid cyst.
2. Dermoid—midline cystic lesion with fat content and capsular calcification. Look for subarachnoid 'fat droplets' to indicate rupture which is associated with chemical meningitis and hydrocephalus.
3. **Teratoma**—multiloculated, heterogeneous mixed soft tissue, fat and calcification.
4. **Lipoma**—fat density/signal lesion, calcification rare in suprasellar location (cf. dermoid and interhemispheric lipomas).
5. **Arachnoid cyst**—well-defined cyst of variable size. Isointense to CSF, nonenhancing, noncalcified.

13.30 CAVERNOUS SINUS (CS)/ PARASELLAR MASS

Extension from pituitary lesion

1. Pituitary macroadenoma—can invade the CS via lateral extension, causing bulging of the CS. Signal difference most appreciable on pre- and postcontrast T1. Tumour extension beyond the intercarotid line suggestive of invasion. ICA encased but not typically narrowed (cf. meningioma). May invade skull base, mimicking a primary bone lesion.

Dural

1. Meningioma—avidly enhancing mass with thickened dural tail; other meningiomas may be present. More often associated with venous congestion, and if ICA is encased it is often narrowed (cf. macroadenoma).
2. Granulomatous/inflammatory infiltration
   (a) Sarcoidosis*—additional dural and nerve deposits, signs of systemic sarcoid in lungs.
   (b) TB*—with basal meningitis ± tuberculomas.
   (c) Idiopathic orbital inflammatory syndrome—also known as orbital pseudotumour. Most commonly involves extraocular muscles with rapid onset unilateral proptosis. Mass is ill-defined and T2 hypointense due to fibrosis (cf. lymphoma, which is more lobular with intermediate T2 signal). Involvement of the orbital apex and cavernous sinus with painful ophthalmoplegia is termed Tolosa-Hunt syndrome; may also narrow the ICA and extend to superior orbital fissure. Linked to many autoimmune diseases, including:

    (i) **IgG4-related disease***—associated with pachymeningitis, hypophysitis and salivary/lacrimal gland enlargement.
    (ii) **Wegener's***—look for sinonasal disease with abnormal soft tissue, osseous erosions and nasoseptal perforation.
    (iii) **Churg-Strauss***—with lung involvement.
3. **Defect**—meningocoele/encephalocoele. Often due to raised intracranial pressure (ICP), clues include a partially empty sella (from arachnoid herniation flattening pituitary) and enlarged Meckel's caves.
4. **Invasive fungal sinusitis**—*Aspergillus;* immunocompromised and diabetic patients. Extension from paranasal sinuses. Hyperdense opacification of paranasal sinus on CT, with susceptibility signal dropout on T2-weighted MRI.

Cavernous sinus metastases

1. Haematogenous.
    (a) Lymphoma*—homogeneous enhancement and restricted diffusion (more than pseudotumour).
    (b) Metastases—irregular, heterogeneous infiltrative enhancing tissue.
2. Direct extension—from malignant sphenoid sinus and nasopharyngeal tumours, with osseous erosion.
3. **Perineural spread**—squamous cell and adenoid cystic carcinomas; review skull base spaces, fissures and optic pathways. Abnormally thickened and enhancing nerve.

Neurogenic

1. **Schwannoma**—may involve CPA, Meckel's cave and pterygomaxillary fissure. Variably solid and cystic, 'dumbbell' shaped, avidly enhancing with skull base remodelling.

Vascular

1. Carotico-cavernous fistula—look for associated venous congestion in/around orbit (± proptosis, muscle swelling and chemosis clinically) and central skull base. May be direct, due to rupture of intracavernous ICA (e.g. traumatic or aneurysmal), or indirect, due to small AV shunts (associated with venous sinus thrombosis and subsequent revascularization).
2. Aneurysm—traumatic (pseudoaneurysm) and nontraumatic; prominent flow void and phase artefacts. May be partially thrombosed ± fistula.
3. Cavernous sinus thrombosis—nonenhancing thrombus in enlarged sinus ± adjacent dural enhancement and venous congestion. Often due to orbitofacial sepsis.

4. **Cavernous haemangioma**—multilobular, well-defined, very T2 bright heterogeneous mass, which can expand/erode into the adjacent sphenoid sinus without hyperostosis. May show gradual filling enhancement on dynamic contrast imaging.

Skull base

1. **Chordoma**—older males, in midline at sphenooccipital synchondrosis. Well-defined, very T2 bright + septa. Encases vessels without narrowing.
2. **Chondrosarcoma**—osseous erosion with calcified chondroid matrix. Greater risk of ophthalmoplegia (cf. chordoma).
3. **Myeloma/metastases/lymphoma***—lytic/sclerotic lesion with variable soft-tissue component.

13.31 OPTIC NERVE ABNORMAL SIGNAL

The optic nerve has four main segments:

- Intraocular—at the point it emerges through the scleral opening.
- Intraorbital—longest segment, has a surrounding optic nerve sheath (ONS) which contains CSF.
- Intracanalicular—segment in the bony optic canal along with ophthalmic artery; ONS adherent to optic canal.
- Prechiasmatic—intracranial segment in suprasellar cistern.

1. **Optic neuritis**—triad of visual impairment, pain and abnormal colour vision. T2 hyperintensity within optic nerve substance (cf. optic perineuritis).
   (a) **Inflammatory**.
      (i) **MS**—usually unilateral retrobulbar optic neuritis and papillitis with variable enhancement and classical WM lesions in the brain (see Section 13.20).
      (ii) **NMO**—usually bilateral with longer segment abnormal signal and enhancement and clinically more severe visual loss (cf. MS). Fewer intracranial WM lesions.
      (iii) **SLE/sarcoid/Wegener's***—optic perineuritis > neuritis (see later). SLE also associated with acute ischaemic optic neuropathy (abrupt severe visual loss).
   (b) **Infective**—herpes zoster, Lyme disease, syphilis and TB.
   (c) **Post vaccination**—ADEM (see Section 13.20).
   (d) **Radiation-induced.**
2. **Optic perineuritis**—idiopathic, SLE, sarcoid, Wegener's, infective. Characterized by thickening of the ONS ('doughnut' sign) in the

intraorbital segment with surrounding fat stranding and less/no abnormal signal in the optic nerve (cf. optic neuritis).

3. Ischaemic optic neuropathy.
   (a) **Anterior (AION)**—intraocular segment/optic nerve head; associated with papilloedema, suggested by flattening or bulging of the optic nerve head on MRI. Imaging generally not indicated.
      (i) **Arteritic**—due to giant cell/temporal arteritis. >70 years, history of jaw claudication and polymyalgia rheumatica. Greater risk of bilateral involvement. Temporal artery wall thickening + periarterial enhancing fat stranding.
      (ii) **Non-arteritic**—associated with vascular risk factors (hypertension, diabetes mellitus, smoking), >50 years, no optic nerve enhancement.
   (b) **Posterior (PION)**—all segments of optic nerve posterior to intraocular. No papilloedema. Watershed ischaemia due to hypoxia and/or hypovolaemia. Intracanalicular segment most severely affected due to optic nerve swelling and compartment syndrome within bony canal.
4. Traumatic.
   (a) **Direct**—direct nerve disruption, e.g. penetrating injury or fracture fragment (especially in the optic canal).
   (b) **Indirect**—transmitted forces cause shear stress on the nerve. The intracanalicular segment is most susceptible as the ONS at this point is tightly adherent to the periosteum of the optic canal.
5. Neoplastic.
   (a) Optic nerve glioma—rare, typically in children, often with NF1. Intraorbital segment most commonly involved and expanded with central isointense (to WM) signal + perineural high signal due to arachnoidal gliomatosis. Variable enhancement; may extend to optic chiasm ± hypothalamus.
   (b) Optic nerve sheath meningioma—'tram-track' sign: avidly enhancing mass surrounding a nonenhancing optic nerve, ± calcification ± adjacent bony hyperostosis. Adults > children, associated with NF2.
   (c) **Leukaemia/lymphoma***—optic nerve and ONS are important review areas for potential CNS deposits.
6. **Extrinsic compression**—from adjacent lesion in the orbit, orbital apex, optic canal or suprasellar cistern.

13.32 PINEAL REGION MASS

Pineal gland

1. **Pineal cyst**—common incidental finding, well-defined CSF intensity unilocular cyst, often slightly T1 hyperintense with incomplete FLAIR suppression ± slight rim enhancement. Rarely haemorrhagic.
2. **Pineal germ cell tumours**—all tend to 'engulf' normal pineal calcification; associated with CSF seeding.
   (a) **Germinoma (85%)**—children and young adults; homogeneous hyperdense enhancing mass. Presence of pineal calcification in children is suspicious.
   (b) **Others**—e.g. mixed (commonest), teratoma (fat, calcification and cysts), embryonal carcinoma, choriocarcinoma and yolk sac tumour. All heterogeneously enhancing. Elevated αFP and/or ß-hCG, depending on type.
3. **Pineal parenchymal tumours**—tend to disperse ('explode') pineal calcification.
   (a) **Pineocytoma**—typically adults; well-defined noninvasive enhancing mass. May be entirely cystic mimicking a benign pineal cyst; any nodular enhancement is suggestive.
   (b) **Pineoblastoma**—typically children; large, aggressive, locally invasive mass with CSF seeding. Hyperdense on CT (hypercellular), heterogeneous signal with restricted diffusion on MRI. Associated with retinoblastoma.

Cystic

1. **Pineal cyst**—see earlier. Located below internal cerebral veins.
2. **Cavum velum interpositum (CVI)**—enlarged CSF space behind the foramen of Monro, beneath the columns of the fornices and above the internal cerebral veins (cf. pineal cyst).
3. **Cyst of the velum interpositum**—when the CVI is >1 cm in axial dimensions with convex bowed margins and mass effect.

Posterior brainstem

1. **Tectal glioma**—low grade astrocytoma in childhood, expands tectal plate and causes hydrocephalus.
2. **Infarct**—prominent restricted diffusion.
3. **Metastasis**—heterogeneous enhancement + vasogenic oedema.
4. **Demyelination**—NMO (see Section 13.20).

Vascular lesions

1. **Vein of Galen malformation**—presents in neonatal period with high output cardiac failure; dilated median prosencephalic vein, which appears as a large midline posterior vessel.

2. Internal cerebral vein thrombosis—hyperdense vein, loss of normal flow void on MRI, surrounding oedema/infarct ± haemorrhage.

Other

1. Meningioma—displaces pineal calcification rather than engulfing or dispersing it. Homogeneous enhancement ± calcification.

Further reading

Smith, A.B., Rushing, E.J., Smirniotopoulos, J.G., 2010. From the archives of the AFIP: lesions of the pineal region: radiologic–pathologic correlation. Radiographics 30 (7), 2001–2020.

13.33 INTRAVENTRICULAR MASS IN ADULTS

Differential guided by location and origin of lesion. Check for complicating hydrocephalus.

Choroid plexus lesion

Distribution follows location of choroid; lateral > fourth ventricle.

1. Xanthogranuloma—degenerative cyst common in elderly. May be hyperintense on T1, FLAIR and DWI due to protein, lipid and blood products.
2. Cyst—CSF signal.
3. Papilloma—lobulated, frond-like avidly enhancing intraventricular mass with hydrocephalus (either obstructive or due to CSF overproduction).
4. Carcinoma—young children; variable-appearing lesion with heterogeneous enhancement, necrosis, calcification and local parenchymal invasion.
5. Metastasis—renal, melanoma, breast, lymphoma. Local invasion ± additional parenchymal/dural metastases.

Tumours of the ventricular wall

1. Central neurocytoma—young adults. In lateral ventricle, arises from septum pellucidum near foramen of Monro. Hyperdense, calcified and T2 bright bubbly mass with heterogeneous enhancement.
2. Meningioma—usually lateral ventricle. Avidly enhancing mass ± calcification.
3. Ependymoma—rare in adults; see Section 13.11.
4. Subependymoma—elderly, fourth ventricle; see Section 13.11.
5. Subependymal giant cell astrocytoma—young patient with tuberous sclerosis; see Section 13.6.
6. CNS lymphoma*—periventricular hypercellular mass with homogeneous enhancement and restricted diffusion.

Nonchoroid cyst-like lesions

1. Colloid cyst—anterior roof of third ventricle. Well-defined nonenhancing cyst, hyperdense on CT. More likely to be symptomatic if >1 cm.
2. **Ependymal cyst**—often CSF intensity with mass effect.
3. **Neurocysticercosis**—in ventricles or parenchyma; see Part 2.

Others

1. **Intraventricular haemorrhage**—haematomas can form solid casts of the ventricles.
2. **Epidermoid**—CSF-like signal intensity on MRI except for restricted diffusion and incomplete suppression on FLAIR.
3. **Cavernous malformation**—rare; T2 hyperintense, mildly T1 hyperintense globular lesion with blood degradation products on SWI/T2* imaging.

Further reading

Smith, A.B., Smirniotopoulos, J.G., Horkanyne-Szakaly, I., 2013. From the Radiologic Pathology Archives: intraventricular neoplasms: radiologic–pathologic correlation. Radiographics 33 (1), 21–43.

13.34 CEREBELLOPONTINE ANGLE MASS

1. Vestibular schwannoma—ovoid, intracanalicular, heterogeneous T2 bright mass with avid enhancement. Small lesions solid, larger lesions may be cystic and haemorrhagic. Expands internal auditory meatus. Bilateral schwannomas diagnostic for NF2.
2. Meningioma—solid uniformly enhancing mass ± calcification and dural tail.
3. Epidermoid—CSF signal on T1 and T2, incomplete suppression on FLAIR + restricted diffusion. Multilobular lesion, no enhancement.
4. **Ependymoma**—usually plastic-like extension from fourth ventricle, but can be purely in CPA; see Section 13.11.
5. **Arachnoid cyst**—isointense to CSF on all sequences.
6. **Vascular.**
   (a) **Aneurysm**—variable signal depending on degree of thrombosis.
   (b) **Ectasia**—tortuous, dilated vascular flow void.
7. **Other schwannomas.**
   (a) **Trigeminal**—enhancing lesion in Meckel's cave extending into CPA.
   (b) **Facial**—same location as vestibular schwannoma, along the path of CN VII.
8. **Lipoma**—isointense to fat; may encase facial nerve.
9. **Dural/leptomeningeal metastasis.**

10. **Granuloma**—dural sarcoid, TB, and Wegener's.
11. **Neurenteric cyst**—usually prepontine, lobular mass. Slightly denser than CSF, variable signal (proteinaceous material). No enhancement or restricted diffusion.
12. **Paraganglioma**—hypervascular mass extending from jugular foramen with erosive changes in skull base on CT and MRI. Flow voids and foci of blood degradation products give 'salt and pepper' appearance on MRI.

13.35 CORTICAL HYPERINTENSITY ON T2/FLAIR

1. **Cortical ischaemia/infarction**—cortical high T2 signal and restricted diffusion, caused by arterial occlusions or hypoxic/hypotensive episodes (watershed areas).
2. **Encephalitis**.
   (a) **HSV**—mesial temporal lobes ± insula and lateral temporal lobe involvement, haemorrhage common (cf. autoimmune). Fever and rapid course.
   (b) **Autoimmune**—mesial temporal lobes + basal ganglia involvement, haemorrhage rare (cf. HSV). Subacute to gradual onset.
   (c) **Paraneoplastic**—indolent onset, other features of malignancy.
3. **Encephalopathy**—drugs, toxic, metabolic and vasculopathic. Multifocal cortical T2 hyperintensities ± restricted diffusion. Includes hypoglycaemia, PRES and hypertensive encephalopathy.
4. **Post ictal/status epilepticus**—GM or subcortical WM signal change ± restricted diffusion. Rapid onset and quick resolution of imaging findings.
5. **Cortical contusion**—blood degradation products. Typically in orbitofrontal and anterior temporal regions.
6. **Cortical-based tumour**—look for mass effect; see Section 13.10.
7. **Cortical malformations**—e.g. focal cortical dysplasia, cortical tubers; see Section 13.10.
8. **CJD**—gyriform cortical T2 hyperintensity and persistent restricted diffusion. vCJD is also associated with bithalamic abnormal signal ('pulvinar' and 'hockey stick' sign).

13.36 SULCAL FLAIR HYPERINTENSITIES

Hyperintensities on FLAIR sequences can be seen in leptomeningeal and/or CSF pathology. If sulcal FLAIR hyperintensity is localized check adjacent structures for a possible underlying source, e.g. mastoiditis and secondary meningitis.

Changes to CSF content

1. Subarachnoid haemorrhage—hyperdense blood on CT, SWI signal dropout.
2. Ruptured dermoid—fat droplets, high T1 signal.

Meningeal

1. Bacterial meningitis—leptomeningeal enhancement, purulent exudate also shows restricted diffusion; check for ventriculitis.
2. Aseptic meningitis—sarcoid, Wegener's and rheumatoid arthritis.
3. Leptomeningeal carcinomatosis.
   (a) **Primary CNS**—glioblastoma, medulloblastoma, ependymoma.
   (b) **Metastatic**—breast, lung, melanoma, lymphoma, leukaemia.
4. **Meningeal melanomatosis**—rare primary melanocytic tumour of the CNS, associated with cutaneous melanocytic lesions and hydrocephalus; hyperdense leptomeninges with high T1 signal.

Vascular

1. Thrombosis of cortical veins—hyperdense vein and loss of flow void + local cerebral swelling from venous congestion.
2. **Dilated leptomeningeal perforators**—Moyamoya (see Section 13.19).
3. **Slow flow in sulcal arteries**—secondary to stenoses/occlusions.

Artefactual/Iatrogenic

1. **Hyperoxygenation.**
2. **CSF flow and pulsation artefact.**
3. **Recent gadolinium administration**—especially if there is adjacent pathology causing breakdown of the blood-brain barrier.

13.37 CAUSES OF HIGH T1 SIGNAL

1. Fat—e.g. lipid-laden macrophages in cortical laminar necrosis, fat-containing lesions (see Section 13.40).
2. Methaemoglobin—subacute haemorrhage, thrombus and cavernoma.
3. Proteinaceous material—colloid cyst, posterior pituitary (normal), mucinous adenocarcinoma metastases, Rathke's cleft cyst and craniopharyngioma.
4. Gadolinium enhancement—look for normal mucosal and vascular enhancement.
5. Melanin—melanoma metastases, meningeal melanomatosis.
6. Minerals—manganese (hepatic encephalopathy), copper (Wilson's), iron (NBIA).

7. **Calcification**—only with diamagnetic calcium salts (see Section 13.7), especially in Fahr disease.
8. **Flow artefact**—CSF or slow vascular flow.

Further reading

Zimny, A., Zińska, L., Bladowska, J., et al., 2013. Intracranial lesions with high signal intensity on T1-weighted MR images – review of pathologies. Pol. J. Radiol. 78 (4), 36–46.

13.38 CAUSES OF LOW T2 SIGNAL

1. **Turbulent/rapid flow**—vessels, aneurysms, CSF flow. Absent normal vascular flow voids may reflect thrombosis or stenosis.
2. **Air**—paranasal sinuses, mastoid air cells and pneumocephalus.
3. **Cortical bone**.
4. **Metallic prosthesis**.
5. **Haemoglobin breakdown products**—see following table.
6. **Proteinaceous material**—colloid cyst, Rathke's cleft cyst, sinus secretions. T2 signal reduces with increasing protein concentration.
7. **Highly cellular lesions**—medulloblastoma, lymphoma, high grade gliomas.
8. **Minerals**—calcium, copper and iron deposition.
9. **Melanin**—melanoma metastases, meningeal melanomatosis.
10. **Fungal hyphae**—invasive fungal sinusitis.
11. **Gadolinium**—causes T2 relaxation. Applied in dynamic susceptibility contrast enhanced perfusion imaging.

MRI signal characteristics of haemorrhage

Phase of bleeding (days)	Haemoglobin breakdown products	T1 signal	T2 signal
Hyperacute (<1)	Oxyhaemoglobin	Low/iso	High
Acute (1–3)	Deoxyhaemoglobin	Low/iso	**Low**
Early subacute (3–7)	Intracellular methaemoglobin	**High**	**Low**
Late subacute (7–14)	Extracellular methaemoglobin	**High**	High
Chronic (>14)	Hemosiderin	Low	**Low**

Further reading

Zimny, A., Neska-Matuszewska, M., Bladowska, J., Sąsiadek, M.J., 2015. Intracranial lesions with low signal intensity on T2-weighted MR images – review of pathologies. Pol. J. Radiol. 80, 40–50.

13.39 CAUSES OF RESTRICTED DIFFUSION

Cortical/subcortical

1. Hypoxic-ischaemic
   (a) **Acute cerebral infarction**—variable distribution: vascular territorial, watershed and lacunar patterns. Causes: thrombotic, embolic or vasculitic.
   (b) **Hypoxic ischaemic injury**—due to global hypoperfusion or hypoxia, e.g. cardiac arrest and drowning. Watershed and DGM infarcts.
2. Post ictal—cortex and hippocampi.
3. PRES—parietooccipital and superior frontal gyri.
4. **Encephalitis/cerebritis**—see Section 13.35.
5. **DAI**—GWMJ, splenium and middle cerebellar peduncles + microhaemorrhages.
6. **Hypoglycaemia**—bioccipital and splenium.
7. **CJD**—insula and pulvinar (see Section 13.35).
8. **MR artefact**—due to susceptibility artefact; affects cortex close to skull, paranasal sinuses and mastoid air cells.

Focal lesion

1. Infection.
   (a) **Abscess**—ring-enhancing, 'dual rim' sign on SWI and T2 (hypointense outer rim and hyperintense inner rim).
   (b) **Empyema**—extraaxial collection + rim enhancement.
   (c) **Ventriculitis**—pus dependent in ventricles (occipital horns).
2. **Hypercellular neoplasms**.
   (a) **Lymphoma***—periventricular, homogeneous enhancement.
   (b) **Medulloblastoma**—fourth ventricle/cerebellum, in children.
   (c) **Germinoma**—children/young adults. Avid enhancement, midline.
   (d) **Glioblastoma**—high grade components show restricted diffusion.
3. **Acute demyelination**—active lesions only; restricted diffusion typically conforms to the incomplete ring enhancement.
4. **Epidermoid**—lobular, insinuating cisternal lesion. Restricted diffusion is the main feature differentiating this from arachnoid cyst.
5. **Mucoid degeneration**—e.g. choroid plexus cyst, Rathke's cleft cyst.
6. **Haemorrhage/haematoma**—blood degradation products induce signal changes on DWI due to susceptibility effect.
7. **Osmotic myelinolysis**—central pons.

13.40 FAT-CONTAINING INTRACRANIAL LESIONS

1. Lipoma—interhemispheric fissure (± callosal dysgenesis) > suprasellar > pineal region > CPA.
2. Dermoid cyst—midline fatty mass with chemical shift artefact ± calcification. Can rupture causing chemical meningitis.
3. Teratoma—midline multiloculated cystic mass with fat, soft-tissue and calcified components.
4. Postsurgical fat plugs—e.g. following pituitary surgery.
5. **White epidermoids**—rare variant containing triglycerides causing T1 hyperintensity (normally CSF signal). Restricts diffusion (cf. dermoid).
6. **Lipomatous degeneration of tumours**—rare, has been reported in meningiomas and small round blue cell tumours, e.g. medulloblastoma.

13.41 CYST-LIKE POSTERIOR FOSSA LESIONS

1. Mega cisterna magna—enlarged retrocerebellar CSF space communicating with fourth ventricle and basal CSF spaces. Normal vermis, cerebellum and fourth ventricle.
2. Dandy-Walker spectrum—variable hypoplasia of vermis, cystic dilatation of fourth ventricle (displacing cerebellar hemispheres anterolaterally) ± enlarged posterior fossa with torcula-lambdoid inversion (torcula above lambdoid suture). If all features are present, it is termed a Dandy-Walker malformation.
3. Blake's pouch cyst—posterior diverticulum of the fourth ventricle due to failed opening of the foramen of Magendie in utero, resulting in hydrocephalus of all four ventricles. Cyst communicates with fourth ventricle but not with cisterna magna. Vermis is of normal size but is displaced superiorly.
4. Arachnoid cyst—CSF signal + mass effect on vermis, which is of normal size. Hydrocephalus is rare.
5. Epidermoid cyst—restricted diffusion and incomplete suppression on FLAIR.
6. Pilocytic astrocytoma—in children; cystic cerebellar mass + enhancing mural nodule and walls.
7. Cerebellar hemangioblastoma—in adults; cystic cerebellar mass + enhancing mural nodule, but no wall enhancement. Surrounding abnormal vessels.
8. **Trapped fourth ventricle**—secondary to haemorrhage or ventriculitis. Typically noted after persistent fourth ventricular dilatation despite successful shunting of lateral ventricles. Associated with diplopia and ataxia.

9. **Neuroglial/neurenteric cyst**—CSF signal parenchymal cyst. No enhancement or restricted diffusion.
10. **Neurocysticercosis**—most commonly in fourth ventricle; can cause obstructive hydrocephalus (see Part 2).

13.42 CEREBRAL VOLUME LOSS

Generalized

1. Normal ageing—0.5% total brain volume loss per year is normal, >1.0% is likely abnormal.
2. Cerebrovascular disease—background of small-vessel disease (see Section 13.20).
3. Drugs.
   (a) Alcohol—additional cerebellar vermian atrophy.
   (b) **Steroids**—short use: transient reduced volume, which recovers. Chronic use: irreversible volume loss.
4. **Postinflammatory**—MS and other inflammatory WM diseases; lesions with WM volume loss and variable cavitation related to chronic lesions (see Section 13.20).
5. **Posttraumatic**—if severe and especially if widespread DAI.
6. **Whole brain radiotherapy**—can also be regional if radiotherapy is confined; ± coexistent radiotherapy-induced meningiomas and cavernomas (see Section 13.20).
7. **HIV encephalopathy**—diffuse symmetric periventricular abnormal WM signal and volume loss.

Focal

1. Postinfarction—wedge-shaped cortical and subcortical volume loss, limited to vascular territory.
2. Posttraumatic—contusion or haematom in typical locations (orbitofrontal and anterior temporal regions).
3. **Postinfective**—encephalitis and meningitis.

Regional pattern

1. Alzheimer's disease.
   (a) **Classical**—old age onset (70–80s), memory impairment with hippocampal and temporoparietal atrophy.
   (b) **Posterior cortical atrophy**—usually younger age onset (50–60s). Visual agnosia and apraxia with occipitoparietal volume loss.
2. Parkinson disease—tremor, rigidity, bradykinesia ± dementia. NB: in dementia with Lewy bodies, cognitive decline and visual hallucinations precede parkinsonism. Generalized cerebral atrophy and atrophy of substantia nigra with relative sparing of hippocampi. Increased putaminal iron (reduced T2 signal).

Loss of normal 'swallowtail' appearance of substantia nigra on SWI.

3. Frontotemporal lobar degeneration—inappropriate behaviour and apathy with frontotemporal atrophy.
4. **Progressive supranuclear palsy**—reduced cognition, supranuclear vertical gaze palsy. Reduced area of midbrain relative to pons in sagittal plane. Midbrain has 'mickey mouse' appearance on axial and 'hummingbird' sign on sagittal imaging (the latter is subjective and of limited utility).
5. **Corticobasal degeneration**—apraxia and dystonia. Asymmetric atrophy of superior parietal lobules and paracentral gyri.
6. **MSA-P**—reduced putamen volume with reduced T2 signal relative to GP. High T2 rim surrounding putamen ('putaminal rim sign').
7. **Huntington's disease**—autosomal dominant, progressive choreoathetoid movements with atrophy of caudate heads.
8. **Post encephalitis**—chronic volume loss in regions affected, e.g. mesial temporal lobes in both HSV and autoimmune limbic encephalitis.

Further reading

Murray, A.D., 2012. Imaging approaches for dementia. AJNR Am. J. Neuroradiol. 33, 1836–1844.

Vernooij, M.W., Smits, M., 2012. Structural neuroimaging in aging and Alzheimer's disease. Neuroimaging Clin. N. Am. 22 (1), 33–55.

13.43 CEREBELLAR VOLUME LOSS

1. Normal ageing.
2. Chronic alcoholism.
3. Drugs—phenytoin, chemotherapy, lithium, benzodiazepines.
4. Chronic vertebrobasilar ischaemia/insufficiency—posterior circulation steno-occlusive disease with multiple infarcts.
5. **Chronic temporal lobe epilepsy**—independent of antiseizure medication.
6. **Cerebellitis**—in children, post infection/vaccination. Acute: generalized cerebellar swelling with cortical T2 hyperintensity + obstructive hydrocephalus. Chronic: generalized cerebellar volume loss.
7. **MSA-C**—'hot cross bun' sign in pons; see Section 13.26.
8. **Olivopontocerebellar atrophy**—atrophy of olivary nuclei and cerebellar peduncles, associated with MSA-C.
9. **Superficial siderosis**—recurrent SAH with haemosiderin depositions associated with deafness and ataxia. Susceptibility-related signal dropout lining cerebellar folia, best seen on SWI.
10. **Post radiation therapy.**

11. **Inherited ataxias.**
    (a) **Friedreich ataxia**—AR, adolescent onset. Dorsal cervical cord volume loss + hypertrophic cardiomyopathy.
    (b) **Ataxia telangiectasia**—AR; multiple telangiectasia, ataxia and lung infections. Vermian volume loss and cerebral WM T2 hyperintensities.
    (c) **Spinocerebellar ataxia syndromes**—wide range of inherited syndromes characterized by atrophy of the spinal cord and cerebellum.
12. **Paraneoplastic cerebellar degeneration**—lung, breast and ovarian cancer.
13. **Gluten ataxia**—gluten sensitivity, improves with gluten-free diet.
14. **Crossed cerebellar diaschisis**—unilateral, due to contralateral supratentorial gliosis.

13.44 BRAINSTEM ATROPHY

Diffuse

1. Radiotherapy.
2. Inflammatory.
    (a) MS—midbrain/pons > medulla.
    (b) NMO—medulla > midbrain/pons.
    (c) **Behçet's***—oedematous lesions + perivascular enhancement.
3. Wallerian degeneration—atrophy and signal change downstream of a supratentorial lesion (e.g. infarct, haemorrhage, demyelination). Diffuse or focal depending on extent of insult.
4. **Infectious rhombencephalitis**—encephalitis of the hindbrain (brainstem and cerebellum), e.g. by *Listeria* or enterovirus. Acute: swollen with enhancing WM lesions and cranial nerve enhancement. Chronic: generalized volume loss.
5. **Infarction.**
6. **Spinocerebellar ataxia**—see Section 13.43.
7. **Inherited leukoencephalopathies**—rare, child/young adult onset.

Regional

1. **Midbrain**—progressive supranuclear palsy, Wilson's disease.
2. **Pons**—MSA-C.
3. **Medulla**—hypertrophic olivary degeneration (late feature), adult onset Alexander's disease.

13.45 SKULL VAULT LUCENCY WITHOUT SCLEROTIC EDGE

Normal

1. **Parietal foramina**—usually bilateral and symmetrical, anterior to lambdoid suture. If enlarged (>5 mm) then may be linked to genetic syndromes and other intracranial anomalies.
2. **Normal ageing calvarium**.
3. **Fontanelle**—anterior (closes <18 months), posterior (closes <3 months), anterolateral ×2, posterolateral ×2.

Neoplastic (adults)

1. **Myeloma**—multiple lytic lesions (pepper pot skull); can involve mandible (where metastases are very rare).
2. **Metastases**—e.g. lung, breast, renal, thyroid and leukaemia.
3. **Paget's sarcoma**—osteosarcoma, chondrosarcoma, fibrosarcoma. Lytic, blastic or mixed lesion with cortical destruction and soft-tissue component on a background of Paget's disease. Usually little/no periosteal reaction; suspect in an area of Paget's that has undergone rapid change on serial imaging.

Neoplastic (children)

1. **Metastases**—neuroblastoma, leukaemia and sarcoma.
2. **Langerhans cell histiocytosis***—especially parietal bone; may be an isolated well-defined lesion with a beveled edge due to unequal involvement of inner and outer tables (also known as eosinophilic granuloma), or multiple coalescent lesions with a geographic appearance (LCH). May contain central sequestrum of residual bone. Enhances avidly.

Traumatic

1. **Fracture**—easy to mistake for normal suture. If involving suture, check for diastasis.
2. **Leptomeningeal cyst**—also known as growing fracture. Skull fracture with trapped meninges; CSF pulsation causes progressive widening and scalloping. Usually in young children.
3. **Burr hole**—typically a perfect circle, often frontal or parietal location, ± evidence of gliosis in the subjacent brain parenchyma.

Metabolic

1. **Osteoporosis**—generalized reduced bone density most appreciable on CT. Vertebral insufficiency fractures common.
2. **Hyperparathyroidism***—multiple foci of lucency and sclerosis ('salt and pepper' skull) ± a discrete brown tumour: expansile lytic

lesion, which causes cortical thinning without cortical destruction or periosteal reaction, ± fluid-fluid levels on MRI.

Infective

1. **Acute pyogenic osteomyelitis**—from sinusitis (frontal bones), mastoiditis (temporal bones), penetrating head trauma or postsurgical. Look for cortical breach of the inner table to suggest intracranial involvement. Complications: intracranial empyema, abscess, meningitis, cerebritis, venous thrombophlebitis (especially with mastoiditis extending into sigmoid sinus).
2. **TB***—rare, punched-out lesion with sequestrum + an overlying soft-tissue component.
3. **Hydatid cyst**—expansile loculated lesion centered in the diploic space.
4. **Syphilis***—moth-eaten appearance.

Vascular

1. **Haemangioma**—expansile lesion with 'sunburst' pattern of radiating spicules, avid enhancement.
2. **Sinus pericranii**—congenital, traumatic or spontaneous venous malformation of the scalp characterized by an abnormally enlarged skull emissary vein, which connects the dural venous sinuses and extracranial veins. Soft tissue mass + an underlying serpiginous vascular channel in the skull.

Others

1. **Osteoporosis circumscripta**—lytic phase of Paget's disease; usually a large, well-defined lytic lesion most commonly in the inferior frontal or occipital bones (rarer at vertex); can cross sutures, ± separate regions of sclerosis reflecting later stage of Paget's.
2. **Neurofibroma**—can be secondary to both mesodermal dysplasia and skull erosion by an adjacent neurofibroma.
3. **Intradiploic arachnoid cyst**—very rare, CSF density/signal.

13.46 SKULL VAULT LUCENCY WITH SCLEROTIC EDGE

Normal

1. **Venous channels**—transcalvarial serpiginous channels containing emissary veins connecting venous sinuses to extracranial veins.
2. **Venous lakes**—enlarged veins with a round or ovoid morphology, avid enhancement post contrast. Often connect to venous channels.

3. <u>Arachnoid granulations</u>—arachnoid projections into skull; round, well-defined lucencies often in region of venous sinuses with disruption of inner table. CSF signal on MRI. Generally a normal variant but if multiple consider chronically raised ICP.

Developmental

1. <u>Epidermoid</u>—intradiploic rare; well-defined, scalloped margins, similar to CSF on T1/T2 but with restricted diffusion and incomplete FLAIR suppression.
2. <u>Meningocoele/encephalocoele</u>—protrusion of meninges ± brain through skull defect. Can be congenital, following trauma/surgery or related to chronically raised ICP.

Neoplastic

1. <u>Langerhans cell histiocytosis</u>*—in healing phase; see Section 13.45.
2. <u>Treated lytic metastasis</u>—see Section 13.45.

Infective

1. <u>Chronic osteomyelitis</u>—staphylococci, pseudomonas and fungal. Same locations and risks as acute osteomyelitis (see Section 13.45). Greater association with soft-tissue masses and dural thickening.
2. **Frontal sinus mucocoele**—completely opacified and expanded frontal sinus containing mucus with variable signal due to protein content. Thinning of sinus walls with variable resorption.

Others

1. <u>Fibrous dysplasia</u>—variable appearance, commonly exhibits a ground-glass matrix but can be an entirely lytic, expanded, well-defined lesion with preserved overlying bone. Monostotic > polyostotic.

13.47 GENERALIZED INCREASE IN SKULL VAULT DENSITY

1. <u>Paget's disease</u>*—in the elderly. Multiple islands of dense bone, loss of clarity of inner and outer tables, thickened skull vault, ± basilar impression.
2. <u>Sclerotic metastases</u>—breast (especially post treatment), prostate.
3. <u>Fibrous dysplasia</u>—younger age group than Paget's; see Section 13.46.
4. <u>Myelofibrosis</u>—diffuse sclerosis without architectural distortion. Associated with extramedullary haematopoiesis, intracranially this may be indicated by dural thickening.
5. <u>Renal osteodystrophy</u>*—osteosclerosis in 25%; mimics Paget's.

6. Acromegaly*—enlarged frontal sinuses, prognathism and thickened skull vault, ± an enlarged sella due to the underlying pituitary adenoma.
7. Chronic haemolytic anaemias—expansion of medullary spaces due to red marrow hyperplasia causing 'hair-on-end' appearance (see Section 13.51); variable sclerosis also related to hyperplastic red marrow (as opposed to bone infarcts).
8. **Sclerosing bone dysplasia.**
   (a) **Osteopetrosis**—infantile (AR) and adult (AD) forms. Infantile form more severe with life expectancy <10 years. Diffusely sclerotic and thickened skeleton with fractures. Associated with narrowing of skull foramina with compression of traversing CNs and vessels. Orbital crowding + proptosis. Poorly pneumatized paranasal sinuses.
   (b) **Pyknodysostosis**—especially skull base; multiple wormian bones, wide sutures from delayed closure, frontoparietal bossing.
   (c) **Craniometaphyseal dysplasia**—diffusely thickened skull with compromise of foramina (like osteopetrosis), flared metaphyses in long bones.
9. **Prolonged phenytoin treatment**—skull thickening and osteosclerosis + cerebellar volume loss (see Section 13.43).
10. **Fluorosis**—due to excessive fluoride ingestion. Osteosclerosis and ossification of tendons/ligaments.

13.48 LOCALIZED INCREASE IN SKULL VAULT DENSITY

Within bone

1. Hyperostosis frontalis interna—older females; benign symmetrical overgrowth of the inner table of the frontal bone, often lobulated. Can involve other skull bones and be diffuse.
2. Tumour.
   (a) Sclerotic metastasis—prostate (men), breast (women) and neuroblastoma (children).
   (b) Osteoma—benign well-defined bone lesion. Two main types: ivory (homogeneously very dense) and mature (has central marrow). Also commonly seen in paranasal sinuses (associated with Gardner syndrome).
   (c) Treated lytic metastasis.
   (d) **Treated brown tumour of hyperparathyroidism***.
3. Paget's disease*—see Section 13.45.
4. Fibrous dysplasia—see Section 13.46.
5. **Depressed fracture**—abrupt cortical irregularity and depression.

Adjacent to bone

1. Meningioma—hyperostosis of adjacent bone is common and usually reactive, though occasionally associated with osseous invasion (look for abnormal enhancement extending into the skull).
2. **Calcified cephalohaematoma**—infants with history of traumatic birth. Well-defined peripherally calcified crescentic lesion overlying outer table of skull.
3. **Calcified epidermoid cyst**—usually still contains more typical cystic components (see Section 13.46).

13.49 THICKENED SKULL

Overlap with sclerotic/hyperostotic processes (see Sections 13.47 and 13.48).

Generalized

1. Normal variant.
2. Prolonged phenytoin treatment.
3. Acromegaly*.
4. Chronic haemolytic anaemia—see Section 13.51.
5. **Microcephaly**.
6. **Shunted hydrocephalus**—secondary to chronic low ICP.

Focal

1. Normal variant—including hyperostosis frontalis interna.
2. Paget's disease*.
3. Fibrous dysplasia.
4. Meningioma—due to reactive hyperostosis or osseous invasion.
5. Osteoma.
6. Sclerotic metastasis—prostate.

13.50 THIN SKULL

Generalized

1. Hyperparathyroidism*—see Section 13.45.
2. Chronically raised intracranial pressure—other signs of raised ICP, e.g. 'empty sella', multiple arachnoid herniations, hydrocephalus. May produce a 'copper-beaten skull' appearance.
3. **Osteogenesis imperfecta**—associated with wormian bones. Characteristic features: osteoporosis, fractures, blue sclera, dental fragility and hearing impairment.
4. **Rickets***—frontal bossing, delayed fusion of cranial sutures and closure of fontanelles.

5. **Hypophosphatasia**—rare metabolic deficiency of alkaline phosphatase, variable severity and age of presentation. Generalized osteoporosis and premature fusion of cranial sutures.
6. **Lacunar skull**—bone dysplasia of membranous skull, associated with Chiari 2 malformation. Indentations or pits in frontal and parietal regions that may be full-thickness; defects separated by thin rims of bone; usually resolves by 6 months. Not associated with raised ICP.

Focal

1. **Normal variant**.
2. **Osteoporosis circumscripta**—see Section 13.45.
3. **Large intracranial cyst**—arachnoid, porencephalic. Causes bony remodelling with smooth, scalloped thinning of the adjacent skull.
4. **Slow-growing tumour in cerebral cortex**—DNET, ganglioglioma. Also associated with gradual bony remodelling.

13.51 'HAIR-ON-END' SKULL VAULT

Appearance of thickened trabeculae in expanded diploic space.

Haemolytic anaemias

All related to red marrow hyperplasia. Dural extramedullary hematopoiesis may also be present.

1. **Thalassaemia***—marrow hyperplasia more marked in this than other anaemias.
2. **Sickle cell anaemia**—initially in frontal region but can involve the whole skull where diploic space (marrow cavity) is present, i.e. above level of internal occipital protuberance.
3. **Hereditary spherocytosis and elliptocytosis.**
4. **Pyruvate kinase deficiency.**
5. **Glucose-6-phosphate dehydrogenase deficiency.**

Other causes of red marrow hyperplasia

1. **Cyanotic heart disease.**
2. **Severe childhood iron deficiency anaemia.**

Neoplastic

Usually more focal than red marrow hyperplasia.

1. **Haemangioma***—'sunburst' spicules; see Section 13.45.
2. **Meningioma**—more suggestive of skull invasion rather than reactive thickening; look for abnormal skull enhancement to support this. Also seen in primary intraosseous meningioma (see Section 13.54).
3. **Metastases.**

13.52 PLATYBASIA AND BASILAR INVAGINATION/IMPRESSION

Platybasia: abnormal asymptomatic flattening of skull base, basal angle >143 degrees.

Basilar invagination: dens telescopes through normal FM.

Basilar impression: dens telescopes through abnormal FM due to bone softening or destruction.

Both basilar invagination and impression are associated with symptoms of spinal cord/brainstem compression ± hydrocephalus.

Congenital

1. **Achondroplasia***—rhizomelic dwarfism.
2. **Chiari malformations.**
   (a) **Chiari 1**—peg-shaped cerebellar tonsils extending >5 mm below FM (excluding those caused by raised ICP) ± syrinx ± hydrocephalus.
   (b) **Chiari 2**—medulla, fourth ventricle and cerebellar vermis displaced through FM; small posterior fossa, beaked tectum. Nearly always associated with a lumbar myelomeningocoele.
   (c) **Chiari 3**—like Chiari 2 but with occipital encephalocoele.
3. **Osteogenesis imperfecta**—wormian bones.

Acquired

1. **Rheumatoid arthritis***—ligamentous softening, erosion of dens and atlantoaxial subluxation.
2. **Paget's**—bone softening (see Section 13.45).
3. **Osteomalacia**—bone softening.
4. **Hyperparathyroidism***—bone softening.
5. **Localized bone destruction**—lytic metastases and destructive infection (e.g. TB).

13.53 J-SHAPED SELLA

Flattened tuberculum sellae with a prominent sulcus chiasmaticus.

1. **Normal variant.**
2. **Optic chiasm glioma**—if chiasmatic sulcus very depressed (W- or omega-shaped sella), glioma may be bilateral.
3. **Neurofibromatosis***.
4. **Achondroplasia***.
5. **Mucopolysaccharidoses***.
6. **Chronic hydrocephalus**—enlarged anterior aspect of third ventricle causes remodelling of sella.

13.54 SCALP MASS

Skin

These all arise from and contact the skin on imaging.

1. **Epidermal inclusion cyst**—also known as 'sebaceous' cyst (misnomer as they do not arise from sebaceous glands). Well-defined, usually of homogeneous fluid density on CT ± calcification. Commonly seen on the scalp, face and neck. If multiple, consider Gardner syndrome.
2. **Trichilemmal cyst**—also known as pilar cyst, originates from hair follicle so common on the scalp. Similar in appearance to epidermal inclusion cyst but calcifies more frequently.
3. **Skin tags**—pedunculated mass arising from skin; normal subcutaneous layer.
4. **Carcinoma**—squamous and basal cell, melanoma. Infiltrating, ulcerating soft-tissue mass with variable enhancement. Gorlin-Goltz syndrome: multiple BCCs and odontogenic keratocysts.
5. **Skin calcification**—associated with acne.

Subcutaneous tissue

1. **Lipoma**—encapsulated fatty mass, often does not contact skin. If internal soft-tissue component, multiple septations or large (>5 cm) then consider liposarcoma.
2. **Haemangioma**—early infancy, rapidly grow then involute before adolescence. High T2 signal, avid enhancement and intrinsic flow voids.

Subgaleal plane

1. **Subgaleal haematoma**—post trauma in adults or children; crescentic haematoma beneath galeal aponeurosis but superficial to periosteum, not confined by cranial sutures.
2. **Cephalohaematoma**—following birth trauma; subperiosteal lentiform haematoma confined by cranial sutures. Parietal region most common.
3. **Dermoid**—most commonly midline, associated with sinus tracts. Fat density mass ± remodelling of underlying skull.
4. **Plexiform neurofibroma**—diagnostic of NF1. Thickening of the nerve sheath across multiple fascicles. Diffuse soft-tissue mass with a branching appearance. High T2 signal with central low signal ('target' sign). 10% undergo sarcomatous degeneration.
5. **Cirsoid aneurysm**—rare AVM of scalp usually fed by the superficial temporal artery.

Bone lesions

1. **Osteoma**—dense bone lesion projecting out from skull with no effect on diploic space.

2. **Malignancy**—metastasis (lytic or sclerotic), plasmacytoma (expansile and lytic), lymphoma (soft-tissue mass often on both sides of skull with relatively little bone destruction), sarcoma.
3. **Pott's puffy tumour**—subperiosteal abscess from frontal bone osteomyelitis secondary to frontal sinusitis or trauma. Opacified frontal sinus with overlying subperiosteal collection and inflammatory stranding.
4. **Haemangioma**—frontal and parietal bones, outer table involved with sparing of inner table, high T1 and T2 signal + flow voids.
5. **Intraosseous meningioma**—expands inner and outer tables of skull, dural component not always present.
6. **Intraosseous epidermoid**—fluid density with variable calcification on CT, high T2 signal and characteristic restricted diffusion.
7. **Encephalocoele**—defect in the skull and dura with extracranial herniation of intracranial structures. Directly related to trauma/surgery or secondary to chronic raised ICP.
8. **Sinus pericranii**—see Section 13.45.
9. **Paget's disease***—skull thickening with expansion of the diploic space and variable sclerosis and lysis.

Paediatrics

Musa Kaleem, Susan Shelmerdine, Thomas Semple

14.1 RETARDED SKELETAL MATURATION

Chronic ill-health

1. **Congenital heart disease**—particularly cyanotic.
2. **Renal failure.**
3. **Inflammatory bowel disease*.**
4. **Malnutrition.**
5. **Rickets*.**
6. **Maternal deprivation.**

Endocrine disorders

1. **Hypothyroidism**—severe retardation (≥5 standard deviations below the mean) with granular, fragmented epiphyses.
2. **Steroid therapy/Cushing's disease**—see Part 2.
3. **Hypogonadism**—including older patients with Turner syndrome.
4. **Hypopituitarism**—panhypopituitarism, growth hormone deficiency and Laron dwarfism (insensitivity to growth hormone).

Congenital disorders

1. **Chromosome disorders**—e.g. trisomy 21, trisomy 18 (severe), Turner syndrome.
2. **Skeletal dysplasias involving the epiphyses**—e.g. multiple epiphyseal dysplasia, pseudoachondroplasia, diaphyseal dysplasia, metatropic dysplasia.

14.2 GENERALIZED ACCELERATED SKELETAL MATURATION

In general, children that display accelerated early skeletal growth will also display earlier closures of their physes and reduced resultant final height.

Endocrine disorders

1. **Idiopathic precocious puberty.**
2. **Hypothalamic dysfunction**—e.g. due to mass lesions (hamartoma, astrocytoma, craniopharyngioma, optic chiasm glioma), hydrocephalus or encephalitis.
3. **Adrenal and gonadal tumours**—e.g. androgen-producing neoplasms.
4. **Hyperthyroidism.**

Congenital disorders

1. **McCune-Albright syndrome**—polyostotic fibrous dysplasia + precocious puberty.
2. **Cerebral gigantism (Sotos syndrome).**
3. **Lipodystrophy.**
4. **Pseudohypoparathyroidism***—premature fusion of cone-shaped epiphyses.
5. **Acrodysostosis**—premature fusion of cone-shaped epiphyses.

Others

1. **Large or obese children.**
2. **Familial tall stature.**

Further reading

Fahmy, J.L., Kaminsky, C.K., Kaufman, F., et al., 2000. The radiological approach to precocious puberty. Br. J. Radiol. 73 (869), 560–567.

Martin, D.D., Wit, J.M., Hochberg, Z., et al., 2011. The use of bone age in clinical practice – Part 1. Horm. Res. Paediatr. 76 (1), 1–9.

Martin, D.D., Wit, J.M., Hochberg, Z., et al., 2011. The use of bone age in clinical practice – Part 2. Horm. Res. Paediatr. 76 (1), 10–16.

14.3 PREMATURE CLOSURE OF A GROWTH PLATE

1. <u>Local hyperaemia</u>—juvenile idiopathic arthritides, infection, haemophilia or arteriovenous malformation.
2. <u>Trauma</u>—especially Salter-Harris fractures.
3. <u>Vascular occlusion</u>—postmeningococcal septicaemia, infarcts and sickle cell anaemia.
4. <u>Radiotherapy</u>.
5. **Thermal injury**—burns, frostbite.
6. **Multiple exostoses or enchondromatosis.**
7. **Hypervitaminosis A**—now more commonly via vitamin A analogue treatment for dermatological conditions rather than dietary overdosage.
8. **Skeletal dysplasias**—e.g. Albright's hereditary osteodystrophy, acrodysostosis, acromesomelic dysplasia (Maroteaux type) and

trichorhinophalangeal syndrome; all with premature fusion of cone-shaped epiphyses in the hand.

9. **Iatrogenic**—for leg length discrepancies surgical epiphysiodesis can be performed to artificially fuse or slow the growth of a normal leg to allow the shorter leg to grow.

Further reading

Piddo, C., Reed, M.H., Black, G.B., 2000. Premature epiphyseal fusion and degenerative arthritis in chronic recurrent multifocal osteomyelitis. Skeletal Radiol. 29 (2), 94–96.

14.4 ASYMMETRICAL MATURATION

NB: normal children may have minor asymmetry.

Hemihypertrophy or localized gigantism

1. **Vascular anomalies**.
   (a) **Parkes-Weber syndrome**—fast-flow vascular malformations with arteriovenous shunting, port-wine stain and limb overgrowth.
   (b) **Klippel-Trénaunay syndrome***—triad of anomalous veins (varicosities or slow-flow malformations), port-wine stain and limb overgrowth.
   (c) **Capillary malformation (port-wine stain)**—associated with congenital hypertrophy.
2. **Chronic hyperaemia**—e.g. juvenile idiopathic arthritides and haemophilia.
3. **Hemihypertrophy**—M>F; R>L. May be a presenting feature of Beckwith-Wiedemann syndrome (hemihypertrophy, macroglossia, hypoglycaemia and umbilical hernia). Increased risk of Wilms tumour.
4. **Neurofibromatosis* (NF1)**.
5. **Macrodystrophia lipomatosa**—bony and fatty overgrowth of one or more digits.
6. **Russell-Silver dwarfism**—evident from birth. Triangular face with down-turned corners of the mouth, frontal bossing, asymmetrical growth and skeletal maturation.
7. **Proteus syndrome**—hamartomatous disorder with multiple and varied manifestations including vascular and lymphatic malformations, macrocephaly and cranial hyperostosis.
8. **WAGR syndrome**—Wilms tumour, aniridia, genitourinary anomalies and mental retardation.

Hemiatrophy or localized atrophy

1. **Paralysis**—with osteopenia and overtubulation of long bones.
2. **Radiation treatment in childhood**.
3. **Pure venous malformation involving skin, muscle and bone.**

Further reading

Enjolras, O., Chapot, R., Merland, J.J., 2004. Vascular anomalies and the growth of limbs: a review. J. Pediatr. Orthop. B 13 (6), 349–357.

14.5 SKELETAL DYSPLASIAS

With predominant metaphyseal involvement

1. Achondroplasia*—see Part 2. NB: hypochondroplasia is due to mutations in the same gene, fibroblast growth factor receptor 3, with milder features.
2. **Metaphyseal chondrodysplasias.**
   (a) **Jansen**—severe rickets-like changes with short stature.
   (b) **Schmid**—milder than Jansen. Bowed legs.
   (c) **McKusick**—immune deficiency and haematological problems.
   (d) **Shwachman-Diamond**—with pancreatic insufficiency and neutropenia.
   (e) **Hypophosphatasia**—severe forms are lethal. V-shaped metaphyseal defects. Diaphyseal spurs.
   (f) **Jeune's asphyxiating thoracic dystrophy**—short ribs with irregular costochondral junctions, renal cysts and short hands.
   (g) **Ellis-van Creveld syndrome**—short ribs with congenital heart disease and polydactyly.

With predominant epiphyseal involvement

1. **Multiple epiphyseal dysplasia**—irregular epiphyseal ossification. Epiphyses may be small and round or flat, depending on type. Normal metaphyses, mild spine changes, mild short stature.
2. **Pseudoachondroplasia**—more severe epiphyseal dysplasia with short stature; proportions resemble achondroplasia but with a normal face. Spinal radiographic changes, but usually preserved spinal height.
3. **Diastrophic dysplasia**—flattened epiphyses with joint contractures (e.g. club feet) and kyphoscoliosis. Cauliflower ear in infancy. Hypoplastic proximally placed 'hitch-hiker's' thumb is characteristic.

Mesomelic dysplasias (short forearms ± shanks)

1. **Dyschondrosteosis (Leri-Weill)**—short radius + Madelung deformity and dorsal subluxation of distal ulna.
2. **Langer mesomelic dysplasia**—more severe mesomelic shortening.
3. **Acromesomelic dysplasia (Maroteaux type)**—short upper limbs with shortening more severe from distal to proximal. Associated spinal abnormalities.

Acromelic dysplasias (short hands and feet)

1. Pseudo- and pseudopseudo-hypoparathyroidism—metacarpal ± phalangeal shortening. Soft-tissue/basal ganglia calcifications and exostoses in some.
2. **Brachydactyly types A–E**—abnormal hands and feet only.
3. **Acrodysostosis**—very short metacarpals and phalanges with cone epiphyses. Similar to acromesomelic dysplasia on imaging.
4. **Trichorhinophalangeal syndrome**—multiple short phalanges with cone epiphyses. Sparse hair and typical facial appearances. Type 2 associated with exostoses.

Dysplasias with major involvement of the spine

1. **Type 2 collagen disorders**—includes spondyloepiphyseal dysplasia congenita, Kniest and Stickler type 1. Delayed appearance of epiphyseal ossification centres with progressive platyspondyly and spinal deformity. Associated ear and eye problems and micrognathia in many. Hands and feet near normal.
2. **Metatropic dysplasia**—'changing form'. In infancy manifests as short-limbed dysplasia, evolving into short spine dysplasia over childhood. Epiphyseal ossification delay with marked metaphyseal flare. Characteristic pattern of platyspondyly with wide flat vertebral bodies. Some patients have a tail. Spondylometaphyseal dysplasia (Kozlowski type) is a milder form.

14.6 LETHAL NEONATAL DYSPLASIA

1. Thanatophoric dysplasia—short ribs; severe platyspondyly with wafer-thin vertebral bodies; small square iliac wings; severe limb shortening. Curved femora and humeri ('telephone handle') in type 1; craniosynostosis in type 2.
2. Osteogenesis imperfecta type 2—deficient skull ossification; numerous fractures resulting in crumpled long bones and beaded ribs.
3. Achondrogenesis—absent or poor ossification, especially of vertebral bodies; small chest; very short long bones.
4. **Hypochondrogenesis**—milder form of achondrogenesis, but still lethal.
5. **Short rib polydactyly syndromes**—extremely short ribs; polydactyly in most with variable acromesomelic shortening depending on type.
6. **Fibrochondrogenesis**—short long bones with metaphyseal flaring and diamond-shaped vertebrae.
7. **Campomelic dysplasia**—bowed femora and tibiae. Deficient ossification of thoracic pedicles and severe hypoplasia of scapular blades are most characteristic features. Eleven ribs.

8. **Chondrodysplasia punctata**—see Section 14.15.
9. **Lethal hypophosphatasia**—severely deficient skull ossification. Absent pedicles in spine. Missing bones. Variable metaphyseal defects. Some bones look normal.

Further reading

Hall, C.M., Offiah, A.C., Forzano, F., 2012. Fetal and Perinatal Skeletal Dysplasias, an Atlas of Multimodality Imaging. Radcliffe, Milton Keynes.
Spranger, J.W., Brill, P.W., Poznanski, A., 2012. Bone Dysplasias, an Atlas of Genetic Disorders of Skeletal Development, third ed. OUP, New York.

14.7 CONDITIONS EXHIBITING DYSOSTOSIS MULTIPLEX

Whereas dysplasia refers to abnormal bone growth and can change in distribution over time, dysostosis refers to abnormal bone formation in early pregnancy and the distribution of involved bones remains static. Dysostosis multiplex is a constellation of findings, which are seen totally or partially in a number of lysosomal storage diseases. These findings include:

(a) Abnormal bone texture.
(b) Large skull vault with calvarial thickening.
(c) J-shaped sella + poor pneumatization of paranasal sinuses.
(d) Odontoid hypoplasia + atlantoaxial subluxation.
(e) Anterior beak of upper lumbar vertebrae + gibbus deformity.
(f) Inferior tapering of iliac bones + steep acetabula + coxa valga.
(g) Widened diaphyses, e.g. ribs (oar-shaped), clavicles, small tubular bones.
(h) Tilting of distal radius and ulna towards each other.
(i) Pointing of the proximal ends of the metacarpals.

Diseases exhibiting dysostosis multiplex include:

1. **Mucopolysaccharidoses***—see Part 2.
2. **Mucolipidoses types I–III.**
3. **Fucosidosis types I and II.**
4. **GM1 gangliosidosis.**
5. **Mannosidosis.**
6. **Aspartylglucosaminuria.**

14

Further reading

Sing, M., Parker, E.I., Moreno-De-Luca, A., et al. Radiological and clinical characterization of the lysosomal storage disorders: non-lipid disorders.

Stevenson, D.A., Steiner, R.D., 2013. Skeletal abnormalities in lysosomal storage diseases. Pediatr. Endocrinol. Rev. 10 (Suppl2), 406–416.

14.8 GENERALIZED INCREASED BONE DENSITY

NB: infants in the first few months of life can exhibit 'physiological' bone sclerosis which regresses spontaneously.

Dysplasias

1. **Osteopetrosis**—diffuse bony sclerosis due to reduced osteoclast activity, with a 'bone-in-bone' appearance and 'rugger jersey' spine. Increase risk of fractures.
2. **Pyknodysostosis**—short stature, hypoplastic lateral ends of clavicles, hypoplastic terminal phalanges, bulging cranium and delayed closure of the anterior fontanelle.
3. **Dysosteosclerosis**—thought to be an osteoclast-poor form of osteopetrosis in infancy, but does not cause 'bone-in-bone' appearance. Progressive spinal involvement with endplate irregularity, and marked undertubulation of long bones with submetaphyseal lucencies.
4. **Progressive diaphyseal dysplasia (Camurati-Engelmann syndrome)**—diffuse symmetrical cortical thickening in diaphyses of long bones (especially femur and tibia) ± skull or spine involvement.
5. **Melorheostosis**—undulating periosteal ± endosteal hyperostosis with a characteristic 'dripping candle wax' appearance. Involves one or more bones in a single limb, in a sclerotomal distribution.
6. **Wnt-pathway disorders**—including endosteal hyperostosis, hyperostosis corticalis generalisata, sclerosteosis and osteopathia striata.

Metabolic

1. **Renal osteodystrophy***—rarely renal osteodystrophy causes bone sclerosis, typically seen as a 'rugger jersey' spine. Oxalosis may also cause renal failure and bone sclerosis.

Poisoning

1. **Lead**—dense metaphyseal bands. Cortex and flat bones may also be slightly dense. Modelling deformities later, e.g. flask-shaped femora.
2. **Fluorosis**—more common in adults. Thickened cortex at the expense of the medulla. Periosteal reaction. Ossification of ligaments, tendons and interosseous membranes.
3. **Hypervitaminosis D**—slightly increased density of skull and vertebrae early, followed later by osteoporosis. Soft-tissue

calcification. Dense metaphyseal bands and widened zone of provisional calcification.

4. Chronic hypervitaminosis A—not <1 year of age. Cortical thickening of long and tubular bones, especially in the feet. Subperiosteal new bone. Normal epiphyses, reduced metaphyseal density. The mandible is not affected (cf. Caffey's disease).

Idiopathic

1. Caffey's disease (infantile cortical hyperostosis)—see Section 14.11.
2. **Idiopathic hypercalcaemia of infancy**—probably a manifestation of hypervitaminosis D. Generalized increased density or dense metaphyseal bands. Increased density of skull base.

Further reading

Herman, T.E., McAlister, W.H., 1991. Inherited diseases in bone density in children. Radiol. Clin. North Am. 29 (1), 149–164.

Ihde, L.L., Forrester, D.M., Gottsegen, C.J., et al., 2011. Sclerosing bone dysplasias: review and differentiation from other causes of osteosclerosis. Radiographics 31 (7), 1865–1882.

Boulet, C., Madani, H., Lenchik, L., et al., 2016. Sclerosing bone dysplasias: genetic, clinical and radiology update of hereditary and non-hereditary disorders. Br. J. Radiol. 89, 20153049.

14.9 PAEDIATRIC TUMOURS THAT METASTASIZE TO BONE

1. Neuroblastoma.
2. Leukaemia.
3. Lymphoma*.
4. Renal clear cell sarcoma.
5. Rhabdomyosarcoma.
6. **Retinoblastoma.**
7. **Ewing sarcoma**—lung metastases much more common.
8. **Osteosarcoma**—lung metastases much more common.

14.10 'MOTH-EATEN BONE' IN A CHILD

See figure in Section 1.15.

Neoplastic

1. Neuroblastoma metastases.
2. Leukaemia—consider when there is diffuse involvement of an entire bone or a neighbouring bone with low T1 and high T2/STIR signal on MRI.
3. Long bone sarcomas—Ewing sarcoma and osteosarcoma.
4. Lymphoma of bone.
5. Langerhans cell histiocytosis (LCH)*.

Infective

1. Acute osteomyelitis.

Further reading

Blickman, J.G., van Die, C.E., de Rooy, J.W., 2004. Current imaging concepts in pediatric osteomyelitis. Eur. Radiol. 14 (Suppl. 4), L55–L64.

14.11 PERIOSTEAL REACTIONS—BILATERALLY SYMMETRICAL IN CHILDREN

1. Normal infants—diaphyseal, not extending to the growth plate, bilaterally symmetrical and a single lamina. Frequently involves femur, tibia and humerus. Very unusual >4 months of age. A mimicker of trauma; sometimes difficult to differentiate from child abuse when seen incidentally on skeletal survey.
2. Juvenile idiopathic arthritis*—in ~25% of cases. Most common in the periarticular regions of phalanges, metacarpals and metatarsals. When it extends into the diaphysis it will eventually result in enlarged, rectangular tubular bones.
3. Acute leukaemia—associated with prominent metaphyseal bone resorption ± a dense zone of provisional calcification. Osteopenia. Metastatic neuroblastoma can look identical.
4. Rickets*—the presence of uncalcified subperiosteal osteoid mimics a periosteal reaction because the periosteum and ossified cortex are separated.
5. Caffey's disease—first evident <5 months of age. Mandible, clavicles and ribs show cortical hyperostosis and a diffuse periosteal reaction. The scapulae and tubular bones are affected less often and tend to be involved asymmetrically.
6. Scurvy*—subperiosteal haemorrhage is most frequent in the femur, tibia and humerus. Periosteal reaction is particularly evident in the healing phase. Age ≥6 months.
7. **Prostaglandin E_1 therapy**—in infants with ductus-dependent congenital heart disease. Severity is related to duration of therapy. Other features include pseudowidening of cranial sutures and bone-in-bone appearance.
8. **Congenital syphilis***—an exuberant periosteal reaction can be due to infiltration by syphilitic granulation tissue (diaphyseal) or healing of osteochondritis by callus (metaphyseal-epiphyseal junction).

14.12 SYNDROMES AND BONE DYSPLASIAS FEATURING MULTIPLE FRACTURES

With reduced bone density

1. Osteogenesis imperfecta.
2. Rickets*—usually only in presence of severe rachitic change and clear demineralization.
3. Hypophosphatasia.
4. **Juvenile idiopathic osteoporosis**—2–4 years duration, age of onset 2–13 years.
5. **Gerodermia osteodysplastica**—osteopenia and wormian bones associated with wrinkly skin (cutis laxa) and hip dislocation.
6. **Osteoporosis-pseudoglioma syndrome**—blindness in infancy + bony fragility.
7. **Mucolipidosis II**—osteopenia and periosteal 'cloaking' in infancy, evolving into dysostosis multiplex.
8. **Cushing's syndrome.**

With normal bone density

1. Cleidocranial dysplasia*.
2. Fibrous dysplasia.

With increased bone density

1. Osteopetrosis.
2. Pyknodysostosis—see Section 14.8.

14.13 PSEUDARTHROSIS IN A CHILD

1. Nonunion of a fracture—including pathological fracture.
2. Congenital—in the mid-lower third of the tibia ± fibula. 50% present in the first year. Later there may be cupping of the proximal bone end and pointing of the distal bone end.
3. Neurofibromatosis*—identical to congenital tibial pseudarthrosis.
4. Osteogenesis imperfecta.
5. **Cleidocranial dysplasia***—congenitally in the femur.
6. **Fibrous dysplasia.**
7. **Proximal focal femoral deficiency**—at the site of the femoral defect.

Further reading

Pannier, S., 2011. Congenital pseudarthrosis of the tibia. Orthop. Traumatol. Surg. Res. 97 (7), 750–761.

14.14 'BONE WITHIN A BONE' APPEARANCE

1. **Normal neonate**—especially in the spine.
2. **Growth arrest/recovery lines.**
3. **Bisphosphonate therapy**—similar to growth arrest lines.
4. **Osteopetrosis.**
5. **Sickle cell anaemia.**
6. **Gaucher disease*.**
7. **Heavy metal poisoning.**
8. **Prostaglandin E_1 therapy**—see Section 14.11.

Further reading

Frager, D.H., Subbarao, K., 1983. The 'bone within a bone'. JAMA 249, 77–79.

14.15 IRREGULAR OR STIPPLED EPIPHYSES

1. **Normal**—particularly in the distal femur.
2. **Avascular necrosis**—single, e.g. Perthes' disease (although 10% are bilateral), or multiple, e.g. sickle cell anaemia.
3. **Congenital hypothyroidism**—not present at birth. Delayed appearance and growth of ossification centres. Appearance varies from slightly granular to fragmentation. The femoral capital epiphysis may be divided into inner and outer halves.
4. **Morquio syndrome**—irregular ossification of the femoral capital epiphyses results in flattening.
5. **Multiple epiphyseal dysplasia**—see Section 14.5.
6. **Meyer dysplasia**—resembles multiple epiphyseal dysplasia but limited to the femoral heads.
7. **Chondrodysplasia punctata**—punctate calcifications of developing epiphyses in fetus and infant which resolve in first few years of life, with disturbance of growth of affected bones. Cause may be genetic or maternal during pregnancy (e.g. mixed connective tissue disease, hyperemesis gravidarum, vitamin K deficiency and warfarin embryopathy).
8. **Trisomy 18 and 21.**
9. **Prenatal infections.**
10. **Zellweger syndrome (cerebrohepatorenal syndrome).**
11. **Fetal alcohol syndrome**—mostly calcaneum and lower extremities.

14.16 SOLITARY RADIOLUCENT METAPHYSEAL BAND

Apart from point 3, this is a nonspecific sign which represents a period of poor endochondral bone formation.

1. Normal neonate.
2. Any severe illness.
3. Metaphyseal fracture—especially in nonaccidental injury. Depending on the radiographic projection there may be the additional appearance of a 'corner' or 'bucket-handle' fracture.
4. Healing rickets*.
5. Leukaemia, lymphoma* or metastatic neuroblastoma.
6. Congenital infections.
7. Intrauterine perforation.
8. Scurvy*.

14.17 ALTERNATING RADIOLUCENT AND DENSE METAPHYSEAL BANDS

1. Growth arrest lines—Harris or Park lines.
2. Bisphosphonate therapy—'zebra stripes' appearance.
3. Rickets*—especially those types that require prolonged treatment such as vitamin D-dependent rickets.
4. Osteopetrosis.
5. Chemotherapy.
6. Chronic anaemias—sickle cell and thalassaemia.
7. Treated leukaemia.

14.18 SOLITARY DENSE METAPHYSEAL BAND

1. Normal infants.
2. Lead poisoning—dense line in the proximal fibula is said to differentiate from normal. Other poisons include bismuth, arsenic, phosphorus, mercury fluoride and radium.
3. Radiation.
4. Congenital hypothyroidism.
5. Osteopetrosis.
6. Hypervitaminosis D.

Further reading

Raber, S.A., 1999. The dense metaphyseal band sign. Radiology 211, 773–774.

14.19 DENSE VERTICAL METAPHYSEAL LINES

1. Congenital rubella—celery stalk appearance. Less commonly in congenital CMV.
2. Osteopathia striata—± exostoses.
3. Hypophosphatasia.
4. Localized metaphyseal injury.

14.20 FRAYING OF METAPHYSES

1. Rickets*.
2. Hypophosphatasia—similar features as rickets.
3. **Chronic stress**—in the wrists of young gymnasts; wide, irregular, asymmetrical widening of the distal radial growth plate and metaphyseal sclerosis.
4. **Copper deficiency.**

14.21 CUPPING OF METAPHYSES

Often associated with fraying.

1. Normal—especially distal ulna and proximal fibula of young children. No fraying.
2. Rickets*—with widening of the growth plate and fraying.
3. Trauma—to the growth plate/metaphysis. Localized changes.
4. **Bone dysplasias**—e.g. achondroplasia, pseudoachondroplasia, metatropic dwarfism, diastrophic dwarfism, the metaphyseal chondrodysplasias, hypophosphatasia.
5. **Scurvy***—usually after fracture.
6. **Menkes disease**—Copper deficiency can have similar appearances.

14.22 ERLENMEYER FLASK DEFORMITY

An Erlenmeyer flask is a wide-necked glass container used in chemical laboratories. The shape of the flask is used to describe the distal expansion of the long bones, particularly the femora, which is observed in a number of sclerosing skeletal dysplasias and other afflictions of bone.

Dysplasias

1. Osteopetrosis—in infantile and juvenile forms. Particularly striking in the similar disorder of dysosteosclerosis.
2. Craniotubular disorders—e.g. metaphyseal dysplasia, craniometaphyseal dysplasia, craniodiaphyseal dysplasia, progressive diaphyseal dysplasia.
3. **Others**—otopalatodigital syndrome type 1, Melnick-Needles syndrome and frontometaphyseal dysplasia.

Haematological

1. **Thalassaemia***.

Depositional disorders

1. Gaucher disease*.
2. **Niemann-Pick disease***.

Poisoning

1. Lead poisoning—thick transverse dense metaphyseal bands are the classic manifestation of chronic infantile and juvenile lead poisoning. There may also be flask-shaped femora, which can persist for years before resolving.

Further reading

Faden, M.A., Krakow, D., Ezgu, F., et al., 2009. The Erlenmeyer flask bone deformity in the skeletal dysplasias. Am. J. Med. Genet. A 149A (6), 1334–1345.

14.23 FOCAL RIB LESION (SOLITARY OR MULTIPLE) IN A CHILD

Neoplastic

1. Metastases—typically neuroblastoma.
2. Ewing sarcoma—can arise from bone or chest wall (Askin tumour).
3. Benign—e.g. osteochondroma, enchondroma.
4. Langerhans cell histiocytosis*.

Nonneoplastic

1. Healed rib fracture.
2. Fibrous dysplasia.
3. Osteomyelitis—bacterial, tuberculous or fungal.

Further reading

Guttentag, A.R., Salwen, J.K., 1999. Keep your eyes on the ribs: the spectrum of normal variants and diseases that involve the ribs. Radiographics 19, 1125–1142.

14.24 WIDENING OF THE SYMPHYSIS PUBIS

>10 mm in the newborn, >9 mm at 3 years, >8 mm at 7 years and over.

Acquired

1. Trauma.
2. Infection—low-grade osteomyelitis mimics osteitis pubis.

Congenital

With normal ossification

1. Bladder exstrophy—marked widening; 'manta ray' sign.
2. **Cloacal exstrophy.**

3. **Epispadias**—degree of widening correlates well with severity of epispadias.
4. **Hypospadias.**
5. **Imperforate anus with rectovaginal fistula.**
6. **Urethral duplication.**
7. **Prune-belly syndrome.**
8. **Sjögren–Larsson syndrome.**
9. **Goltz syndrome.**

Poorly ossified cartilage

1. **Cleidocranial dysplasia*.**
2. **Achondrogenesis/hypochondrogenesis.**
3. **Campomelic dysplasia.**
4. **Chondrodysplasia punctata.**
5. **Hypophosphatasia.**
6. **Congenital hypothyroidism.**
7. **Spondyloepiphyseal dysplasia congenita.**
8. **Spondyloepimetaphyseal dysplasia.**
9. **Pyknodysostosis.**
10. **Larsen syndrome.**
11. **Wolf-Hirschhorn syndrome.**
12. **Chromosome 9(p+) trisomy syndrome.**

Further reading

Muecke, E.C., Currarino, G., 1968. Congenital widening of the symphysis pubis. Associated clinical disorders and roentgen anatomy of affected bony pelves. AJR Am. J. Roentgenol. 103, 179–185.

Patel, K., Chapman, S., 1993. Normal symphysis pubis width in children. Clin. Radiol. 47, 56–57.

Taybi, H., Lachman, R.S., 2007. Radiology of Syndromes, Metabolic Disorders, and Skeletal Dysplasias, fifth ed. Mosby, St Louis, MO, p. 1234.

14.25 'SHEETS' OF CALCIFICATION IN A CHILD

1. **Fibrodysplasia ossificans progressiva**—manifests in childhood. Initially neck and trunk muscles involved. Short first metacarpal and metatarsal.
2. **Juvenile dermatomyositis.**

14.26 DIFFERENTIAL DIAGNOSIS OF SKELETAL LESIONS IN NONACCIDENTAL INJURY*

Disease	Shaft fractures	Abnormal metaphysis	Osteopenia	Periosteal reaction	Comments
<u>Nonaccidental injury</u>	+	+	–	+	
<u>Accidental trauma</u>	+	–	–	Callus	
<u>Birth trauma</u>	+	±	–	±	Clavicle, humerus and femur are most frequent fractures
<u>Osteogenesis imperfecta</u>	+	±	+	–	Highly unlikely in the absence of blue sclerae, osteopenia, wormian bones, dentinogenesis imperfecta or a relevant family history
Osteomyelitis	–	+	Localized	+	May be multifocal
Rickets	+	+	+	+	↑ Alkaline phosphatase and parathyroid hormone. Fractures in nonmobile infant in absence of florid rachitic change unlikely to be due to vitamin D deficiency
Scurvy	–	+	+	+	Not before 6 months of age
Congenital syphilis	–	+	–	+	
Congenital insensitivity to pain	+	+	–	+	Charcot joints
Paraplegia	+	+	+	With fractures	Lower limb changes only
Prostaglandin E_1 therapy	–	–	–	+	
Menkes syndrome	–	+	+	+	Males only. Abnormal hair. Retardation. Wormian bones
Copper deficiency	+	+	+	±	See note[a]

[a] *Copper deficiency: rare. Unlikely in the absence of at least one risk factor: prematurity, total parenteral nutrition, malabsorption or a low-copper diet. Unlikely in full-term infants <6 months of age. Microcytic, hypochromic anaemia. Leukopenia. Normal serum copper and caeruloplasmin do not exclude the diagnosis. Skull fracture never recorded in copper deficiency. Rib fractures only recorded in premature infants.*

Further reading

Bilo, R.A.C., Robben, S.G.F., van Rijn, R.R., 2009. Forensic Aspects of Paediatric Fractures. Springer, Berlin.

Carty, H., Pierce, A., 2002. Non-accidental injury: a retrospective analysis of a large cohort. Eur. Radiol. 12 (12), 2919–2925.

Chapman, S., Hall, C.M., 1997. Non-accidental injury or brittle bones. Pediatr. Radiol. 27, 106–110.

Kleinman, P., 1998. Diagnostic Imaging of Child Abuse, second ed. Mosby, St Louis, MO.

Offiah, A., van Rijn, R.R., Perez-Rossello, J.M., et al., 2009. Skeletal imaging of child abuse (non-accidental injury). Pediatr. Radiol. 39 (5), 461–470.

14.27 PLATYSPONDYLY IN CHILDHOOD

This sign describes a uniform decrease in the distance between the upper and lower vertebral endplates and should be differentiated from wedge-shaped vertebrae. Platyspondyly may be generalized (all vertebral bodies), multiple (some vertebral bodies) or localized (one vertebral body, i.e. vertebra plana).

Congenital platyspondyly

1. Thanatophoric dwarfism—inverted 'U'- or 'H'-shaped vertebrae with markedly increased disc space/body height ratio. Telephone handle-shaped long bones.
2. Metatropic dwarfism—flat-appearing vertebral bodies, but large disc spaces mean that overall spinal height is near normal in infancy. As childhood progresses, relative spinal height reduces.
3. Osteogenesis imperfecta—type IIA.
4. **Homozygous achondroplasia.**

Platyspondyly in later childhood

1. Morquio syndrome.
2. **Spondyloepiphyseal dysplasia congenita/tarda.**
3. **Kniest syndrome.**

Acquired platyspondyly

1. Scheuermann's disease—irregular endplates and Schmorl's nodes in the thoracic spine of children and young adults. Disc-space narrowing. May progress to a severe kyphosis.
2. Langerhans cell histiocytosis*—the spine is more frequently involved in eosinophilic granuloma and Hand-Schüller-Christian disease than in Letterer-Siwe disease. The thoracic and lumbosacral spine are the usual sites of disease. Disc spaces are preserved.
3. Osteogenesis imperfecta—multiple spinal compression fractures, resulting in loss of height and spinal deformity.
4. Sickle cell anaemia—characteristic step-like depression in the central part of the endplates ('H-shaped' vertebrae).

Further reading

Kozlowski, K., 1974. Platyspondyly in childhood. Pediatr. Radiol. 2 (2), 81–87.

14.28 ANTERIOR VERTEBRAL BODY BEAKS

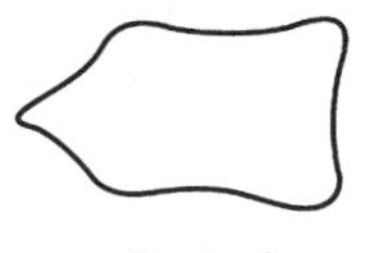

Central

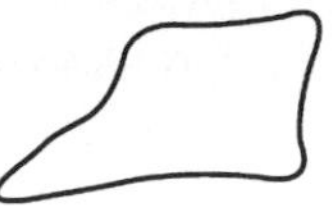

Lower third

Involves 1–3 vertebral bodies at the thoracolumbar junction, usually associated with a kyphosis. Hypotonia is probably the common denominator, leading to an exaggerated thoracolumbar kyphosis, anterior herniation of the nucleus pulposus and subsequently an anterior vertebral body defect.

1. **Mucopolysaccharidoses***—with platyspondyly in Morquio; this is probably a more useful distinguishing characteristic than the position of the beak (inferior or middle), which is variable.
2. **Achondroplasia***.
3. **Mucolipidoses.**
4. **Pseudoachondroplasia.**
5. **Congenital hypothyroidism.**
6. **Down's syndrome*.**
7. **Neuromuscular diseases.**

Further reading

Levin, T.L., Berdon, W.E., Lachman, R.S., et al., 1997. Lumbar gibbus in storage diseases and bone dysplasias. Pediatr. Radiol. 27 (4), 289–294.
Swischuk, L.E., 1970. The beaked, notched or hooked vertebra. Its significance in infants and young children. Radiology 95, 661–664.

14.29 MULTIFOCAL BONE MARROW LESIONS ON MRI

Similar to causes that result in multifocal lytic/destructive bone lesions. Best detected on nonfat saturated T1 sequences as low-signal lesions. Haematogenously disseminated metastases and infection favour metaphyses and equivalent sites in children >2 years old.

Malignancy

1. **Metastases**—commonly from neuroblastoma, leukaemia, lymphoma, clear cell sarcoma, rhabdomyosarcoma, retinoblastoma, osteosarcoma and Ewing sarcoma.

2. Langerhans cell histiocytosis*—low T1 signal, high signal on T2 fatsat sequences, variable enhancement pattern.

Dysplasias

1. Hereditary multiple osteochondromas.
2. Enchondromatosis.
3. Polyostotic fibrous dysplasia—isointense with focal low signal areas on T1, heterogeneous on T2, patchy variable enhancement.

Infection/inflammatory

1. Multifocal osteomyelitis—may present with nonenhancing fluid collections and rim-enhancing abscesses in bone, joint effusions and cartilaginous involvement.
2. Chronic recurrent multifocal osteomyelitis—idiopathic, noninfective, inflammatory disorder. Diagnosis of exclusion. Tends to occur at epiphyseal/metaphyseal regions in long bones, especially the clavicles (rare for haematogenous osteomyelitis).

Trauma/infarction

1. Multiple stress fractures—as seen in gymnasts and young athletes from repetitive strain.
2. Multifocal infarction/avascular necrosis—children prone to this include those with sickle cell disease, corticosteroid exposure, storage disorders and inflammatory arthritis. May also occur secondary to radiotherapy.

Further reading

Raissaki, M., Demetriou, S., Spanakis, K., et al., 2017. Multifocal bone and bone marrow lesions in children – MRI findings. Pediatr. Radiol. 47, 342–360.

14.30 SOFT-TISSUE TUMOURS AND MASSES

Vascular lesions are the most common category of all soft-tissue masses in children and comprise two distinct types: tumours and malformations.

Vascular tumours

1. Infantile haemangioma—usually solitary, first noticed around time of birth with a period of proliferation before involution (90% will have involuted by 9 years).
2. **Congenital haemangioma**—similar appearance to infantile type, but does not grow after birth; depending on subtype they can involute.
3. **Kaposiform haemangioendothelioma**—associated with Kasabach-Merritt syndrome.

Vascular malformations (can also occur in combination with each other)

1. **Arteriovenous malformation**—high flow lesion, 60% are diagnosed at birth.
2. **Venous malformations**—low flow lesion, phleboliths commonly present.
3. **Lymphatic malformation**—previously referred to as cystic hygromas.
4. **Capillary malformations**—usually do not require imaging to diagnose.

Fat-containing soft-tissue lesions

1. **Lipoma**—usually no vascularity, can have a fibrous capsule that may enhance, but should not internally enhance on MRI. Uncommon in children.
2. **Lipoblastoma**—benign tumour, exclusively found within first 3 years of life. Slightly lower T1 signal compared to normal fat.
3. **Angiolipoma**—slow growing, painful, ± vascular flow (in 25%).
4. **Lipomatosis**—infiltrative adipose tissue involving multiple layers (muscle, skin and bone). Usually <2 years of age.
5. **Fibrous hamartoma of infancy (FHI)**—>90% occur in infancy, most common around shoulder or inguinal region. Subcutaneous location. Contains fat and T1/T2 hypointense strands of fibrous tissue.
6. **Lipofibromatosis**—benign tumour of young children, most common in hands and feet (in contrast to FHI). Contains fat and fibrous tissue, often infiltrative.

Fibrous soft-tissue lesions

1. **Rhabdomyosarcoma**—most common soft-tissue sarcoma in children. Can occur anywhere (not just in skeletal muscle), e.g. orbit, pharynx, sinuses, paratesticular, bladder, etc. Nonspecific imaging features.
2. **Synovial sarcoma**—usually in adolescents, most commonly in soft tissues near the knees. Calcification, if present, is suggestive.
3. **Infantile myofibroma**—typically <2 years of age. Benign, usually solitary and subcutaneous, but can be multiple (myofibromatosis) and deep, involving muscle, bone or viscera (the latter is rare and conveys a poor prognosis). Bone lesions are typically metaphyseal and well-defined. Often regresses spontaneously if viscera are not involved.
4. **Fibrous hamartoma of infancy**—contains fat; see above.
5. **Lipofibromatosis**—contains fat; see above.
6. **Nodular fasciitis**—see Section 4.4. Can occur in children, usually adolescents (except cranial fasciitis that occurs <2 years of age).

7. **Desmoid tumour**—see Section 4.4. May be the first sign of Gardner syndrome ('Gardner fibroma').
8. **Inflammatory pseudotumour**—can occur anywhere, most commonly lung, mesentery and omentum. Variable imaging appearance.
9. **Fibromatosis colli**—<6 months of age, benign fibroblastic proliferation specific to the sternocleidomastoid muscle. Unilateral fusiform muscle thickening is characteristic.
10. **Fibroma of tendon sheath**—typically involves tendons of the hands. T2 hypointense, no/minimal enhancement.
11. **Infantile digital fibroma**—<3 years of age, subcutaneous nodule in dorsolateral aspect of digits.
12. **Infantile fibrosarcoma**—typically <2 years of age. Large painless mass, rapid growth. Heterogeneous and hypervascular on US/MRI, can cause adjacent bone erosion.
13. **Low-grade fibromyxoid sarcoma**—can occur in children. Alternating T2 hyper- and hypointense areas due to mixture of myxoid and fibrous components.

Soft-tissue tumour mimics

1. Posttraumatic lesions—e.g. contusion, fat necrosis, foreign body reaction or cellulitis. Typically painful and ill-defined on imaging.
2. Subcutaneous granuloma annulare—rapidly growing painless subcutaneous nodule, typically in children <5 years of age. Most common on extensor surface of extremities (especially pretibial) or in scalp. Nonspecific ill-defined lesion on US/MRI. Resolves spontaneously.
3. **Pilomatricoma**—often calcified; see Section 4.2.
4. **Microcystic lymphatic malformation**—appears solid on US ± enhancement on MRI.

Further reading

Navarro, O.M., 2011. Soft tissue masses in children. Radiol. Clin. North Am. 49 (6), 1235–1259.

Johnson, C.M., Navarro, O.M., 2017. Clinical and sonographic features of pediatric soft-tissue vascular anomalies. Pediatr. Radiol. 47 (9), 1184–1208.

Sheybani, E.F., Eutsler, E.P., Navarro, O.M., 2016. Fat-containing soft-tissue masses in children. Pediatr. Radiol. 46 (13), 1760–1773.

Sargar, K.M., Sheybani, E.F., Shenoy, A., et al., 2016. Pediatric fibroblastic and myofibroblastic tumours: a pictorial review. Radiographics 36 (4), 1195–1214.

14.31 PAEDIATRIC PHYSEAL INJURIES: SALTER-HARRIS CLASSIFICATION

These fractures are very common and occur exclusively in children due to the presence of a physis—a naturally occurring weak area of the bone. The classification is commonly used in paediatric radiology reporting even though more complex classifications exist.

MRI is most helpful in determining occult Salter-Harris 1 (SH1) injuries as these can be very subtle on radiographs.

- **Salter-Harris 1**—manifests as either widening of the physis or displacement of the epiphysis, e.g. slipped capital femoral epiphysis.
- **Salter-Harris 2**—fracture of the metaphysis extending into the physis.
- **Salter-Harris 3**—fracture of the epiphysis extending into the physis (common in distal tibia).
- **Salter-Harris 4**—fracture through the epiphysis and metaphysis.
- **Salter-Harris 5**—physeal plate compression/crush injury; least common type, worst prognosis.

14.32 OSTEOCHONDRITIS DISSECANS (OSTEOCHONDRAL DEFECTS)

Uncertain aetiology, possibly related to microtrauma. Damage to subchondral bone ± cartilage can lead to detachment of an osteochondral fragment (loose body). Important to differentiate stable versus unstable lesions on MRI (T2/STIR). Different criteria for instability exist for children compared to adults. Features for stability include intact cartilage surface and lack of bone marrow oedema. Features for instability in children include:

- Multiple adjacent bone cysts at margin of defect, or a single cyst >5 mm
- Fluid separating bone fragment from adjacent bone (fluid rim)
- Multiple disruptions in subchondral plate

Common locations

- Arms: capitellum of humerus, radial head.
- Legs: anteromedial talar dome, lateral aspect of medial femoral condyle.

Further reading

Jans, L.B., Ditchfield, M., Anna, G., et al., 2012. MR imaging findings and MR criteria for instability in osteochondritis dissecans of the elbow in children. Eur. J. Radiol. 81 (6), 1306–1310.

O'Dell, M.C., Jaramillo, D., Bancroft, L., et al., 2016. Imaging of sports related injuries of the lower extremity in pediatric patients. Radiographics 36, 1807–1827.

14.33 ACUTE UPPER AIRWAY OBSTRUCTION IN A CHILD

Most common in infants because of the small calibre of their upper airways. Small- or normal-volume lungs with distension of the upper airway proximal to the obstruction during inspiration.

1. **Laryngotracheobronchitis (croup)**—most common 6 months–3 years. Narrowing of the glottic and subglottic airway. Ballooning of hypopharynx on lateral view. 'Steepling' of upper airway on frontal view.
2. **Acute epiglottitis**—the epiglottis is swollen ± shortened. Other components of the supraglottic region (aryepiglottic folds, arytenoids, uvula and prevertebral soft tissues) are also swollen. The hypopharynx and pyriform sinuses are distended with air.
3. **Abscess**—retropharyngeal is more common <2 years as retropharyngeal nodes atrophy thereafter. Enlarged prevertebral soft tissues ± gas or air-fluid level. Rim enhancement seen post contrast on CT or MRI. Role for US in diagnosis and follow-up. Peritonsillar is more common in teenagers and young adults.
4. **Oedema**—caused by angioedema (allergic, anaphylactic or hereditary), inhalation of noxious gases or trauma. Predominantly laryngeal oedema.
5. **Foreign body**—more commonly occludes a major bronchus rather than the upper airway.
6. **Choanal atresia**—most common congenital nasal abnormality; bilateral (33%) or unilateral (R>L), bony (90%) or membranous, complete or incomplete. When bilateral and complete, it presents with severe respiratory distress at birth (infants are primarily nasal breathers until 6 weeks–6 months of age). Incomplete obstruction is associated with respiratory difficulty during feeding. Diagnosis is determined by failure to pass a catheter through the nose, nasopharyngography or CT.
7. **Retropharyngeal haemorrhage**—due to trauma, neck surgery, direct carotid arteriography or bleeding disorders. Widened retropharyngeal soft-tissue space.

Further reading

Adil, E., Huntley, C., Choudhary, A., et al., 2012. Congenital nasal obstruction: clinical and radiologic review. Eur. J. Pediatr. 171 (4), 641–650.

Pfleger, A., Eber, E., 2016. Assessment and causes of stridor. Paediatr. Respir. Rev. 18, 64–72.

14.34 CHRONIC UPPER AIRWAY OBSTRUCTION IN A CHILD

May be associated with overinflation of the lungs.

Nasal

1. **Choanal atresia**—see Section 14.33.
2. **Juvenile nasopharyngeal angiofibroma**—nearly always in adolescent males. Symptoms of nasal obstruction and/or recurrent atraumatic epistaxis. Benign but locally aggressive, causing bony remodelling. Avid enhancement on CT/MRI. Plain films may show:
   (a) Anterior bowing of the posterior wall of the maxillary antrum.
   (b) Deviation of the nasal septum.
   (c) A nasopharyngeal soft-tissue mass with erosion of contiguous bony structures.
3. **Antrochoanal polyp.**

Supraglottic

1. **Grossly enlarged tonsils and adenoids.**
2. **Laryngomalacia**—presents at or shortly after birth, persists for several months and usually resolves by 2 years. Diagnosis is confirmed by direct laryngoscopy, but fluoroscopy reveals anterior motion of aryepiglottic folds and distension of hypopharynx.
3. **Micrognathia**—e.g. in Pierre Robin syndrome.
4. **Cysts**—of the epiglottis or aryepiglottic folds. The degree of obstruction depends on size and location.

Glottic

1. **Laryngeal polyp, papilloma or cyst.**

Subglottic and tracheal

1. **Tracheomalacia**—weakness of tracheal wall, may be:
   (a) Primary—e.g. premature infants; also in cartilage disorders, e.g. polychondritis, chondromalacia, mucopolysaccharidoses.
   (b) Secondary.
      (i) Following prolonged intubation.
      (ii) With tracheoesophageal fistula/oesophageal atresia.
      (iii) With vascular ring or other extrinsic vascular compression.
      (iv) With long-standing external compression by tumour, etc.
2. **Vascular ring.**
   (a) Double aortic arch.
   (b) Right arch with left-sided duct/ductal ligament.
   (c) Pulmonary artery sling—often coexists with intrinsic airway narrowing from complete cartilage rings.
   (d) Anomalous subclavian artery ± large Kommerell diverticulum.

3. **Following prolonged inflammation**—e.g. prolonged tracheal intubation (may be fixed stenosis or malacia) or chronic aspiration (laryngeal cleft, H-type tracheoesophageal fistula, etc.).
4. **External compression from other structures**—e.g. adenopathy, foregut duplication cyst, teratoma, lymphovascular malformation, enlarged heart or pulmonary trunk (especially in tetralogy of Fallot with absent pulmonary valve or severe pulmonary hypertension).
5. **Subglottic haemangioma**—the most common subglottic soft-tissue mass in infancy. Occurs <6 months. 50% have associated cutaneous haemangiomas. Characteristically produces an asymmetrical narrowing of the subglottic airway.
6. **Intrinsic congenital obstruction**—e.g. tracheal stenosis due to complete cartilage rings, webs, etc. Can result in congenital high airway obstruction syndrome (CHAOS).
7. **Respiratory papillomatosis**—occurs anywhere from the nose to the lungs; most cases are limited to the larynx. Irregular soft-tissue masses ± cavitation of lung lesions.

Further reading

Chess, M.A., Chaturveda, A., Stanescu, A.L., et al., 2012. Emergency pediatric ear, nose, and throat imaging. Semin. Ultrasound CT MR 33 (5), 449–462.

Mok, Q., 2017. Airways problems in neonates – A review of the current investigation and management strategies. Front Pediatr. 5, 60.

Semple, T., Calder, A., Owens, C.M., Padley, S., 2017. Current and future approaches to large airways imaging in adults and children. Clin. Radiol. 72 (5), 356–374.

14.35 NEONATAL RESPIRATORY DISTRESS

Pulmonary causes

With no mediastinal shift

1. **Respiratory distress syndrome (RDS)**—surfactant deficiency disorder, occurs in premature infants. Symptomatic soon after birth but maximum radiographic findings develop at 12–14 hours. Fine granular pattern throughout both lungs, air bronchograms, and later, obscured heart and diaphragm outlines. Small lung volumes due to diffuse microatelectasis. Often cardiomegaly. May progress to a complete 'white-out'. Frequent ventilator-associated complications include pulmonary interstitial emphysema, pneumomediastinum and pneumothorax, all of which can lead to mediastinal displacement. Patchy clearing of infiltrate occurs after exogenous surfactant therapy. As oxygenation improves, bidirectional or left-to-right shunting through the patent ductus arteriosus may lead to pulmonary oedema, cardiomegaly and occasionally pulmonary haemorrhage.

2. **Transient tachypnoea of the newborn (TTN)**—prominent interstitial markings and vessels, thickened septa, small effusions and occasionally mild cardiomegaly. May mimic RDS, MAS or neonatal pneumonia, but resolves within 2–3 days.
3. **Meconium aspiration syndrome (MAS)**—predominantly in term and postmature babies. Coarse linear and irregular opacities of uneven size, generalized hyperinflation and focal areas of collapse. Spontaneous pneumothorax in 20%. Pleural effusion in up to 2/3; supposedly never seen in RDS. No air bronchograms. High risk of superimposed infection.
4. **Pneumonia**—in <1% of newborns. Risk factor: prolonged rupture of membranes. Most commonly group B streptococcus. Segmental or lobar consolidation. Pleural effusions may be large, and suggest diagnosis. May resemble RDS or MAS, but should be suspected if unevenly distributed.
5. **Pulmonary haemorrhage**—75% are <2.5 kg. Onset at birth or delayed several days. May occur after surfactant therapy, probably due to left-to-right shunting. Resembles MAS or RDS.
6. **Upper airway obstruction**—e.g. choanal atresia, micrognathia.
7. **Abnormal thoracic cage.**
   (a) Neuromuscular disorders—often with thin ribs and clavicles.
   (b) Skeletal dysplasias—e.g. Jeune's asphyxiating thoracic dysplasia, thanatophoric dwarfism, osteogenesis imperfecta and metatropic dwarfism.
   (c) Pulmonary hypoplasia—e.g. due to fetal renal failure (Potter sequence) or primary (rare).
   (d) Major abdominal wall defects (exomphalos/gastroschisis)—short, down-sloping ribs with 'long' chest.
8. **Infant-onset childhood interstitial lung disease** (chILD)—wide variety of rare pathologies (see Section 14.37). Variable appearance from complete bilateral white-out to normal.

With mediastinal shift away from the abnormal side

1. **Diaphragmatic hernia**—six times more common on the left side. Multiple lucencies due to gas-containing bowel in the chest. Herniated bowel may appear solid if X-rayed too early, but there will still be a paucity of gas in the abdomen. Liver herniation present in large hernias, bad prognostic sign. Displaces umbilical venous catheters.
2. **Congenital lobar overinflation (CLO)**—left upper > right middle > right upper lobe, with compression of the lung base (cf. pneumothorax which produces generalized compression). CT is useful, particularly to exclude extrinsic compression of a bronchus by an aberrant vessel or foregut duplication cyst.
3. **Large congenital pulmonary airway malformation (CPAM)**—translucencies of various shapes and sizes scattered throughout an

area of opaque lung with well-defined margins. Types 0–IV, varying from cystic to apparently solid. Generally asymptomatic unless very large or superadded infection.

4. Pneumothorax—may complicate resuscitation or positive pressure ventilation, or may be spontaneous. Spontaneous pneumothorax is associated with pulmonary hypoplasia, e.g. in Potter sequence. In the supine neonate, pleural air collects anteriorly and may not collapse the lung medially. In the absence of a lung edge, other signs include:
   (a) Sharp ipsilateral heart border.
   (b) Depression or inversion of the ipsilateral hemidiaphragm with a deep lateral sulcus.
   (c) Sharp ipsilateral parietal pleura in the upper medial part of the hemithorax. If there is tension this may herniate across the superior mediastinum.
   (d) Medial deviation of the ipsilateral compressed thymic lobe.
   (e) Mediastinal shift to the contralateral side.
5. Pleural fluid—effusion (especially in congenital heart disease), chylothorax (especially in Noonan and Turner syndromes), empyema (rare).

With mediastinal shift towards the abnormal side

1. Atelectasis—most commonly due to incorrect placement of an endotracheal tube down a major bronchus. Other causes include extrinsic compression (e.g. large duplication cyst, aberrant vasculature), intrinsic causes (e.g. tracheobronchomalacia), luminal obstruction by a large mucus plug or, rarely, primary atelectasis without another abnormality.
2. **Pulmonary agenesis/aplasia**—rare. May be difficult to differentiate from collapse but other congenital defects, especially hemivertebrae, are often present. Agenesis = no bronchus; aplasia = rudimentary bronchus present.
3. **Unilateral pulmonary hypoplasia**—most commonly due to compression, e.g. by diaphragmatic hernia. May also be associated with vascular anomalies, e.g. absent pulmonary artery and anomalous venous drainage (scimitar syndrome).

Other causes

1. Cardiac causes—e.g. congenital heart diseases.
2. Cerebral causes—e.g. haemorrhage, oedema, drugs. After cardiopulmonary causes, these account for 50% of the remainder.
3. **Metabolic causes**—metabolic acidosis, hypoglycaemia and hypothermia.
4. **Abdominal causes**—massive organomegaly, e.g. polycystic kidneys, elevating the diaphragms.

Further reading
Liszewski, M.C., Stanescu, A.L., Phillips, G.S., et al., 2017. Respiratory distress in neonates: underlying causes and current imaging assessment. Radiol. Clin. North Am. 55 (4), 629–644.
Agrons, G.A., Courtney, S.E., Stocker, J.T., et al., 2005. From the archives of the AFIP: lung disease in premature neonates: radiologic–pathologic correlation. Radiographics 25 (4), 1047–1073.
Schwartz, D.S., Reyes-Mugica, M., Keller, M.S., 1999. Imaging of surgical diseases of the newborn chest. Radiol. Clin. North Am. 37 (6), 1067–1078.

14.36 RING SHADOWS IN A CHILD

Neonate

1. **Diaphragmatic hernia**—unilateral.
2. **Pulmonary interstitial emphysema (PIE)**—secondary to ventilator therapy. Linear lucencies, unilateral or bilateral. Usually transient, but may persist.
3. **CPAM**—Stocker types I/IV (at least one cyst >2 cm) and type II (all cysts <2 cm). Unilateral focal lucency/lucencies. Type III is microcystic and appears solid.
4. **Bronchopulmonary dysplasia (BPD)**—aka chronic lung disease of prematurity. Bilateral, diffuse 'bubbly lung' appearances, with alternating areas of overinflation and atelectasis.
5. **Cystic lung disease in chromosomal disorders**—especially Down's.

Older child

1. **Bronchiectasis**—postinfective, cystic fibrosis, primary ciliary dyskinesia, immunodeficiency, etc.
2. **Pneumatocoeles**—e.g. postinfective, ventilation-induced.
3. **Respiratory papillomatosis**—multiple cystic lesions with nodular walls on CT. Laryngeal and tracheal involvement is usually also present.
4. **Pleuropulmonary blastoma (type 1)**—indistinguishable from type I/IV CPAM on imaging and similar histologically to type IV CPAM.
5. **Langerhans cell histiocytosis***—lung involvement very rare in children.
6. **Neurofibromatosis***—upper zone cysts/bullae.

Further reading
Liszewski, M.C., Stanescu, A.L., Phillips, G.S., et al., 2017. Respiratory distress in neonates: underlying causes and current imaging assessment. Radiol. Clin. North Am. 55 (4), 629–644.
Semple, T., Akhtar, M., Owens, C.M., 2017. Imaging bronchopulmonary dysplasia – a multimodality update. Front Med. 4, 88.

14.37 INTERSTITIAL LUNG DISEASE UNIQUE TO CHILDHOOD

Very rare conditions divided into infant or later onset.

1. **Disorders of infancy.**
   (a) Diffuse developmental disorders—e.g. congenital alveolar dysplasia, alveolar capillary dysplasia with misalignment of pulmonary veins.
   (b) Lung growth abnormalities—e.g. pulmonary hypoplasia, chronic BPD, cystic disease in Down's.
   (c) Conditions of undefined origin—e.g. pulmonary interstitial glycogenosis, neuroendocrine hyperplasia of infancy.
   (d) Genetic surfactant dysfunction disorders—most commonly surfactant protein B/C or ABCA3 mutations.
2. **Disorders not specific to infancy.**
   (a) Normal host—e.g. postinfective constrictive obliterative bronchiolitis.
   (b) Systemic disease processes—e.g. storage disorders (Gaucher, Niemann-Pick).
   (c) Immunocompromise—e.g. lymphocytic interstitial pneumonitis in HIV (rare but much more common in children with AIDS versus adults with AIDS).
   (d) Masqueraders of interstitial lung disease—e.g. pulmonary hypertension, lymphatic disorders.

Further reading

Semple, T., Ashworth, M., Owens, C.M., 2017. Interstitial lung disease in children made easier...well almost. Radiographics 37 (6), 1679–1703.

Copley, S.J., Padley, S.P., 2001. High-resolution CT of paediatric lung disease. Eur. Radiol. 11, 2564–2575.

Owens, C.M., 2004. Radiology of diffuse interstitial pulmonary disease in children. Eur. Radiol. 14 (Suppl. 4), L2–L12.

14.38 THE NORMAL THYMUS

The normal thymus is a bilobed anterosuperior mediastinal structure. It is only visible on plain films of infants and young children, and is inconsistently visible after 2–3 years of age. On plain films three radiological signs aid diagnosis—the 'sail' sign (a triangular projection to one, usually right, or both sides of the mediastinum), the 'wave' sign (a rippled thymic contour due to indentations by the anterior rib ends) or the 'notch' sign (an indentation at the junction of thymus and heart). A large normal thymus may be seen:

(a) In well-nourished children.
(b) Following recovery from illness (rebound overgrowth in 25% after previous involution).
(c) In hyperthyroidism or euthyroid children under treatment for hypothyroidism.

It has the following CT characteristics:

1. **Incidence**—decreases in size over lifetime, identifiable in 100% <30 years of age, decreasing to 17% >49 years.
2. **Shape**—quadrilateral shape in childhood usually with convex, undulating margins. After puberty, two separate lobes (ovoid, triangular or semilunar) or an arrowhead (triangle). The normal thymus is never multilobular.
3. **Size**—progressive enlargement during childhood. Maximum absolute size is reached in the 12–19-year age group, but relative to body size it is largest in infancy. Left lobe nearly always larger than right lobe. Becomes narrower with increasing age with a more triangular outline and convex borders. Maximum thickness (perpendicular to the long axis) of one lobe in those >20 years is 1.3 cm. In those >40 years there may be linear or oval soft-tissue densities but they are never >7 mm in size and never alter the lateral contour of the mediastinal fat.
4. **Density**—homogeneous, iso- or hyperdense relative to chest wall musculature in childhood. After puberty, becomes inhomogeneous and progressively lower in attenuation due to fatty infiltration. The majority >40 years will have total fatty involution.

On MRI the normal thymus is:

1. Larger than on CT (probably because the study is undertaken during quiet respiration rather than with suspended full inspiration).
2. Homogeneous in childhood (T1-weighted slightly greater than muscle, T2-weighted similar to fat).
3. Heterogeneous in adults (T1-weighted and T2-weighted similar to fat).

Further reading

Manchanda, S., Bhalla, A., Jana, M., Gupta, A., 2017. Imaging the pediatric thymus: clinicoradiologic approach. World J. Clin. Pediatr. 6 (1), 10.

Goldstein, A., Oliva, I., Honarpisheh, H., Rubinowitz, A., 2015. A tour of the thymus: a review of thymic lesions with radiologic and pathologic correlation. Can. Assoc. Radiol. J. 66 (1), 5–15.

14.39 ANTERIOR MEDIASTINAL MASSES IN CHILDHOOD

The mediastinum is the most common site of a chest mass in a child. 45% of these occur in the anterior mediastinum.

Congenital

1. Normal thymus—see Section 14.38.
2. **Lymphangioma**—nearly all extend into the mediastinum from the neck. Cystic.
3. **Morgagni hernia**—anterior, usually on the right side.

Neoplastic

1. Lymphoma* and leukaemia—most common cause of an anterior mediastinal mass in children. The majority are due to Hodgkin disease. At presentation, enlarged mediastinal lymph nodes (LN) are seen in 85% of Hodgkin, 50% of non-Hodgkin and 5%–10% of leukaemias. The lymphadenopathy is usually confluent and homogeneous on CT. Comparing mediastinal involvement in Hodgkin versus non-Hodgkin lymphoma:

Hodgkin lymphoma	Non-Hodgkin lymphoma
Usually >10 years old	Any age in children
Mostly localized. Paratracheal > hilar > subcarinal LN. Hilar LN without mediastinal LN is rare	Disseminated disease in >75% at presentation
Displacement of other mediastinal structures rather than compression	Tracheal compression is more likely
Lung involvement in 10% at diagnosis—direct spread from lymph nodes	Lung involvement and pleural effusion more common

   After lymphoma treatment, a residual anterior mediastinal mass may present a diagnostic dilemma. If CT shows this to be homogeneous and there is no other lymphadenopathy then a tumour is unlikely to be present. PET-CT is currently used to risk stratify and determine whether radiotherapy is needed.
2. Germ cell tumours—5%–10% of germ cell tumours arise in the mediastinum. Two age peaks: at 2 years and in adolescence. 60% are benign teratomas. Endodermal sinus (yolk sac) tumours are more aggressive. Seminomas rare. Tumours may contain calcification (including teeth), fat and cystic/necrotic areas. Large

size, marked mass effect and local infiltration suggest an aggressive lesion.

3. Thymic cysts—either congenital, or in young children with LCH, or in HIV/EBV-driven lymphoproliferative disease.
4. Thymolipoma—contains fat and thymic tissue.
5. **Thymoma**—1%–2% of mediastinal tumours in childhood. Most occur >10 years of age. Linear calcification in 10%. Only rarely associated with myasthenia gravis.

Inflammatory

1. Lymphadenopathy—less common than neoplasia. Most frequent causes are TB and histoplasmosis. Involved nodes typically show central necrosis.

Further reading

Ranganath, S.H., Lee, E.Y., Restrepo, R., Eisenberg, R.L., 2012. Mediastinal masses in children. AJR Am. J. Roentgenol. 198 (3), W197–W216.

14.40 MIDDLE MEDIASTINAL MASSES IN CHILDHOOD

20% of paediatric mediastinal masses occur at this site. Excluding cardiovascular anomalies, e.g. double aortic arch:

Neoplastic

Most middle mediastinal tumours are extensions of those which arise primarily in the anterior mediastinum (see Section 14.39).

Inflammatory

1. Lymphadenopathy—TB, histoplasmosis and sarcoidosis (NB: pulmonary sarcoid is very rare before early teens).

Congenital

1. Foregut duplication cysts—account for 10%–20% of paediatric mediastinal masses. The spectrum of abnormalities includes:
   (a) Bronchogenic cyst—abnormal lung budding and development of ventral foregut during first trimester. Round/oval, well-defined, unilocular and homogeneous mass; usually 0–20 HU, but can be up to 100 HU due to mucus, haemorrhage or even milk of calcium contents. There may be airway obstruction and secondary infection, both within the cyst and in the surrounding lung. May rarely communicate with the tracheobronchial tree, resulting in a cavity ± infection.

14

Most commonly attached to the carina, but can be located anywhere along tracheobronchial tree, e.g. paratracheal, hilar, intrapulmonary, paraoesophageal.

(b) Oesophageal duplication cyst—abnormal development of the posterior division of the embryonic foregut. Less common than bronchogenic cysts, usually larger and along the upper third of the oesophagus, situated to the right of the midline extending into the posterior mediastinum. May produce symptoms related to oesophageal or tracheobronchial tree compression. May contain ectopic gastric mucosa (+ve ^{99m}Tc-pertechnetate scan), which causes ulceration, haemorrhage or perforation. Communication with the oesophageal lumen is rare.

(c) Neurenteric cyst—failure of separation of gastrointestinal tract from primitive neural crest. Located in the middle or posterior mediastinum, contains neural tissue and maintains a connection with the spinal canal. R>L. Vertebral body anomalies (hemivertebra, butterfly vertebra and scoliosis) are usually superior to the cyst.

2. **Lymphangioma**—5% of lymphangiomas in the neck extend into the mediastinum. Most are present at birth. Cystic ± solid components on imaging.
3. **Congenital hiatus hernia**—less common than other congenital diaphragmatic hernias.
4. **Achalasia**—rare in children.

Further reading

Ranganath, S.H., Lee, E.Y., Restrepo, R., Eisenberg, R.L., 2012. Mediastinal masses in children. AJR Am. J. Roentgenol. 198 (3), W197–W216.

Manson, D.E., 2013. MR imaging of the mediastinum, chest wall and pleura in children. Acta Radiol. 54, 1075–1085.

14.41 POSTERIOR MEDIASTINAL MASSES IN CHILDHOOD

30%–40% of paediatric mediastinal masses are in this location, and 95% of these are of neurogenic origin. All right-sided paravertebral soft-tissue shadows are abnormal. Left-sided paravertebral soft tissues wider than the width of the adjacent pedicle are abnormal, especially on radiographs taken in the upright position.

Neoplastic

1. Ganglion cell tumours—neuroblastoma (most malignant, usually <5 years), ganglioneuroblastoma (malignant potential, age 5–10

years) and ganglioneuroma (benign, usually >10 years). Imaging features of all three types are similar but metastases do not occur with ganglioneuroma. Plain films show a paravertebral soft-tissue mass with calcification in 30%. Thinning/separation of posterior ribs and enlargement of intervertebral foramina may be seen. CT shows calcification in 90%. Both CT and MRI may show extradural extension.

2. **Nerve sheath tumours**—benign (schwannoma, neurofibroma) or malignant peripheral nerve sheath tumour.

Congenital

1. **Bochdalek hernia**—most present at, or shortly after, birth with respiratory distress, but 5% present after the neonatal period. Rarely it may complicate group B streptococcal infection. A herniated liver/kidney may mimic a mass or pleural effusion, and a herniated bowel may mimic a pneumothorax, pneumatocoeles or CPAM. Bochdalek hernias include:
   (a) Persistence of the pleuroperitoneal canal with a posterior lip of diaphragm.
   (b) Larger defects with no diaphragm.
   (c) Herniation through the costolumbar triangles.

Other

1. **Extramedullary haematopoiesis**—in children, usually related to thalassaemia or sickle cell disease. Single or multiple paravertebral masses with features of the underlying cause.

Further reading

Donnelly, L.F., Frush, D.P., Zheng, J.Y., et al., 2000. Differentiating normal from abnormal inferior thoracic paravertebral soft tissues on chest radiography in children. AJR Am. J. Roentgenol. 175, 477–483.

14.42 SOLITARY PULMONARY MASS IN CHILDHOOD

Pseudomass lesions

1. **Round pneumonia**—may contain air-bronchograms. Rarer >8 years.
2. **Encysted pleural effusion**—usually an elliptiform mass in right midzone. Lateral film confirms.
3. **Mucus plug in cystic fibrosis**—can be large. CT confirms location.
4. **Vasculitis.**

Nonneoplastic lesions

1. Pulmonary sequestration—focal area of lung that does not communicate with the bronchial tree or pulmonary arteries, appearing as a nonaerated mass with systemic arterial supply (usually from descending aorta). Two types:
   (a) Intralobar—most common type. No separate pleural covering, usually has pulmonary venous drainage. Typically in lower lobes (L>R). Usually presents in older children or adolescents with recurrent infection.
   (b) Extralobar—has its own separate pleural covering, usually has systemic venous drainage. Typically in left lower lobe, but can be subdiaphragmatic. Usually presents in neonates with respiratory distress. Often associated with other congenital anomalies.
2. Intrapulmonary bronchogenic cyst—well-defined rounded lesion that may contain air–fluid level, particularly if a previous infection.
3. CPAM—type III is microcystic and appears solid. Type I/II are fluid-filled at birth and gradually become air-filled (often reimaged at 3 months). Note that CPAM-sequestration hybrid lesions can occur (looks like CPAM but has systemic arterial supply).
4. Granuloma—most common after TB or histoplasmosis. Usually small and calcified.
5. Pulmonary AVM—may visualize draining vein.
6. Bochdalek hernia—due to defect in posterior diaphragm; located at lung base, well-defined cranial margin. May contain abdominal viscera, e.g. kidney.

Neoplastic lesions

Lung neoplasms are less common than mediastinal masses in children. Metastases are much more common than primary lung neoplasms. Malignant > benign neoplasms.

Malignant

1. Solitary metastasis—most commonly Wilms tumour and sarcomas. Note that ~one-third of lung nodules in children with a known primary tumour are NOT metastases, e.g. drug reaction, intrapulmonary lymph node, etc. Lung metastases are rarely an incidental finding in children.
2. Neuroendocrine tumour—80% are carcinoids. Usually malignant, frequently endobronchial, causing lobar collapse or overinflation. Carcinoid syndrome less common in pulmonary carcinoids than tumours elsewhere.
3. Pleuropulmonary blastoma (PPB)—may be cystic (type I, mimics CPAM), mixed (type II) or solid (type III). Can be very large, often peripheral and locally invasive.
4. **Bronchogenic carcinoma**—most commonly mucoepidermoid carcinoma.

Benign

1. **Inflammatory myofibroblastic tumour**—neoplastic subset of inflammatory pseudotumours. Most common primary lung neoplasm in children. Usually benign but can be malignant. Variable size, usually peripheral. Calcified in 25%.
2. **Hamartoma**—occasionally calcified. Slow-growing, well-defined.
3. **Chondroma**—e.g. in Carney triad.

Further reading

Newman, B., 2011. Thoracic neoplasms in children. Radiol. Clin. North Am. 49, 633–664.

LeBlanc, C., Baron, M., Desselas, E., et al., 2017. Congenital pulmonary airways malformations: state-of-the-art review for pediatrician's use. Eur. J. Pediatr. 1-13.

14.43 MULTIPLE PULMONARY NODULES IN A CHILD

Benign

1. **Miliary TB*/other granulomatous infection**—miliary pattern of haematogenous spread should be distinguished from 'tree-in-bud' pattern of endobronchially disseminated TB.
2. **Septic emboli**—frequently cavitary.
3. **Wegener's granulomatosis***—may cavitate.
4. **Respiratory papillomatosis**—represents pulmonary seeding of laryngeal papillomas, occurring in 1% of cases. Nodular and cystic lesions. Poor prognosis. Risk of malignant transformation.
5. **Prior varicella infection**—can result in multiple small calcified granulomas.
6. **Multiple AVMs**—2/3 associated with HHT. Multiple in most cases, usually lower lobes.

Malignant

1. **Multiple pulmonary metastases**—Wilms tumour and sarcomas (calcified nodules in osteosarcoma) are the most common primary sites. Multiple nodules are more likely to be malignant than a single nodule.
2. **Lymphoma* or PTLD**.

14.44 SITUS AND CARDIAC MALPOSITIONS

Assess the position of the cardiac apex first, and then the position of the aortic arch, main and upper lobe bronchi, stomach bubble, liver and spleen.

Cardiac apex

1. **Levocardia**—cardiac apex on the left (i.e. normal position).
2. **Mesocardia**—cardiac apex midline.
3. **Dextrocardia**—cardiac apex on the right (i.e. reverse of normal).

NB: this accounts only for the position of the apex. Atrial position supposedly follows visceral position and is described as 'situs'.

Visceral situs

1. **Situs solitus**—normal position, i.e. liver on the right, gastric bubble on the left and normal airway anatomy.
2. **Situs inversus**—completely switched positions, i.e. liver on the left, stomach bubble on the right, inverted airway anatomy (i.e. earlier take-off of the left-sided upper lobe bronchus).
3. **Left atrial isomerism (LAI)**—bilateral left-sidedness, i.e. long main bronchi passing inferior to the pulmonary arteries with late upper-lobe take-off (as per a normal left bronchus), bilateral bilobed lungs, azygous continuation of the IVC (absent intrahepatic IVC with resultant large azygous venous system) and polysplenia. Associated with complex congenital heart disease.
4. **Right atrial isomerism (RAI)**—bilateral right-sidedness, i.e. bilateral short main bronchi with early upper-lobe take-off (as per a normal right bronchus), bilateral trilobed lungs, ± asplenia. Associated with more severe cardiac and extracardiac malformations than left atrial isomerism.

For simplicity, the isomerisms can be grouped together as conditions of 'visceral heterotaxy' and the individual site of each organ then described in turn.

Further reading

Bierhals, A.J., Rossini, S., Woodard, P.K., Gutierrez, F.R., 2014. Segmental analysis of congenital heart disease: putting the "puzzle" together with computed tomography. Int. J. Cardiovasc. Imaging 30, 1161–1172.

14.45 CONGENITAL HEART DISEASES

Some have characteristic radiographic appearances:

- Ebstein's anomaly—markedly enlarged right heart (RA).
- Transposition of the great arteries (TGA)—narrow superior mediastinum ('egg on a string').
- Tetralogy of Fallot—raised apex (RV enlargement) and cardiomegaly ('boot-shaped heart').

However, these signs are not specific or sensitive and the preferred method of assessment is to start with the lung vasculature—increased (plethoric), decreased (oligaemic) or normal—then to examine the heart size and shape; see table below.

Plethoric		Oligaemic	Normal
Acyanotic (L→R shunt)	*Cyanotic (mixed shunt)*	*Cyanotic (R→L shunt)*	*Acyanotic (no shunt)*
VSD ASD AVSD APW	d-TGA TAPVD Truncus arteriosus HLHS Tricuspid atresia + TGA Single ventricle	Tetralogy of Fallot Ebstein's anomaly Tricuspid atresia Pulmonary atresia	Aortic stenosis Coarctation of aorta Pulmonary stenosis

VSD = ventricular septal defect, ASD = atrial septal defect, AVSD = atrioventricular septal defect, APW = aortopulmonary window, d-TGA = dextro-transposition of the great arteries, TAPVD = total anomalous pulmonary venous drainage, HLHS = hypoplastic left heart syndrome

14.46 CARDIOVASCULAR INVOLVEMENT IN SYNDROMES

Syndrome	Involvement
Down's	AV canal, VSD, PDA, ASD, aberrant right subclavian artery
Ehlers-Danlos	Mitral valve prolapse, aortic root dilatation, dissecting aortic aneurysm, intracranial aneurysm
Ellis-van Creveld	ASD, common atrium
Friedreich ataxia	Hypertrophic cardiomyopathy
Holt-Oram	ASD, VSD
Homocystinuria	Medial degeneration of aorta and pulmonary artery causing dilatation. Arterial and venous thromboses
Hurler/Hunter	Intimal thickening of coronary arteries and valves
Kartagener's	Situs inversus and lower lobe predominant bronchiectasis

Continued

Syndrome	Involvement
Loeys-Dietz	Increased arterial tortuosity and predisposition to aneurysm formation
Marfan	Cystic medial necrosis of aortic wall ± pulmonary artery, leading to dilatation ± dissection. Aortic and mitral regurgitation
Morquio	Late onset of aortic regurgitation
Noonan	Pulmonary valve stenosis, branch stenosis of pulmonary arteries, septal defects
Osteogenesis imperfecta	Aortic and mitral regurgitation, ruptured chordae
Rubella	VSD, ASD, PDA, pulmonary artery branch stenoses, myocardial disease
Trisomy 13	VSD, ASD, PDA, dextroposition
Trisomy 18	VSD, ASD, PDA
Tuberous sclerosis	Cardiomyopathy, cardiac rhabdomyoma
Turner	Aortic coarctation, bicuspid aortic valve stenosis
William	Peripheral pulmonary stenosis, supravalvular aortic stenosis, hypertension

Further reading

Schweigmann, G., Gassner, I., Maurer, K., 2006. Imaging the neonatal heart – essentials for the radiologist. Eur. J. Radiol. 60, 159–170.

14.47 ABDOMINAL MASS IN A CHILD

Renal (55%)

1. **Renal tumours**—see Sections 14.57–14.58.
2. **Hydronephrosis**—see Section 14.59.
3. **Cysts**—see Section 9.15.

Non-renal retroperitoneal (23%)

See also Section 9.32.

1. **Neuroblastoma** (21%)—most common solid extracranial childhood malignancy. 90% <5 years, median age 2 years. Accounts for 50% of all neonatal tumours. 70% are metastatic at presentation.
   - **(a)** Site—adrenal (40%), abdominal sympathetic chain (25%), posterior mediastinal sympathetic chain (15%), neck (5%), pelvis (5%) and unknown (10%).

(b) Clinical presentation.
   (i) Local effects—pain, mass, spinal cord compression, dyspnoea, dysphagia.
   (ii) Effects of metastases—blueberry muffin syndrome (skin metastases), scalp masses, limping, bone pain, weight loss, anaemia, fatigue, etc.
   (iii) Effects of hormone secretion—severe diarrhoea (due to vasoactive intestinal peptides), hypertension, flushing and sweating.
   (iv) Opsomyoclonus—jerky eye movements, myoclonic jerks and cerebellar ataxia; 50% will have neuroblastoma, therefore must investigate thoroughly.

(c) Plain films—calcification (in 2/3), loss of psoas outline, bony metastases, enlarged intervertebral foramina, and in the chest, abnormal posterior ends of ribs.

(d) US—heterogeneous echogenic mass + vascularity ± calcification.

(e) CT—heterogeneous soft-tissue mass with calcification in nearly all. Encasement rather than displacement of major vessels. Paravertebral fat plane is often obliterated ± intraspinal extension via the intervertebral foramina.

(f) MRI—heterogeneously T1 hypointense and T2 hyperintense. Calcification is not as readily recognized as on CT, but MRI is superior for lymph-node metastases, liver metastases and extradural spread of tumour.

(g) Nuclear imaging—bone scan (for cortical disease) and MIBG scan (for medullary disease) are complementary techniques to identify skeletal metastases.

2. **Lymphoma***—uncommon in the absence of mediastinal disease. NHL > Hodgkin disease in children <5 years.
3. **Germ cell tumours**—usually represent a metastasis from a gonadal primary. The most common primary retroperitoneal GCT in children is benign teratoma; typically it contains variable amounts of fluid, soft tissue, fat and calcification.
4. **Other ganglion cell tumours**—i.e. ganglioneuroma (benign, usually >10 years) and ganglioneuroblastoma (malignant potential, age 5–10 years). Similar imaging features to neuroblastoma, but ganglioneuroma does not metastasize, is less commonly calcified and may have a characteristic whorled appearance on MRI.
5. **Other adrenal masses**—see Section 14.56.
6. **Other neurogenic tumours**—schwannoma, neurofibroma (multiple in NF1, may mimic lymphadenopathy), paraganglioma (hypervascular).
7. **Sarcomas**—most commonly rhabdomyosarcoma. Heterogeneous, often with areas of necrosis, but calcification is rare (in contrast to neuroblastoma).

8. **Lipoblastoma**—contains fat. NB: lipomas and liposarcomas are very rare in children.
9. **Intraabdominal pulmonary sequestration**—pyramidal suprarenal solid-cystic mass, separate from adrenal. Has its own arterial supply, usually from aorta.

Gastrointestinal (18%)

1. **Appendix mass/abscess** (10%)—particularly spreads to pouch anterior to rectum.
2. **Hepatoblastoma**—see Section 14.53.
3. **Haemangioma**—commonly multiple, involving entire liver; may also involve mesentery. Large haemangiomas may bleed and appear heterogeneous, but shrink with time. Rarely calcify. May be associated with congestive heart failure and cutaneous haemangiomas.
4. **Choledochal cyst**—the classic triad of mass, pain and jaundice is only present in 10%. Dynamic radionuclide scintigraphy (HIDA scan) is diagnostic. See Section 14.55.
5. **Enteric duplication cyst.**
6. **Mesenteric cyst.**
7. **Meconium pseudocyst**—complication of meconium peritonitis in newborns, forming a rim-calcified pseudocyst in the peritoneal cavity. Other peritoneal calcifications may also be present.

Genital (4%)

1. **Ovarian cysts or teratoma**.
2. **Urogenital sinus-associated cyst.**
3. **Fetus in fetu**—malformed parasitic fetus located inside the body of its viable twin.

Further reading

Haddad, M.C., Birjawi, G.A., Hemadeh, M.S., et al., 2001. The gamut of abdominal and pelvic cystic masses in children. Eur. Radiol. 11, 148–166.

Hoffer, F.A., 2005. Magnetic resonance imaging of abdominal masses in the pediatric patient. Semin. Ultrasound CT MR 26 (4), 212–223.

Xu, Y., Wang, J., Peng, Y., Zeng, J., 2010. CT characteristics of primary retroperitoneal neoplasms in children. Eur. J. Radiol. 75 (3), 321–328.

14.48 ABDOMINAL CYST IN A FETUS OR NEONATE

1. **Ovarian**—most common cyst in a female infant; occasionally cystic teratoma.
2. **Bowel**—enteric duplication cyst, mesenteric/omental cysts and atresias.

3. Renal—hydronephrosis (± urinoma), multicystic dysplastic kidney and autosomal recessive polycystic kidney disease (markedly enlarged kidneys + microcysts).
4. Liver/biliary tree—choledochal cyst, hydatid cyst, mesenchymal hamartoma (cystic) and umbilical vein varix.
5. **Peritoneum**—meconium pseudocyst.
6. **Bladder**—urachal cyst and megacystis.
7. **Genital tract**—urogenital sinus.
8. **Spleen**—simple cyst and hydatid.
9. **Adrenal**—endothelial/epithelial cysts, hydatid and following haemorrhage.
10. **Spine**—anterior meningocoele and sacrococcygeal teratoma.
11. **Pulmonary sequestration**—intraabdominal suprarenal location.

Further reading

Cramer, B., Pushpanathan, C., Kennedy, R., 1993. Nonrenal cystic masses in neonates and children. Can. Assoc. Radiol. J. 44 (2), 93–98.

Silva, C.T., Engel, C., Cross, S.N., et al., 2014. Postnatal sonographic spectrum of prenatally detected abdominal and pelvic cysts. AJR Am. J. Roentgenol. 203 (6), W684–W696.

McEwing, R., Hayward, C., Furness, M., et al., 2003. Foetal cystic abdominal masses. Australas. Radiol. 47 (2), 101–110.

14.49 INTESTINAL OBSTRUCTION IN A NEONATE

1. It is usually impossible to differentiate small from large bowel in a neonate.
2. Not all gaseously distended bowel is obstructed. Resuscitation and positive pressure ventilation may lead to significant bowel distension. Rule of thumb: bowel that is wider than the width of a lumbar vertebral body is dilated.
3. Ileus is characterized by uniform bowel dilatation. It is found in sepsis, necrotizing enterocolitis (NEC) and electrolyte imbalance. Infants with sepsis and NEC are sick; those with uncomplicated bowel obstruction are otherwise usually well.
4. Bowel obstruction should be considered as 'high' (as far down as the jejunum) or 'low' (for more distal obstructions). The former presents with vomiting and is investigated by upper GI contrast study, whereas the latter presents with delayed passage of meconium and may require a contrast enema.

High intestinal obstruction

1. Duodenal atresia/stenosis/web—marked dilatation of the proximal duodenum with the 'double bubble' sign, which may also be seen on US of the fetus (50% have a history of polyhydramnios). No gas distally when there is atresia, but a

variable amount of gas in the distal bowel when there is stenosis. Duodenal web may produce a 'windsock' appearance as web balloons into distal duodenum. Bile-stained vomiting in the majority. Associated with annular pancreas, Down's syndrome, cardiac anomalies, oesophageal atresia and other anomalies of GI tract. A preduodenal portal vein may be seen—this is associated with intrinsic duodenal obstruction (the vein is not the direct cause of obstruction).

2. **Malrotation and volvulus**—sudden onset of bile-stained vomiting. Few radiological signs if the obstruction is recent, intermittent or incomplete. Due to its acute nature, the duodenum is not dilated. If not recognized, progresses to bowel ischaemia, infarction and death. A contrast study should show the normal C-shaped duodenal loop terminating to the left of the left-sided pedicle at the same level as the duodenal cap. In malrotation without volvulus the duodenojejunal flexure is abnormal, to the right of and below its normal position. Volvulus with incomplete obstruction leads to a 'corkscrew' jejunum. With complete obstruction, the distal duodenum terminates as a beak.
3. **Malrotation with obstructing Ladd's bands**—these fibrous bands connect the malrotated caecum to the right posterolateral abdominal wall and typically cross the duodenum (D2). They can cause obstruction even in the absence of volvulus.
4. **Jejunal atresia**—constitutes 50% of small bowel atresias, and 50% are associated with other atretic sites distally (ileum > colon). AXR demonstrates three ('triple bubble') or more dilated, air-filled loops. Colon is usually normal in calibre.
5. **Pyloric atresia**—rare.
6. **Pyloric or prepyloric membrane/antral web**—gastric outlet obstruction with a normal pylorus and the appearance of two duodenal caps. The web may be identified by US.

Low intestinal obstruction

1. **Meconium ileus**—mottled lucencies ('soap bubble' appearance) due to gas trapped in meconium but only few fluid levels (since it is very viscous). Bowel loops of variable calibre. Rapid appearance of fluid levels suggests volvulus. Peritoneal calcification (due to perforation in utero) is seen in 30%. Secondary microcolon on contrast enema, which also shows meconium pellets in the distal ileum. Cystic fibrosis in the majority.
2. **Hirschsprung's disease**—multiple dilated loops of bowel. Diagnosis is made by contrast enema, which shows normal or small size of aganglionic distal bowel with a transition zone at the junction with proximal dilated ganglionic bowel; classically reversed rectosigmoid ratio. The rectum may have a serrated corkscrew appearance. Total colonic aganglionosis may lack a transition zone and present as diffuse microcolon.

3. **Ileal atresia**—50% of small bowel atresia, may be multiple ± jejunal atresia. Multiple dilated loops with fluid levels. Secondary microcolon.
4. **Incarcerated inguinal hernia**.
5. **Small left colon syndrome (SLCS)**—due to functional colonic immaturity; 50% associated with maternal diabetes. Small colon on enema up to level of splenic flexure, ± meconium plugs. Infants should be followed up to exclude Hirschsprung's.
6. **Meconium plug syndrome**—meconium plugs in distal colon. Overlaps with SLCS. May be a presenting feature of Hirschsprung's or cystic fibrosis (but note this is not the same as meconium ileus).
7. **Inspissated milk**—presents from 3 days to 6 weeks of age. Dense, amorphous intraluminal masses frequently surrounded by a rim of air, ± mottled lucencies internally. Usually resolves spontaneously.
8. **Colonic atresia**—5%–15% of intestinal atresias. AXR may be similar to other distal bowel obstructions but some infants show a huge, disproportionately dilated loop (between the atretic segment and a competent ileocaecal valve).
9. **Anorectal malformation/imperforate anus**.
   (a) High—± sacral agenesis/hypoplasia and gas in the bladder (due to a rectovesical or rectourethral fistula). Currarino triad = anorectal malformation, sacral dysgenesis and sacrococcygeal teratoma variant/meningocoele.
   (b) Low—± perineal or urethral fistula.

Further reading

Applegate, K.E., Anderson, J.M., Klatte, E.C., 2006. Intestinal malrotation in children: a problem-solving approach to the upper gastrointestinal series. Radiographics 5, 1485–1500.

Berrocal, T., Torres, I., Gutierrez, J., et al., 1999. Congenital anomalies of the upper gastrointestinal tract. Radiographics 19, 855–872.

Berrocal, T., Lamas, M., Gutierrez, J., et al., 1999. Congenital anomalies of the small intestine, colon, and rectum. Radiographics 19, 1219–1236.

Carty, H., Brereton, R.J., 1983. The distended neonate. Clin. Radiol. 34, 367–380.

14.50 INTRAABDOMINAL CALCIFICATIONS IN THE NEWBORN

1. **Meconium peritonitis**—antenatal bowel perforation results in aseptic peritonitis, which rapidly calcifies. Calcification occurs in the peritoneum itself most commonly, but also in the bowel wall and in the scrotum and may be punctate, linear or plaque-like. The most common causes are meconium ileus and ileal atresia, but any cause of bowel obstruction may be associated.
2. **Meconium pseudocyst**—cyst-like mass with peripheral calcification resulting from walling-off of extruded meconium after perforation.

3. **Bowel calcification**—intramural lymphatic or intraluminal meconium calcification in cases of distal bowel obstruction, particularly meconium ileus, total colonic aganglionosis and anorectal malformations. Occasionally a duodenal duplication cyst may calcify and appear as a spherical upper abdominal calcification.
4. **Hepatic calcification**—see Section 14.54.
5. **Adrenal calcification**—following adrenal haemorrhage; rarely in Wolman disease.

Further reading

Beasley, S.W., de Campo, M., 1986. Intraluminal calcification in the newborn: diagnostic and surgical implications. Pediatr. Surg. 1, 249.

Miller, J.P., Smith, S.D., Sukarochana, K., 1988. Neonatal abdominal calcification: is it always meconium peritonitis? J. Pediatr. Surg. 23, 555.

14.51 ABNORMALITIES OF BOWEL ROTATION

1. **Exomphalos**—total failure of the bowel to return to the abdomen from the umbilical cord. Bowel is contained within a sac.
2. **Gastroschisis**—bowel protrudes through a defect in the abdominal wall without a sac, classically in a right paraumbilical position.
3. **Nonrotation**—usually an asymptomatic condition with the small bowel on the right side of the abdomen and the colon on the left side. Small and large bowel lie on either side of the SMA with a common mesentery. Imaging shows the SMV lying to the left of the SMA (opposite of normal arrangement).
4. **Malrotation**—the duodenojejunal flexure lies to the right and caudad to its usual position. The caecum is usually more cephalad than normal, but is normally sited in 5%. Malrotation is a frequent feature of diaphragmatic hernia, abdominal wall defects and visceral heterotaxy. CT/US shows the SMV to the left of the SMA. A normal US does not, however, exclude malrotation (3% false-negative rate); upper GI contrast study remains the gold standard. At risk of life-threatening volvulus.
5. **Reverse rotation**—rare. Colon lies dorsal to the SMA with jejunum and duodenum anterior to it.
6. **Paraduodenal hernia**—rare.
7. **Cloacal exstrophy**—rare. No rotation of the bowel, and the ileum and colon open separately onto the extroverted area in the midline below the umbilical cord. Associated with 'open-book pelvis' and split genitalia.

Further reading

Applegate, K.E., Anderson, J.M., Klatte, E.C., 1992. Intestinal malrotation in children: a problem-solving approach to the upper gastrointestinal series. Radiographics 26 (5), 1485–1500.

Strouse, P.J., 2004. Disorders of intestinal rotation and fixation ('malrotation'). Pediatr. Radiol. 34, 837–851.

14.52 GAS IN THE PORTAL VEINS

1. Necrotizing enterocolitis—seen in 10%. Necrotic bowel wall allows gas or gas-forming organisms into the portal circulation.
2. Umbilical vein catheterization—with inadvertent injection of air.
3. **Postoperative**—e.g. after liver transplant or corrective bowel surgery.
4. **Haemolytic disease of the newborn.**
5. **Neonatal viral gastroenteritis.**

14.53 HEPATIC MASSES IN CHILDREN

Account for ~5% of all childhood abdominal masses.

Malignant tumours (two-thirds)

1. Metastases—from neuroblastoma or Wilms tumour.
2. Hepatoblastoma—M>F, usually <5 years old (peak 18-24 months). Serum αFP usually raised. Typically a large well-defined heterogeneous mass ± vascular invasion ± areas of necrosis, haemorrhage and calcification. Metastasizes to lungs, abdominal nodes and bones. Associated with Beckwith-Wiedemann syndrome, hemihypertrophy and FAP.
3. Hepatocellular carcinoma—similar features to hepatoblastoma, but occurs in an older age group (>5 years, peak 12-14 years with a smaller peak at 2-4 years), is more likely to be multifocal, and has a worse prognosis. Associated with chronic liver disease (cirrhosis, glycogen storage disease 1, tyrosinaemia, biliary atresia, chronic hepatitis, alpha-1 antitrypsin deficiency).
4. **Undifferentiated embryonal sarcoma of the liver**—rare; majority are 6–10 years of age.
5. **Teratoma.**

Benign tumours (one-third)

1. Infantile hepatic haemangioma—most common benign tumour. Often presents in the newborn period with hepatomegaly and congestive cardiac failure ± skin haemangiomas (50%) ± consumptive coagulopathy (thrombocytopenia). Unifocal or multifocal, well-defined or diffuse. Typical enhancement pattern on CT with early peripheral enhancement + variable delayed centripetal filling over 30 minutes. On MRI the lesions have a nonspecific T1 hypointense and T2 hyperintense appearance with variable areas of hypointensity corresponding to fibrosis and haemosiderin deposition. ^{99m}Tc-labelled red cells will accumulate in

this tumour. In the neonate, this and cavernous haemangioma may be considered together.
2. **Mesenchymal hamartoma**—second most common benign tumour. <2 years of age. May be (multi)cystic or stromal, with a 'Swiss cheese' appearance. Solid components may enhance.
3. **Adenoma**—uncommon in paediatric population. Solitary or multiple, occurring spontaneously or complicating glycogen storage disease, Fanconi anaemia treated with anabolic steroids, and teenagers on the oral contraceptive pill. See Chapter 8.

Other lesions

1. **Cysts**—simple, choledochal or hydatid.
2. **Focal nodular hyperplasia**—2%–6% of hepatic lesions in childhood. See Chapter 8.
3. **Abscess**.

Further reading

Burrows, P.E., Dubois, J., Kassarjian, A., 2001. Pediatric hepatic vascular anomalies. Pediatr. Radiol. 3, 533–545.
Faingold, R., Albuquerque, P.A., Carpineta, L., 2011. Hepatobiliary tumors. Radiol. Clin. North Am. 49 (4), 679–687.

14.54 FETAL OR NEONATAL LIVER CALCIFICATION

Peritoneal surface of liver

1. **Meconium peritonitis**—solid or cystic masses with calcified walls.
2. **Plastic peritonitis due to ruptured hydrometrocolpos**—similar appearance to meconium peritonitis but US may show a dilated, fluid-filled uterus and vagina.

Parenchymal

1. **Congenital infections**—TORCH complex (toxoplasmosis, rubella, CMV, herpes simplex) and varicella. Randomly scattered nodular calcification. Often calcification elsewhere and other congenital abnormalities.
2. **Tumours**—haemangioma, hamartoma, hepatoblastoma, teratoma and metastatic neuroblastoma. Complex mass on US.
3. **Haematoma**—following vascular catheter injury, or haemorrhage in a vascular mass such as haemangioma.

Vascular

1. **Portal vein thromboemboli**—subcapsular branching calcification.
2. **Ischaemic infarcts**—branching calcifications but distributed throughout the liver.

14.55 JAUNDICE IN INFANCY

1. Neonatal cholestasis—due to breastfeeding, maternal diabetes, drugs and total parenteral nutrition. Usually transient.
2. Haemolytic anaemias—hereditary, ABO or Rhesus incompatibilities. Unconjugated hyperbilirubinaemia (unlike the other causes on this list).
3. Biliary atresia—type 1 involves CBD only; type 2a involves CHD only; type 2b involves CHD, CBD and cystic duct; type 3 involves all extrahepatic ducts including left and right hepatic ducts (>90% of cases). May be associated with congenital anomalies, e.g. polysplenia, intestinal malrotation, azygos continuation of IVC, situs inversus and preduodenal portal vein. On US, the 'triangular cord' sign (band of echogenic fibrous tissue at the porta hepatis replacing the bile duct) is highly specific. An absent or small irregular gallbladder (gallbladder 'ghost') is seen in types 2b and 3. A prominent hepatic artery may also support the diagnosis, but cannot be used in isolation. A normal-sized gallbladder that contracts after a fatty meal excludes the diagnosis. On HIDA scan, normal uptake by hepatocytes but no excretion into the bowel suggests the diagnosis (though alpha-1 antitrypsin may look similar). Operative cholangiography is definitive.
4. Neonatal hepatitis—often idiopathic but some cases are viral (e.g. hepatitis A–C, rubella, CMV). Liver may be enlarged or hyperechoic on US, and the gallbladder may be small due to poor hepatocyte function. HIDA scan may show delayed hepatocyte uptake, but excretion into bowel is usually normal.
5. Choledochal cyst—may present in the neonatal period or at a later age. See Chapter 8. On US: anechoic structure separate from the gallbladder, which communicates with the biliary tree. On HIDA scan: photopenic area, which accumulates tracer on delayed images. Complications include calculi, infection, pancreatitis, biliary cirrhosis, portal hypertension and malignancy.
6. **Alagille syndrome**—hypoplasia of intrahepatic bile ducts, cardiovascular abnormalities (especially pulmonary stenosis), dysmorphic facies, eye abnormalities, butterfly vertebrae, radioulnar synostosis.
7. **Metabolic defects**—e.g. alpha-1 antitrypsin deficiency, galactosaemia, tyrosinaemia and glucose-6-phosphate dehydrogenase enzyme deficiency.

Further reading

Humphrey, T.M., Stringer, M.D., 2007. Biliary atresia: US diagnosis. Radiology 244, 845–851.

Santiago, I., Loureiro, R., Curvo-Semedo, L., et al., 2012. Congenital cystic lesions of the biliary tree. AJR Am. J. Roentgenol. 198 (4), 825–835.

14.56 ADRENAL MASS IN CHILDHOOD

NB: in neonates the adrenals are normally large in size with a hyperechoic medulla and hypoechoic cortex. This involutes over the first few months of life.

Neoplastic

Medullary

1. **Neuroblastoma, ganglioneuroblastoma, ganglioneuroma**—see Section 14.47.
2. **Phaeochromocytoma**—uncommon. Mean age 11 years, 25% bilateral. Associated with MEN type 2, NF1 and vHL.

Cortical

1. **Adrenocortical neoplasms**—differentiating benign (adenoma) from malignant (carcinoma) lesions not possible in childhood. Usually hormonally active and most patients <5 years of age.
2. **Malignant rhabdoid tumour**—rare, highly aggressive.

Nonneoplastic—rare beyond infancy

1. **Hyperplasia**—e.g. congenital adrenal hyperplasia (characteristic cerebriform appearance). Typically bilateral.
2. **Haemorrhage**—blunt trauma, bleeding diathesis and meningococcal sepsis. Avascular on US.
3. **Cyst**—rare, usually a lymphatic malformation or haemorrhagic pseudocyst.
4. **Abscess**—rare; haematogenous or direct intraperitoneal spread.
5. **Calcification**—Wolman disease; bilateral enlarged calcified adrenals.

Conditions that can mimic adrenal lesions

1. **Subdiaphragmatic extralobar pulmonary sequestration.**
2. **Extramedullary hematopoiesis.**
3. **Diaphragmatic lesions.**

Further reading

Bittman, M.E., Lee, E.Y., Restrepo, R., Eisenberg, R.L., 2013. Focal adrenal lesions in pediatric patients. Am. J. Roentgenol. 200 (6), W542–W556.

14.57 PRIMARY RENAL NEOPLASMS IN CHILDHOOD

1. **Wilms tumour**—accounts for 87% of pediatric renal masses. Peak incidence at 3–4 years of age, 80% present <5 years. Bilateral in 5%. Associated abnormalities: cryptorchidism, hypospadias, hemihypertrophy, sporadic aniridia. Associated syndromes:

Denys-Drash, WAGR, Beckwith-Wiedemann (10% will develop Wilms tumour). Metastasizes to lungs and liver. 5% have a tumour thrombus in the IVC or right atrium. Hypertension in 25% (renin-induced). Screening in patients with associated syndromes should begin at 6 months of age, mainly by serial US every 3 months up to 7 years of age.

(a) Plain film—bulging flank, loss or enlargement of renal outline, displacement of bowel gas, loss of psoas outline, calcification (10%).
(b) US—large, well-defined mass, similar or greater echogenicity than liver. Solid with haemorrhage/necrosis. Lack of IVC narrowing on inspiration suggests occlusion.
(c) CT—large, well-defined, heterogeneous with foci of low attenuation necrosis. Minimal enhancement compared with the residual rind of functioning renal tissue. Claw sign (rim of preserved renal tissue clawing at the tumour mass).
(d) MRI—heterogeneous, low T1 signal, high T2 signal. Inhomogeneous enhancement compared with residual renal tissue.

2. **Nephroblastomatosis**—nephrogenic rests which maintain the potential for malignant induction to Wilms tumour. Seen in up to 40% of unilateral and 99% of bilateral Wilms tumours. May be perilobar (most common, at the lobar surface), intralobar (anywhere in the cortex or medulla) or combined. Hypoechoic on US, similar signal to renal cortex on MRI. Nonenhancing on CT/MRI, therefore best seen on postcontrast images.
3. **Congenital mesoblastic nephroma**—most common solid renal tumour in the newborn. May contain cystic, haemorrhagic or necrotic areas. Mean age at diagnosis is 3.5 months. Often indistinguishable from Wilms tumour on imaging, but different age group.
4. **Multilocular cystic nephroma**—presents at 3 months to 4 years. Multiple cysts of varying size, thin septa only. May contain variable signal on MRI due to haemorrhage or protein content. Thick septa, nodules or a large solid component suggest Wilms tumour with cystic degeneration. Resection is curative, local recurrence is rare. Differential diagnosis is a multicystic dysplastic kidney, but this typically affects the entire kidney.
5. **Angiomyolipoma (AML)**—in children, nearly always associated with tuberous sclerosis, and typically multiple and bilateral. Lesions >3 cm carry increased risk of bleeding. Surveillance with US or MRI is recommended 1–2 times yearly if lesions are <3 cm and annually if they are bigger. Characteristically contain fat on imaging (NB: fat may also occasionally be identified within Wilms tumour).
6. **Clear cell sarcoma**—presents at 3–5 years. Poor prognosis with early metastases to bone (usually lytic but may be sclerotic). Never

bilateral. Imaging features often similar to Wilms (but different pattern of metastases).

7. **Rhabdoid tumour of kidney**—presents at 3 months to 4.5 years (50% in first year). Most malignant renal tumour with poorest prognosis. Extrarenal extension or haematogenous metastases (to brain or bone) often present at diagnosis. Associated with midline posterior cranial fossa tumours. Similar on imaging to Wilms tumour; however, areas of necrosis or calcification outlining tumour lobules may suggest rhabdoid tumour.
8. **Renal cell carcinoma**—rare. Differentiating features from Wilms tumour are: older age (mean 11–12 years), calcification is more common (25%), more homogeneous, smaller at the time of diagnosis and haematuria is more common. Poorer prognosis compared with Wilms tumour. Similar imaging findings. Associated with von Hippel-Lindau disease and tuberous sclerosis.
9. **Ossifying renal tumour of infancy (ORTI)**—rare benign tumour of infancy, which mimics a staghorn calculus. Presents with gross hematuria and a calcified mass in the pelvicalyceal system.

Further reading

Geller, E., Kochan, P.S., 2011. Renal neoplasms of childhood. Radiol. Clin. North Am. 49 (4), 689–709, vi.

McHugh, K., 2007. Renal and adrenal tumours in children. Cancer Imaging 7, 41–51.

Lowe, L.H., Isuani, B.H., Heller, R.M., et al., 2000. Pediatric renal masses: Wilms tumor and beyond. Radiographics 20 (6), 1585–1603.

14.58 RENAL MASS IN THE NEWBORN AND YOUNG INFANT

1. <u>**Hydronephrosis**</u>—unilateral or bilateral. The most common cause of an abdominal mass in the first 6 months of life.
2. <u>**Multicystic dysplastic kidney**</u>—unilateral, but 30% have an abnormal contralateral kidney (mostly reflux or PUJ obstruction). On imaging, presents as multiple cysts replacing the renal parenchyma with intervening fibrous tissue.
3. <u>**Polycystic kidneys (autosomal recessive)**</u>—bilateral. Large and highly echogenic on US.
4. <u>**Renal vein thrombosis**</u>—unilateral or bilateral.
5. <u>**Renal neoplasms**</u>—e.g. congenital mesoblastic nephroma, multilocular cystic nephroma, rhabdoid tumour and ORTI (see Section 14.57).
6. <u>**Nephroblastomatosis**</u>.

Further reading

Geller, E., Kochan, P.S., 2011. Renal neoplasms of childhood. Radiol. Clin. North Am. 49 (4), 689–709, vi.

14.59 HYDRONEPHROSIS IN A CHILD

1. **PUJ obstruction**—L>R, 20% bilateral. Due to stricture, neuromuscular incoordination or aberrant vessels. Contralateral kidney may be dysplastic or absent.
2. **Primary vesicoureteric reflux without obstruction**—usually idiopathic. Common in the lower moiety of a duplex system.
3. **Vesicoureteric junction (VUJ) obstruction**—may be secondary to bladder hypertrophy/neurogenic dysfunction or obstructive ureterocoele (e.g. upper moiety of a duplex kidney). Primary type is more common in males and on the left side. May be bilateral.
4. **Primary megaureter**—represents ureteral atony. Sometimes associated with UTI; may be nonobstructive and nonrefluxing.
5. **Bladder outflow obstruction**—usually due to posterior urethral valves (in males), causing bilateral upper tract dilatation.

Further reading

Riccabona, M., 2004. Assessment and management of newborn hydronephrosis. World J. Urol. 22 (2), 73–78.

Berrocal, T., López-Pereira, P., Arjonilla, A., Gutiérrez, J., 2002. Anomalies of the distal ureter, bladder, and urethra in children: embryologic, radiologic, and pathologic features. Radiographics 22 (5), 1139–1164.

14.60 BLADDER OUTFLOW OBSTRUCTION IN A CHILD

Assessed by micturating cystourethrogram (MCUG). The most common cause is posterior urethral valves (in males) and ectopic ureterocoele (in females). Results in a distended bladder with incomplete emptying, or reduced bladder volume with trabeculation if long-standing obstruction, ± bilateral upper tract dilatation ± upper tract cystic dysplasia.

Causes (from proximal to distal)

1. **Vesical diverticulum**—posteriorly behind the bladder base. It fills during micturition and compresses the bladder neck and proximal urethra. M>F.
2. **Bladder neck obstruction**—e.g. by an ectopic ureterocoele or rhabdomyosarcoma.
3. **Ectopic ureterocoele**—80% are associated with the ectopic upper moiety ureter of a duplex kidney. 15% are bilateral. F>M. Ectopic ureter may open into the urethra, bladder neck or vestibule. Ureterocoele may be largely outside the bladder, elevating the bladder base, or may prolapse into the urethra.

4. <u>Posterior urethral valves</u>—on MCUG, posterior urethra is dilated and the distal urethra is small. Almost exclusively males.
5. **Urethral stricture**—posttraumatic strictures (e.g. instrumentation or catheterization) are most commonly at the penoscrotal junction.
6. **Cowper's syringocoele**—dilatation of the main duct of the bulbourethral (Cowper's) glands; males only. Filling of Cowper's ducts may be a normal finding. When dilated, occasionally presents with haematuria, infection or urethral obstruction.
7. **Anterior urethral diverticulum/valve**—a saccular wide-necked, ventral expansion of the anterior urethra, usually at the penoscrotal junction. The proximal lip of the diverticulum may show as an arcuate filling defect and during micturition the diverticulum expands with urine and obstructs the urethra.
8. **Prune-belly and megacystis-microcolon syndromes.**
9. **Calculus or foreign body.**
10. **Meatal stenosis**—males only; usually a clinical diagnosis, but may be detected on MCUG; voiding images should include the meatus (external urethral opening).
11. **Phimosis**—clinical diagnosis.

14.61 VESICOURETERIC REFLUX

Congenital = primary reflux

1. <u>Simple congenital reflux</u>—due to VUJ incompetence secondary to abnormal tunnelling of distal ureter through bladder. 10% of normal Caucasian babies and 30% of children with a first episode of UTI. Usually disappears in 80%. Medium- to high-grade reflux can lead to renal damage in association with UTI.
2. <u>Reflux associated with duplex kidneys</u>—usually occurs into lower-moiety ureter, which has a normal position but abnormal tunnelling. Reflux may also occur into a ureterocoele if this everts during filling or voiding.

Acquired = secondary reflux

1. <u>Hutch diverticulum</u>—congenital bladder diverticulum at the VUJ.
2. <u>Cystitis</u>—in 50%.
3. <u>Neurogenic bladder</u>.
4. <u>Urethral obstruction</u>—most commonly posterior urethral valves (see Section 14.60). L>R.

5. Prune-belly syndrome—almost exclusively males. High mortality. Bilateral hydronephrosis and hydroureters with a distended bladder. Associated with undescended testes, hypoplasia of the anterior abdominal wall and urethral obstruction.

Further reading

Riccabona, M., Avni, F.E., Blickman, J.G., et al., 2008. Imaging recommendations in paediatric uroradiology: minutes of the ESPR workgroup session on urinary tract infection, fetal hydronephrosis, urinary tract ultrasonography and voiding cystourethrography, Barcelona, Spain, June 2007. Pediatr. Radiol. 38 (2), 138–145.

14.62 RETINOBLASTOMA AND ITS DIFFERENTIALS

Rare but most common intraocular tumour of childhood; usually presents <5 years. An aggressive malignant tumour, accounts for ~10% of all cancers in the first year of life. Bilateral or multifocal tumours occur in patients with heritable retinoblastoma (~30–60% of cases). If bilateral heritable retinoblastomas occur with a primary intracranial neuroblastic tumour (usually pineal or parasellar), the syndrome is called 'trilateral retinoblastoma'. Leukocoria and strabismus are the most common presenting symptoms.

Differential diagnosis of retinoblastoma

Greater than 50% of children presenting with a clinical diagnosis of retinoblastoma have another diagnosis, commonly persistent hyperplastic primary vitreous (PHPV), Coat's disease or toxocariasis. Calcification (95% on CT) is the most important feature that differentiates retinoblastoma from other tumour-like lesions. None of the conditions in the following table show calcification <3 years, but above that age some may do so, e.g. retinal astrocytoma, retinopathy of prematurity and toxocariasis.

Further reading

Brennan, R.C., Wilson, M.W., Kaste, S., et al., 2012. US and MRI of pediatric ocular masses with histopathological correlation. Pediatr. Radiol. 42 (6), 738–749.

Chung, E.M., Specht, C.S., Schroeder, J.W., 2007. From the archives of the AFIP: pediatric orbit tumors and tumorlike lesions: neuroepithelial lesions of the ocular globe and optic nerve. Radiographics 27 (4), 1159–1186.

	Clinical features	Age	Radiology
Persistent hyperplastic primary vitreous (PHPV)	Unilateral leukocoria	At or soon after birth	Microphthalmia. Small irregular lens; shallow anterior chamber. No calcification. Increased attenuation of the vitreous. Enhancement of abnormal intravitreal tissue. Triangular retrolental density with its apex on the posterior lens and base on the posterior globe. Fluid level on decubitus scanning
Coat's disease	A vascular anomaly of telangiectatic vessels, which leak proteinaceous material into the subretinal space. Usually boys; unilateral. Present at birth but usually asymptomatic until the retina detaches and vision deteriorates	4–8 years	Appearances of retinal detachment. Indistinguishable from noncalcified retinoblastoma on CT. High T1/T2 signal subretinal effusion on MRI
Retinopathy of prematurity	Unilateral or bilateral leukocoria. Previous history of prematurity and oxygen therapy	7–10 weeks	No calcification (but may calcify in the older child). Microphthalmia
Toxocariasis	Close contact with dogs. No systemic symptoms. Positive ELISA	Mean 6 years	Opaque vitreous or a localized, irregular retinal mass. No contrast enhancement
Chronic retinal detachment	Rare. Presentation late. More common in developmentally abnormal eyes and dysmorphic syndromes		No enhancement or calcification
Retinal astrocytoma (astrocytic hamartoma)	In 40% of patients with tuberous sclerosis or less commonly NF1, retinitis pigmentosa or as an isolated abnormality		Multiple small retinal masses, may be bilateral. May calcify in the older child
Retinal dysplasia	Bilateral leukocoria	At or soon after birth	Bilateral retrolental masses. No calcification

ELISA = enzyme-linked immunosorbent assay.

14.63 PREVERTEBRAL SOFT-TISSUE MASS ON THE LATERAL CERVICAL X-RAY

NB: anterior buckling of the trachea with an increase in the thickness of the retropharyngeal tissues may occur as a normal phenomenon in expiration during the first 2 years of life and is due to laxity of the retropharyngeal tissues. These soft tissues may contain a small collection of air, trapped in the inferior recess of the laryngeal pharynx above the contracted upper oesophageal sphincter. An ear lobe may also mimic a prevertebral mass.

1. Trauma/haematoma—± associated fracture.
2. Abscess—± gas lucencies within it. Unlike the normal variant described above, these lucencies are constant and persist during deep inspiration. A sharp foreign body may be visible within the collection.
3. Neoplasms—e.g. lymphangioma, lymphoma, nasopharyngeal rhabdomyosarcoma, neuroblastoma and LCH (with vertebra plana).

14.64 NECK MASSES IN INFANTS AND CHILDREN

US is a valuable first imaging modality. MRI is generally preferred to CT. Different classification systems, e.g. soft versus firm; midline versus lateral; or:

Congenital

1. Lymphovascular malformations—soft. Lymphangiomas are uni- or multilocular and often involve multiple neck spaces. Infantile haemangiomas are solid and hypervascular, and typically resolve spontaneously.
2. Cysts—firm.
   (a) Thyroglossal—midline position.
   (b) Branchial cleft—lateral position. Second branchial arch remnant most common, lying posterior to the submandibular gland, lateral to the carotid space and anteromedial to the sternomastoid muscle.
   (c) Lingual—including ranula.
   (d) **Thymic**—rare, remnant of thymopharyngeal duct. Located close to carotid sheath, often extends into mediastinum.
   (e) **Dermoid/epidermoid/teratoma**—midline, often contains fat and calcification (except epidermoid, which only contains fluid).
3. **Ectopic cervical thymic lobe.**

Acquired

1. Infective/reactive lymphadenopathy—e.g. viral, bacterial, mycobacterial and cat-scratch disease. Nonviral nodal infections can lead to suppuration/abscess formation.
2. Malignant neoplasms—e.g. lymphoma, neuroblastoma (secondary > primary), rhabdomyosarcoma, LCH (disseminated disease in infants) and thyroid cancer (rare, usually papillary).
3. Benign neoplasms—e.g. lipoma, neurofibroma (in NF1), pilomatricoma (arises from skin, often calcified), thyroid cyst or nodule.
4. Fibromatosis colli—unilateral enlargement of sternocleidomastoid muscle in young infants ± torticollis. Thought to be related to birth trauma.
5. **Trauma/haematoma.**
6. **Diffuse thyroid enlargement**—e.g. Graves' disease, multinodular goitre and Hashimoto's thyroiditis.
7. **Parotitis**—e.g. bacterial (unilateral), HIV (bilateral) and Sjögren's (bilateral).

Further reading

Friedman, E.R., John, S.D., 2011. Imaging of pediatric neck masses. Radiol. Clin. North Am. 49 (4), 617–632, v.

14.65 CAUSES OF STROKE IN CHILDREN AND YOUNG ADULTS

1. Emboli—cyanotic heart disease (due to R→L intracardiac shunt), cardiomyopathies, mitral valve prolapse, HHT (due to pulmonary AVMs).
2. Arterial wall abnormalities.
   (a) Dissection—may be traumatic (including nonaccidental injury), spontaneous, or secondary to Marfan syndrome, Ehlers-Danlos syndrome or homocystinuria.
   (b) Vasculitis/vasculopathy—e.g. due to Moyamoya disease, fibromuscular dysplasia (also vessel stenoses and saccular dilatations, intracranial aneurysms), NF1, Kawasaki, SLE and sarcoidosis.
   (c) Reversible cerebral vasoconstriction syndrome—due to vasospasm, presents with 'thunderclap' headache (adolescents > children). Can cause watershed infarcts. Associated with pregnancy (including preeclampsia and puerperium), drugs (e.g. cocaine and amphetamines) and migraine.
3. Cerebral venous sinus thrombosis—pregnancy, postpartum, oral contraceptive pill, skull base/intracranial sepsis, IBD, SLE, Behçet's disease and malignancy.

4. <u>Infection</u>—purulent meningitis may cause arterial and venous strokes. Viral infection can cause a vasculitis, usually of the proximal MCA, leading to infarction of the basal ganglia with sparing of the cortical territories.
5. <u>Blood disorders</u>—sickle cell anaemia, polycythaemia, protein C and S deficiency and antiphospholipid syndrome.
6. **MELAS**—**M**itochondrial **E**ncephalomyopathy with **L**actic **A**cidosis and **S**troke-like episodes.
7. **Idiopathic**—in many cases, a cause is not found.

14.66 LARGE HEAD IN INFANCY

1. **Benign familial macrocephaly**—usually associated with parental large head and large head circumference at birth.
2. **Benign enlargement of subarachnoid space (BESS)**—also called 'external hydrocephalus'. Benign, self-limiting. Increased risk of subdural haematoma either spontaneously or after minor accidental trauma, which may mimic nonaccidental injury.
3. **Hydrocephalus.**
4. **Chronic subdural haematoma.**
5. **Brain tumours.**
6. **Neurofibromatosis* type 1.**
7. **Mucopolysaccharidoses*.**
8. **Hemimegalencephaly.**
9. **Leukodystrophy.**
   (a) **Alexander's disease**—typically involves the frontal lobes early in its course.
   (b) **Canavan's disease**—typically affects the subcortical arcuate fibres, but often involves the entire cerebral white matter.
10. **Overgrowth syndromes**—e.g. Sotos, Simpson-Golabi-Behmel, Beckwith-Wiedemann.
11. **Hydranencephaly.**

Further reading

Williams, C.A., Dagli, A., Battaglia, A., 2008. Genetic disorders associated with macrocephaly. Am. J. Hum. Genet. 146A, 2023–2037.

Tucker, J., Choudhary, A.K., Piatt, J., 2016. Macrocephaly in infancy: benign enlargement of the subarachnoid spaces and subdural collections. J. Neurosurg. Pediatr. 18 (1), 16–20.

14.67 WIDE CRANIAL SUTURES

>10 mm at birth; >3 mm at 2 years; >2 mm at 3 years.

1. <u>Raised intracranial pressure</u>—e.g. due to intracranial tumour, subdural haematoma or hydrocephalus. Only seen in children <10 years.

2. **Infiltration of sutures**—e.g. by neuroblastoma (± skull vault lucencies and 'sunray' spiculation), leukaemia or lymphoma.
3. **Metabolic disease**—rickets, hypoparathyroidism, lead toxicity or bone dysplasias with defective mineralization (e.g. hypophosphatasia).
4. **Traumatic diastasis of the sutures.**
5. **Recovery from illness**—rapid rebound growth of the brain following chronic illness, deprivational dwarfism, prematurity or hypothyroidism.

14.68 MULTIPLE WORMIAN BONES

Intrasutural ossicles common in infancy (lambdoid, posterior sagittal and temporosquamosal). Considered abnormal if large (≥6 x 4 mm) and multiple (>10), and arranged in a general mosaic pattern.

1. **Idiopathic.**
2. **Down's syndrome***.
3. **Pyknodysostosis.**
4. **Osteogenesis imperfecta.**
5. **Rickets***.
6. **Cleidocranial dysplasia***.
7. **Kinky hair (Menkes) syndrome.**
8. **Hypophosphatasia.**
9. **Hypothyroidism.**
10. **Otopalatodigital syndrome.**
11. **Primary acroosteolysis (Hajdu-Cheney syndrome).**
12. **Pachydermoperiostosis.**
13. **Gerodermia osteodysplastica**—see Section 14.12.
14. **Progeria.**

Further reading

Cremin, B., Goodman, H., Spranger, J., et al., 1982. Wormian bones in osteogenesis imperfecta and other disorders. Skeletal Radiol. 8, 35–38.

14.69 CRANIOSYNOSTOSIS

Premature closure of one or more sutures. May occur as an isolated primary abnormality, as part of a more complex syndrome or secondary to systemic disease. Fusion of a suture arrests growth of the calvarium. Raised intracranial pressure may occur with closure of multiple sutures. Volumetric CT with 3D reformatting offers the best evaluation of the skull sutures and also demonstrates the intracranial contents (e.g. malformations, hydrocephalus and arrested brain growth).

Primary craniosynostosis

1. **Sagittal synostosis**—elongated narrow 'boat-shaped' skull (scaphocephaly).
2. **Unilateral coronal synostosis**—oblique appearance of the craniofacial structures (frontal plagiocephaly) with harlequin orbit.
3. **Bilateral coronal synostosis**—'short head' (brachycephaly), often seen with synostosis of other sutures.
4. **Metopic synostosis**—triangular-shaped head (trigonocephaly) with orbital hypotelorism.
5. **Unilateral lambdoid synostosis**—asymmetric occipital plagiocephaly.
6. **Bilateral lambdoid synostosis**—occipital plagiocephaly with flattened occiput. Beware postural flattening of the occiput due to infants being placed to sleep on their backs (no sutural fusion in these cases).
7. **Cloverleaf skull**—'trilobular skull' due to synostosis of multiple paired sutures.

Syndromic craniosynostosis

Most commonly seen in acrocephalosyndactylies (e.g. Apert, Carpenter and Pfeiffer syndromes). Each syndrome exhibits synostosis of multiple sutures with severe calvarial and facial malformations. Crouzon syndrome differs in that there is no syndactyly.

Secondary

1. **Brain damage or malformation**—following hypoxic ischaemic encephalopathy, holoprosencephaly, microcephaly.
2. **Iatrogenic**—shunted hydrocephalus.
3. **Metabolic**—rickets, hyperthyroidism, hypophosphatasia.
4. **Inborn errors of metabolism**—Hurler and Morquio syndromes.
5. **Haematological disease**—thalassaemia and sickle cell.

Further reading

Aviv, R.I., Rodger, E., Hall, C.M., 2002. Craniosynostosis. Clin. Radiol. 57, 93–102.

14.70 CYSTIC LESIONS ON CRANIAL US IN NEONATES AND INFANTS

Normal variants

1. **Coarctation of the lateral ventricles**—aka connatal cysts: small cysts at the superolateral margin of the frontal horns.
2. **Cavum septum pellucidum/vergae/velum interpositum**—common, particularly in premature neonates.

Infratentorial cysts

1. Mega cisterna magna—as an isolated finding, probably a normal variant. Intact vermis.
2. Dandy-Walker malformation/variant—vermian hypoplasia + cystic dilatation of posterior fossa in communication with the fourth ventricle.
3. Arachnoid cyst—one-quarter occur in the posterior fossa, most commonly retrocerebellar.

Supratentorial cysts

1. Subependymal cysts—located in subependymal region around the caudothalamic notch. Most commonly represent previous germinal matrix haemorrhage. May be congenital, probably reflecting germinolysis, particularly in association with CMV infection.
2. Choroid plexus cysts—usually located within body of choroid plexus. Weak markers of aneuploidy, particularly if large and bilateral. No clinical significance if detected after birth.
3. Cystic periventricular leukomalacia—white matter necrosis in preterm infant. Hyperechoic lesions dorsal and lateral to external angles of lateral ventricles, developing into cysts in severe cases.
4. Porencephalic cyst—an area of cystic encephalomalacia filled with CSF, often following haemorrhage or infection, communicating with the ventricular system.
5. Arachnoid cyst—most commonly in the sylvian fissure, usually incidental. Suprasellar cysts are more frequently symptomatic.
6. Vein of Galen malformation—not a cyst, but may appear so on US. Colour Doppler flow confirms.

Further reading

Epelman, M., Daneman, A., Blaser, S.I., 2006. Differential diagnosis of intracranial cystic lesions at head US: correlation with CT and MR imaging. Radiographics 26 (1), 173–196.

14.71 DISORDERS OF NEURONAL MIGRATION

The neuronal population of the normal cerebral cortex arrives by a process of outward migration from the periventricular germinal matrix between the 8th–16th weeks of gestation. This complex process can be interfered with by many causes, sporadic and unknown, chromosomal or genetic.

1. Agyria-pachygyria—poorly formed gyri and sulci, the former being more severe. Focal pachygyria may cause focal epilepsy. Polymicrogyria may coexist with pachygyria. Pachygyria may also

be seen in Zellweger syndrome and prenatal CMV infection. Extreme cases with a smooth brain = lissencephaly. Complete lissencephaly = agyria. Several distinct forms.

(a) Type I lissencephaly—small brain with few gyri; smooth, thickened four-layer cortex resembling that of a 13-week fetus with diminished white matter and shallow vertical sylvian fissures ('figure-of-eight' appearance on axial images) ± agenesis of corpus callosum. Severe mental retardation, diplegia, seizures, microcephaly and limited survival. Some infants have specific dysmorphic features: Miller-Dieker syndrome and Norman-Roberts syndrome.

(b) Type II lissencephaly (Walker-Warburg syndrome)—smooth cobblestone cortex, cerebellar hypoplasia, vermian aplasia and hydrocephalus (in 75%) due to cisternal obstruction by abnormal meninges or aqueduct stenosis. Eye abnormalities including microphthalmia and buphthalmos due to increased pressure and cataract.

2. **Polymicrogyria**—the neurons reach the cortex but are distributed abnormally. Macroscopically the surface of the brain appears as multiple small bumps. Localized abnormalities are more common than generalized and often involve arterial territories, especially the MCA. Most common location is around the sylvian fissure. The cortex is isointense to grey matter but in 20% the underlying white matter has high T2 signal. Linear flow voids, due to anomalous venous drainage, may be present. Polymicrogyria may be present in the vicinity of a porencephalic cyst, and may be associated with heterotopic grey matter, agenesis of corpus callosum or signs of fetal infection (e.g. intracranial calcification). The majority have mental retardation, seizures and neurological signs.
3. **Schizencephaly**—clefts that extend through the full thickness of the cerebral mantle from ventricle to subarachnoid space. The cleft is lined by heterotopic grey matter and microgyria, indicating that it existed prior to the end of neuronal migration. Unilateral or bilateral (usually asymmetrical) and usually near the sylvian fissure. May be associated with absence of the septum pellucidum or, less commonly, dysgenesis of the corpus callosum. Variable clinical manifestations, from profound retardation to isolated partial seizures.
4. **Heterotopic grey matter**—collections of neurons in a subependymal location, i.e. at the site of the germinal matrix or arrested within the white matter on their way to the cortex. Isointense to normal grey matter on all imaging sequences. Nodules or bands, ± mass effect. Often a part of complex malformation syndromes, or when isolated, may be responsible for focal seizures (amenable to surgical treatment).

5. Cortical dysplasia—focal disorganization of the cerebral cortex. A single enlarged gyrus resembling focal pachygyria. Usual presentation is with partial epilepsy.

Further reading

Barkovich, A.J., Raybaud, C., 2011. Pediatric Neuroimaging, fifth ed. Lippincott Williams & Wilkins, Philadelphia, PA.

14.72 SUPRATENTORIAL TUMOURS IN CHILDHOOD

Primary CNS tumours are the second most common malignancy in children after leukaemia. Overall, supratentorial and infratentorial tumours occur with equal incidence.

1. Hemispheric astrocytoma—solid ± necrotic centre, or cystic with a mural nodule. Usually large at presentation and can involve basal ganglia and thalami. Most are low grade. Enhancement with contrast medium does not correlate with histological grade. Associated with NF1.
2. Craniopharyngioma—>50% of all craniopharyngiomas occur in children (8–14 years). Cystic/solid partially calcified suprasellar mass presenting with headache, visual disturbance and endocrine abnormalities.
3. Optic pathway glioma—low grade but infiltrative pilocytic astrocytomas associated with NF1. Solid enhancing tumours that extend along the length of the anterior optic pathways and may invade adjacent structures (e.g. hypothalamus) and extend posteriorly into the optic tracts and radiations.
4. Giant cell subependymal astrocytoma—occurs in tuberous sclerosis; slow-growing partially cystic, partially calcified tumour located at the foramen of Monro. Presents with obstructive hydrocephalus.
5. **Germ cell tumours**—germinoma and teratoma.
6. **Primitive neuroectodermal tumour (PNET)**—large heterogeneous hemispheric mass presenting in neonates and infants. Necrosis, haemorrhage and enhancement are common.
7. **Dysembryoplastic neuroepithelial tumour (DNET)**—benign cortical tumour often presenting with seizures. Cortical (temporal) mass, usually small ± internal cysts and calcification.
8. **Ganglioglioma**—well-defined peripheral tumour that often presents with seizures. Cystic tumour with mural nodule ± calcification.
9. **Choroid plexus papilloma**—presents in young children with hydrocephalus. Most occur in the atrium of the lateral ventricle (fourth ventricle in adults) and appear as a well-defined

multilobulated avidly enhancing intraventricular mass ± calcification. Invasion of brain suggests choroid plexus carcinoma.

10. **Ependymoma**—often in the frontal lobe adjacent to the frontal horn, but not usually intraventricular.

Further reading

Barkovich, A.J., Raybaud, C., 2011. Pediatric Neuroimaging, fifth ed. Lippincott Williams & Wilkins, Philadelphia, PA.

14.73 INFRATENTORIAL TUMOURS IN CHILDHOOD

The majority arise from the cerebellum. Cerebellar astrocytomas, medulloblastomas and ependymomas present with symptoms of obstructive hydrocephalus and ataxia. Brainstem gliomas involve the cranial nerve nuclei and long tracts at an early stage.

1. **Cerebellar astrocytoma**—most common posterior fossa tumour in children ≥5 years. Vermis (50%), hemispheres (20%) or both (30%). Calcification in 20%. Large mass displacing (or invading) the fourth ventricle. 80% are juvenile pilocytic astrocytomas with an excellent prognosis. 50% are cystic with an enhancing mural nodule. 40% are solid with central necrosis. 10% are purely solid (usually smaller than the other types). Usually no restricted diffusion.
2. **Medulloblastoma**—most common posterior fossa tumour in children <5 years. Short history (aggressive). 80% located in the vermis, often extending into the fourth ventricle through its roof; 30% extend into the brainstem. Moderately well-defined mass, slightly hyperdense to surrounding cerebellum on CT + rim of oedema. Calcification in 10%. Small cystic or necrotic areas can be seen. Variable enhancement. Heterogeneous T2 signal on MRI. Marked restricted diffusion is typical. Tumour disseminates through CSF into the subarachnoid space (including spinal canal) and ventricular system. Extracranial metastases to bone, lymph nodes or soft tissues.
3. **Ependymoma**—15% of posterior fossa tumours. Usually a long clinical history. Most commonly arises from the floor of the fourth ventricle. On CT, typically an iso- or hyperdense mass with punctate calcifications, small cysts and heterogeneous enhancement. Calcification in a fourth ventricular mass or adjacent to the fourth ventricle = ependymoma. Heterogeneous on MRI, with less restricted diffusion than medulloblastoma. Tumour extension through the foramina of Luschka or Magendie is characteristic.

4. **Brainstem glioma**—insidious onset because of its location and tendency to infiltrate cranial nerve nuclei and long tracts without producing CSF obstruction until late. Four subgroups: medullary, pontine (most common), mesencephalic and those associated with NF1 (slower progression). Tumours may also be diffuse (>50%–75% of the brainstem in the axial plane, most common in pons) or focal (<50%, most common in tectal plate). Calcification rare. Typically T2 hyperintense on MRI, with no/minimal restricted diffusion or enhancement.
5. **Atypical teratoid/rhabdoid tumour (ATRT)**—rare but aggressive, with high potential for CNS dissemination. Usually in children <3 years. On MRI, ATRT often shows heterogeneous signal with diffusion restriction, similar to medulloblastoma, but has a higher propensity for calcification (~50%), haemorrhage, necrosis and cystic change.

Further reading

Barkovich, A.J., Raybaud, C., 2011. Pediatric Neuroimaging, fifth ed. Lippincott Williams & Wilkins, Philadelphia, PA.

14.74 INTRAVENTRICULAR MASS IN CHILDREN

Solid mass

Lateral ventricles

1. **Choroid plexus papilloma/carcinoma**—see Section 14.72.
2. **Astrocytomas**—usually arise from subependymal tissue and protrude into ventricle.
3. **Ependymoma**—less common than in fourth ventricle.
4. **Primitive neuroectodermal tumour**—see Section 14.72.
5. **Meningioma**—rare in children except in NF2.
6. **Choroid plexus enlargement**—NF1, Sturge-Weber.
7. **Teratoma.**
8. **Arteriovenous malformation**—enlarged draining veins.
9. **Subependymal heterotopia**—nodules of ectopic grey matter.
10. **Metastatic seeding**—e.g. medulloblastoma, ependymoma.
11. **ATRT.**

Foramen of Monro

1. **Subependymal giant cell astrocytoma**—see Section 14.72.
2. **Central neurocytoma**—well-defined heterogeneous mass arising from septum pellucidum close to foramen of Monro. Often contains calcification and cystic change.

Third ventricle

1. **Craniopharyngioma**—arises from the suprasellar region (see Section 14.72); may mimic a third ventricle mass if large.

2. **Glioma**—hypothalamic or chiasmatic pilocytic astrocytomas.
3. **Germinoma**—pineal or suprasellar; see Chapter 13.
4. **Teratoma**—usually posterior, in the pineal region.
5. **Langerhans cell histiocytosis***—arises from the floor of the third ventricle or suprasellar region.
6. **Choroid plexus papilloma**—see Section 14.72.
7. **Metastatic seeding.**

Fourth ventricle

1. **Medulloblastoma**—see Section 14.73.
2. **Ependymoma**—see Section 14.73.
3. **Choroid plexus papilloma**—see Section 14.72.
4. **Exophytic brainstem/cerebellar glioma**—see Section 14.73.
5. **ATRT**—see Section 14.73.

Cystic mass

1. **Choroid plexus cyst/xanthogranuloma**—typically in the trigone of the lateral ventricles, often bilateral. Usually incidental.
2. **Colloid cyst**—characteristic location in the anterosuperior aspect of the third ventricle, close to the foramina of Monro ± obstructive hydrocephalus. Typically contains proteinaceous material, appearing hyperdense on unenhanced CT and causing variable (but homogeneous) T1 and T2 signal on MRI. No enhancement.
3. **Intraventricular simple cysts**—e.g. ependymal cyst, arachnoid cyst. Follows CSF on all MRI sequences, thin/imperceptible wall and no enhancement. Distorts ventricle outline when large (may be the only sign of its presence).
4. **Cysticercosis***—appearance varies depending on stage. Often causes ventriculitis leading to aqueduct stenosis and hydrocephalus.
5. **Hydatid cyst**—rare.

Nuclear medicine

Clare Beadsmoore, Nabil Hujairi

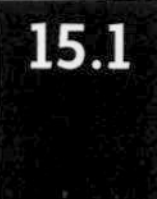

15.1 DIFFUSE INCREASED UPTAKE ON WHOLE-BODY BONE SCANS ('SUPERSCAN')

Definition: diffuse increased uptake in the axial skeleton ± proximal long bones with almost no uptake in soft tissues and kidneys, though bladder activity may still be present.

1. **Widespread bone metastases**—most common sources include prostate and breast. Uptake is diffuse but often patchy/asymmetrical. Long bones less commonly involved.
2. **Metabolic bone disorders**—osteomalacia, hyperparathyroidism and renal osteodystrophy. Uptake is diffuse and symmetrical. Proximal long bones usually involved, with prominent uptake in the skull and mandible. May have focal areas of very high uptake due to brown tumours in hyperparathyroidism.
3. **Myeloproliferative disorders**—e.g. myelofibrosis, mastocytosis, leukaemia, lymphoma and Waldenstrom's macroglobulinaemia.
4. **Widespread polyostotic Paget's disease or fibrous dysplasia**—usually multifocal rather than diffuse.

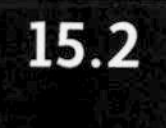

15.2 FOCAL INCREASED UPTAKE ON WHOLE-BODY BONE SCANS

Neoplastic

1. **Metastatic**—multiple randomly scattered lesions especially in the axial skeleton. Solitary lesions in typical locations, e.g. sternum in breast cancer, pelvis/sacrum/lower lumbar spine in prostate cancer.
2. **Hypertrophic pulmonary osteoarthropathy**—tramline sign: linear, symmetrical uptake along the periphery of the long bones (distal > proximal). Corresponds to the periosteal reaction seen on plain film. See Section 1.24 for a list of causes.
3. **Primary bone tumours**—e.g. Ewing sarcoma, osteosarcoma. Solitary, but may also have distant bone metastases.

4. **Erdheim-Chester disease***—skeletal involvement in 96%, typically femur, tibia and fibula. Less commonly ulna, radius and humerus. Bilateral symmetrical increased metadiaphyseal uptake corresponding to osteosclerosis on plain film.
5. **Eosinophilic granuloma/Langerhans cell histiocytosis***—variable uptake (increased or decreased). Most common sites include skull, pelvis and femur. Less common sites include ribs, humerus, mandible and spine.

Joint disease

1. Degenerative—most common sites include:
   (a) Cervical and lumbar spine—facet joint arthropathy is often best seen on posterior views, in the lumbar spine appearing to lie between two adjacent vertebrae. Arthropathy at the intervertebral disc is often best seen on anterior views due to cervical and lumbar lordosis.
   (b) Hips and knees—most commonly seen in the superior aspect of the hip joints and medial compartment of the knees at the site of maximal load.
   (c) Shoulders—three potential sites of focal arthropathic uptake: glenohumeral joint, acromioclavicular joint and greater tuberosity (due to rotator cuff impingement).
   (d) Other common sites—sternoclavicular joints, hands, ankles and feet.
2. **Inflammatory arthropathies**—uptake is related to increased blood flow to the affected joint, resulting in diffuse tracer accumulation surrounding the joint rather than the focal uptake associated with degenerative change. Distribution depends on the underlying arthropathy.

Fractures

1. Traumatic—80% of fractures demonstrate tracer uptake on bone scan 24 hours after injury (may be delayed in elderly/osteoporotic patients). By 1 week, 100% of fractures are visible on bone scan. Aligned fractures in ribs are always traumatic (i.e. not pathological). With single lesions elsewhere, always ask if history of trauma ± correlate with plain film. As the fracture evolves, the bone scan appearances change with three distinct phases:
   (a) Phase 1—0 to 4 weeks: diffuse increased uptake at the fracture site ± fracture line.
   (b) Phase 2—4 to 12 weeks: intense linear uptake at the fracture site.
   (c) Phase 3—12 weeks to 2 years: gradual reduction in uptake.
2. Stress—caused by abnormal stress on a normal bone. Bone scans are commonly used in their detection and can be combined with SPECT-CT when evaluating smaller bones, e.g. hallux, sesamoids

and pars defects. Bone scans can differentiate between tibial stress fractures (focal uptake usually at the junction of the mid-distal thirds of the tibia) and shin splints (periostitis at the insertion of tibialis and soleus muscles causing longitudinal linear increased uptake involving ≥ one-third of the posterior tibial cortex). Enthesopathy and periosteal reactions related to stress will all show increased uptake, e.g. plantar fasciitis shows focal uptake at the inferior aspect of the calcaneum.
3. **Insufficiency**—caused by normal stress on an abnormal bone, e.g. osteoporosis, metabolic bone disorders. Common sites include tibial plateau, calcaneum, sacrum (H-shaped 'Honda' sign), lesser trochanter of femur (especially in metabolic bone disorders) and vertebral bodies (compression fractures).
4. **Nonaccidental injury***—bone scans can detect radiologically occult fractures and may be considered if the clinical suspicion is high.

Post surgery

Increased uptake is seen in relation to any orthopaedic implant. See Section 15.3.

Paget's disease

Can affect any bone, but most commonly seen in the spine (especially lower lumbar spine), femora, skull and pelvis. Characterized by diffuse increased uptake within the affected bone, often starting from one end and progressing until the entire bone is involved. The associated bony expansion and flame-shaped advancing edge may also be visible on bone scan.

The exception to this rule is in the skull, where the increased uptake starts in the skull base and progresses to the vertex during the lytic/active phase of the disease, corresponding to the classic 'osteoporosis circumscripta' on plain film.

70% of patients have polyostotic disease. On a bone scan the intensity of tracer uptake can vary depending on the phase and treatment of the disease. Complications—bone deformity, fracture and malignant degeneration (e.g. osteosarcoma)—are often well seen on bone scan due to the increased uptake in the underlying Pagetic bone.

Infection

1. **Periprosthetic infection**—see Section 15.3.
2. **Dental infection/sinusitis**—including Garre's sclerosing osteomyelitis of the mandible. Focal uptake in the mandible or maxilla.
3. **CRMO/SAPHO**—multifocal areas of uptake; CRMO usually occurs in children or adolescents and favours metaphyses of long bones

(especially femur and tibia, also clavicle); SAPHO usually occurs in adults and favours sternoclavicular joints (commonest site of involvement, bull's head sign), manubriosternal joint, costochondral joints, spine (paravertebral hyperostosis) and sacroiliac joints (often unilateral).

4. **Paediatric polyostotic osteomyelitis**—6.8% of osteomyelitis in infants is polyostotic (up to 22% in neonates) due to haematogenous spread of infection. Bone scan is largely replaced by MRI (whole-body STIR) but can still be useful in patients unable to tolerate MRI.

Benign lesions

1. **Osteomas**—skull and mandible; also ivory osteomas in paranasal sinuses.
2. **Fibrous cortical defect/nonossifying fibroma**—variable uptake, increased in healing or fracture.
3. **Bone island**—usually no uptake; low-grade uptake has been reported in larger lesions.
4. **Osteoid osteoma**—increased uptake on blood pool images and late (bone phase) images, ± a central intense focus of uptake corresponding to the nidus on anatomical imaging, surrounded by less intense uptake corresponding to the surrounding sclerosis.
5. **Fibrous dysplasia**—persistent increased uptake on bone scan; 20%–30% polyostotic, commonly unilateral and monomelic (one limb).
6. **Melorheostosis**—monostotic or polyostotic, monomelic, commonly involves long bones.
7. **Osteochondroma**—increased uptake in an adult suggests growth or malignant degeneration.
8. **Enchondroma.**
9. **Heterotopic bone formation.**

Avascular necrosis (AVN)

Bone scan is more sensitive than plain film, but less sensitive than MRI. Many different causes (see Section 1.26). The pattern of uptake depends on the time following insult and can be divided into four stages:

1. **<1 month**—photopenia at the site of AVN.
2. **1–4 months**—increased uptake around the area of AVN due to peripheral revascularization (e.g. 'donut' sign in the hip).
3. **4–10 months**—diffuse increase at the site of AVN as healing occurs.
4. **>10 months**—either the scan returns to normal (uncomplicated healing) or there is increased uptake due to sclerosis and secondary degenerative changes.

15.3 INCREASED UPTAKE ON LOCAL VIEW BONE SCANS

1. **Joint replacement**—two-phase bone scans (blood pool and late) are used to look for evidence of loosening or infection. Normal scans have a high negative predictive value, but a significant number of normal prosthetic joints continue to accumulate tracer years after surgery.
   (a) **Loosening**—typically shows increased uptake only on the late phase images with normal uptake on the blood pool phase.
      (i) **Hips**—focal increased uptake in the greater and lesser trochanters and at the tip of the femoral prosthesis suggests loosening.
      (ii) **Knees**—normal uptake can persist for up to 4 years. Uptake at the femoral prosthesis normalizes first, followed by the lateral tibial prosthesis, with the medial tibial prosthesis normalizing last. Any focal uptake not conforming to this pattern is suspicious for loosening.
   (b) **Infection**—increased uptake surrounding the prosthesis on both the blood pool and late phase images.
   (c) **Synovitis/capsulitis**—following knee replacement. Increased uptake in the synovium/capsule on the blood pool phase only.
2. **Complex regional pain syndrome**—two- or three-phase (dynamic flow, blood pool and late) bone scan. Increased uptake in the affected limb on all three phases in a periarticular distribution. Over time this increased uptake normalizes; in chronic cases decreased uptake may be seen on all phases.

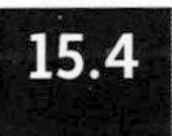

15.4 INCREASED UPTAKE ON BONE SCANS NOT DUE TO SKELETAL ABNORMALITY

Artefacts

1. **Urine contamination**—can be anywhere.
2. **Extravasated injection in the arm/leg**—± uptake in the draining sentinel node.
3. **Post surgery**—increased uptake due to hyperaemia.
4. **Arterial injection**—increased uptake in the injected arm distal to the injection site.
5. **Tracer preparation problems.**
   (a) **Free pertechnetate**—uptake in stomach, thyroid, GI tract and salivary glands.
   (b) **Colloid formation due to aluminium**—liver uptake, reduced bone uptake.
   (c) **High pH**—uptake in liver, gallbladder and GI tract.

6. **Equipment.**
   (a) **Edge effect**—apparent increased uptake at the edges of the field.
   (b) **Distance from camera/rotation of patient**—bones closer to the camera will appear to show increased uptake.
   (c) **Summation artefact**—contamination of the collimator/camera.

Physiological variants

1. **Epiphyses.**
2. **Calcification of costal cartilages.**
3. **Bladder diverticulum.**
4. **Nipples.**
5. **Renal anomalies.**
6. **Hyperostosis frontalis.**

Soft-tissue uptake

1. **Calcification**—e.g. myositis ossificans, dermatomyositis, hyperparathyroidism, calcified tumours/metastases, vascular calcification, calcific tendonitis, tumoural calcinosis, calcified abscess and alveolar microlithiasis.
2. **Others (noncalcified):**
   (a) Infarcts—cardiac, cerebral.
   (b) Renal uptake—long term antibiotics, chemotherapy, hypercalcaemia and hypercalciuria.
   (c) Malignant pleural effusions and ascites.
   (d) Metastases—commonly liver metastases from colon, breast or small cell carcinoma.
   (e) Amyloidosis—cardiac uptake.
   (f) Tumour—e.g. inflammatory breast cancer.
   (g) Hypercalcaemia with metastatic calcification—uptake in lungs and stomach.
   (h) Amiodarone lung.

15.5 PHOTOPENIC AREAS ON BONE SCANS

1. **Artefacts**—the most common cause.
   (a) External—metal objects, e.g. coins, belts, lockets and buckles.
   (b) Internal—joint prostheses, pacemakers.
2. **Lytic metastases**—e.g. renal, thyroid and lung.
3. **Avascular lesions**—e.g. bone cysts.
4. **Spinal haemangiomas**—occasionally slightly increased uptake.
5. **Radiotherapy fields**—nonanatomical, usually oblong in shape.
6. **Multiple myeloma***—bone scan often normal due to the lack of osteoblastic activity; larger lesions may be photopenic or show increased uptake.

15.6 VENTILATION-PERFUSION MISMATCH ON V/Q SCANS

Mismatched perfusion defects

Perfusion defect > ventilation defect.

1. **Pulmonary embolus**—especially if multiple and segmental.
2. **Bronchial carcinoma**—but more commonly matched.
3. **Tuberculosis***—typically affects an apical segment.
4. **Vasculitis**—polyarteritis nodosa, SLE, etc.
5. **Tumour/fat embolus.**
6. **Post radiotherapy.**
7. **Pulmonary hypertension.**
8. **Pulmonary artery narrowing.**

Mismatched ventilation defects

Ventilation defect > perfusion defect. Caused by airway obstruction with normal blood supply.

1. **Chronic obstructive pulmonary disease (COPD).**
2. **Pneumonia.**
3. **Lung collapse**—of any cause.
4. **Pleural effusion.**
5. **Bronchial carcinoma**—the rarest appearance.

Further reading

Carvandho, P., Lavender, J.P., 1988. Incidence and aetiology of the reverse (V/Q) mismatch defect. Nucl. Med. Commun. 9, 167.

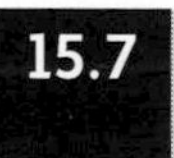

15.7 MATCHED VENTILATION-PERFUSION DEFECTS ON V/Q SCANS

Multiple

1. **Chronic bronchitis.**
2. **Pulmonary infarct/chronic pulmonary embolus (PE)**—do not confuse with the mismatched perfusion defect of acute PE.
3. **Asthma or acute bronchitis**—may also show mismatched ventilation or perfusion defects.
4. **Bullae**—long-standing bullae have scarce vessels and hypoventilation results in vascular constriction.
5. **Collagen vascular disease.**
6. **Lymphangitis carcinomatosa.**
7. **Pulmonary hypertension.**
8. **Sarcoidosis*.**
9. **Intravenous drug abuse.**

Solitary

1. Pneumonia—results in hypoventilation and compensatory hypoperfusion with a corresponding area of opacification on CXR (triple match). This cannot be distinguished from a pulmonary infarct on V/Q scan or CXR alone.
2. **Bulla.**
3. **Pulmonary infarct.**

15.8 ARTEFACTS ON V/Q SCANS

1. Breast prostheses—matched defect.
2. Cardiomegaly—matched defect.
3. Pacemaker—matched defect.
4. Clumping—technical problem causing focal areas of increased uptake on perfusion images due to clumping of tracer particles.
5. Central airways deposition—areas of focal increased uptake seen centrally on ventilation images due to precipitation of aerosol, secondary to turbulent air flow in the major bronchi, commonly in COPD.
6. **Right to left cardiac shunt**—uptake seen in the brain and abdominal viscera on the perfusion images.
7. **Renal uptake on the ventilation images**—in pneumonitis or smokers.

15.9 CAUSES OF A PERFUSION DEFECT ON A MYOCARDIAL PERFUSION SCAN

1. **Inducible/reversible ischaemia.**
2. **Infarction.**
3. **Hibernating myocardium**—often reduced activity during stress and at rest.
4. **Breast-related artefact**—particularly anterior defects.
5. **Inferior wall defects**—may result from diaphragmatic motion or the increased distance of this wall from the camera.
6. **Apical thinning.**

15.10 SCINTIGRAPHIC LOCALIZATION OF GI BLEEDING

Technique

^{99m}Tc-labelled red blood cells. Labelling efficiency is important, as false-positive scans can result from accumulations of free pertechnetate. Can detect a bleeding rate of >0.1 mL/min.

Common sites

1. Ulcers—benign or malignant.
2. Vascular lesions—angiodysplasia (most common in right colon), varices (oesophageal or gastric), fistula (including aortoenteric), telangiectasia (e.g. in HHT, vasculitis, scleroderma), intramural haematoma.
3. Tumours—malignant (primary or metastatic) and benign (e.g. adenoma, leiomyoma).
4. Inflammatory lesions—gastritis, duodenitis.
5. Diverticula—e.g. colonic or Meckel's.
6. Surgical anastomosis.
7. **Intussusception.**
8. **False-positive scintigraphy**—uptake may be seen in renal tract, liver, spleen (including splenunculi), uterus, bone marrow and hypervascular small bowel.

15.11 MECKEL'S SCAN

Positive scan

1. Meckel's diverticulum containing ectopic gastric mucosa—note that the timing of tracer uptake in the diverticulum should match the timing of normal gastric uptake.

False positive scan

1. **Duplication cyst containing ectopic gastric mucosa.**
2. **Bowel inflammation or obstruction**—including intussusception.
3. **GI bleeding**—e.g. peptic ulcer.
4. **Vascular lesions with increased blood pool.**
5. **Radioactive tracer in the renal collecting systems**—including tracer in a bladder diverticulum.

False negative scan

1. **Meckel's containing no gastric mucosa**—or nonfunctioning gastric mucosa.
2. **Meckel's hiding behind the bladder**—may be masked by normal bladder uptake.
3. **Technical problem with the scan**—always check for normal gastric uptake.

15.12 HIDA SCAN

Delayed uptake

Any cause of hepatocellular failure/dysfunction.

Delayed excretion into the biliary tree

1. Infants—biliary atresia.
2. Adults—biliary obstruction; if there is focal dilatation of the bile duct this may be due to a choledochal cyst.

Abnormal gallbladder uptake/ejection fraction

Gallbladder uptake is normally seen within 1 hour, and after a fatty meal the gallbladder ejection fraction should be >40%.

1. **Acute cholecystitis**—no gallbladder uptake.
2. **Chronic cholecystitis**—delayed tracer uptake by the gallbladder with poor gallbladder ejection fraction.
3. **Gallbladder dyskinesia**—normal gallbladder uptake with poor ejection fraction. Also consider acalculous cholecystitis.

Pooling of tracer within the liver parenchyma

1. Biloma—HIDA scan can be used to diagnose postoperative bile leaks.
2. **Focal biliary dilatation/choledochal cyst.**

Other findings

1. **Sphincter of Oddi dysfunction**—delayed passage of tracer into the bowel.
2. **Biliary reflux**—tracer passes from the duodenum into the stomach.

15.13 PHOTOPENIC DEFECTS ON RADIONUCLIDE (DMSA) RENAL IMAGES

1. Scars—note that defects present during infection may resolve later, hence imaging is routinely delayed until 3 months after the acute infective episode.
2. **Hydronephrosis**—central defect.
3. **Focal renal lesions**—cysts, tumours (e.g. RCC, lymphoma, Wilms tumour, metastases) and abscesses.
4. **Trauma**—subcapsular or intrarenal.
5. **Infarct/ischaemia.**

Further reading

Fogelman, I., Maisey, M., 1988. An Atlas of Clinical Nuclear Medicine. Martin Dunitz, London, pp. 217–373.

Mettler, F.A., Jr., Guiberteau, M.J., 2012. Essentials of Nuclear Medicine Imaging, sixth ed. Elsevier Saunders, Philadelphia, PA, (Chapter 9).

15.14 ABNORMAL RADIONUCLIDE RENOGRAM (MAG3)

Delayed tracer uptake

1. Renal artery stenosis.
2. Poor renal function.
3. Dehydration—particularly children.
4. **Renal tubular acidosis.**
5. **Renal transplant rejection.**

Delayed excretion

1. **All of the above.**
2. **Nephritis.**
3. **Obstruction**—together with delayed drainage.

Delayed drainage

1. **Obstruction**—including PUJ and ureteric obstruction.
2. Baggy renal pelvis – drains with posture/diuretic.
3. **Nephritis.**
4. **Megaureter.**

15.15 PHOTOPENIC AREAS ON RADIONUCLIDE THYROID IMAGING

Localized

1. Colloid cyst.
2. Nonfunctioning adenoma.
3. Carcinoma—papillary, follicular; medullary may be bilateral.
4. Multinodular goitre.
5. **Marine-Lenhart syndrome**—cold thyroid stimulating hormone (TSH)-dependent nodule in the presence of Graves disease.
6. **Vascular.**
7. **Abscess.**
8. **Artefact.**

Generalized

1. Concurrent medication for hyperthyroidism.
2. Hypothyroidism.
3. Thyroiditis—e.g. acute (infectious), De Quervain's, Riedel's and Hashimoto's (later stages). Shows diffusely reduced/absent uptake.
4. **Ectopic hormone production**—e.g. ectopic thyroid tissue.
5. **Amiodarone induced thyroiditis type 2**—subacute inflammatory thyroiditis.

15.16 INCREASED UPTAKE ON RADIONUCLIDE THYROID IMAGING

Focal increased uptake

1. **Toxic nodule**—± suppression of the rest of the gland.
2. **Artefact**—e.g. swallowed tracer activity in the oesophagus.

Diffuse increased uptake

1. **Graves disease**—very hot, uniform and both lobes.
2. **Multinodular goitre**—mildly increased, heterogeneous.
3. **Hashimoto's thyroiditis**—in the early stages.
4. **Amiodarone-induced thyrotoxicosis type 1**—exacerbation of a preexisting thyroid condition by amiodarone. May be normal or show diffuse increased uptake.
5. **Lithium therapy.**

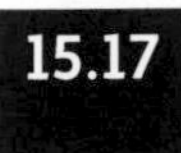

15.17 FOCAL INCREASED UPTAKE ON A PARATHYROID SESTAMIBI SCAN

Physiological

1. **Salivary glands.**
2. **Oral cavity**—due to secretions from the salivary glands.
3. **Thyroid gland.**
4. **Heart.**
5. **Liver.**
6. **Bone marrow.**
7. **Thymus.**
8. **Brown fat.**
9. **Uptake in the arm vein used for injection.**

Pathological

1. **Parathyroid adenoma.**
2. **Parathyroid carcinoma.**
3. **Thyroid adenoma/carcinoma.**
4. **Other malignancies**—adenocarcinoma (e.g. lung), squamous cell cancers (e.g. head and neck), bronchial carcinoid, lymphoma and breast cancer.
5. **Sarcoidosis*.**
6. **Parathyroid hormone secreting paraganglioma.**

15.18 BRAIN DATSCAN

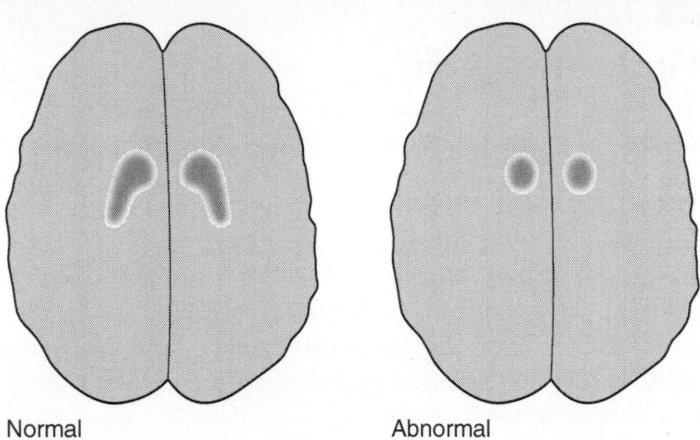

Normal

1. Normal patient.
2. Drug-induced or vascular Parkinsonism.
3. Essential tremor.
4. **Drug interactions**—e.g. cocaine, anti-ADHD (attention-deficit hyperactivity disorder) drugs and antidepressants. These can cause a false negative scan.

Abnormal

Bilateral symmetrically reduced putaminal uptake with relative sparing of the caudate, reflecting an underlying Parkinsonian syndrome including:

1. Parkinson's disease.
2. **Multiple system atrophy.**
3. **Progressive supranuclear palsy.**
4. **Corticobasal degeneration.**
5. **Lewy body dementia.**

Asymmetrical/unilateral reduced uptake

1. Early Parkinson's disease—NB: other Parkinsonian syndromes (see earlier) are less likely to be asymmetrical.
2. **Cerebral infarct**—causes punched-out defects.
3. **Brain tumour.**

15.19 DEMENTIA IMAGING BY FDG PET-CT

1. **Alzheimer's disease**—temporoparietal reduced uptake, starts in mesotemporal and posterior cingulate gyrus.
2. **Lewy body dementia**—same as in Alzheimer's disease, except it can also involve the occipital lobes.
3. **Frontotemporal dementia**—disproportionate frontal reduced uptake.
4. **Vascular dementia**—patchy reduced uptake.

15.20 MIBG SCINTIGRAPHY

^{131}I-MIBG uptake occurs in organs with adrenergic innervation or those that process catecholamines for excretion.

Normal uptake

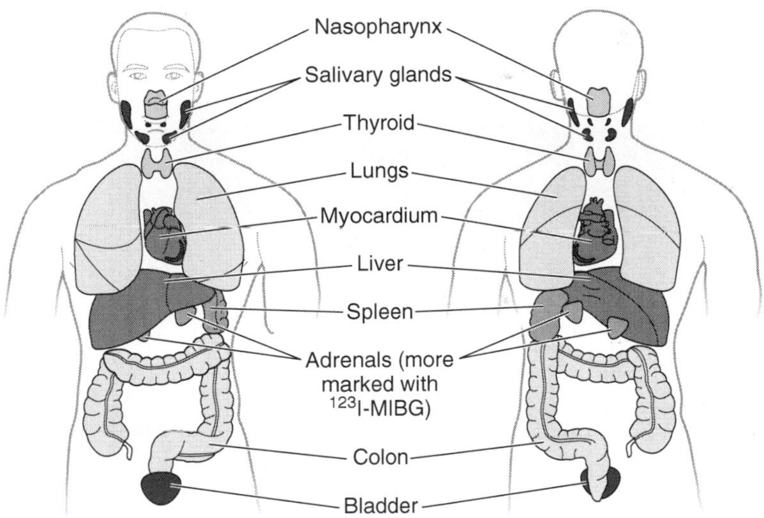

NB: the darker the organ, the higher the uptake

Abnormal uptake

1. Phaeochromocytoma.
2. Neuroblastoma—in children.
3. Paraganglioma.
4. **Medullary thyroid carcinoma.**
5. **Ganglioneuroma.**
6. **Neuroendocrine neoplasms**—less avid than with SRS (see Section 15.21).

Further reading

Chen, C.C., Carrasquillo, J.A., 2012. Molecular imaging of adrenal neoplasms. J. Surg. Oncol. 106 (5), 532–542.

Standalick, R.C., 1992. The biodistribution of metaiodobenzylguanidine. Semin. Nucl. Med. 22, 46–47.

15.21 SOMATOSTATIN RECEPTOR SCINTIGRAPHY (OCTREOTIDE SCAN)

Normal uptake

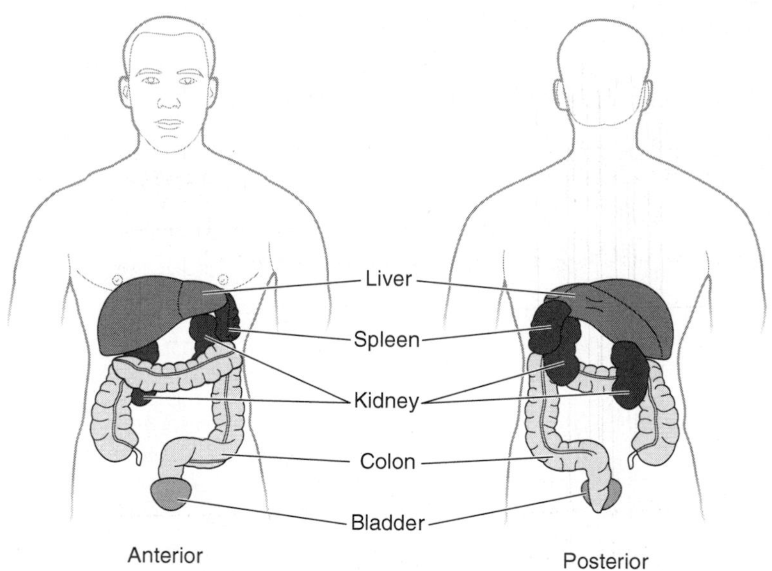

NB: the darker the organ, the higher the uptake

Abnormal uptake

1. <u>**Neuroendocrine neoplasms**</u>—carcinoid tumours, pancreatic NETs.
2. <u>**Inflammation**</u>—e.g. sarcoidosis, rheumatoid arthritis and IBD.
3. <u>**Scar tissue**</u>—e.g. postsurgical.
4. **Phaeochromocytoma**—less avid than with MIBG.
5. **Neuroblastoma**—less avid than with MIBG.
6. **Paraganglioma**—less avid than with MIBG.
7. **Medullary thyroid carcinoma**—less avid than with MIBG.

15.22 FDG PET-CT

Normal distribution of FDG

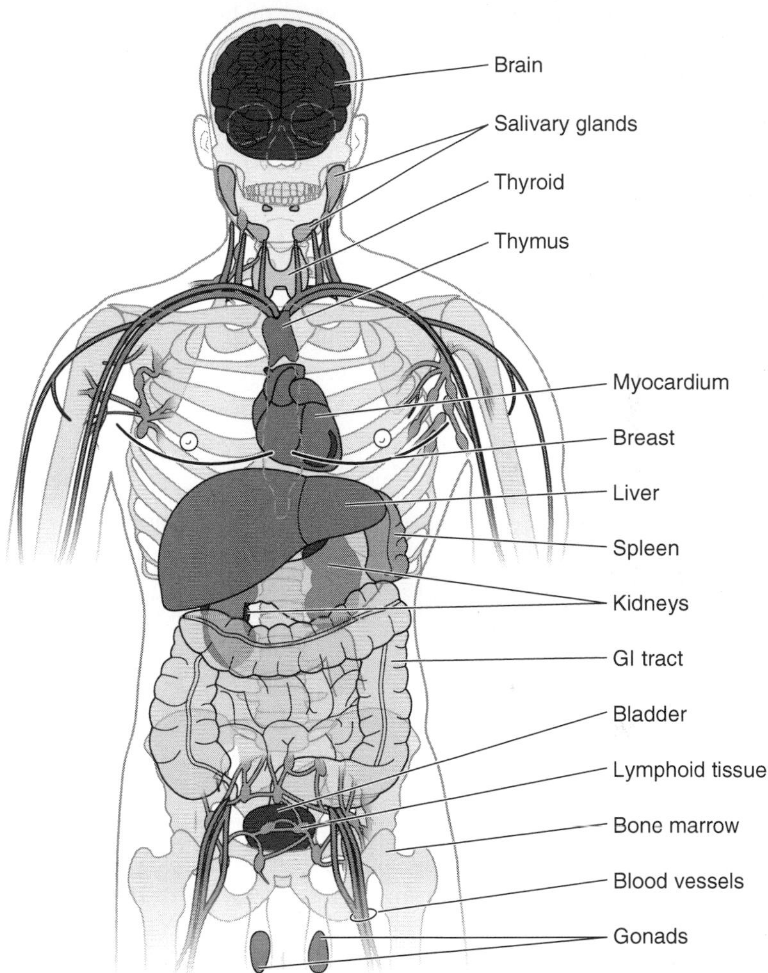

NB: the darker the organ, the higher the uptake

Causes of nonmalignant FDG uptake on PET-CT

1. **Physiological uptake**—liver, spleen, kidneys, bowel, urine, endometrium (ovulatory and menstrual phases) and ovaries/corpus luteum (ovulatory phase).
2. **Skeletal uptake**—degenerative, fractures, Paget's disease, inflammatory arthropathy and reactive bone marrow (GCSF, anaemia, infection etc.).

3. Inflammation—e.g. recent surgery (especially <6 weeks), foreign body reaction, diverticulitis, gastritis, pancreatitis and retroperitoneal fibrosis.
4. Granulomatous disease—e.g. TB, sarcoidosis and sarcoid-like tumour reaction (immune phenomenon by host's defense against tumour cells, most common in mediastinal and hilar nodes).
5. Infection/abscesses.
6. Fat.
   (a) Brown fat—common in young thin women; seen in supraclavicular fossae, posterior thorax, mediastinum and upper abdomen. Also in hibernoma (benign tumour of brown fat).
   (b) Lipomatous hypertrophy of the interatrial septum—1%–8% of the population.
   (c) **Fat necrosis.**
7. Metformin—diffuse increased GI tract uptake.
8. **Benign tumours**—e.g. adrenal adenoma (5%), pituitary adenoma and parathyroid adenoma.
9. **Uterine fibroid**—18% show uptake.
10. **Thyroid nodules**—2.1% incidence; 36% malignant, the rest are benign.
11. **Parotid nodules**—0.5% incidence; 50% benign, commonly Warthin tumours or pleomorphic adenomas.
12. **Venous thrombosis.**
13. **Attenuation correction artefacts.**

Malignancies with poor FDG PET avidity

The majority of malignancies are FDG PET avid; those with poor uptake include:

1. HCC—up to 50% show no uptake.
2. Lymphoma* subtypes—e.g. MALT.
3. Necrotic or mucinous adenocarcinoma.
4. Renal cell carcinoma—around 60% sensitivity.
5. Early-stage pancreatic cancer.
6. Prostate cancer—but may take up choline.
7. Well-differentiated neuroendocrine tumours—e.g. carcinoid; gallium-based tracers such as DOTATOC are useful.
8. Well-differentiated thyroid malignancy.

Further reading

McDermott, S., Skehan, S.J., 2010. Whole-body imaging in the abdominal cancer patient: pitfalls of PET–CT. Abdom. Imaging 35 (1), 55–69.

15.23 CHOLINE PET-CT

Normal distribution

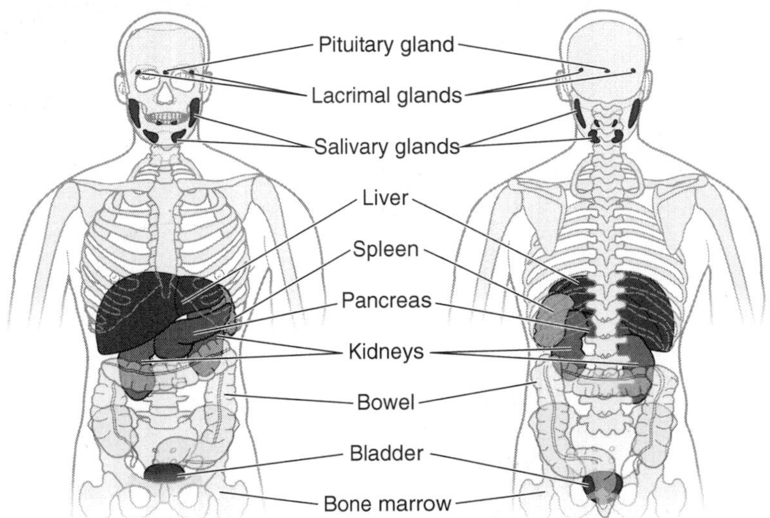

NB: the darker the organ, the higher the uptake

Causes of malignant uptake

1. Prostate cancer—main indication for the scan.
2. **Lymphoma***.
3. **Mucinous adenocarcinoma.**
4. **Lung cancer**—small cell and adenocarcinoma (including low-grade tumours that only show minimal uptake on FDG PET).

Causes of nonmalignant uptake

1. **Skeletal uptake**—same as with FDG (see Section 15.22).
2. **Inflammation**—same as with FDG (see Section 15.22).
3. **Granulomatous disease**—same as with FDG (see Section 15.22).
4. **Infection/abscesses.**
5. **Benign tumours**—e.g. adrenal adenoma (5%), pituitary macroadenoma (larger focus of uptake than normal pituitary uptake) and parathyroid adenoma.

15.24 GALLIUM-68 DOTA PET-CT

Normal distribution (somatostatin receptors)

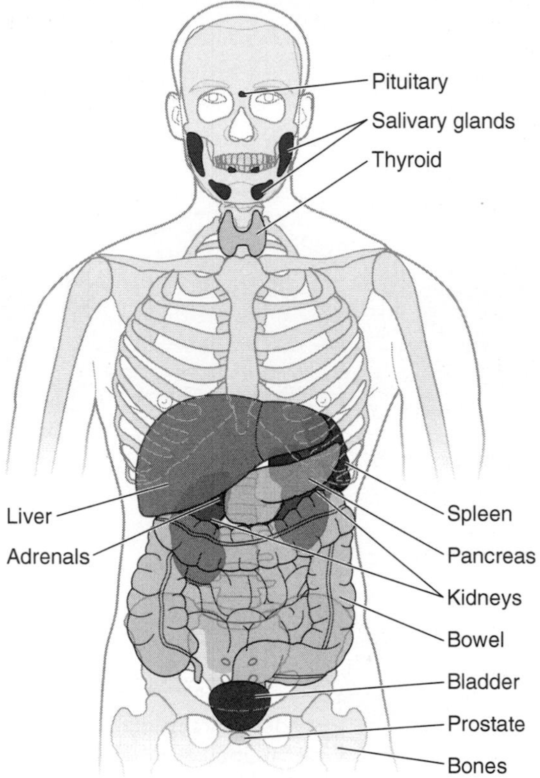

NB: the darker the organ, the higher the uptake

Causes of malignant uptake

1. <u>Neuroendocrine tumours</u>—main indication for the scan. Higher avidity with well-differentiated tumours (the opposite of FDG PET). Includes pancreatic NETs (insulinoma, glucagonoma, gastrinoma, VIPoma), ACTH-secreting carcinoids and Merkel cell tumours.
2. **Phaeochromocytoma and paraganglioma.**
3. **Medullary and iodine negative thyroid carcinomas.**
4. **Small-cell lung cancer.**
5. **Meningioma.**
6. **Medulloblastoma.**
7. **Invasive lobular breast cancer.**
8. **Benign phosphaturic mesenchymal tumour**—causes oncogenic osteomalacia (see Section 1.19).

Causes of nonmalignant uptake

1. **Skeletal uptake**—seen in osteoblastic processes, e.g. degenerative, fractures, Paget's disease, inflammatory arthropathy, epiphyseal growth plates, haemangioma and enchondroma.
2. **Inflammation**—white blood cells (including leukocytes and macrophages) express somatostatin receptors. Seen in recent surgery (especially <6 weeks), foreign body reaction, diverticulitis, gastritis, pancreatitis, prostatitis, post radiotherapy and reactive nodes.
3. **Infection/abscesses.**
4. **Splenunculi and splenosis.**

Part 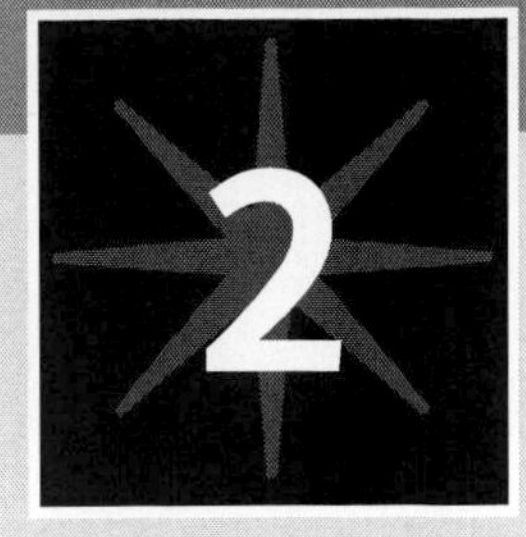

ACHONDROPLASIA

An AD (80% new mutation rate) skeletal dysplasia due to impaired enchondral bone growth.

Skull

1. Large skull. Small base. Small sella. Steep clivus. Small, funnel-shaped foramen magnum.
2. Hydrocephalus of variable severity.

Thorax

1. Thick, stubby sternum.
2. Short ribs with deep concavities to the anterior ends.

Axial skeleton

1. Decreasing interpedicular distance caudally in lumbar spine.
2. Short pedicles with a narrow sagittal diameter of the lumbar spinal canal.
3. Posterior scalloping.
4. Anterior vertebral body beak at T12/L1/L2 associated with gibbus deformity when sitting. Gibbus may reverse and develop into hyperlordosis of lumbar spine when walking.

Pelvis

1. Square iliac wings.
2. 'Champagne-glass' pelvic cavity.
3. Short, narrow sacrosciatic notch.
4. Horizontal sacrum articulating low on the ilia.

Appendicular skeleton

1. Rhizomelic micromelia with bowing of long bones.
2. Widened metaphyses.
3. Ball-and-socket epiphyseal/metaphyseal junction.
4. Broad and short proximal and middle phalanges.
5. Trident-shaped hands. Increased angle between middle and ring fingers.

ACQUIRED IMMUNE DEFICIENCY SYNDROME

Widespread use of highly active antiretroviral therapy (HAART) has significantly changed the patterns of presentation of HIV-related disease in adults in developed nations. Opportunistic infections are less common, whereas non-AIDS-defining cancers and disorders related to immune reconstitution are being seen with greater frequency. In nondeveloped countries without widespread access to HAART, the profile of AIDS-related diseases has changed little.

Chest

Many patients present acutely with chest presentations. The likely causes of chest infection will vary with CD4 count: between 200 and 500 cells/μL, bacterial, mycobacterial and candidal infections predominate. CD4 <200 predisposes patients to pneumocystis pneumonia; with CD4 <100, viral, protozoal and other fungal infections become common. CXR/CT changes rarely provide definitive diagnosis.

Opportunistic infections

1. *Pneumocystis jirovecii*—most common opportunistic (fungal) infection. With effective chemoprophylaxis and antiretroviral treatment, incidence has fallen. CXR may be normal at presentation but typically progresses to show bilateral perihilar or diffuse GGO and reticulation. Without treatment, there is rapid progression to air-space opacification. Diffuse GGO, thickened interlobular septa and consolidation are the key findings on HRCT. Thin-walled cysts (± pneumothorax) may also be present and aid differentiation from viral infections (e.g. CMV). Less common imaging features include:
   (a) Asymmetrical upper lobe disease—in patients on prophylactic therapy; may be confused with TB.
   (b) Miliary nodules or solitary nodule ± cavitation.
   (c) Pleural effusions.
2. *Mycobacterium tuberculosis*—an important infection in HIV-positive patients, and diagnosis is difficult. Imaging features depend on severity of immune compromise: depressed but near-normal CD4 levels are associated with similar radiological features to immunocompetent patients (upper lobe nodules ± cavitation). With more severe depression, more atypical patterns (non–upper lobe predilection; lower propensity for cavitation) and disseminated infection are likely.

Neoplasms

1. Kaposi sarcoma—decreasing incidence with advent of HAART. Lung involvement is less common than cutaneous or visceral disease. Perihilar bronchocentric nodules or masses are the typical imaging findings—'flame-shaped' opacities may be seen on CT.
2. Pulmonary lymphoma—increasingly common, especially NHL.
3. Lung cancer.

Other parenchymal lung diseases

1. NSIP—variable prevalence. Clinical presentation and imaging features may mirror those seen in patients with PCP, but CD4 counts tend to be higher in patients with NSIP.
2. Lymphocytic interstitial pneumonia—most common in children, associated with EBV infection. Nonspecific imaging appearances (GGO, small nodules, thin-walled cysts, mild bronchiectasis).
3. Obliterative bronchiolitis—in adolescents with vertically transmitted infection.
4. Emphysema.

Abdomen and GI tract

Infections

Dependent on level of immunocompromise: CD4 <400—TB, *Candida*; CD4 <200—*Candida, Histoplasma, Cryptosporidium, Pneumocystis*; CD4 <100—CMV, herpes simplex, MAC.

1. Primary HIV—oesophageal ulceration.
2. *Candida*—usually oropharynx and oesophagus. AIDS-defining. Mucosal plaques, fold thickening, 'shaggy' oesophagus on barium swallow.
3. Herpes—discrete ulcers on barium swallow.
4. CMV—most common GI infection. Can occur anywhere but usually lower GI tract. Oesophagus—large midoesophageal ulcer; CMV gastritis, enteritis and colitis—superficial or deep ulceration, extensive bowel wall thickening on CT; lymphadenopathy not prominent.
5. TB—ileocaecal and jejunoileal most common sites (upper GI tract less common). Segmental ulcers, wall thickening, strictures and mass-like lesions of the caecum and terminal ileum. Regional low-attenuation necrotic lymphadenopathy. Hepatosplenomegaly ± focal lesions.
6. *Chlamydia trachomatis*—causes lymphogranuloma venereum. Generally in men who have sex with men as an HIV coinfection. Introduced anally and causes proctitis ± large necrotic inguinal lymph nodes.
7. *Mycobacterium avium* complex—usually small bowel; mural thickening and mild dilatation. Mesenteric lymphadenopathy ± central necrosis. Hepatosplenomegaly ± focal lesions.
8. *Cryptosporidium*—diffuse mural thickening. No lymphadenopathy.
9. *Bartonella henselae*—causes peliosis hepatis: blood-filled cystic spaces which enhance avidly post contrast. Liver > spleen > other organs.

10. PCP—liver, spleen, kidneys: hypoechoic/hypoattenuating masses or multiple tiny calcified foci.

Malignancy

1. Kaposi sarcoma—CD4 count typically <200.
   (a) Liver/spleen—multifocal hyperechoic nodules (5–12 mm) adjacent to portal veins on US. CT: enhancing nodules (may mimic haemangiomas).
   (b) GI tract—usually with cutaneous involvement. Can occur anywhere, duodenum most common. Submucosal masses (0.5–3 cm) ± ulceration. Hyperattenuating lymphadenopathy.
2. Lymphoma—usually aggressive form of NHL. Peripheral nodes are present in 50% and extranodal involvement is common, especially bowel, viscera and marrow.

Other abdominal manifestations

1. Retroperitoneal/mesenteric lymphadenopathy.
   (a) Progressive generalized lymphadenopathy—adenopathy in ≥2 sites persisting for >3 months with no obvious cause. Biopsy reveals benign hyperplasia, and CT shows clusters of small nodes <1 cm in the mesentery and retroperitoneum.
   (b) Kaposi sarcoma—hyperattenuating nodes, hypervascular post contrast.
   (c) Lymphoma—typically homogeneous and confluent.
   (d) *Mycobacterium*/TB—typically necrotic.
2. AIDS cholangiopathy—due to infection by CMV or *Cryptosporidium*. GB wall thickening, pericholecystic fluid, intrahepatic and extrahepatic bile duct strictures, diverticula, intraluminal filling defects and strictures of the juxtaampullary PD.
3. HIV nephropathy—proteinuria and rapidly progressive renal failure. Usually globally enlarged and echogenic kidneys.
4. Pyelonephritis and renal abscesses.

CNS

HIV can affect the brain directly or can predispose to opportunistic infection (commonest toxoplasma, *Cryptococcus*, progressive multifocal leukoencephalopathy). Increased incidence of intracerebral lymphoma.

Viral

1. HIV—progressive dementia and atrophy due to subacute encephalitis. Diffuse/patchy white matter hypoattenuation (CT) and high T2 signal (MRI), may involve basal ganglia. Mass effect and contrast enhancement usually absent.

2. CMV—signal abnormalities typically seen in periventricular distribution.
3. Progressive multifocal leukoencephalopathy—JC virus infection. MRI: multifocal or confluent, asymmetrical increased T2 signal in white matter; no/minimal mass effect, grey matter spared, no atrophy.

Fungal

1. *Cryptococcus*—meningitis spreading along perivascular spaces. MRI: multifocal areas of increased T2 signal in basal ganglia and brainstem.
2. *Aspergillus* and *Candida*—rare in HIV; commoner in other immunocompromised groups, e.g. bone marrow transplant recipients.

Protozoal

1. *Toxoplasma*—multiple small nodules or ring-enhancing lesions in basal ganglia, thalami and grey–white junction. May mimic lymphoma but multiple lesions favours toxoplasma.

Bacterial

1. Typical pyogenic infections.
2. TB—meningitis with leptomeningeal thickening, hydrocephalus, perforating vessel infarcts, cerebritis and abscess.

Tumour

1. Lymphoma—periventricular location with subependymal spread suggests lymphoma instead of toxoplasmosis. Lymphoma in HIV can cavitate prior to treatment and be ring-enhancing (cf. immunocompetent patients).

Musculoskeletal

Infection

Opportunistic and nonopportunistic. Commonest organism is *Staphylococcus aureus*, but also TB, *Mycobacterium avium*, *Nocardia*, *Cryptococcus*, *Toxoplasma*, *Salmonella*. Can cause cellulitis, necrotizing fasciitis, pyomyositis, osteomyelitis or septic arthritis.

Inflammatory

1. Arthritides
   (a) HIV-associated (1–6 weeks).
   (b) Painful articular syndrome (48 hours).
   (c) Seronegative, e.g. reactive arthritis.
2. Polymyositis—bilateral symmetrical proximal muscle weakness and raised creatine kinase.

Neoplasms

1. NHL.
2. Kaposi sarcoma.

Miscellaneous

1. Osteonecrosis.
2. Osteoporosis.
3. Rhabdomyolysis.
4. Hypertrophic osteoarthropathy.
5. Anaemia—T1 hypointense bone marrow (red marrow reconversion).

Further reading

Boiselle, P.M., Crans, S.A., Jr., Kaplan, M.A., 1999. The changing face of *Pneumocystis carinii* pneumonia in AIDS patients. AJR Am. J. Roentgenol. 172, 1301–1309.

Burns, J., Shaknovich, R., Lau, J., Haramati, L.B., 2007. Oncogenic viruses in AIDS: mechanisms of disease and intrathoracic manifestations. AJR Am. J. Roentgenol. 189, 1082–1087.

Ferrand, R.A., Desai, S.R., Hopkins, C., et al., 2012. Chronic lung disease in adolescents with delayed diagnosis of vertically-acquired HIV infection. Clin. Infect. Dis. 55, 145–152.

Guihot, A., Couderc, L.J., Rivaud, E., et al., 2007. Thoracic radiographic and CT findings of multicentric Castleman disease in HIV-infected patients. J. Thorac. Imaging 22, 207–211.

Kuhlman, J.E., 1999. Imaging pulmonary disease in AIDS: state of the art. Eur. Radiol. 9, 395–408.

Logan, P.M., Finnegan, M.M., 1998. Pictorial review: pulmonary complications in AIDS: CT appearances. Clin. Radiol. 53, 567–573.

Major, N.M., Tehranzadeh, J., 1997. Musculoskeletal manifestations of AIDS. Radiol. Clin. North Am. 35, 1167–1190.

Provenzale, J.M., Jinkins, J.R., 1997. Brain and spine imaging findings in AIDS patients. Radiol. Clin. North Am. 35, 1127–1166.

Redvanly, R.D., Silverstein, J.E., 1997. Intra-abdominal manifestations of AIDS. Radiol. Clin. North Am. 35, 1083–1126.

Reeders, J.W., Goodman, P.C., 2001. Radiology of AIDS. Springer.

Reeders, J.W., Yee, J., Gore, R.M., et al., 2004. Gastrointestinal infection in the immunocompromised (AIDS) patient. Eur. Radiol. 14 (Suppl. 3), E84–E102.

Restrepo, C., Lemos, D., Gordillo, H., 2004. Imaging findings in musculoskeletal complications of AIDS. Radiographics 24, 1029–1049.

Restrepo, C.S., Ocazionez, D., 2011. Kaposi's sarcoma: imaging overview. Semin. Ultrasound CT MR 32 (5), 456–469.

Richards, P.J., Armstrong, P., Parkin, J.M., Sharma, A., 1998. Chest imaging in AIDS. Clin. Radiol. 53, 554–566.

Spencer, S.P., Power, N., Reznek, R.H., 2009. Multidetector computed tomography of the acute abdomen in the immunocompromised host: a pictorial review. Curr. Probl. Diagn. Radiol. 38 (4), 145–155.

ACQUIRED IMMUNE DEFICIENCY SYNDROME (AIDS) IN CHILDREN

The majority are due to transmission from an infected mother. Infection from transfusions (in the neonatal period or because of diseases such as thalassaemia and haemophilia) is rare in the West but still occurs in developing countries. 50% of those infected congenitally will present in the first year of life. Prognostic factors: severity of disease in the mother, age of onset, severity at onset. AIDS in children differs from AIDS in adults in the following ways:

1. Shorter incubation period.
2. More likely to have serious bacterial infections or CMV.
3. More commonly develop pulmonary lymphoid hyperplasia (PLH) and lymphocytic interstitial pneumonia (LIP).
4. Almost never develop Kaposi sarcoma.
5. Less likely to be infected with *Toxoplasma*, TB, *Cryptococcus* and *Histoplasma*.
6. Two patterns of presentation and progression can be recognized:
   (a) In the first year of life—serious infections and encephalopathy. Poor prognosis.
   (b) Preschool and school age—bacterial infections and lymphoid tissue hyperplasia. Survival is longer, to adolescence.

Generalized features

Failure to thrive, weight loss, fever, generalized lymphadenopathy, hepatosplenomegaly, recurrent infections, chronic diarrhoea, parotitis (hypoechoic nodules, hyperechoic striae and lymphoepithelial cysts on US).

Chest

1. PCP—may be localized initially but typically progresses rapidly to diffuse lung shadowing, which is a mixed alveolar and interstitial infiltrate. 50% occur at age 3–6 months. Often the first and only infective episode.
2. CMV pneumonia.
3. LIP/PLH—in 50% of patients. Insidious onset. CXR shows a diffuse, symmetrical reticulonodular or nodular pattern (2–3 mm), best seen at the lung bases and peripheries, ± hilar or mediastinal adenopathy. The nodules consist of collections of lymphocytes and plasma cells without any organisms. Children with LIP are more likely to have generalized lymphadenopathy, salivary gland enlargement (especially parotid) and finger clubbing than those with opportunistic chest infections, and the prognosis for LIP is

better. Chronic LIP may result in lower lobe bronchiectasis or cystic lung disease.

4. Mediastinal or hilar adenopathy may be secondary to PLH, TB, MAC, CMV, lymphoma or fungal infection.
5. Cardiomyopathy, dysrhythmias and unexpected cardiac arrest.

Abdomen

1. Hepatosplenomegaly—due to chronic active hepatitis, hepatitis A/B, CMV, EBV, TB, generalized sepsis, tumour (fibrosarcoma of the liver) or congestive cardiac failure.
2. Oesophagitis—*Candida*, CMV or herpes simplex.
3. Chronic diarrhoea—in 40%–60% of children. Infectious agents (e.g. *Candida*, CMV and *Cryptosporidium*) are only infrequently found. Imaging findings are nonspecific and include a malabsorption-type pattern with bowel wall thickening and dilatation.
4. Pneumatosis coli.
5. Mesenteric, paraaortic and retroperitoneal lymphadenopathy—due to MAC, lymphocytic proliferation, NHL or (rarely) Kaposi sarcoma.
6. HIV nephropathy—children may present with proteinuria, fluid and electrolyte imbalances and/or acute or chronic renal failure. US shows enlarged echogenic kidneys, CT shows enlarged pyramids ± simple cysts.
7. UTI—in up to 50% of AIDS patients. May be due to common organisms or unusual agents, e.g. CMV, *Cryptococcus, Candida, Aspergillus, Mycobacterium* and *Pneumocystis*.

Brain

1. HIV encephalopathy—divided into two types (see following). Imaging may show cerebral atrophy (worse with progressive encephalopathy) or nonenhancing white matter lesions in the frontal lobes, periventricular regions and centrum semiovale.
   - **(a)** Progressive encephalopathy—comparable to adult AIDS dementia complex, associated with severe immune deficiency. Stepwise deterioration of mental status and higher functions.
   - **(b)** Static encephalopathy—associated with better higher functions but failure to reach appropriate milestones.
2. Intracranial calcifications—in up to 33% of HIV-infected children. Usually bilateral and symmetrical and most common in the globus pallidus and putamen; less commonly in the subcortical frontal white matter and cerebellum. Usually not seen <10 months of age; early calcifications are more likely due to congenital TORCH infections.
3. Malignancy—most commonly high-grade B-cell lymphoma associated with EBV.

4. Cerebral infarcts.
5. Infections:
   (a) Progressive multifocal leukoencephalopathy—hard to distinguish from HIV encephalopathy, but tends to be more focal, asymmetrical and commoner in the posterior parietal lobes.
   (b) Toxoplasmosis—enhancing mass lesions with surrounding oedema in basal ganglia and corticomedullary junction.
   (c) Meningitis—due to fungi, *Mycobacteria* spp. and *Nocardia*, in addition to the more usual causes of meningitis.
   (d) CMV.
6. Chronic otitis media and sinusitis.

Further reading

Haller, J.O., 1997. AIDS-related malignancies in pediatrics. Radiol. Clin. North Am. 35 (6), 1517–1538.

Haller, J.O., Cohen, H.L., 1994. Pediatric HIV infection: an imaging update. Pediatr. Radiol. 24, 224–230.

Martinoli, C., Pretolesi, F., Del Bono, V., et al., 1995. Benign lymphoepithelial parotid lesions in HIV-positive patients: spectrum of findings at gray-scale and Doppler sonography. AJR Am. J. Roentgenol. 165 (4), 975–979.

Miller, C.R., 1997. Pediatric aspects of AIDS. Radiol. Clin. North Am. 35, 1191–1222.

Safriel, Y.I., Haller, J.O., Lefton, D.R., Obedian, R., 2000. Imaging of the brain in the HIV-positive child. Pediatr. Radiol. 30, 725–732.

Stoane, J.M., Haller, J.O., Orentlicher, R.J., 1996. The gastrointestinal manifestations of pediatric AIDS. Radiol. Clin. North Am. 34 (4), 779–790.

Zinn, H.L., Haller, J.O., 1999. Renal manifestations of AIDS in children. Pediatr. Radiol. 29, 558–561.

ACROMEGALY

Caused by a pituitary adenoma producing excess growth hormone. Main imaging manifestations are musculoskeletal.

Skull

1. Thickened skull vault.
2. Enlarged paranasal sinuses and mastoids.
3. Enlarged pituitary fossa due to the adenoma.
4. Prognathism (protruding mandible).

Thorax and spine

1. Increased sagittal diameter of the chest with a kyphosis.
2. Increased AP and transverse diameters of the vertebral bodies with posterior scalloping.

Appendicular skeleton

1. Increased width of bones but unaltered cortical thickness.
2. Tufting of the terminal phalanges, giving an 'arrowhead' appearance.
3. Prominent muscle attachments.
4. Widened joint spaces—especially the MCP joints, due to cartilage hypertrophy.
5. Premature osteoarthritis.
6. Increased heel-pad thickness (>21.5 mm in women; >23 mm in men).
7. Generalized osteoporosis.

Extraskeletal manifestations

1. Cardiac hypertrophy (early) and dilated cardiomyopathy (late).
2. Visceromegaly—e.g. liver, spleen, kidneys, prostate, thyroid, salivary glands.
3. Tracheal cartilage calcification.
4. Diabetes.

ALKAPTONURIA

The absence of homogentisic acid oxidase leads to the accumulation of homogentisic acid and its excretion in sweat and urine. The majority of cases are AR.

Axial skeleton

1. Osteoporosis.
2. Intervertebral disc calcification—especially in the lumbar spine.
3. Disc space narrowing with vacuum phenomenon.
4. Marginal osteophytes and endplate sclerosis.
5. Symphysis pubis—joint space narrowing, chondrocalcinosis, subchondral sclerosis and, rarely, ankylosis.

Appendicular skeleton

1. Large joints show joint space narrowing, bony sclerosis, articular collapse and fragmentation, and intraarticular loose bodies.
2. Calcification of bursae and tendons.

Extraskeletal

Ochronotic deposition in other organs may result in:

1. CVS—atherosclerosis, myocardial infarction, calcification of aortic and mitral valves.
2. Genitourinary (GU) system—renal calculi, nephrocalcinosis, prostatic enlargement + calculi.
3. Upper respiratory tract—glottic narrowing.

ALPHA-1 ANTITRYPSIN DEFICIENCY

Hereditary metabolic disorder; main manifestations are in the lungs and liver.

1. Lungs—panlobular emphysema with a basal predominance. Commonest clinical presentation, usually in young/middle aged adults. Bronchiectasis may also be seen.
2. Liver—cirrhosis in 15% of adult patients. May also cause cholestasis in neonates.
3. Aneurysms—especially intracranial.
4. Subcutaneous necrotizing panniculitis.
5. Other associations—pancreatitis, IBD, vasculitis (e.g. Wegener's), hypothyroidism, glomerulonephritis.

AMYLOIDOSIS

Group of diseases characterized by deposition of amyloid proteins which can occur in any organ or tissue. Usually presents in older adults. Many different types:

1. Systemic—involves multiple organs or tissues.
   - (a) Amyloid light chain (AL)—produced by an abnormal clonal population of plasma cells, e.g. in multiple myeloma, B-cell lymphoma or Waldenström's macroglobulinaemia.
   - (b) Serum amyloid A (AA)—secondary to chronic inflammatory disorders, e.g. rheumatoid arthritis, Crohn's disease, seronegative spondyloarthropathies, Sjögren's syndrome, dermatomyositis, vasculitis, SLE, familial Mediterranean fever, chronic infections such as osteomyelitis, TB or bronchiectasis, and some tumours (e.g. RCC).
   - (c) Amyloid transthyretin (ATTR)—two subtypes:
     - (i) Wild-type ATTR—also known as senile systemic amyloidosis. Almost exclusively in older men; mainly involves the heart ± carpal tunnel syndrome.
     - (ii) Mutant ATTR— also known as familial amyloid polyneuropathy. Hereditary (AD), usually presenting in young adults. Primarily involves peripheral and autonomic nerves.
   - (d) Amyloid β_2 microglobulin (Aβ_2M)—seen in patients on long-term haemodialysis; mainly involves joints.
2. Localized—less common. Amyloid protein (typically AL) is deposited in a specific organ or tissue, most commonly respiratory tract, skin or urinary tract. Not associated with a generalized plasma cell dyscrasia. Cerebral amyloid angiopathy and Alzheimer's disease can also be considered as localized forms of amyloidosis (Aβ).

General imaging features

1. Amyloid deposits may be focal (amyloidoma) or diffuse, and are typically hypovascular on postcontrast CT/MRI, though delayed enhancement can be seen.
2. CT—calcification is common and suggestive when present.
3. MRI—amyloid deposits are typically T1 and T2 hypointense.

Amyloidosis in specific organs and tissues

1. Heart—major cause of mortality in systemic AL amyloidosis (better prognosis in ATTR). Manifests as restrictive cardiomyopathy ± pericardial effusion. On MRI, there is typically diffuse myocardial thickening with global subendocardial or transmural LGE; all chambers can be involved.
2. Larynx, trachea and bronchi—usually localized amyloidosis. May manifest as diffuse circumferential airway thickening or multifocal plaques/masses ± calcification.
3. Lung parenchyma—localized amyloidosis usually manifests as single or multiple lung nodules (amyloidomas) which often contain calcification. Systemic AL/AA disease usually manifests as interlobular septal thickening, reticulation, micronodules, consolidation and punctate calcification with a basal and peripheral predominance, ± pleural effusions or thickening. AA disease may also be associated with LIP.
4. Mediastinum—usually systemic amyloidosis. Manifests as lymphadenopathy ± calcification, or as a focal mass.
5. GI tract—very common in systemic amyloidosis; may present with dysmotility, GI bleeding, diarrhoea, obstruction or perforation. Duodenum > stomach > rest of GI tract. On CT, luminal dilatation and diffuse/nodular wall thickening ± calcification may be seen. Focal amyloidomas are rare.
6. Liver and spleen—common in systemic amyloidosis. Typically causes diffuse organomegaly ± punctate calcifications. The liver may be hypoattenuating on unenhanced CT, and the spleen often shows poor arterial enhancement. The gallbladder may be thick-walled. Focal amyloidomas are rare.
7. Pancreas—usually localized amyloidosis, causing type 2 diabetes. Diffuse pancreatic infiltration ± enlargement with loss of normal T1 hyperintensity on MRI, ± punctate calcification mimicking chronic pancreatitis.
8. Renal parenchyma—very common in systemic amyloidosis, causing nephrotic syndrome and renal failure. Kidneys may be enlarged and echogenic in early disease ± focal masses, with atrophy in chronic disease ± amorphous calcification. Infiltration of the renal sinus fat may also be seen.
9. Urothelium—usually localized amyloidosis; bladder > ureter > renal pelvis > urethra. Manifests as focal urothelial thickening,

stricture or mass ± calcification. Isolated seminal vesicle involvement can also occur, manifesting as diffuse wall thickening.

10. Adrenals and testes—usually systemic amyloidosis. Diffuse infiltration ± enlargement is typical and may cause organ dysfunction.
11. Mesentery and retroperitoneum—usually systemic amyloidosis, manifesting as diffuse infiltrative soft tissue replacing the normal fat, often with progressive calcification. Lymphadenopathy can also be seen and may be of low attenuation. Ascites is usually absent.
12. Joints (amyloid arthropathy)—usually in Aβ_2M amyloidosis. Manifests as a bilateral erosive polyarthropathy involving wrists, shoulders, hips and knees, with T1/T2 hypointense synovial thickening on MRI (without blooming—cf. PVNS) + joint effusions, but usually without joint space narrowing. The surrounding muscles may be diffusely swollen (e.g. 'shoulder pad' sign), suggesting the diagnosis. Spine involvement is destructive and most common in the C-spine.
13. Bones and soft tissues—usually systemic AL amyloidosis, manifesting as focal soft-tissue masses. Osseous lesions are lytic. Muscle involvement can cause pseudohypertrophy or may mimic an inflammatory myopathy. Breast involvement mimics carcinoma.
14. Peripheral nerves—usually in mutant ATTR or AL amyloidosis, causing diffuse nerve enlargement ± enhancement on MRI. Isolated carpal tunnel syndrome can occur in wild-type ATTR or Aβ_2M amyloidosis.
15. CNS—localized Aβ amyloidosis. Manifestations include:
    (a) Alzheimer's disease—most common. Causes cerebral atrophy especially of the parietal and mesial temporal lobes.
    (b) Cerebral amyloid angiopathy—common. Typically causes multiple microhaemorrhages in a subcortical distribution. Larger intracerebral or subarachnoid haemorrhages can also occur. Focal areas of inflammation (vasogenic oedema) may rarely be seen.
    (c) Cerebral amyloidoma—rare. Enhancing nodular masses + surrounding vasogenic oedema.
    (d) Pituitary—amyloid deposits can be seen in pituitary adenomas.
16. Head and neck:
    (a) Orbits—usually localized disease; can involve any part of orbit, especially lacrimal glands.
    (b) Nasal cavity and paranasal sinuses—usually localized disease; focal mass which may obstruct drainage pathways.
    (c) Oral cavity—usually systemic disease; macroglossia is characteristic.
    (d) Thyroid and salivary glands—usually systemic disease; may cause organ dysfunction.

Further reading

Czeyda-Pommersheim, F., Hwang, M., Chen, S.S., et al., 2015. Amyloidosis: modern cross-sectional imaging. Radiographics 35 (5), 1381–1392.

Georgiades, C.S., Neyman, E.G., Barish, M.A., Fishman, E.K., 2004. Amyloidosis: review and CT manifestations. Radiographics 24 (2), 405–416.

Kawashima, A., Alleman, W.G., Takahashi, N., et al., 2011. Imaging evaluation of amyloidosis of the urinary tract and retroperitoneum. Radiographics 31 (6), 1569–1582.

Özcan, H.N., Haliloğlu, M., Sökmensüer, C., et al., 2017. Imaging for abdominal involvement in amyloidosis. Diagn. Interv. Radiol. 23 (4), 282–285.

Siakallis, L., Tziakouri-Shiakalli, C., Georgiades, C.S., 2014. Amyloidosis: review and imaging findings. Semin. Ultrasound CT MR 35 (3), 225–239.

Takahashi, N., Glockner, J., Howe, B.M., et al., 2016. Taxonomy and imaging manifestations of systemic amyloidosis. Radiol. Clin. North Am. 54 (3), 597–612.

ANKYLOSING SPONDYLITIS

A seronegative spondyloarthropathy manifesting as an inflammatory arthritis affecting the sacroiliac joints and entire spine, eventually resulting in ankylosis. Onset 20–40 years; M>F.

Axial skeleton

1. Involved initially in 70%–80%. Initial changes in the SIJs followed by thoracolumbar and lumbosacral regions. The entire spine may be involved eventually. MRI is the most sensitive technique for detecting early disease (oedema) and all changes except syndesmophytes.
2. Spondylitis—anterior and posterior erosion of vertebral endplate corners (Romanus lesion) due to enthesitis of annulus fibrosus. Then sclerosis causing a 'shiny corner' (osteitis).
3. Discovertebral—involvement of intervertebral discs and central portion of vertebral endplates (Andersson lesion).
4. Syndesmophytes—vertical bony outgrowths from vertebral margins.
5. Squaring of vertebrae—due to bone proliferation.
6. Synovial joints—facet, costovertebral and costotransverse joints (synovitis, erosion, ankylosis).
7. Enthesitis—interspinous ligaments with osteitis.
8. Ankylosis—fusion of spine, leading to 'bamboo spine'.
9. Insufficiency fracture—in ankylosed spine, especially at cervicothoracic and thoracolumbar junctions.
10. Osteoporosis—with longstanding disease.
11. Kyphosis.
12. Arachnoiditis—rare and late. Arachnoid diverticula, laminar erosions, dural calcification.

Appendicular skeleton

1. Hip—axial migration, concentric joint space narrowing, cuff-like femoral osteophytes, acetabular protrusio. Symptoms may be dominant, leading to flexion contracture and ankylosis.
2. Shoulder—narrowing of glenohumeral and acromioclavicular joints. Hatchet erosion at greater tuberosity.
3. Knee—tricompartmental narrowing and erosion.
4. Hands and feet—asymmetric involvement; small erosions and osseous proliferation.

Extraskeletal

1. Anterior uveitis—in 20%; more frequent with a peripheral arthropathy.
2. Lungs—upper lobe fibrosis and bullous change (may mimic a cavitating lesion). Uncommonly lung nodules, pleural thickening, organizing pneumonia. Restrictive lung function due to costotransverse and costosternal joint involvement.
3. CVS—aortic valve incompetence, arrhythmias, pericarditis, aortitis.
4. Inflammatory bowel disease.
5. Amyloidosis—rare.

Further reading

Jang, J.H., Ward, M.M., Rucker, A.N., et al., 2011. Ankylosing spondylitis: patterns of radiographic involvement – a re-examination of accepted principles in a cohort of 769 patients. Radiology 258 (1), 192–198.

Lambert, R.G., Dhillon, S.S., Jaremko, J.L., 2012. Advanced imaging of the axial skeleton in spondyloarthropathy: techniques, interpretation, and utility. Semin. Musculoskelet. Radiol. 16 (5), 389–400.

ASBESTOS-RELATED DISEASES

Lung and/or pleural disease caused by the inhalation of asbestos fibres. Long latency (>20–30 years) between exposure and lung/pleural disease. Pleural disease alone in 50%; pleura + lung disease 40%; lung disease alone 10%.

Pleura

1. Pleural plaques—commonest manifestation, developing 20–30 years after exposure. Typically seen on parietal pleura on undersurface of ribs, diaphragmatic pleura and next to spine; virtually pathognomonic. Sharply angulated 'holly-leaf' opacities on CXR. Discrete appearance at CT.
2. Benign pleural effusion—most common 'early' (<10 years) manifestation; occurs in <10%. May be unilateral or bilateral ± followed by residual benign diffuse pleural thickening.
3. Diffuse pleural thickening—less specific for asbestos exposure than plaques.

4. Round atelectasis—peripheral rounded mass with adjacent pleural thickening and parenchymal bands/distortion ('comet tail' appearance).
5. Malignant mesothelioma—long latency (30–40 years). Lobulated pleural thickening involving mediastinal pleura ± large pleural effusion but minimal mediastinal shift.

Lung parenchyma

1. Asbestosis—long latency (30–40 years). Histological and radiological appearances very similar to UIP. Subpleural lines paralleling the chest wall are an early feature and may suggest the diagnosis.
2. Lung cancer—increased risk even in the absence of a smoking history or asbestosis.

Other associations

1. Peritoneal mesothelioma.
2. Laryngeal carcinoma.
3. Ovarian cancer.

Further reading

Peacock, C., Copley, S.J., Hansell, D.M., 2000. Asbestos-related benign pleural disease. Clin. Radiol. 55, 422–432.

BEHÇET'S DISEASE

Chronic multisystem vasculitis involving vessels of variable size. Most common in young adult men, especially in eastern Mediterranean and eastern Asia. Presents clinically with oral and genital ulcers, ocular inflammation (e.g. uveitis and retinal vasculitis) and skin lesions (e.g. erythema nodosum). Imaging features include:

1. Venous thrombosis—commonest feature; can involve lower and upper limb veins, SVC, IVC, hepatic, portal and renal veins. SVC obstruction can also be caused by fibrosing mediastinitis.
2. Arteritis—can involve the aorta, aortic root, pulmonary arteries, coronary and peripheral arteries (femoral, subclavian and popliteal), causing characteristic saccular aneurysms, stenoses and occlusions. Pulmonary artery aneurysms in particular are highly suggestive.
3. Cardiac—pericarditis, myocarditis, endocarditis, myocardial infarction, endomyocardial fibrosis, intracardiac thrombosis.
4. Lungs—pulmonary emboli, infarcts and haemorrhage due to vasculitis, ± pleural effusions or nodules. Airway ulceration and occlusion can rarely be seen.

5. GI tract—ulcers are the typical feature, most common in the ileocaecal region. On CT/MRI there is mural thickening ± perforation or fistulation ± mesenteric fat wrapping, mimicking Crohn's disease (though perforation is more common in Behçet's and strictures are less common). Inflammatory polypoid lesions can also be seen.
6. Kidneys—glomerulonephritis, renal failure, infarcts, amyloidosis.
7. CNS—focal T2 hyperintense lesions with variable enhancement; brainstem > basal ganglia > thalamus > cerebral white matter and spinal cord. In atypical cases these may appear mass-like. Dural venous sinus thrombosis and cerebral arterial aneurysms/occlusions can also occur.
8. Rhinosinusitis ± bone erosions.
9. Arthritis—usually a subacute self-limiting nondeforming oligoarthropathy, most commonly involving the knee, ankle and SIJs. Manifests as periarticular osteopenia, soft-tissue swelling and joint space narrowing ± erosions.
10. Myositis—rare. Diffuse, patchy or nodular involvement.

Further reading

Ceylan, N., Bayraktaroglu, S., Erturk, S.M., et al., 2010. Pulmonary and vascular manifestations of Behçet disease: imaging findings. AJR Am. J. Roentgenol. 194, W158–W164.

Chae, E.J., Do, K.H., Seo, J.B., et al., 2008. Radiologic and clinical findings of Behçet disease: comprehensive review of multisystemic involvement. Radiographics 28 (5), e31.

Chung, S.Y., Do, K.H., Seo, J.B., et al., 2001. Radiologic findings of Behçet syndrome involving the gastrointestinal tract. Radiographics 21 (4), 911–924.

Mehdipoor, G., Davatchi, F., Ghoreishian, H., Arjmand Shabestari, A., 2018. Imaging manifestations of Behcet's disease: key considerations and major features. Eur. J. Radiol. 98, 214–225.

BIRT-HOGG-DUBÉ SYNDROME

Hereditary (AD) disorder characterized by:

1. Multiple lung cysts with a lower lobe predominance ± pneumothoraces.
2. Multiple bilateral renal tumours—especially oncocytomas and chromophobe RCCs.
3. Skin features—especially fibrofolliculomas (hair follicle hamartomas).
4. Other possible associations—benign and malignant tumours of the breast, colon, skin, lung, thyroid, parathyroid, parotid, peripheral nerves and fat (lipomas).

BLUE RUBBER BLEB NAEVUS SYNDROME

Rare syndrome characterized by multiple venous malformations. On MRI, these lesions are markedly T2 bright and show avid homogeneous enhancement ± thrombi and phleboliths. Any part of the body can be involved; common sites include:

1. Skin—commonest site, giving rise to the so-called 'blue rubber bleb' naevi. Usually visible at birth.
2. GI tract—very common, especially in the small bowel; causes GI bleeding ± intussusception.
3. Musculoskeletal—skin lesions may extend into underlying muscles, bones and/or joints. Lesions can also arise from within deep soft tissues. Joint involvement can cause recurrent haemarthrosis and secondary arthritis. Bone involvement can cause cortical remodelling or focal lytic lesions. Limb overgrowth, undergrowth or bowing may also be seen.
4. Others—e.g. solid abdominal viscera, lung, heart, head and neck.

CARNEY COMPLEX

Hereditary (AD) multiple endocrine neoplasia syndrome, characterized by:

1. Skin lesions—pigmented spots, blue naevi, cutaneous myxomas.
2. Cardiac myxomas—often multiple.
3. Breast myxomas (in women and men), ductal adenomas and myxoid fibroadenomas.
4. Endocrine tumours:
   (a) Pituitary hyperplasia or adenoma—secreting growth hormone or prolactin.
   (b) Thyroid cysts, adenomas or carcinoma.
   (c) Primary pigmented nodular adrenocortical disease—causes Cushing's syndrome.
   (d) Testicular tumours—especially large cell calcifying Sertoli cell tumours (microcalcification is characteristic).
   (e) Ovarian cysts, cystadenoma or teratoma.
5. Psammomatous melanotic schwannoma—can arise anywhere in the CNS or PNS; commonest sites are the GI tract (including liver), paraspinal sympathetic chain and chest wall. Melanin content may cause T1 hyperintensity and T2 hypointensity on MRI. Often calcified.
6. Osteochondromyxomas of bone—most common in the diaphysis of long bones (tibia and radius) and sinonasal bones. Variable appearances—may be well-defined or permeative, lytic or mixed density.

Further reading

Correa, R., Salpea, P., Stratakis, C., 2015. Carney complex: an update. Eur. J. Endocrinol. 173 (4), M85–M97.

CARNEY TRIAD

Rare syndrome, most common in young women. Characterized by the triad of:

1. Extraadrenal paraganglioma—e.g. retroperitoneal, mediastinal, intraspinal, carotid body.
2. GIST—usually gastric, often multifocal.
3. Pulmonary chondroma—lung nodule containing chondroid calcification. Usually multiple.

CHAGAS DISEASE

Tropical protozoan infection (*Trypanosoma cruzi*) endemic in Central and South America, transmitted by triatomine insects. Characteristic imaging features mostly result from chronic infection, and include:

1. Myocarditis—acute and chronic phase, resulting in dilated cardiomyopathy. On MRI, myocardial thinning is typically seen in the apex and inferolateral wall with midwall or subepicardial LGE ± apical aneurysm formation.
2. GI tract dysmotility and dilatation—especially affecting the oesophagus (mimicking achalasia), but large and small bowel can also be involved. Always consider Chagas disease in young patients from endemic areas with diffuse oesophageal dilatation (megaoesophagus) and cardiomegaly.
3. Ureteric dilatation—occasionally.
4. CNS—meningoencephalitis can rarely occur if a chronically infected patient becomes immunocompromised. MRI shows multiple enhancing brain and spinal cord lesions.

CHURG-STRAUSS SYNDROME

Also known as eosinophilic granulomatosis with polyangiitis. Small–medium vessel vasculitis, most common in young–middle-aged adults. Nearly all patients have asthma and peripheral eosinophilia. Other clinical features include mononeuritis multiplex, skin rash/purpura, arthralgia and glomerulonephritis. Imaging features include:

1. Lungs—most common site. Transient/migratory peripheral multifocal patchy consolidation and GGO ± interlobular septal

thickening ± noncavitary nodules ± bronchial wall thickening or dilatation ± small pleural effusions.
2. Heart—common cause of mortality. Pericarditis, valve insufficiency, myocardial infarction or endomyocarditis ± intracardiac thrombosis can occur. MRI may show mural LGE with variable patterns.
3. Allergic rhinosinusitis ± polyposis.
4. GI tract—eosinophilic gastroenteritis/oesophagitis, vasculitic bowel ischaemia (± perforation or stricture formation), GI bleeding, peritonitis/ascites, omental granulomatous nodules or haematoma.
5. HPB—hepatic artery aneurysms and infarcts, Budd-Chiari syndrome, eosinophilic hepatitis, acalculous eosinophilic cholecystitis, pancreatitis.
6. CNS—infarcts, haemorrhage or, rarely, granulomatous masses of the meninges or choroid plexus.
7. Orbits—optic neuritis, central retinal artery occlusion, inflammatory pseudotumour.

CLEIDOCRANIAL DYSPLASIA

AD. One-third are new mutations.

Skull

1. Brachycephaly, wormian bones, frontal and parietal bossing.
2. Wide sutures and fontanelles with delayed closure.
3. Broad mandible, small facial bones, delayed eruption and supernumerary teeth.
4. Platybasia.

Thorax

1. Aplasia or hypoplasia of the clavicles, more commonly in the lateral two-thirds.
2. Small, deformed scapulae.

Pelvis

1. Absent or delayed ossification of the pubic bones, producing apparent widening of the symphysis pubis.

Appendicular skeleton

1. Short or absent fibulae.
2. Coxa vara or coxa valga.
3. Congenital pseudarthrosis of the femur.
4. Hands:
   (a) Long 2nd and 5th metacarpals with short middle phalanges.
   (b) Cone-shaped epiphyses.
   (c) Tapered distal phalanges.
   (d) Supernumerary ossification centres.

COELIAC DISEASE

Common autoimmune disease affecting the GI tract, triggered by gluten intolerance. Treatment is a gluten-free diet; patients who do not respond to this are classified as having refractory disease and are at higher risk of complications. Imaging features include:

1. Dilated and fluid-filled small bowel with reversal of jejunoileal fold patterns ± transient intussusceptions. In severe refractory cases mural thickening and ulceration can be seen (ulcerative jejunoileitis), which can lead to haemorrhage, perforation, stricture formation and lymphoma.
2. Mesenteric lymphadenopathy is common. Rarely, in refractory disease, nodes may cavitate ± fat–fluid levels (cavitating mesenteric lymph node syndrome).
3. Increased risk of small bowel T cell lymphoma (especially terminal ileum; only in those with refractory disease) and adenocarcinoma (especially jejunum), as well as oesophageal SCC.

Extraintestinal associations include:

1. Splenic atrophy and hyposplenism—often accompanies cavitating mesenteric lymph node syndrome.
2. Other autoimmune disorders—autoimmune hepatitis, PBC, sclerosing cholangitis, type 1 diabetes, autoimmune thyroiditis, Sjögren's syndrome.
3. Cardiovascular—pericardial effusion, autoimmune myocarditis, cardiomyopathy, thromboembolism, accelerated atherosclerosis.
4. Dermatitis herpetiformis—papulovesicular skin rash.
5. Osteopenia and osteomalacia.
6. Lane-Hamilton syndrome—coeliac disease + idiopathic pulmonary haemosiderosis.
7. CEC syndrome—coeliac disease + bilateral occipital lobe calcifications ± epilepsy.

CUSHING'S SYNDROME

Cushing's syndrome results from increased endogenous or exogenous cortisol. Causes include:

1. Iatrogenic—high doses of corticosteroids. Most common cause.
2. Pituitary disease (Cushing's disease)—typically due to a microadenoma, which may be hard to visualize on MRI due to its small size. Both adrenals usually appear hyperplastic.
3. Adrenal disease—adenoma or carcinoma. The contralateral adrenal appears atrophic.
4. Ectopic ACTH—e.g. from lung cancer.

Effects

1. Clinical: striae, easy bruising, proximal myopathy, hypertension, diabetes, growth retardation (in children).
2. Central obesity—mediastinal, retroperitoneal and epidural lipomatosis can also be seen.
3. Osteoporosis.
4. Pathological fractures which show excessive callus formation and sclerosis during healing, especially vertebral endplate fractures.
5. Avascular necrosis of bone.
6. Increased incidence of infection—e.g. osteomyelitis, septic arthritis (most often involving the knee).
7. Oedema—due to water retention.

CUTIS LAXA

Heterogeneous group of rare inherited and acquired disorders characterized by loose and redundant skin with reduced elasticity. Other elastic tissues can also be involved, resulting in:

1. Lungs—emphysema, bronchiectasis.
2. Abdominal hernias—including hiatus hernia.
3. Diverticulosis—of the pharynx, GI tract and urinary tract.
4. Arterial aneurysms and pulmonary artery stenosis.

CYSTIC FIBROSIS

AR condition, with carrier rate of 1:25 in Caucasians, affecting 1:2000 live births. Basic defect is of highly viscid secretions. Main complications are pulmonary.

Thoracic findings

1. Peribronchial thickening and bronchial dilatation/bronchiectasis.
2. Mucus plugging—in central bronchi this may appear as nodules or filling-in of airways. In peripheral bronchi this appears as centrilobular nodules, often with a 'tree-in-bud' pattern.
3. Air-trapping—may result in generalized overinflation of the lungs with diaphragmatic flattening. Mosaic attenuation on inspiratory CT, accentuated on expiratory phase.
4. Cystic changes—unusual in early disease. Not true cysts, but represent either areas of localized emphysema or cystic bronchiectasis.
5. Pulmonary hypertension.
6. Hilar enlargement—due to lymphadenopathy or pulmonary arterial dilatation.

Gastrointestinal findings

1. Meconium ileus—in 10%. Presents in neonates.
2. Distal intestinal obstruction syndrome—meconium ileus equivalent that occurs in older children and young adults. Distal ileal obstruction due to a large volume of thick inspissated mucofaeculent bowel contents. NB: the appendix may be distended but the risk of appendicitis is actually reduced in CF.
3. Intussusception—may be ileocolic or more proximal.
4. Colonic wall thickening, jejunization (due to an increase in folds) or fibrosing colonopathy.
5. Pneumatosis intestinalis.
6. Gastrooesophageal reflux.
7. Rectal prolapse—due to chronic coughing and hard faeces.
8. Increased risk of GI tract cancers.

Hepatobiliary/pancreatic

1. Pancreatic changes and exocrine insufficiency. On imaging:
   (a) Fatty replacement—may be partial or complete ('invisible pancreas' on CT).
   (b) Features of chronic pancreatitis—calcifications, atrophy, cysts.
   (c) Pancreatic fibrosis—low T1/T2 signal on MRI.
2. Liver disease—hepatomegaly, steatosis, periportal echogenicity, multilobular cirrhosis and portal hypertension.
3. Biliary—microgallbladder, gallstones, biliary obstruction, sclerosing cholangitis.

Renal

1. Renal stones.
2. Parenchymal disease—IgA nephropathy, secondary amyloidosis.

Skeletal

1. Retarded skeletal maturation.
2. Clubbing and hypertrophic osteoarthropathy.

Head and neck

1. Chronic sinusitis, nasal polyps and mucocoeles.

Further reading

Aziz, Z.A., Davies, J.C., Alton, E.W., et al., 2007. Computed tomography and cystic fibrosis: promises and problems. Thorax 62 (2), 181–186.

King, L.J., Scurr, E.D., Murugan, N., et al., 2000. Hepatobiliary and pancreatic manifestations of cystic fibrosis: MR imaging appearances. Radiographics 20 (3), 767–777.

Lavelle, L.P., McEvoy, S.H., Ni Mhurchu, E., et al., 2015. Cystic fibrosis below the diaphragm: abdominal findings in adult patients. Radiographics 35 (3), 680–695.

Ruzal-Shapiro, C., 1998. Cystic fibrosis. An overview. Radiol. Clin. North Am. 36 (1), 143–161.

CYSTICERCOSIS

Parasitic infection caused by the pork tapeworm *Taenia solium*; endemic in Central and South America, Africa and Asia. Cysticerci may involve any tissue or organ, most commonly:

1. Soft tissues—especially subcutaneous and intramuscular. Usually seen in the chronic calcified stage, as multiple discrete rice/cigar-shaped soft-tissue calcifications.
2. CNS (neurocysticercosis)—usually involves the brain but the spine, eyes and pituitary may also be involved. Lesions can be seen in subarachnoid spaces, brain parenchyma and ventricles. Complications include arachnoiditis, encephalitis, hydrocephalus (especially if ventricular involvement) and stroke (if vascular involvement). Lesions pass through four stages, each of which has a characteristic appearance:
   1. Vesicular (viable)—small nonenhancing cyst, often with a characteristic eccentric 'dot' (scolex). If subarachnoid in location, may be large and clustered (racemose) without a scolex, mimicking an arachnoid cyst.
   2. Colloidal (early degeneration)—cyst shows ring enhancement with surrounding oedema. Scolex may also enhance. This stage is often triggered by initiating treatment. Seizures are most common in this stage.
   3. Granular (late degeneration)—enhancing wall retracts, becomes thicker and starts becoming calcified. May show solid enhancement. Variable oedema.
   4. Calcified (dead)—small nodular calcification with no fluid, oedema or enhancement.

Further reading

Kimura-Hayama, E.T., Higuera, J.A., Corona-Cedillo, R., et al., 2010. Neurocysticercosis: radiologic-pathologic correlation. Radiographics 30 (6), 1705–1719.

DOWN'S SYNDROME (TRISOMY 21)

Head and neck

1. Brachycephaly and microcephaly.
2. Hypoplasia of facial bones and sinuses + hypotelorism.
3. Wide sutures and delayed closure. Multiple wormian bones.
4. Dental abnormalities.
5. Cystic hygroma (lymphangioma).

Central nervous system

1. Bilateral basal ganglia calcification.
2. Cerebellar and vermian hypoplasia.
3. Moyamoya syndrome.

Axial skeleton

1. Atlantoaxial or atlantooccipital subluxation—may cause cord compression.
2. Hypoplastic posterior arch of C1.
3. Increased height and decreased AP diameter of lumbar vertebrae with incomplete fusion of the vertebral arches.

Pelvis

1. Flared iliac wings with small acetabular angles resulting in an abnormal iliac index (iliac angle + acetabular angle).

Hands

1. Short tubular bones, clinodactyly and hypoplasia of the middle phalanx of the little finger.

Chest

1. Congenital heart disease—endocardial cushion defects, VSD, aberrant right subclavian artery.
2. Eleven pairs of ribs.
3. Two ossification centres for the manubrium (90%).
4. Congenital diaphragmatic hernia.
5. Congenital chylous pleural effusion.
6. Subpleural lung cysts.

Gastrointestinal

1. Duodenal atresia/stenosis/annular pancreas.
2. Coeliac disease.
3. Omphalocoele.
4. Hirschsprung's disease.
5. Anorectal malformation.

Further reading

James, A.E., Jr., Merz, T., Janower, M.L., Dorst, J.P., 1971. Radiological features of the most common autosomal disorders: trisomy 21–22 (mongolism or Down's syndrome), trisomy 18, trisomy 13–15, and the cri-du-chat syndrome. Clin. Radiol. 22 (4), 417–433.

Stein, S.M., Kirchner, S.G., Horev, G., Hernanz-Schulman, M., 1991. Atlanto-occipital subluxation in Down syndrome. Pediatr. Radiol. 21, 121–124.

EHLERS-DANLOS SYNDROME (EDS)

A group of hereditary collagen disorders; many subtypes of varying severity. General clinical features include skin hyperelasticity and fragility, joint hypermobility and blood vessel fragility resulting in bleeding tendency. General imaging features include:

1. Soft tissues—subcutaneous calcification (due to fat necrosis) and heterotopic ossification.
2. Joint instability due to ligament laxity—can manifest as dislocations, joint effusions and haemarthroses, abnormal angulations, atlantoaxial and craniocervical instability, pes planus, early osteoarthritis.
3. Tendinopathy ± tendon rupture.
4. Spine—kyphoscoliosis, spondylolisthesis, dural ectasia.
5. Abdominal and diaphragmatic hernias, pelvic floor prolapse, visceroptosis.
6. GI tract—diverticula, dysmotility and dilatation, gastric volvulus and reflux.
7. Mitral valve prolapse.
8. Bladder diverticula.

EDS type IV

Also known as vascular EDS, this is the most severe form (though skin features tend to be mild) and is associated with additional important complications:

1. Fragility of large and medium-sized arteries—typically affecting the aorta and its major branches, resulting in multiple aneurysms (and associated rupture), spontaneous dissection and occlusion (causing cerebral or visceral infarcts), and spontaneous caroticocavernous fistula. There is an especially high risk of vessel dissection or rupture related to interventional procedures, so these must be avoided where possible.
2. GI tract—spontaneous perforation (especially sigmoid, even without diverticulosis), intramural haematoma and GI bleeding.
3. Spontaneous uterine rupture during pregnancy.
4. Spontaneous rupture of the liver, spleen and gallbladder.
5. Lungs—haemorrhagic cavities, bullae and haemopneumothoraces.

ENDOMETRIOSIS

Common disorder characterized by ectopic endometrial tissue outside the uterus. Nearly always occurs in premenopausal women. Cyclical (catamenial) symptoms are characteristic. Endometriotic deposits may be:

1. Cystic (endometrioma)—usually unilocular with diffuse low-level echoes on US ± echogenic avascular foci adherent to the wall. On MRI, the contents show uniform T1 hyperintensity and reduced T2 signal (uniform or layered). The cyst wall is usually T2 dark (due to haemosiderin) + signal voids on SWI ± an adherent nonenhancing T2 dark mural nodule. NB: an enhancing mural nodule would be suspicious for malignant transformation to clear cell or endometrioid carcinoma.
2. Solid—spiculate fibrotic mass or plaque tethered to or invading adjacent structures. Usually T1 and T2 hypointense on MRI ± tiny hyperintense foci on T1 (blood products) or T2 (endometrial glands). Enhances post contrast. Associated adhesions may cause obstruction of fallopian tubes, ureters or bowel.

Typical locations for endometriotic deposits include:

1. Ovaries—usually cystic, often multiple and bilateral.
2. Pelvic peritoneum—usually solid.
   (a) Pouch of Douglas—often obliterates the pouch and may extend inferiorly into rectovaginal septum ± invasion of posterior vaginal fornix or rectum. Often draws the ovaries together ('kissing ovaries' sign).
   (b) Surface of rectosigmoid colon—may invade the wall and mimic a colonic tumour on CT. On MRI, an intact T2 hyperintense submucosal layer is usually seen overlying the mural deposit, giving a 'mushroom cap' appearance.
   (c) Fallopian tubes—causes hydro- or haematosalpinx.
   (d) Surface of bladder dome in uterovesical pouch—may invade wall and project into lumen.
   (e) Parametrium—may obstruct distal ureters.
   (f) Round ligament—R>L, may extend into the groin/labia via the canal of Nuck.
3. Abdominal wall—typically at a caesarean-section scar, usually solid. Due to implantation of endometrial tissue during surgery, so usually occurs without evidence of endometriosis in the pelvis. Can mimic a desmoid tumour.

Less common sites include:

1. Extrapelvic peritoneum—e.g. on the serosal surface of bowel (appendix > caecum > terminal ileum > other loops). May cause strictures, mimicking Crohn's disease or malignancy. Appendiceal involvement may cause appendicitis or mucocoele formation. Peritoneal deposits may also rarely occur within hernias, in the subphrenic space (R>L), mesentery, omentum or on the surface of the stomach, gallbladder, liver or spleen.

2. Thorax—uncommon, nearly always occurs in the presence of chronic pelvic disease.
   (a) Pleura—nearly always right-sided. Causes cyclical haemopneumothorax.
   (b) Lung parenchyma—rare; causes cyclical haemoptysis and lung nodules.
   (c) Tracheobronchial tree—rare; causes cyclical haemoptysis and endoluminal nodules.
   (d) Pericardium—rare; causes cyclical pericardial effusions.
3. Cervix—post surgery (e.g. cone biopsy). Rare.
4. Perineum—at an episiotomy scar. Rare.
5. Umbilicus—rare; may be primary or secondary (e.g. laparoscopy port site).
6. Pelvic nerves—sacral plexus, pudendal or sciatic nerves. Can cause cyclical sciatica. Very rare.
7. Within solid abdominal viscera—e.g. liver, pancreas, kidneys, adrenals. Very rare; usually cystic.
8. Other rare sites—e.g. breast, skin, muscle, bone, lymph nodes, nasal cavity, eyes, brain, spinal canal.

Further reading

Chamié, L.P., Ribeiro, D.M.F.R., Tiferes, D.A., et al., 2018. Atypical sites of deeply infiltrative endometriosis: clinical characteristics and imaging findings. Radiographics 38 (1), 309–328.

Gui, B., Valentini, A.L., Ninivaggi, V., et al., 2017. Shining light in a dark landscape: MRI evaluation of unusual localization of endometriosis. Diagn. Interv. Radiol. 23 (4), 272–281.

ERDHEIM-CHESTER DISEASE

Rare non-Langerhans cell histiocytosis with multisystem manifestations which are often characteristic on imaging. Usually presents in middle age.

1. Bones—involved in nearly all patients. Characteristically causes bilateral symmetrical metadiaphyseal sclerosis in the medulla of long bones, especially femora and tibiae. Other bones may also be involved, e.g. skull and facial bones.
2. Retroperitoneum—soft-tissue cuffing of the aorta ('coated aorta') and kidneys ('hairy kidneys') is almost pathognomonic if both are present. Tends to spare the IVC and ureters (cf. retroperitoneal fibrosis), though the renal pelvises and adrenals may be involved.
3. Orbits—bilateral retrobulbar inflammatory pseudotumours, usually intraconal.
4. CNS—variable manifestations: infiltration and enhancement of the pituitary and its stalk (causing diabetes insipidus), enhancing T2 hypointense dural masses or thickening, intracerebral lesions/

masses or periarterial masses. Intracranial disease nearly always occurs in the presence of orbital or facial bone involvement.

5. Lungs—most commonly causes interlobular septal thickening, but other findings, e.g. GGO, centrilobular nodules, lung cysts, pleural thickening and effusions may be seen.
6. Cardiovascular—pericardial thickening and effusion ± infiltrative soft-tissue mass involving the myocardium (especially right atrium and AV groove). Soft-tissue cuffing of the thoracic aorta and its branches may be seen.
7. Other rare sites—skin, breasts, lymph nodes, thyroid, testes, other abdominal viscera.

Further reading

Dion, E., Graef, C., Haroche, J., et al., 2004. Imaging of thoracoabdominal involvement in Erdheim-Chester disease. AJR Am. J. Roentgenol. 183, 1253–1260.

Drier, A., Haroche, J., Savatovsky, J., et al., 2010. Cerebral, facial, and orbital involvement in Erdheim-Chester disease: CT and MR imaging findings. Radiology 255 (2), 586–594.

Kumar, P., Singh, A., Gamanagatti, S., et al., 2018. Imaging findings in Erdheim-Chester disease: what every radiologist needs to know. Pol. J. Radiol. 83, e54–e62.

FAMILIAL MEDITERRANEAN FEVER

Inherited (AR) inflammatory serositis mainly affecting young adults of Mediterranean heritage. Most commonly presents with recurrent episodes of peritonitis ± skin rash. Imaging findings include:

1. Peritonitis—peritoneal thickening and ascites without another cause, ± mesenteric adenopathy and fat stranding ± hepatosplenomegaly.
2. Synovitis—joint effusion and soft-tissue swelling; may be mono- or polyarticular, lower > upper limbs. Usually nonerosive.
3. Pleuritis—pleural effusions.
4. Pericarditis—rare.
5. Complications of chronic disease—encapsulating peritonitis with cyst formation, peritoneal mesothelioma, systemic amyloidosis.
6. Possible associations—vasculitis, multiple sclerosis, haemolytic anaemia.

Further reading

Ishak, G.E., Khoury, N.J., Birjawi, G.A., et al., 2006. Imaging findings of familial Mediterranean fever. Clin. Imaging 30 (3), 153–159.

GAUCHER DISEASE

Commonest hereditary (AR) lysosomal storage disease, most common in Ashkenazi Jews. Results in the accumulation of glucosylceramide-filled macrophages (Gaucher cells) in the bone marrow, spleen and liver. May present in infants, children or young adults depending on subtype.

1. Bones—most commonly spine and long bones. Features include:
   - (a) Osteopenia, remodelling (Erlenmeyer flask), lytic lesions and pathological fractures.
   - (b) Bone infarcts and avascular necrosis with resultant sclerosis, H-shaped vertebrae and femoral/humeral head collapse.
   - (c) On MRI: diffuse T1 hypointense marrow replacement + bone infarcts.
   - (d) Increased risk of osteomyelitis.
2. Splenomegaly—typically massive ± focal infarcts. Focal masses are also common, comprising of Gaucher cells or extramedullary haematopoiesis.
3. Hepatomegaly—less marked than splenomegaly. Focal nodules may be seen.
4. Lungs—uncommon, typically in the presence of severe bone and visceral disease. Interlobular septal thickening, GGO, consolidation and bronchial wall thickening may be seen.

Further reading

Simpson, W.L., Hermann, G., Balwani, M., 2014. Imaging of Gaucher disease. World J. Radiol. 6 (9), 657–668.

GENERALIZED LYMPHATIC ANOMALY

Also known as lymphangiomatosis. Rare congenital disease usually presenting in childhood, characterized by widespread lymphangiomas which can involve nearly any organ or tissue except the CNS. Most common sites include:

1. Bones—especially axial and proximal appendicular skeleton. Numerous well-defined cysts with thin sclerotic margins and preserved cortex.
2. Soft tissues—including skin, mediastinum, retroperitoneum, mesentery and neck.
3. Spleen—multiple lymphatic cysts.
4. Pleural and pericardial effusions and ascites—often chylous.
5. Lungs (diffuse pulmonary lymphangiomatosis)—thickening of interlobular septa and bronchovascular bundles ± GGO.

Related conditions include:

1. Cystic angiomatosis—less aggressive, usually presenting in adolescence or adulthood.
2. Kaposiform lymphangiomatosis—more aggressive, with more severe and infiltrative thoracic involvement and poorer prognosis. Also associated with thrombocytopenia, resulting in haemorrhagic effusions.
3. Gorham-Stout disease—also known as vanishing bone disease. Progressive osteolysis also involving cortex without a periosteal reaction. Usually limited to one bone, though the process can spread to adjacent bones and soft tissues. Splenic cysts may also be seen.

Further reading

Joshi, M., Phansalkar, D.S., 2015. Simple lymphangioma to generalized lymphatic anomaly: role of imaging in disclosure of a rare and morbid disease. Case Rep. Radiol. 2015, 603859.

Ozeki, M., Fujino, A., Matsuoka, K., et al., 2016. Clinical features and prognosis of generalized lymphatic anomaly, Kaposiform lymphangiomatosis, and Gorham-Stout disease. Pediatr. Blood Cancer 63, 832–838.

GORLIN-GOLTZ SYNDROME

Also known as basal cell naevus syndrome. Hereditary (AD) neurocutaneous syndrome characterized by:

1. Multiple cutaneous basal cell carcinomas at a young age—NB: patients are highly sensitive to ionizing radiation (especially radiotherapy), which can trigger the formation of skin tumours.
2. Multiple odontogenic keratocysts in the mandible and/or maxilla.
3. Dense calcification of the falx, tentorium and diaphragma sellae.
4. Rib anomalies (especially 3rd–5th)—bifid, fused, splayed or hypoplastic.
5. Palmoplantar pits or keratosis.
6. Increased risk of medulloblastoma, meningioma, ovarian/cardiac fibroma, fetal rhabdomyoma, mesenteric and pleural cysts.
7. Other skeletal anomalies—vertebral anomalies, pectus excavatum/carinatum, Sprengel deformity, poly/syndactyly, flame-shaped lucencies in hands and feet.
8. Other CNS anomalies—ventriculomegaly, cavum septum pellucidum, corpus callosum dysgenesis, colloid cyst.
9. Other clinical features—macrocephaly, hypertelorism, frontal bossing, cleft lip, high-arched palate, ocular anomalies, dermal cysts.

Further reading

Kimonis, V.E., Mehta, S.G., Digiovanna, J.J., et al., 2004. Radiological features in 82 patients with nevoid basal cell carcinoma (NBCC or Gorlin) syndrome. Genet. Med. 6 (6), 495–502.

GRAFT-VERSUS-HOST DISEASE (GvHD)

Common and serious immunologic complication of allogeneic haematopoietic stem cell transplantation. May be acute (10–100 days post transplant) or chronic (>100 days)—each has different imaging features. NB: GvHD does not usually occur <10 days post transplant (unlike many infectious complications) since the transplanted marrow has not yet started functioning.

Acute GvHD

Usually develops <100 days post transplant, though some cases may persist beyond 100 days; rarely, late-onset acute GvHD may develop >100 days. A skin rash is usually the first manifestation, then progressing to involve GI tract and liver.

1. GI tract—dilated fluid-filled bowel with diffuse wall thickening, oedema and mucosal hyperenhancement, mesenteric vascular engorgement ± mesenteric fat stranding and ascites. Both small and large bowel are often involved, though small bowel involvement is usually more marked. The extent of inflammation is more than with other causes of acute enteritis in these patients (e.g. neutropenic enterocolitis, CMV and other viruses).
2. Hepatobiliary—usually in the presence of bowel involvement. Imaging features are nonspecific and include hepatosplenomegaly, periportal and gallbladder wall oedema, and biliary dilatation, wall thickening and enhancement. It can be difficult to distinguish hepatic GvHD from venoocclusive disease (another complication of bone marrow transplantation), though the presence of small-calibre hepatic veins and absence of bowel involvement suggests venoocclusive disease.
3. Lungs—rare. May cause nonspecific interstitial and alveolar opacities similar to pulmonary oedema.

Chronic GvHD

Usually develops >100 days post transplant, but can rarely occur earlier and is not always preceded by acute GvHD. Skin involvement often occurs first, manifesting as a scleroderma-like skin reaction which may also involve the mouth and genitalia.

1. GI tract—oesophageal webs or strictures; fibrotic strictures of small or large bowel.

2. Hepatobiliary—thickening and enhancement of bile ducts and gallbladder ± intra- and extrahepatic ductal strictures similar to PSC.
3. Lungs—common; can manifest as obliterative bronchiolitis, organizing pneumonia or interstitial fibrosis. Rarely, in patients with obliterative bronchiolitis, spontaneous pneumomediastinum, pneumothorax or pulmonary interstitial emphysema may occur ('air-leak syndrome').
4. Neuromuscular—fasciitis, muscle contractures, polymyositis, autoimmune neuropathy (e.g. Guillain-Barré), myasthenia gravis. Rare.
5. CNS—cerebral vasculitis, demyelination, encephalitis. Rare.

Further reading

Grauer, O., Wolff, D., Bertz, H., et al., 2010. Neurological manifestations of chronic graft-versus-host disease after allogeneic haematopoietic stem cell transplantation: report from the consensus conference on clinical practice in chronic graft-versus-host disease. Brain 133 (10), 2852–2865.

Lubner, M.G., Menias, C.O., Agrons, M., et al., 2017. Imaging of abdominal and pelvic manifestations of graft-versus-host disease after haematopoietic stem cell transplant. AJR Am. J. Roentgenol. 209 (1), 33–45.

Peña, E., Souza, C.A., Escuissato, D.L., et al., 2014. Noninfectious pulmonary complications after haematopoietic stem cell transplantation: practical approach to imaging diagnosis. Radiographics 34 (3), 663–683.

HAEMOCHROMATOSIS

1. Primary—AR disorder of iron metabolism. Results in iron deposition in the liver, pancreas, heart, pituitary, thyroid and synovium.
2. Secondary—two causes:
   (a) Increased hepatic iron uptake—due to cirrhosis or chronic anaemias (e.g. thalassaemia, myelodysplasia). Iron deposition in liver ± pancreas and thyroid.
   (b) Iron overload—due to multiple blood transfusions (e.g. for thalassaemia) or chronic iron supplementation (oral or IV). Iron deposition in spleen, bone marrow and liver.
3. Clinical—cirrhosis, skin pigmentation, diabetes, arthropathy and, later, ascites and cardiac failure.
4. Liver biopsy can aid assessment of patients without typical haemochromatosis-associated *HFE* genotypes who have serum ferritin concentrations >1000 μg/L, because many such patients have an inflammatory disease, not iron overload.

Bones and joints

1. Osteoporosis.
2. Chondrocalcinosis—due to CPPD deposition.

3. Arthropathy—resembles CPPD arthropathy but shows a predilection for the MCP joints (especially 2nd and 3rd), midcarpal joints and CMC joints. It also exhibits distinctive beak-like osteophytes and is less rapidly progressive.

Liver and spleen

1. Liver fibrosis and cirrhosis. Increased risk of HCC.
2. Mottled increased density of liver on CT (≥72 HU) and reduced T2 signal on MRI (lower than paraspinal muscles) due to iron deposition. The liver usually shows signal loss on in-phase T1 sequences (opposite to steatosis).

Others

1. Cardiomyopathy.
2. Hypogonadism.

Further reading

Adams, P.C., Barton, J.C., 2007. Haemochromatosis. Lancet 370, 1855–1860.
Queiroz-Andrade, M., Blasbalg, R., Ortega, C.D., et al., 2009. MR imaging findings of iron overload. Radiographics 29 (6), 1575–1589.

HAEMOLYTIC-URAEMIC SYNDROME

Multisystem thrombotic microangiopathy typically triggered by gut infection with Shiga toxin-producing *E. coli*. Most common in young children; presents initially with bloody diarrhoea and a triad of thrombocytopenia, haemolytic anaemia and AKI. Causes microvascular ischaemia of:

1. Kidneys—most common site. Increased cortical echogenicity on US with reduced blood flow in renal parenchyma and high resistance Doppler waveform in renal arteries. CT may show patchy infarcts, diffuse cortical necrosis or generalized poor renal enhancement.
2. GI tract—haemorrhagic or ischaemic colitis, or less commonly enteritis.
3. CNS—bilateral areas of increased DWI signal ± haemorrhage, especially in basal ganglia, thalami and deep white matter.
4. Others—necrotizing pancreatitis, hepatic infarcts, myocardial infarction, pulmonary haemorrhage. These features are more common in the atypical form of HUS, which is caused by an underlying genetic predisposition (complement system mutation) together with a trigger (e.g. infection, trauma, surgery, pregnancy, systemic diseases) and can occur in adults; this has a poorer prognosis.

HAEMOPHAGOCYTIC LYMPHOHISTIOCYTOSIS

Immune disorder characterized by abnormal macrophage activation. May be primary (familial) or secondary to infection (especially viruses, e.g. EBV), malignancy (especially haematological), autoimmune disorders (e.g. juvenile idiopathic arthritis, SLE, vasculitis) or immune suppression. Most common in infants and young children. Imaging features include:

1. Lungs—consolidation, pulmonary oedema/haemorrhage, pleural effusions.
2. Abdomen—hepatosplenomegaly, periportal and gallbladder oedema, enlarged echogenic kidneys, ascites, adenopathy.
3. CNS—periventricular T2 hyperintensities, enlarged extraaxial fluid spaces and ventriculomegaly, meningeal enhancement and/or enhancing intraaxial lesions.

Further reading

Fitzgerald, N.E., McClain, K.L., 2003. Imaging characteristics of hemophagocytic lymphohistiocytosis. Pediatr. Radiol. 33 (6), 392–401.

HENOCH-SCHÖNLEIN PURPURA

Multisystem small vessel IgA vasculitis. Typically presents in children with purpura (especially lower limbs). Usually self-limiting. Imaging features include:

1. GI tract—bowel wall oedema and haemorrhage, mural hypervascularity, ascites, mesenteric oedema and adenopathy. Intussusception (especially ileoileal) can occur. Bowel infarction is rare.
2. Joints—synovitis, joint effusions, soft-tissue swelling.
3. Urinary tract—nephritis (enlarged echogenic kidneys); urothelial thickening, strictures or haematomas; penoscrotal oedema, orchitis.
4. Lungs—pulmonary oedema/haemorrhage, pleural effusions. Rare.
5. CNS—cerebral oedema/haemorrhage, venous sinus thrombosis, PRES. Rare.
6. Other rare manifestations—acute pancreatitis, adrenal haemorrhage, myocardial infarction.

HEREDITARY HAEMORRHAGIC TELANGIECTASIA (HHT)

Inherited (AD) disorder characterized by multiple telangiectasias in the skin and mucous membranes and vascular malformations in many organs. Classically presents with recurrent epistaxis.

1. Lungs—AVMs are common and often symptomatic due to haemorrhage, right-to-left shunting and paradoxical emboli (resulting in stroke or cerebral abscesses). Most patients with >1 pulmonary AVM will have HHT.
2. Liver—commonly involved but often asymptomatic. Malformations may be arterioportal, arteriovenous or portovenous. Small malformations (telangiectasias) appear as <1 cm arterially enhancing lesions that equilibrate on the portal phase. Larger malformations appear as tortuous vascular connections or large (>1 cm) confluent vascular masses with persistent enhancement. Arterial enhancement of the liver is often diffusely heterogeneous, with dilated hepatic arteries and veins due to AV shunting + early venous filling ± high-output heart failure. FNH-like lesions may also be seen. Liver enhancement usually becomes homogeneous on the portal phase. Severe arterioportal shunting or NRH may lead to portal hypertension. Rarely, an ischaemic or necrotizing cholangiopathy may occur if severe AV shunting 'steals' oxygenated blood from the bile ducts.
3. GI tract—telangiectasias and/or AVMs may occur at any point along the GI tract causing recurrent bleeding, but only the larger malformations are visible on imaging.
4. CNS—intracranial or spinal AVMs (usually small and superficial), arteriovenous fistulas, capillary telangiectasias and developmental venous anomalies may be seen.
5. Other rare sites—pancreas, spleen.

Further reading

Carette, M., Nedelcu, C., Tassart, M., et al., 2009. Imaging of hereditary hemorrhagic telangiectasia. Cardiovasc. Intervent. Radiol. 32 (4), 745–757.

Krings, T., Kim, H., Power, S., et al., 2015. Neurovascular manifestations in hereditary hemorrhagic telangiectasia: imaging features and genotype-phenotype correlations. AJNR Am. J. Neuroradiol. 36 (5), 863–870.

Siddiki, H., Doherty, M.G., Fletcher, J.G., et al., 2008. Abdominal findings in hereditary hemorrhagic telangiectasia: pictorial essay on 2D and 3D findings with isotropic multiphase CT. Radiographics 28 (1), 171–184.

HOMOCYSTINURIA

AR inborn error of metabolism resulting in the accumulation of homocysteine.

1. Brain—multiple white matter lesions and infarcts at a young age. Can result in seizures and developmental delay.
2. Tall stature, slim build and arachnodactyly, resembling Marfan syndrome.
3. Pectus excavatum or carinatum, kyphoscoliosis, genu valgum and pes cavus.
4. Osteoporosis (not seen in Marfan syndrome).
5. Aortic root dilatation—due to cystic medial degeneration of elastic arteries.
6. Arterial and venous thromboses.
7. Lens subluxation—usually downward (cf. Marfan syndrome).

HYDATID DISEASE

Parasitic infection caused by the larval stage of the *Echinococcus* tapeworm. Humans become accidental intermediate hosts after ingesting the eggs. The larvae penetrate through the bowel wall and primarily infect the liver, though any organ or tissue can be involved. There are two main types:

Cystic echinococcosis

Caused by *E. granulosus*. Canines are the definitive host; sheep are usually the intermediate host. Infection forms cystic masses that have a characteristic appearance and pattern of evolution—see Section 8.16. When unilocular, these can mimic simple cysts (unless characteristic hydatid 'sand' is seen on US). When multilocular, these can usually be distinguished from other multilocular cysts by the characteristic absence of internal enhancement within septa and solid components (since these are generated by the parasite, not the host). An enhancing fibrous capsule may be seen around the periphery. Internal haemorrhage is very rare (cf. other cystic lesions). Imaging features are similar regardless of which organ is involved. In order of decreasing frequency:

1. Liver—may rupture into the biliary tree (± obstruction) or peritoneal cavity, or may extend through the diaphragm and rupture into the pleural space. A ruptured cyst may become superinfected by bacteria. Involvement of distant extrahepatic sites usually occurs via haematogenous dissemination of liver disease.
2. Lungs—may be seen with or without liver disease. Cysts may grow very large and are usually of the unilocular type. Calcification is very rare. Erosion into the bronchial tree is common, resulting in air entering the cyst ('crescent' sign) ± endocyst collapse ('water lily' sign). The cyst may also rupture

into the lung parenchyma (producing consolidation) or pleural space. The cyst may become completely air-filled, mimicking a bulla. Rarely, cysts may invade the vena cava or pulmonary artery, causing PEs.

3. Peritoneum—nearly always secondary to liver disease, either due to surgery or spontaneous rupture into the peritoneal space. Usually multiple, can occur anywhere in the peritoneal cavity, e.g. on serosal surface of viscera (e.g. spleen, bowel, bladder, ovaries) or within abdominal wall hernias (including the scrotal sac).
4. Spleen—nearly always secondary to liver disease, with a similar appearance.
5. Kidneys—rare. Often solitary, may be large. May rupture into the collecting system ± obstruction of ureter by daughter cysts ± secondary involvement of ureter or bladder.
6. Brain—rare. Usually solitary and unilocular, without surrounding oedema (cf. cerebral abscess). Usually intracerebral, though can rarely be intraventricular or extraaxial.
7. Heart—rare. Most commonly involves LV myocardium. The pericardium may less commonly be involved.
8. Soft tissues—including retroperitoneum, mediastinum and breasts. Rare. Muscle involvement favours the trunk, neck and proximal limbs.
9. Bone—spine (especially thoracic) > pelvis > long bones > ribs > skull > scapula. Unlike in other tissues, bone lesions are not round due to the rigid nature of bone. Lesions are irregular, lytic, expansile and multilocular with cortical thinning and extension into surrounding soft tissues.
10. Spinal canal—usually via epidural extension of vertebral involvement, though intradural and intramedullary lesions can rarely occur.
11. Other rare sites—e.g. pancreas, adrenals, thyroid, orbit.

Alveolar echinococcosis

Rare; caused by *E. multilocularis*. Foxes are usually the definitive host; rodents are the intermediate host. Infection forms microcystic sponge-like hepatic masses that appear mostly solid and infiltrative on imaging, mimicking malignancy. Prominent calcification and lack of internal enhancement or haemorrhage is suggestive. The mass may directly invade adjacent structures, or disseminate via lymphatics or blood vessels to distant sites (most commonly lungs and brain). Extrahepatic lesions have similar imaging features.

Further reading

Kantarci, M., Bayraktutan, U., Karabulut, N., et al., 2012. Alveolar echinococcosis: spectrum of findings at cross-sectional imaging. Radiographics 32 (7), 2053–2070.

Malik, A., Chandra, R., Prasad, R., et al., 2016. Imaging appearances of atypical hydatid cysts. Indian J. Radiol. Imaging 26 (1), 33–39.
Mehta, P., Prakash, M., Khandelwal, N., 2016. Radiological manifestations of hydatid disease and its complications. Trop. Parasitol. 6 (2), 103–112.
Pedrosa, I., Saíz, A., Arrazola, J., et al., 2000. Hydatid disease: radiologic and pathologic features and complications. Radiographics 20 (3), 795–817.
Polat, P., Kantarci, M., Alper, F., et al., 2003. Hydatid disease from head to toe. Radiographics 23 (2), 475–494.

HYPERPARATHYROIDISM, PRIMARY

Results in hypercalcaemia.

Causes

1. Adenoma of one gland (90%)—2% are multiple.
2. Hyperplasia of all four glands (5%)—more likely if there is a family history.
3. Carcinoma of one gland.
4. Ectopic parathormone—e.g. from lung cancer.
5. MEN 1/2A syndromes—hyperplasia or adenoma + other associations (see MEN section).
6. Hyperparathyroidism-jaw tumour syndrome—parathyroid adenoma/carcinoma + ossifying fibromas of the jaw ± renal cysts, hamartomas and Wilms tumours ± uterine tumours.

Bones

1. Osteopenia—when advanced there is loss of the fine trabeculae ± a ground-glass appearance.
2. Subperiosteal bone resorption—especially affecting the radial side of the phalanges, proximal humerus, lateral ± medial ends of clavicles, superior surface of ribs, symphysis pubis, SIJs, ischial tuberosity, medial femoral neck, medial proximal tibia, dorsum sellae and lamina dura of the teeth. Severe disease produces terminal phalangeal resorption and, in children, the 'rotting fence-post' appearance of the proximal femur.
3. Cortical tunnelling—may be diffuse, leading to a 'basketwork' appearance.
4. 'Salt and pepper' skull—mixed foci of lucency and sclerosis (cf. 'pepper pot' skull—purely lytic lesions due to myeloma).
5. 'Rugger-jersey' spine—multilevel linear endplate sclerosis. Rare in primary hyperparathyroidism; usually seen in secondary type.
6. Brown tumours—may be the only sign. Most frequent in the mandible, ribs, pelvis and femora.
7. Bone softening—basilar invagination, wedged or codfish vertebrae, kyphoscoliosis, triradiate pelvis, pathological fractures.

Joints

1. Marginal erosions—especially DIP joints, ulnar side of the base of the 5th metacarpal and the hamate. No joint space narrowing.
2. Weakened subarticular bone, leading to collapse.
3. Chondrocalcinosis (CPPD) and true gout.
4. Periarticular calcification, including capsule and tendons.

Extraosseous manifestations

1. Calcification in soft tissues, pancreas, lungs and arteries—more common in secondary hyperparathyroidism.
2. Renal tract—nephrocalcinosis and calculi.
3. GI tract—peptic ulcer disease, pancreatitis (due to hypercalcaemia).

Further reading

Hayes, C.W., Conway, W.F., 1991. Hyperparathyroidism. Radiol. Clin. North Am. 29 (1), 85–96.

McDonald, D.K., Parman, L., Speights, V.O., Jr., 2005. Best cases from the AFIP: primary hyperparathyroidism due to parathyroid adenoma. Radiographics 25 (3), 829–834.

IgG4-RELATED DISEASE

Multisystem fibroinflammatory disorder characterized by infiltration of various organs and tissues by IgG4-positive plasma cells and fibrosis. Due to the fibrosis, associated mass lesions (inflammatory pseudotumours) tend to be T2 hypointense and hypovascular with homogeneous delayed enhancement on MRI. Most common in men >45 years. Usually responds well to steroids.

Abdomen

1. Autoimmune pancreatitis—commonest manifestation, present in most patients. Usually causes diffuse swelling of the pancreas with loss of normal lobulation ('sausage-like') and a thin discrete halo of fat stranding, but can be focal mimicking a tumour. Hypoechoic on US, T1 hypointense on MRI. The PD is typically narrowed and irregular within diseased areas ± mild upstream dilatation (cf. adenocarcinoma which causes more marked upstream dilatation). Calcification is rare.
2. Sclerosing cholangitis—frequently accompanies autoimmune pancreatitis, but can occur without it. Wall thickening, enhancement and stricturing most commonly involves distal CBD, but can also cause multifocal intra- and extrahepatic strictures mimicking PSC (though strictures tend to be longer vs. PSC). The gallbladder may also be diffusely thick-walled.

3. Renal involvement—most commonly multiple bilateral round or wedge-shaped hypovascular cortical lesions, but can also cause diffuse parenchymal infiltration or soft-tissue thickening of the perinephric space or renal sinus/pelvis.
4. Retroperitoneal fibrosis—see Section 9.33. Most primary cases are now thought to be due to IgG4-related disease. Fibrous soft tissue coating the abdominal aorta (typically sparing its posterior aspect), often tethering and obstructing the ureters ± IVC. May cause an inflammatory AAA.
5. Retractile mesenteritis—infiltrative fibrous mesenteric mass encasing ± narrowing mesenteric vessels ± SBO ± chylous ascites (due to lymphatic obstruction).
6. Prostatitis—diffuse prostatic enlargement.

Head and neck

1. Sclerosing sialadenitis—uni- or bilateral swelling and fibrosis of submandibular, parotid and/or sublingual glands, often with lacrimal gland involvement.
2. Orbital pseudotumour—most commonly involves the lacrimal glands (± salivary glands) but can manifest in any compartment of the orbit.
3. Riedel thyroiditis—focal or diffuse fibrous infiltration of the thyroid and surrounding tissues. Hypoechoic on US, hypovascular on CT. The rare fibrosing subtype of Hashimoto's thyroiditis is also a manifestation of IgG4-related disease, but does not extend beyond the thyroid.
4. Hypophysitis—enlargement and enhancement of pituitary ± stalk.
5. Hypertrophic pachymeningitis—dural thickening and enhancement.
6. Sinusitis—diffuse mucosal thickening or destructive mass.

Other sites

1. Lymphadenopathy—e.g. abdominal, thoracic, cervical, axillary. Common but nonspecific, usually <2 cm in size.
2. Lungs—may manifest as inflammatory pseudotumours, GGO, bronchiectasis or thickening of interlobular septa, bronchovascular bundles or pleura.
3. IgG4-related inflammatory pseudotumours can occur in virtually any organ, e.g. liver, breasts, scrotum.

Further reading

Martinez-de-Alegria, A., Baleato-González, S., García-Figueiras, R., et al., 2015. IgG4-related disease from head to toe. Radiographics 35 (7), 2007–2025.

Thompson, A., Whyte, A., 2018. Imaging of IgG4-related disease of the head and neck. Clin. Radiol. 73 (1), 106–120.

Toyoda, K., Oba, H., Kutomi, K., et al., 2012. MR imaging of IgG4-related disease in the head and neck and brain. AJNR Am. J. Neuroradiol. 33 (11), 2136–2139.

INFLAMMATORY BOWEL DISEASE

Chronic autoimmune inflammatory disorders of the GI tract, most common in young adults. Two main types: Crohn's disease and ulcerative colitis (UC). Extraintestinal manifestations are common.

Crohn's disease

Can involve the entire GI tract (small bowel > colon > stomach > oesophagus), including the mouth and pharynx.

Small bowel

1. Terminal ileum is the commonest site. Asymmetrical wall thickening and skip lesions are characteristic. The disease predominates on the mesenteric border, which can create a 'pseudosacculated' appearance.
2. Aphthoid ulcers—the earliest sign in the TI and colon, best seen on barium follow-through. May be invisible on CT/MRI. Progress to linear fissure ulcers, producing a 'cobblestone' pattern.
3. Blunting, thickening or distortion of valvulae conniventes—earliest sign in jejunal involvement.
4. Transmural inflammation leads to adjacent inflammatory masses, abscess formation, sinuses and fistulae.
5. Fat wrapping around diseased loops—almost pathognomonic for Crohn's.
6. Strictures—short or long, single or multiple. Subacute > acute obstruction.
7. MRI signs of active disease include mural thickening, T2 hyperintensity, early enhancement (especially if trilayered), reduced peristalsis and restricted diffusion.

Colon

1. Similar appearance to small bowel disease—asymmetrical wall thickening and skip lesions, aphthoid ulcers, deeper fissures, strictures, fistulae, abscesses.
2. Inflammatory pseudopolyps—more common in UC.
3. The ileocaecal valve may be thickened, narrowed and ulcerated.
4. Perianal disease—complex fistulae and abscesses. Perianal disease may predominate.

Complications

1. Fistulae—e.g. enterocutaneous, enterocolic, enteroenteric, enterourinary.
2. Perforation—usually localized and results in abscess formation.
3. Toxic megacolon—more common in UC.
4. Carcinoma—colon (less common than in UC) and small bowel (300× increased incidence).
5. Lymphoma.

Ulcerative colitis

Usually limited to the colon.

1. Acute colitis—typically starts in the rectum and extends proximally in a contiguous circumferential fashion. Mucosal oedema causes 'thumbprinting' on AXR. On CT, the wall is thickened and oedematous with mucosal hyperenhancement. Inflammation is limited to the mucosa and submucosa (cf. transmural inflammation in Crohn's). The rectum may appear spared if steroid enemas have been used.
2. Toxic megacolon—severe acute colitis with dilatation >6 cm. High morbidity.
3. Backwash ileitis—pancolonic inflammation can spread into the terminal ileum.
4. Chronic colitis—submucosal fat deposition can be seen on CT, especially in the rectum ± mesorectal fatty proliferation. 'Lead pipe' colon in severe cases due to blunting of haustral folds and luminal narrowing. Benign strictures can occur.
5. Polyps—benign inflammatory pseudopolyps (acute phase), benign worm-like filiform polyps (chronic phase) and premalignant adenomatous polyps.
6. Colon cancer—risk increases with duration and extent of disease; requires endoscopic surveillance. Tumours may be multiple and/or infiltrative (mimicking benign strictures).

Extraintestinal manifestations of IBD

* = more common in Crohn's. † = more common in UC.

1. Clinical—erythema nodosum, pyoderma gangrenosum, oral aphthous ulcers*, episcleritis, scleritis, anterior uveitis, conjunctivitis.
2. Musculoskeletal:
   (a) Inflammatory spondyloarthropathy—mimics ankylosing spondylitis. Activity is independent of bowel disease and may precede it.
   (b) Peripheral oligoarthropathy*—involves <5 joints (most commonly knees), usually asymmetrical, nonerosive and self-limiting. Activity parallels bowel disease.
   (c) Peripheral polyarthropathy*—involves ≥5 joints (most commonly MCPJs), usually symmetrical and persistent ± erosions. Activity is independent of bowel disease.
   (d) Dactylitis—similar to psoriatic arthropathy.
   (e) Osteoporosis.
   (f) Osteonecrosis—due to steroid therapy.
   (g) Hypertrophic osteoarthropathy.
   (h) Osteomyelitis*—due to fistulating Crohn's, e.g. involving sacrum or ilium.

3. Hepatobiliary—steatosis, gallstones, primary sclerosing cholangitis†, autoimmune hepatitis†, pancreatitis*, aseptic abscesses* (in liver and/or spleen).
4. Urinary tract calculi*—oxalate or uric acid types.
5. Bronchiectasis† ± tracheobronchial wall thickening†.
6. Thrombosis—DVT, PE, portal vein thrombosis, Budd-Chiari syndrome.
7. Moyamoya syndrome.

Further reading

Kohli, M.D., Maglinte, D.D., 2009. CT enteroclysis in small bowel Crohn's disease. Eur. J. Radiol. 69 (3), 398–403.

Olpin, J.D., Sjoberg, B.P., Stilwill, S.E., et al., 2017. Beyond the bowel: extraintestinal manifestations of inflammatory bowel disease. Radiographics 37 (4), 1135–1160.

Tolan, D.J., Greenhalgh, R., Zealley, I.A., et al., 2009. MR enterographic manifestations of small bowel Crohn disease. Radiographics 30 (2), 367–384.

JUVENILE IDIOPATHIC ARTHRITIS

A heterogeneous group of conditions which begin in childhood (age <16 years) and involve persistent inflammation of ≥1 joint for ≥6 weeks.

Oligoarticular or monoarticular onset (45%)

1. Most commonly presents at 1–5 years.
2. ≤4 joints involved at onset—knees, ankles and hips, most commonly.

Polyarticular onset (23%)

1. Usually rheumatoid factor negative. F>M; onset >11 years.
2. Arthritis predominates with a similar distribution to the systemic onset, but also including the small joints of the fingers and toes. The cervical spine is involved frequently and early.
3. Prolonged disease leads to growth retardation and abnormal epiphyseal development.

Systemic onset (Still's disease)

1. Most common at 1–5 years. M=F.
2. Severe extraarticular clinical manifestations—pyrexia, rash, adenopathy and hepatosplenomegaly.
3. Joint involvement is late—polyarthritis especially affecting the knees, wrists, carpals, ankles and tarsals.

Other types

1. Psoriatic arthritis—M>F.
2. Enthesitis-related arthritis—HLA B27 positive; affects lumbar spine, SIJs and distal > proximal appendicular joints. >8 years; M>F.

Radiological changes

1. Joint effusion and periarticular soft-tissue swelling—early findings.
2. Osteopenia—juxtaarticular, diffuse or band-like in the metaphyses, the latter especially in the distal femur, proximal and distal tibia and distal radius.
3. Periostitis—common. Mainly periarticular in the phalanges, metacarpals and metatarsals, but when diaphyseal will eventually result in enlarged rectangular tubular bones.
4. Growth disturbances—epiphyseal overgrowth; premature fusion of growth plates; short broad phalanges, metacarpals and metatarsals; hypoplasia of the TMJ; leg length discrepancy.
5. Subluxation and dislocation—common in the wrist and hip (± protrusio acetabuli). Atlantoaxial subluxation is most frequent in seropositive juvenile-onset rheumatoid arthritis.
6. Bony erosions—late manifestation; mainly knees, hands and feet.
7. Joint-space narrowing—late finding; due to cartilage loss.
8. Bony ankylosis—late finding; especially carpus, tarsus and cervical spine.
9. Epiphyseal compression fractures.
10. Lymphoedema.

Further reading

Johnson, K., 2006. Imaging of juvenile idiopathic arthritis. Pediatr. Radiol. 36, 743–758.

Restrepo, R., Lee, E.Y., 2012. Epidemiology, pathogenesis, and imaging of arthritis in children. Orthop. Clin. North Am. 43 (2), 213–225.

KLIPPEL-TRÉNAUNAY SYNDROME

A syndrome characterized by the following features, typically affecting one lower limb:

1. Cutaneous capillary malformations (port wine stain).
2. Congenital varicose veins or venous malformations—look for phleboliths on plain film. NB: if AVMs are also present, this is termed Parkes-Weber syndrome.
3. Localized gigantism—hypertrophy of soft tissues ± bone, due to local hyperaemia from the multiple vascular malformations.

Vascular malformations can also involve:

1. GI tract—especially rectosigmoid. Causes GI bleeding.
2. GU tract—especially bladder (often accompanied by pelvic and genital involvement). Causes macroscopic haematuria.
3. Cavernous haemangiomas may be seen in solid abdominal viscera (e.g. spleen) or in the retroperitoneum or mediastinum.
4. Facial involvement is associated with intracranial vascular malformations, e.g. leptomeningeal and choroid plexus angiomatosis ± cerebral atrophy and calcification similar to

Sturge-Weber syndrome. Macrocephaly and hemimegalencephaly may also be seen.

5. Lungs—pulmonary vein varicosities, recurrent PE ± pulmonary hypertension.

Other associations and complications include:

1. Legs—venous eczema, cellulitis, thrombophlebitis, DVT.
2. Kasabach-Merritt syndrome—consumptive coagulopathy, due to trapping of platelets within the vascular malformations.
3. High-output heart failure—in Parkes-Weber syndrome, if large AVMs are present.
4. Bone anomalies—hip dislocation and scoliosis (due to leg length discrepancy), poly/oligo/syndactyly.

Further reading

Cha, S.H., Romeo, M.A., Neutze, J.A., 2005. Visceral manifestations of Klippel-Trénaunay syndrome. Radiographics 25 (6), 1694–1697.

Elsayes, K.M., Menias, C.O., Dillman, J.R., et al., 2008. Vascular malformation and haemangiomatosis syndromes: spectrum of imaging manifestations. AJR Am. J. Roentgenol. 190 (5), 1291–1299.

Sharma, D., Lamba, S., Pandita, A., Shastri, S., 2015. Klippel-Trénaunay syndrome—a very rare and interesting syndrome. Clin. Med. Insights Circ. Respir. Pulm. Med. 9, 1–4.

Williams, D.W., 3rd, Elster, A.D., 1992. Cranial CT and MR in the Klippel-Trenaunay-Weber syndrome. AJNR Am. J. Neuroradiol. 13, 291–294.

LANGERHANS CELL HISTIOCYTOSIS (LCH)

A disease characterized by clonal proliferation of Langerhans cells, usually seen in children. Variable presentation, from benign single-system disease to life-threatening multisystem disease. NB: the terms 'Hand–Schüller–Christian disease' and 'Letterer–Siwe disease' have been abandoned. LCH is now categorized based on disease extent.

Unifocal unisystem disease (70% of cases)

Typically a single lytic bone lesion (also known as eosinophilic granuloma), though can involve a few bones. Peak age 5–15 years, most common in the flat bones (skull > pelvis > ribs > mandible > scapula and clavicle), femur, humerus and spine. Can appear aggressive (early) or nonaggressive (late) on plain film. In the skull, lesions are usually well-defined with a 'bevelled' edge. In the spine, often presents as vertebra plana with intact discs. In the mandible, there is loss of the lamina dura ('floating teeth'). On MRI, lesions usually show avid enhancement. Excellent prognosis, often self-limiting; biopsy may induce healing. NB: isolated unisystem involvement of the pituitary, skin or lymph nodes can rarely occur.

Multifocal unisystem disease (20% of cases)

Multiple bone lesions with features as above. Peak age 1–5 years; intermediate prognosis, has a chronic course. May rarely also involve the pituitary gland (causing diabetes insipidus) and skin.

Multisystem disease (10% of cases)

Peak age <2 years. Poor prognosis, fulminant course. Disseminated involvement of various sites categorized as:

1. High-risk—bone marrow, spleen, liver. Hepatic and splenic involvement can manifest as diffuse organomegaly or multifocal lesions ± sclerosing cholangitis. Poorest prognosis.
2. CNS-risk—skull base, orbit, brain, meninges, choroid plexus. In the brain, the cerebellum (especially dentate nuclei) and basal ganglia are the commonest sites of involvement. Associated with irreversible neurodegeneration which may be debilitating.
3. Low-risk—bones, skin, lymph nodes, thymus, lungs, pituitary, GI tract.

Pulmonary LCH (adults)

Isolated lung disease strongly related to smoking, peaking at 20–40 years of age. Multiple lung nodules and irregular cysts with an upper-midzone predominance ± pneumothorax ± reticulation ± GGO ± hilar adenopathy. Often resolves spontaneously after smoking cessation.

Further reading

Haupt, R., Minkov, M., Astigarraga, I., et al., 2013. Langerhans cell histiocytosis (LCH): guidelines for diagnosis, clinical work-up, and treatment for patients till the age of 18 years. Pediatr. Blood Cancer 60 (2), 175–184.

Zaveri, J., La, Q., Yarmish, G., Neuman, J., 2014. More than just Langerhans cell histiocytosis: a radiologic review of histiocytic disorders. Radiographics 34 (7), 2008–2024.

LI-FRAUMENI SYNDROME

Hereditary (AD) cancer syndrome. ~50% develop malignancy by age 30 years, including:

1. Sarcomas—rhabdomyosarcoma, osteosarcoma.
2. Early breast cancer.
3. CNS—gliomas, choroid plexus carcinoma, medulloblastoma (and other PNETs).
4. Adrenocortical carcinoma—if this occurs in childhood, it is highly suggestive of the syndrome.
5. Leukaemia.
6. Melanoma.
7. Increased risk of radiation-induced cancers.

Further reading

Monsalve, J., Kapur, J., Malkin, D., Babyn, P.S., 2011. Imaging of cancer predisposition syndromes in children. Radiographics 31 (1), 263–280.

Shinagare, A.B., Giardino, A.A., Jagannathan, J.P., et al., 2011. Hereditary cancer syndromes: a radiologist's perspective. AJR Am. J. Roentgenol. 197 (6), W1001–W1007.

LOEYS-DIETZ SYNDROME

Hereditary (AD) connective tissue disorder with multisystem manifestations and Marfanoid features. Classical triad of:

1. Arterial tortuosity and aneurysms—nearly all patients have an aortic root aneurysm. Most patients will also have aneurysms elsewhere, e.g. rest of aorta, main pulmonary artery and/or coronary, subclavian, carotid, vertebral, intracranial, mesenteric, splenic, iliac and popliteal arteries (these are rare in Marfan). Dissection and rupture are common. Marked tortuosity is characteristic, especially of neck arteries.
2. Bifid uvula or cleft palate.
3. Hypertelorism.

NB: severity of craniofacial features correlates with severity of vascular abnormalities. Other features include:

1. Cardiovascular—ASD, PDA, bicuspid aortic valve, mitral valve prolapse.
2. Craniofacial—craniosynostosis, Chiari I malformation, hydrocephalus, blue sclerae, malar hypoplasia.
3. Musculoskeletal—joint laxity, arachnodactyly, camptodactyly, club foot, pectus deformity.
4. Spine—dural ectasia, scoliosis, cervical instability.

Further reading

Johnson, P.T., Chen, J.K., Loeys, B.L., et al., 2007. Loeys-Dietz syndrome: MDCT angiography findings. AJR Am. J. Roentgenol. 189, W29–W35.

Loughborough, W.W., Minhas, K.S., Rodrigues, J.C.L., et al., 2018. Cardiovascular manifestations and complications of Loeys-Dietz syndrome: CT and MR imaging findings. Radiographics 38 (1), 275–286.

LYMPHANGIOLEIOMYOMATOSIS

Multisystem disorder caused by abnormal smooth muscle proliferation in lymphatics and small airways. Often thought to be a 'forme fruste' of tuberous sclerosis. Almost exclusively seen in premenopausal women. Manifestations include:

1. Lungs—numerous uniformly distributed thin-walled cysts of varying size ± smooth interlobular septal thickening ± pneumothorax ± chylous pleural or pericardial effusion ± areas of pulmonary haemorrhage.

2. Renal AMLs—common. Hepatic or splenic AMLs may also rarely be seen.
3. Lymphatics—dilated thoracic duct, lymphadenopathy, lymphangioleiomyomas (benign cystic masses in mediastinum, retroperitoneum or mesentery—may change in size throughout the day).
4. Chylous ascites—due to rupture of lymphangioleiomyoma.
5. Uterine leiomyomas or AMLs.

Further reading

Abbott, G.F., Rosado-de-Christenson, M.L., Frazier, A.A., et al., 2005. From the archives of the AFIP: lymphangioleiomyomatosis: radiologic-pathologic correlation. Radiographics 25 (3), 803–828.

Avila, N.A., Dwyer, A.J., Moss, J., 2011. Imaging features of lymphangioleiomyomatosis: diagnostic pitfalls. AJR Am. J. Roentgenol. 196, 982–986.

LYMPHOMA

Most commonly involves lymph nodes and spleen, but can involve any site or system. In general it tends to be a soft tumour, encasing vessels and other structures without causing significant obstruction. Typically hypoechoic on US (may appear almost cystic) and of homogeneous soft-tissue attenuation on CT with mild uniform enhancement. Restricted diffusion is typical on MRI due to its high cellularity. PET-CT is superior to CT for staging and treatment response assessment. Low-grade lymphomas (especially follicular lymphoma) can be very indolent, remaining stable for years, and are often not treated if asymptomatic ('watch and wait'); these typically manifest as group(s) of discrete enlarged lymph nodes (>10 mm). Higher grade lymphomas usually manifest as confluent nodal masses ± splenomegaly ± extranodal disease; isolated (primary) involvement of extranodal sites can occur but is less common. Very high-grade cases may show central necrosis and progress rapidly over days to weeks. Calcification is typically not seen unless posttreatment. Classified as:

1. Hodgkin lymphoma—peaks in young adults with a 2nd peak >55 years; usually limited to lymph nodes (most commonly in the neck and mediastinum), though lung involvement can occur. Mediastinal adenopathy tends to be bilateral and asymmetrical.
2. Non-Hodgkin lymphoma (NHL)—wide variety of subtypes, manifestations and patient demographics. Follicular lymphomas are typically indolent, whereas diffuse large B-cell lymphomas are aggressive. Burkitt's lymphoma typically occurs in children or HIV patients, and is highly aggressive. Posttransplant

lymphoproliferative disorder (PTLD) can involve the transplant itself or occur at distant sites.

The spectrum of extranodal disease is described as follows.

Lungs

1. Hodgkin > NHL; usually in the presence of nodal disease. Isolated (primary) lung disease is usually MALT-type NHL.
2. Most frequently one or more large irregular masses (± cavitation) or areas of consolidation (± air bronchograms). Less commonly can manifest as an endobronchial mass (± collapse) or disseminated miliary nodules.
3. Lymphatic obstruction can cause interstitial oedema or lymphangitis carcinomatosa.
4. Pleural and pericardial effusions ± thickening may occur.

Solid abdominal viscera

1. In general, involvement may be diffuse (organomegaly without discrete lesions) or may manifest as single or multiple mass lesions or nodules. Lesions are typically hypovascular relative to the background organ enhancement.
2. Spleen—not considered as an extranodal site. Isolated splenomegaly may be seen with mantle cell lymphoma (aggressive) or marginal zone lymphoma (indolent).
3. Liver—nodules may be disseminated randomly throughout liver or may have a periportal distribution. Biliary dilatation is typically absent.
4. Pancreas—rare; diffuse involvement may mimic pancreatitis (enlargement, peripancreatic fat infiltration, reduced enhancement). Focal involvement may mimic adenocarcinoma but duct dilatation, gland atrophy and vascular occlusion are rare with lymphoma.
5. Renal—rare; most frequent pattern is multiple bilateral 1–3 cm masses. A single renal or perinephric mass may also occur. Diffuse involvement results in enlargement ± areas of reduced enhancement. PTLD may predominantly involve the renal sinus (without causing hydronephrosis).
6. Adrenals—may be unilateral or bilateral. Primary involvement (rare) is typically bilateral, often with adrenal insufficiency.
7. Testes—commonest testicular malignancy in men >60 years. Often multifocal and bilateral.
8. Ovaries—especially in Burkitt's lymphoma. Homogeneous solid masses, often bilateral.
9. Uterus/cervix—diffuse enlargement, usually sparing the endometrium.

Gastrointestinal tract

1. In general, tends to cause a long segment of concentric wall thickening without obstruction, often with a degree of aneurysmal dilatation. The thickening is homogeneous and hypovascular, with loss of normal bowel wall stratification. Local mesenteric adenopathy is usually present.
2. Less common manifestations include single or multiple masses or polyps ± intussusception (if in bowel) ± ulceration or cavitation.
3. Stomach > small bowel > colon > oesophagus. Usually NHL, secondary > primary. Gastric lymphomas are associated with *H. pylori* and are mainly of the MALT type. Coeliac disease is associated with small bowel T cell lymphoma.
4. Associated peritoneal disease can also occur, manifesting as diffuse peritoneal thickening and ascites.

Head and neck

1. Lymph node involvement is most common. Beware of intraparotid nodes mimicking a primary parotid lesion.
2. Commonly involves Waldeyer's ring (lingual, palatine and adenoid tonsils).
3. Sinonasal involvement can be destructive and mimic other processes.
4. Salivary and lacrimal glands—especially in Sjögren's syndrome (MALT lymphoma).
5. Lymphoma is the commonest malignancy in the orbit and has a variety of patterns (see Section 12.30).
6. Thyroid—especially in chronic Hashimoto's thyroiditis (MALT lymphoma). Rapidly enlarging goitre. May be diffuse or a focal hypoechoic mass.

CNS

1. In immunocompetent patients, primary CNS disease usually manifests as a homogeneously enhancing mass or masses, most common in the periventricular region. May cross the corpus callosum or show subependymal extension. The mass is classically hyperattenuating on unenhanced CT due to its cellularity.
2. In immunocompromised patients, primary CNS disease usually manifests as single or multiple ring-enhancing lesions.
3. Can rarely involve the pituitary stalk.
4. If secondary to systemic disease, usually manifests as leptomeningeal or dural involvement.

Bones

1. Most commonly involves axial and/or proximal appendicular skeleton.

2. May be lytic, sclerotic or mixed. The degree of bone destruction is usually less than with other malignant bone lesions. An associated soft-tissue mass is typical and often large—the mass appears to 'walk through' the bone without causing much destruction.

Other rare sites

1. Heart, gallbladder, bladder, prostate, vagina, subcutaneous tissues—nonspecific homogeneous infiltrative mass.
2. Muscle—usually an infiltrative diffusely enhancing mass oriented along muscle fibres, often involving multiple compartments. Usually involves the trunk, thigh or upper limb.
3. Breast—rare; well-defined noncalcified mass on mammography. Also note the rare implant-associated anaplastic large cell lymphoma—consider in any patient with an enlarging intracapsular periimplant effusion occurring >1 year after implantation.

Further reading

Frampas, E., 2013. Lymphomas: basic points that radiologists should know. Diagn. Interv. Imaging 94 (2), 131–144.

Thomas, A.G., Vaidhyanath, R., Kirke, R., Rajesh, A., 2011. Extranodal lymphoma from head to toe: part 1, the head and spine. AJR Am. J. Roentgenol. 197 (2), 350–356.

Thomas, A.G., Vaidhyanath, R., Kirke, R., Rajesh, A., 2011. Extranodal lymphoma from head to toe: part 2, the trunk and extremities. AJR Am. J. Roentgenol. 197 (2), 357–364.

MALARIA

Parasitic infection caused by *Plasmodium* species, transmitted by mosquitos. Parasites invade RBCs, which become sequestered in the microvasculature of the spleen ± brain.

1. Splenomegaly ± infarcts ± abscesses ± splenic rupture. In chronic cases, a perisplenic rim of fibrosis may be seen.
2. Hepatomegaly ± periportal and gallbladder wall oedema ± ascites may also be seen.
3. Cerebral malaria—high mortality. Imaging findings include multifocal small infarcts, microhaemorrhages, nonspecific T2 hyperintensities and diffuse cerebral oedema in severe cases.
4. Lungs—interstitial or alveolar oedema.

Further reading

Kim, E.M., Cho, H.J., Cho, C.R., et al., 2010. Abdominal computed tomography findings of malaria infection with *Plasmodium vivax*. Am. J. Trop. Med. Hyg. 83 (6), 1202–1205.

Potchen, M.J., Kampondeni, S.D., Seydel, K.B., et al., 2012. Acute brain MRI findings in 120 Malawian children with cerebral malaria: new insights into an ancient disease. AJNR Am. J. Neuroradiol. 33 (9), 1740–1746.

MARFAN SYNDROME

A connective tissue disorder transmitted as an AD trait, but with variable expression. 25% spontaneous mutations. Multisystem features due to defective fibrillin, a component of microfibrils which is found in mesenchymal tissues.

Skeletal system

1. Tall stature—upper/lower segment <0.86; or arm span/height ratio >1.05.
2. Arachnodactyly—metacarpal index 8.4–10.4.
3. Joint hypermobility—subluxation and dislocation.
4. Spine—scoliosis (>20 degrees), dural ectasia, vertebral scalloping, atlantoaxial subluxation.
5. Chest—pectus carinatum or excavatum.
6. Pelvis—acetabular protrusio, SUFE.
7. Knees—patella alta.
8. Feet—pes planus.
9. High-arched palate with crowding of teeth.
10. Abnormal facies—dolichocephaly, malar hypoplasia, enophthalmos, retrognathism.
11. Perilunate, hip and sternoclavicular joint dislocations.
12. Rib notching.

Ocular system

1. Ectopia lentis—usually upwards.

Cardiovascular system

1. Ascending aortic dilatation ± aortic regurgitation.
2. Descending thoracic or abdominal aortic dilatation ± dissection.
3. Pulmonary artery dilatation.
4. Mitral valve prolapse and calcification of mitral annulus.

Lungs

1. Pulmonary emphysema and bullae.
2. Spontaneous pneumothorax.

Further reading

Ha, H.I., Seo, J.B., Lee, S.H., et al., 2007. Imaging of Marfan syndrome: multisystemic manifestations. Radiographics 27, 989–1004.

MASTOCYTOSIS

Rare myeloproliferative disorder of mast cells. The cutaneous form usually presents in childhood with a skin rash (urticaria pigmentosa); the less common systemic form usually presents in adulthood and can involve multiple systems (± skin):

1. Bones—commonest site; involved in most patients. Typically causes diffuse heterogeneous sclerosis or osteopenia of the axial and proximal appendicular skeleton, though focal sclerotic or lytic lesions may also occur.
2. Hepatosplenomegaly—due to diffuse mast cell infiltration. Focal lesions (mastocytomas) may be seen. The bile ducts may also be infiltrated, causing irregular strictures. Portal hypertension (ascites and varices) and Budd-Chiari syndrome may also occur.
3. Lymphadenopathy—mesenteric, periportal, retroperitoneal, mediastinal.
4. GI tract—peptic ulcers, diffuse small bowel thickening ± mesenteric and omental stranding.
5. Other rare sites—e.g. ovary (complex mass), lungs (nodules, cysts or diffuse 'crazy paving').

Further reading

Avila, N.A., Ling, A., Worobec, A.S., et al., 1997. Systemic mastocytosis: CT and US features of abdominal manifestations. Radiology 202 (2), 367–372.

Fritz, J., Fishman, E.K., Carrino, J.A., Horger, M.S., 2012. Advanced imaging of skeletal manifestations of systemic mastocytosis. Skeletal Radiol. 41, 887–897.

MICROSCOPIC POLYANGIITIS

Multisystem small vessel vasculitis presenting clinically with constitutional symptoms and skin rash (usually purpura). Manifestations include:

1. Kidneys—rapidly progressive glomerulonephritis occurs in nearly all patients. The kidneys may be enlarged and hyperechoic on US.
2. Lungs—diffuse pulmonary haemorrhage is typical. Chronic recurrent haemorrhage can result in fibrosis.
3. Neurologic—mononeuritis multiplex is common. CNS involvement is less common, manifesting as cerebral infarction, haemorrhage or hypertrophic pachymeningitis.
4. GI tract—low-grade GI bleeding or, rarely, bowel ischaemia can occur.
5. Other rare features—pancreatic necrosis, adrenal haemorrhage.

Further reading

Chung, S.A., Seo, P., 2010. Microscopic polyangiitis. Rheum. Dis. Clin. North Am. 36 (3), 545–558.

MUCOPOLYSACCHARIDOSES

Group of hereditary lysosomal storage disorders presenting in childhood, caused by specific enzyme deficiencies resulting in the accumulation of mucopolysaccharides. Many different types (see table following); nearly all show AR inheritance except Hunter syndrome (X-linked). All are characterized by the following features which vary in severity depending on the type (NB: there is also considerable variation within each type—the table is only a guide):

1. Dysostosis multiplex—constellation of abnormally formed bones (see Section 14.7).
2. Neurological—multifocal or diffuse white matter lesions, dilated perivascular spaces, cerebral atrophy and communicating hydrocephalus.
3. Spinal cord compression—due to atlantoaxial instability.
4. Abdominal—hepatosplenomegaly, hernias.
5. Eyes—optic canal narrowing (resulting in fluid accumulation within the optic nerve sheath and optic nerve atrophy), corneal clouding, glaucoma.
6. ENT—recurrent rhinitis and otitis media, obstructive sleep apnoea (due to macroglossia, tonsillar hypertrophy and TMJ dysfunction).
7. Respiratory—tracheomalacia and restrictive lung function, resulting in recurrent pneumonia.
8. Cardiac—valve dysplasia and insufficiency, cardiomyopathy.

Type	Lifespan	DM	AAI	ND	Other features
IH (Hurler)	<10 years	+++	+++	+++	All of the above. Most severe form
IHS (Hurler-Scheie)	20–40 years	++	++	+	Intermediate form
IS (Scheie)	Normal	+	+	–	Mildest form of type I
II (Hunter)	Variable	++	++	++	Variable features and severity
III (Sanfilippo)	10–40 years	–	–	+++	ND predominates
IV (Morquio)	20–40 years	+++	+++	–	DM predominates. Joint laxity
VI (Maroteaux-Lamy)	10–30 years	++	+++	–	DM predominates. Heart disease
VII (Sly)	Variable	++	++	++	Variable features and severity
IX (Natowicz)	Normal	–	–	–	Synovitis, periarticular masses

DM = dysostosis multiplex; AAI = atlantoaxial instability; ND = neurodegeneration

Further reading

Palmucci, S., Attinà, G., Lanza, M.L., et al., 2013. Imaging findings of mucopolysaccharidoses: a pictorial review. Insights Imaging 4 (4), 443–459.

Rasalkar, D.D., Chu, W.C., Hui, J., et al., 2011. Pictorial review of mucopolysaccharidosis with emphasis on MRI features of brain and spine. Br. J. Radiol. 84 (1001), 469–477.

Reichert, R., Campos, L.G., Vairo, F., et al., 2016. Neuroimaging findings in patients with mucopolysaccharidosis: what you really need to know. Radiographics 36 (5), 1448–1462.

MULTIPLE ENDOCRINE NEOPLASIA SYNDROMES

A group of AD syndromes, each featuring a collection of endocrine tumours.

MEN 1 (Wermer syndrome)

1. Parathyroid adenomas (95%)—usually multiple or diffuse hyperplasia, causing hyperparathyroidism.
2. Pancreatic NET (40%–80%)—especially gastrinomas (may also arise from duodenum) and nonfunctioning NETs, usually multiple; see Section 8.34. Malignant NETs are a major cause of mortality.
3. Pituitary adenoma (30%)—usually functioning (60% are prolactinoma) and locally aggressive.
4. Facial angiofibromas (85%) and collagenomas (70%)—often multiple.
5. Adrenal cortical tumours (40%)—usually adenomas or hyperplasia.
6. Lipomas (10%–30%)—subcutaneous and visceral.
7. Thyroid adenomas (5%–30%).
8. Meningiomas (8%).
9. Foregut carcinoid tumours (2%–5%)—thymus, bronchus, stomach and duodenum.
10. Other rare associations—phaeochromocytoma (1%), visceral leiomyomas, ependymoma, breast cancer, testicular cancer.

MEN 2A (Sipple syndrome)

1. Medullary thyroid carcinoma (>99%)—often aggressive and multifocal. Occurs in adolescents or young adults.
2. Phaeochromocytoma (50%)—bilateral in 50%.
3. Parathyroid hyperplasia (20%–30%).
4. Other associations—Hirschsprung's disease, cutaneous lichen amyloidosis.

MEN 2B (also known as MEN 3)

1. Medullary thyroid carcinoma (>99%)—aggressive and multifocal. Occurs in young children.
2. Marfanoid appearance (>99%).
3. Mucosal neuromas (>99%)—on the lips, tongue, conjunctiva, nose and larynx.
4. Phaeochromocytoma (50%).
5. Intestinal ganglioneuromatosis (40%)—resulting in megacolon.

MEN 4

1. Parathyroid adenoma—hyperparathyroidism in 80%.
2. Pituitary adenoma (37%)—less aggressive than in MEN 1.
3. Neuroendocrine tumours—of lung, GI tract and pancreas.
4. Other rare tumours—adrenal, thyroid.

Further reading

Scarsbrook, A.F., Thakker, R.V., Wass, J.A., et al., 2006. Multiple endocrine neoplasia: spectrum of radiologic appearances and discussion of a multitechnique imaging approach. Radiographics 26, 433–451.

MULTIPLE MYELOMA/PLASMACYTOMA

Plasma cell neoplasms of bone are either solitary (plasmacytoma; 3% of all plasma cell tumours) or multiple/diffuse (94% of all plasma cell tumours). 3% of all plasma cell tumours are solely extraosseous. Plasma cell disorders nearly always occur in patients >40 years, and may be associated with amyloidosis. Staging includes skeletal survey (best for appendicular skeleton) and whole-body MRI ± PET-CT (best for axial skeleton and extraosseous disease).

Plasmacytoma

1. A solitary, well-defined, grossly expansile lytic bone lesion arising most commonly in the spine, pelvis or ribs, ± soft-tissue extension or pathological fracture. Homogeneous mild-moderate enhancement. Low T1 and high T2 fatsat signal + restricted diffusion.
2. May rarely be extramedullary—most common in the upper aerodigestive tract (paranasal sinuses, pharynx, trachea) and GI tract, but can occur anywhere. Manifests as a nonspecific soft-tissue mass.
3. Normal background bone marrow on imaging and biopsy.
4. No paraproteinaemia, anaemia, hypercalcaemia or renal failure.

Monoclonal gammopathy of undetermined significance (MGUS)

1. Serum paraproteinaemia with mild diffuse plasma cell infiltration of bone marrow on biopsy (<10% plasma cells). Commonest plasma cell disorder; can progress to multiple myeloma.
2. No anaemia, hypercalcaemia, renal failure, bone pain or other symptoms.
3. No lytic bone lesions. Normal marrow signal on MRI. Osteoporosis ± vertebral compression fractures may be seen.

Smouldering myeloma

1. Serum paraproteinaemia with diffuse plasma cell infiltration of bone marrow on biopsy (10%–60% plasma cells). Intermediate stage between MGUS and multiple myeloma.
2. No anaemia, hypercalcaemia, renal failure, bone pain or other symptoms.
3. No lytic bone lesions. On MRI, the marrow may be normal or may show diffuse signal change (reduced T1 and increased T2 fatsat signal, restricted diffusion, ± early wash-in and wash-out on dynamic postcontrast sequences) without discrete focal lesions. The signal changes can mimic red marrow, but red marrow is rare in those >40 years.

Multiple myeloma

Commonest primary bone malignancy. Serum paraproteinaemia with diffuse plasma cell infiltration of bone marrow on biopsy; often with anaemia, hypercalcaemia and/or renal failure. Three forms of skeletal involvement:

1. Multiple well-defined lytic lesions disseminated throughout the axial and proximal appendicular skeleton. Usually fairly uniform in size (cf. metastases which are usually of varying size). In the spine, typically involves the vertebral bodies (cf. metastases which have a predilection for the pedicles). In the ribs, tends to be expansile + a soft-tissue component. Pathological fractures are common.
2. Diffuse marrow infiltration—results in diffuse osteopenia on plain film. On MRI, the marrow shows diffuse signal change (similar to smouldering myeloma above) which may be:
   (a) Mild—heterogeneous T1 signal with a 'salt and pepper' appearance.
   (b) Moderate—homogeneous low T1 signal which is still slightly > the discs.
   (c) Severe—homogeneous low T1 signal ≤ the discs.
3. Osteosclerotic myeloma—rare. Multiple sclerotic or mixed lytic/sclerotic bone lesions; lesions may be lytic with a sclerotic rim. Associated with POEMS syndrome:

(a) **P**olyneuropathy—must be present for diagnosis. Bilateral symmetrical motor and sensory neuropathy, starting distally and progressing proximally.
(b) **O**rganomegaly—hepatosplenomegaly, lymphadenopathy (often manifesting as Castleman disease).
(c) **E**ndocrinopathy—may involve pituitary, thyroid, parathyroid, pancreas, adrenals, gonads.
(d) **M**onoclonal gammopathy—must be present for diagnosis. Often manifests as osteosclerotic myeloma.
(e) **S**kin changes—e.g. hyperpigmentation, skin thickening, hypertrichosis.
(f) Other features—fluid overload (oedema, pleural effusions, ascites), papilloedema, raised serum vascular endothelial growth factor (VEGF) levels.

Extraosseous myeloma can involve any part of the body, producing nonspecific soft-tissue masses or diffuse organ infiltration; commonest sites include:

1. Paraskeletal soft tissues.
2. Lymph nodes and spleen.
3. Liver and pancreas.
4. Perinephric fat ± renal involvement.
5. Lungs and pleura.
6. CNS—usually as leptomeningeal disease.

Further reading

Dutoit, J.C., Verstraete, K.L., 2016. MRI in multiple myeloma: a pictorial review of diagnostic and post-treatment findings. Insights Imaging 7 (4), 553–569.

Ferraro, R., Agarwal, A., Martin-Macintosh, E.L., et al., 2015. MR imaging and PET/CT in diagnosis and management of multiple myeloma. Radiographics 35 (2), 438–454.

MURCS ASSOCIATION

Refers to a constellation of congenital findings:

1. **Mü**llerian duct aplasia—absence of uterus, cervix and upper two-thirds of vagina.
2. **R**enal anomalies—e.g. unilateral renal agenesis, hypoplasia, ectopia or horseshoe kidney.
3. **C**ervicothoracic **s**omite dysplasia—i.e. Klippel-Feil syndrome (vertebral fusion ± hemivertebrae ± spina bifida ± omovertebral bone).

NB: if spinal anomalies are absent, consider Mayer-Rokitansky-Küster-Hauser syndrome.

NEUROFIBROMATOSIS

Neurofibromatosis type 1 (NF1)

Commonest phakomatosis; usually presents in childhood. AD inheritance, though 50% are new mutations. Diagnosis requires the presence of ≥2 of the following criteria (the last three can be identified on imaging):

1. First-degree relative with NF1.
2. ≥6 café-au-lait spots >5 mm (prepubertal) or >15 mm (postpubertal).
3. Axillary or inguinal freckles.
4. ≥2 iris hamartomas (Lisch nodules).
5. ≥2 neurofibromas or ≥1 plexiform neurofibroma.
6. Optic pathway glioma—pathognomonic if bilateral.
7. Typical bone lesion, e.g. sphenoid wing dysplasia or tibial pseudarthrosis.

NF1 is a multisystem disorder with numerous manifestations as described below. The presence or absence of these features varies widely between patients.

Neurofibromas

These can occur anywhere, though most arise from superficial nerves in the skin or larger nerves in deeper tissues, e.g. spinal or cranial nerves. On imaging:

1. US—well-defined, hypoechoic, hypovascular on Doppler. An associated peripheral nerve may be seen entering and exiting the lesion, suggesting the diagnosis of a nerve sheath tumour—neurofibromas tend to be fusiform and centrally located, whereas schwannomas tend to be more rounded and eccentric.
2. CT—typically homogeneously hypoattenuating with minimal enhancement. May occasionally mimic cystic lesions. At sites where nerves and lymphatics are adjacent (e.g. neck, axillae, groin, mediastinum, mesentery, retroperitoneum), the low attenuation aids differentiation from lymphadenopathy, which is usually of higher attenuation.
3. MRI—T1 hypointense. T2 hyperintense, often with central hypointensity ('target' sign). Variable enhancement, often central. No restricted diffusion (cf. lymph nodes).

Plexiform neurofibromas are larger, diffusely infiltrating nerves and their branches and adjacent soft-tissue planes, giving a 'bag of worms' appearance. They displace adjacent structures and vessels without invading or occluding them. On MRI, multiple 'target' signs may be seen within. There is a 10% risk of malignant transformation—look for increasing size, internal necrosis or cystic change, peripheral enhancement and perilesional oedema.

Skull

1. Sphenoid wing dysplasia—hypoplastic/absent greater wing ± lesser wing ('bare orbit' sign on plain film) resulting in a posterolateral orbital wall defect ± herniation of middle cranial fossa structures into orbit ± proptosis ± buphthalmos.
2. Enlarged skull base foramina due to bony remodelling by cranial nerve neurofibromas.
3. Enlarged internal auditory meati due to a nerve sheath tumour or dural ectasia.
4. Lucent defects in the calvarium, especially in or near the lambdoid sutures.
5. Macrocephaly.
6. Mandible—may be dysplastic or remodelled by adjacent neurofibromas.

Brain

1. Focal or multifocal T2 hyperintensities without mass effect or enhancement, most often in the white matter, basal ganglia, thalamus, cerebellum (+ peduncles) and brainstem. Present in most children with NF1; usually regress by adulthood.
2. Optic pathway glioma—common; can involve optic nerve and/or optic tract, chiasm or optic radiations. Usually presents in childhood; most children with optic nerve gliomas will have NF1 (pathognomonic if bilateral).
3. Other gliomas—e.g. in brainstem, cerebellum, tectal plate, basal ganglia. These are often pilocytic astrocytomas.
4. Neurofibromas—of the cranial nerves, orbits, head and neck.
5. Hydrocephalus—insidious onset, usually due to aqueduct stenosis caused by gliosis but may be due to a tumour.
6. Arterial abnormalities—ectasia, aneurysm, occlusion, Moyamoya, AV fistula.
7. Arachnoid cyst.

Spine

1. Kyphoscoliosis—typically thoracic. May be isolated (nondystrophic, similar to idiopathic scoliosis) or associated with other spinal abnormalities (dystrophic—these tend to be sharply angulated).
2. Dural ectasia with posterior vertebral body scalloping ± lateral meningocoeles.
3. Absent or hypoplastic pedicles ± spondylolisthesis.
4. Multiple neurofibromas which may have a dumbbell morphology, extending through enlarged intervertebral foramina. Most common in the cervicothoracic region.
5. Paraspinal plexiform neurofibromas.

Thorax

1. Thinned 'ribbon' ribs (due to bone dysplasia) or rib notching ± splaying (due to intercostal neurofibromas).
2. Lung parenchymal disease—upper zone bullae, lower zone fibrosis.
3. Mediastinal mass—neurofibroma, lateral thoracic meningocoele, paraganglioma.

Abdomen

1. Neurofibromas—most commonly involve the lumbosacral plexus ± enlargement of neural foramina. May mimic a psoas collection or mass on CT, though the MRI appearance is usually characteristic. In other locations:
   (a) Paraaortic—can mimic other retroperitoneal masses.
   (b) Mesentery—can mimic low-attenuation adenopathy (e.g. mycobacterial infection, necrotic metastases, Whipple's disease), but neurofibromas typically do not show rim enhancement. May diffusely infiltrate the mesentery.
   (c) Bowel—may manifest as a well-defined exophytic mass (similar to a GIST) or as diffuse mural thickening.
   (d) Liver—most commonly periportal in location.
   (e) Pelvis—often plexiform and very infiltrative, involving bladder and other pelvic organs; may mimic lymphangioma, haemangioma or sarcoma on CT.
2. Neuroendocrine tumours—phaeochromocytoma, paraganglioma.
3. GI tract—periampullary carcinoid, small bowel GIST (may be multiple), small bowel adenocarcinoma, colonic ganglioneuromatosis.
4. Ganglioneuroma—in the paravertebral regions.
5. Rhabdomyosarcoma—in children only, typically involving the GU tract.

Appendicular skeleton and soft tissues

1. Mesodermal dysplasia—abnormal bone formation in the shoulder and pelvic girdles or long bones; manifests as cortical thinning, overtubulation, discrete erosions or lucencies, sclerosis or periostitis. Anterolateral bowing of the tibia is the most common feature, usually evident in the first year and often progressing to fracture and pseudarthrosis. Other long bones (e.g. ulna) may also form a pseudarthrosis.
2. Nonossifying fibromas—often multiple, bilateral and symmetrical.
3. Intraosseous neurofibromas—subperiosteal or cortical lucencies with a smooth expanded outer margin.
4. Soft-tissue neurofibromas—either cutaneous, subcutaneous or intramuscular (usually oriented along muscle fibres).
5. Focal gigantism or limb hemihypertrophy (elephantiasis neuromatosa)—due to the combination of an infiltrative plexiform neurofibroma, soft-tissue hyperaemia and hypertrophy, and

lymphatic insufficiency. The underlying bones may be enlarged, scalloped, deformed or resorbed.

Vascular

1. Stenoses—of the aorta (midaortic syndrome), arch vessels, renal and visceral arteries.
2. Aneurysms—less common than stenoses. Can affect any artery.
3. Pulmonary arterial hypertension.
4. AVMs.

Neurofibromatosis type 2 (NF2)

Less common than NF1; usually presents in young adults. AD inheritance, though 50% are new mutations. Despite the name, NF2 is not usually associated with neurofibromas. Characterized by multiple inherited schwannomas, meningiomas and ependymomas (MISME). Schwannomas most commonly arise from the vestibular nerves but can also arise from other cranial nerves, the spine or other sites. Ependymomas are usually spinal (intramedullary). Meningiomas may be intracranial, spinal or of the optic nerve sheath. The presence of a meningioma in a child should raise the suspicion of NF2. The presence of multiple spinal tumours of different types is also suggestive. Diagnosis requires one of the following criteria to be met:

1. Bilateral vestibular schwannomas.
2. Any two of the following:
   - (a) Unilateral vestibular schwannoma.
   - (b) Any two of: meningioma, nonvestibular schwannoma, glioma (especially ependymoma), neurofibroma or juvenile cataract.
   - (c) First-degree relative with NF2.
3. ≥2 meningiomas + one of the following:
   - (a) Unilateral vestibular schwannoma.
   - (b) Any two of: nonvestibular schwannoma, glioma (especially ependymoma), neurofibroma or juvenile cataract.

Schwannomatosis (NF3)

Rare. Typically presents in adults >30 years (older than NF2). Characterized by multiple nonvestibular schwannomas usually involving the peripheral nerves or spine, though nonvestibular cranial nerves can also be involved.

Further reading

Fortman, B.J., Kuszyk, B.S., Urban, B.A., Fishman, E.K., 2001. Neurofibromatosis type 1: a diagnostic mimicker at CT. Radiographics 21 (3), 601–612.

Levy, A.D., Patel, N., Dow, N., et al., 2005. Abdominal neoplasms in patients with neurofibromatosis type 1: radiologic-pathologic correlation. Radiographics 25 (2), 455–480.

Menor, F., Martí-Bonmatí, L., Mulas, F., et al., 1991. Imaging considerations of central nervous system manifestations in paediatric patients with neurofibromatosis type 1. Pediatr. Radiol. 21, 389–394.
Patel, N.B., Stacy, G.S., 2012. Musculoskeletal manifestations of neurofibromatosis type 1. AJR Am. J. Roentgenol. 199 (1), W99–W106.
Rossi, S.E., Erasmus, J.J., McAdams, H.P., Donnelly, L.F., 1999. Thoracic manifestations of neurofibromatosis-1. AJR Am. J. Roentgenol. 173, 1631–1638.

NIEMANN-PICK DISEASE

A group of hereditary (AR) lysosomal storage diseases predominantly involving the CNS, liver and spleen.

1. Type A—typically presents in infancy with severe hepatosplenomegaly, cerebral atrophy and white matter T2 hyperintensities. Death usually occurs in early childhood.
2. Type B—more indolent course, minimal CNS involvement. Multisystem manifestations:
   (a) Hepatosplenomegaly is nearly always present ± punctate calcifications. Focal splenic lesions may also be seen, typically echogenic on US and hypoattenuating on CT.
   (b) Lungs—interlobular septal thickening ± GGO ± small nodules which may be calcified. Findings usually start at the bases and progress cranially.
   (c) Accelerated atherosclerosis.
   (d) Bones—delayed maturation, osteopenia, diffusely reduced marrow T1 signal on MRI.
   (e) Other rare features—adrenal masses, renal enlargement, lymphadenopathy.
3. Type C—variable age of presentation and prognosis. Progressive CNS involvement, mild hepatosplenomegaly.

Further reading

Simpson, W.L., Jr., Mendelson, D., Wasserstein, M.P., McGovern, M.M., 2010. Imaging manifestations of Niemann-Pick disease type B. AJR Am. J. Roentgenol. 194, W12–W19.

NONACCIDENTAL INJURY (NAI)

Skeletal

1. Fractures—more common in the younger child; >50% of fractures in children <1 year are due to NAI. An implausible explanation for the fracture should raise suspicion. Often multiple, in varying stages of healing. Clues to help dating of fractures:
   (a) Associated soft-tissue swelling—fracture is <14 days old.
   (b) Absent periosteal reaction—fracture is <14 days old.
   (c) Periosteal reaction—develops between 4 and 14 days.

(d) Hard callus bridging the fracture line—usually at ~8 weeks.
(e) Diaphyseal and rib fractures usually heal within 3 months. Metaphyseal fractures heal within 4–6 weeks. Skull fractures fade gradually over several months.
(f) NB: metaphyseal, vertebral and skull fractures do not heal with a periosteal reaction so cannot be reliably dated.

2. Long bone diaphyseal fracture—suspicious in a nonambulatory child. The older the child, the more likely it is accidental.
3. Metaphyseal fractures—almost pathognomonic for NAI after excluding differential diagnoses below. Most common in distal femur, proximal and distal tibia/fibula and proximal humerus. Usually a 'bucket-handle' or 'corner' fracture, but can be transverse through the metaphysis.
4. Rib fractures—5%–27% of all fractures in abused children; most are occult and require a repeat CXR in 2 weeks to look for signs of healing. Specific for NAI (especially if posterior) after excluding differential diagnoses below.
5. Infants and young children—certain fractures have a high specificity for abuse due to their unusual locations, e.g. scapula, sternum, spine and small bones of the hands and feet.
6. Dislocations—rarely encountered in abused children. Malalignment of bones at a joint usually indicates a growth plate injury.
7. Differential diagnosis for NAI: birth trauma (in babies <3 months), major trauma (e.g. RTA), osteogenesis imperfecta (multiple fractures; look for osteopenia, gracile bones, bone remodelling, wormian bones), osteopathy of prematurity, haemophilia (intracranial haemorrhage), Caffey's disease (florid periosteal reaction), rickets, Menkes disease, some skeletal dysplasias (e.g. metaphyseal dysplasias)—the last three cause metaphyseal irregularities which can mimic fractures. See also Section 14.26.

Head injuries

Shaking is the most important mechanism of intracranial injury in NAI. Intracranial injury may be detected even when the skeletal survey and neurological examination are normal.

1. Skull fractures—linear parietal bone fractures are most common but least specific, and may occur following a fall from height of >1 m. More specific for NAI: multiple, bilateral or complex fractures, depressed or diastased fractures, fracture crossing a suture and nonparietal fractures.
2. Subdural haematoma (SDH).
   (a) Features suspicious of NAI: mixed density, multifocal, SDHs of differing ages, no overlying scalp swelling or fracture, parafalcine or supratentorial locations.
   (b) Features suggesting accidental injury: uniformly dense, unifocal at site of impact (i.e. on cerebral convexity) with overlying scalp swelling ± fracture.

   (c) Chronic SDHs with CSF density must be differentiated from benign extracerebral fluid collections of infancy—these are common in babies 3-9 months old (often macrocephalic), and are frontal, bilateral and symmetrical.
   (d) SDH caused by birth trauma typically resolves by 4 weeks after birth.
3. Cortical contusions/shearing injuries, SAH and intraventricular haemorrhage can also be seen in NAI (and significant accidental trauma, e.g. RTA), but not usually in isolation. Isolated SAH suggests a coagulopathy, and isolated intracerebral haemorrhage suggests an underlying vascular anomaly or stroke.
4. Subdural hygromas—tears in the arachnoid may allow CSF to collect within the subdural space, creating a fluid density collection that can mimic a chronic SDH.
5. Cerebral laceration—best seen on US/MRI. Virtually pathognomonic of shaking injury in the first 6 months.
6. Cerebral oedema—effacement of sulci and basal cisterns + loss of normal grey–white matter differentiation.
7. Hypoxia—the cerebellum and thalami appear hyperdense relative to the hypodense cerebral hemispheres as a result of asphyxia (reversal sign).
8. Vascular injuries—dissection of intracranial or cervical vessels. May lead to pseudoaneurysm formation.
9. Late sequelae—hydrocephalus, atrophy, gliosis and growing fractures.
10. Coexistent non-CNS injuries—retinal haemorrhages, skeletal fractures, visceral injuries.

Visceral injuries

Often seen in mobile children. Mortality of 50% for visceral injuries associated with child abuse. The most likely mechanism of injury is a direct blow or the effect of rapid deceleration after being thrown. Most commonly involves the hollow viscera, mesentery, liver and pancreas.

Imaging protocol for suspected NAI

1. Neuroimaging.
   (a) CT head in all premobile children on the day of admission.
   (b) Consider CT head in ambulant small children if there are rib or spinal fractures, retinal haemorrhages or visceral injuries.
   (c) MRI brain and spine (at day 2–5) if abnormal CT, or if persistent neurological signs despite a normal CT.
2. Skull XR.
   (a) AP and lateral ± Towne view for occipital injury.
   (b) Should be taken even if a CT has been performed, as in-plane horizontal fractures can be missed on CT.

3. Body.
   (a) AP chest (including clavicles and shoulders).
   (b) Oblique views of the ribs (left and right).
   (c) AP abdomen covering pelvis and hips.
4. Lateral spine—cervical and thoracolumbar.
5. Limbs.
   (a) AP humeri and forearms.
   (b) Coned lateral elbows and wrists.
   (c) PA hands and wrists.
   (d) AP femora and tibia/fibula.
   (e) Coned lateral knees and ankles.
   (f) Dorsoplantar (DP) feet.

Follow-up imaging—at 11–14 days, in all suspected NAI.

1. AP chest (including clavicles and shoulders).
2. Oblique views of the ribs (left and right).
3. AP humeri and forearms (including shoulders, elbows, wrists).
4. AP femora and tibia/fibula (including hips, knees and ankles).
5. Plus any other areas that were abnormal or suspicious on the initial survey.
6. Plus follow-up MRI brain within 3 months if an initial MRI scan has been done and is abnormal.

Further reading

Paddock, M., Sprigg, A., Offiah, A.C., 2017. Imaging and reporting considerations for suspected physical abuse (nonaccidental injury) in infants and young children. Part 1: initial considerations and appendicular skeleton. Clin. Radiol. 72 (3), 179–188.

Paddock, M., Sprigg, A., Offiah, A.C., 2017. Imaging and reporting considerations for suspected physical abuse (nonaccidental injury) in infants and young children. Part 2: axial skeleton and differential diagnoses. Clin. Radiol. 72 (3), 189–201.

The radiological investigation of suspected physical abuse in children. London: The Royal College of Radiologists and The Society and College of Radiographers; 2017. Available at: https://www.rcr.ac.uk/system/files/publication/field_publication_files/bfcr174_suspected_physical_abuse.pdf (Accessed 13 October 2018).

OXALOSIS

Deposition of calcium oxalate in tissues (dense on CT). May be primary (AR, presents in childhood) or secondary to excessive oxalate intake/absorption. Sites include:

1. Kidneys—calculi and diffuse corticomedullary nephrocalcinosis, due to hyperoxaluria. Usually the first sign. Results in renal failure, leading to calcium oxalate deposition in other tissues.

2. Bones—typically causes dense metaphyseal bands and vertebral endplate sclerosis. Diffuse sclerosis and a 'bone-in-bone' appearance may also be seen. In those with end-stage renal failure, features of renal osteodystrophy may coexist.
3. Joints—chondrocalcinosis.
4. Soft tissues—e.g. tumoural calcinosis, calcification of skin, ligaments and tendons.
5. Vascular calcification—may cause ischaemia and infarction.
6. Heart—diffuse myocardial hyperattenuation on CT.

Further reading

El Hage, S., Ghanem, I., Baradhi, A., et al., 2008. Skeletal features of primary hyperoxaluria type 1, revisited. J. Child. Orthop. 2 (3), 205–210.
Kuo, L.W., Horton, K., Fishman, E.K., 2001. CT evaluation of multisystem involvement by oxalosis. AJR Am. J. Roentgenol. 177 (3), 661–663.

PAGET'S DISEASE

Common condition characterized by excessive abnormal remodelling of bone. Prevalence increases with age; rare in patients <40 years old. The disease predominates in the spine, skull, pelvis and proximal long bones (especially femur). Polyostotic > monostotic. There are three stages.

Active (osteolytic)

1. Skull—osteoporosis circumscripta, especially in the frontal and occipital bones.
2. Long bones—lucency starts in the subarticular region and advances into the shaft with a well-defined flame-shaped margin.

Mixed (osteolytic and osteosclerotic)

1. Skull—osteoporosis circumscripta with focal areas of sclerosis.
2. Pelvis—mixed lytic and sclerotic areas; thickening and sclerosis of iliopectineal and ischiopubic lines.
3. Long bones—epiphyseal and metaphyseal sclerosis with diaphyseal lucency.

Inactive (osteosclerotic)

Three characteristic features are seen in all involved bones: bony expansion, cortical thickening and trabecular coarsening.

1. Skull—thickened vault. 'Cotton wool' areas of sclerotic bone. The facial bones are not usually affected (cf. fibrous dysplasia).
2. Spine—especially lumbar spine. Enlarged 'picture frame' vertebral body (due to cortical thickening) or ivory vertebra (diffuse sclerosis).
3. Pelvis—changes are often widespread and asymmetrical.

4. Long bones—cortical thickening can encroach on the medullary canal. The epiphyseal region is nearly always involved.

Complications

1. Bone softening—bowed long bones, basilar invagination, 'Tam O'Shanter' skull and protrusio acetabuli.
2. Fractures—transverse, with a predilection for the convex aspect of the bone. Usually only partially traverses the bone.
3. Sarcomatous change—in 1% of patients (5%–10% if widespread disease), most commonly to osteosarcoma; less commonly fibrosarcoma or chondrosarcoma. Most common in the femur, pelvis and humerus. Predominantly lytic + soft-tissue mass. Giant cell tumours can also occur.
4. Osteoarthritis—most frequent in the hip and knee.
5. Osteomyelitis.
6. Neurological complications—nerve entrapment (e.g. cranial nerves in skull base, especially CN VIII) and spinal cord compression.
7. High-output cardiac failure—if widespread disease.
8. Hyperparathyroidism.
9. Extramedullary haematopoiesis.
10. Pagetic vertebral ankylosis—this only occurs if Paget's disease coexists with DISH or ankylosing spondylitis. The presence of bridging osteophytes or syndesmophytes allows the Paget's disease to spread from one vertebra to adjacent vertebrae, and can eventually involve the whole spine.

Further reading

Theodorou, D.J., Theodorou, S.J., Kakitsubata, Y., 2011. Imaging of Paget disease of bone and its musculoskeletal complications: review. AJR Am. J. Roentgenol. 196 (Suppl. 6), S64–S75.

PARANEOPLASTIC SYNDROMES

Non-metastatic systemic or remote effects of tumours.

Endocrine disorders

1. Cushing's syndrome—lung cancer, malignant epithelial thymoma, islet cell carcinoma, small cell carcinoma, medullary thyroid carcinoma, ovarian carcinoma.
2. Hypercalcaemia—osseous metastases; lung cancer, oesophageal carcinoma, squamous carcinomas of the head and neck, lymphoma and leukaemia.
3. Hypocalcaemia and osteomalacia—nonossifying fibroma, giant cell tumour, osteoblastoma, fibrous dysplasia, neurofibromatosis and melorheostosis.

4. Hypoglycaemia—insulinoma, sarcomas, mesothelioma, lymphoma, GI tract carcinomas, adrenocortical carcinoma.
5. Hyperglycaemia—glucagonoma, enteroglucagon-producing RCC.
6. SIADH (syndrome of inappropriate antidiuretic hormone secretion)—lung cancer, GI tract adenocarcinomas.
7. Carcinoid syndrome—carcinoid tumours, pancreatic adenocarcinoma, islet cell tumours, small cell carcinoma of the lung, medullary carcinoma of the thyroid, APUD (amine precursor uptake and decarboxylation) tumours.
8. Gynaecomastia—nonseminomatous testicular tumours, HCC, RCC, lung cancer.
9. Hyperthyroidism—hydatidiform mole or choriocarcinoma, nonseminomatous testicular tumours.
10. Hypertension—phaeochromocytoma, neuroblastoma, aldosterone-secreting tumours, renal tumours (Wilms tumour, RCC, solitary fibrous tumour).

Haematological disorders

1. Polycythaemia—renal tumours (Wilms tumour, RCC), HCC, cerebellar haemangioblastoma, uterine fibroids, renal cystic disease.
2. Red cell aplasia—thymoma, carcinomas of the lung, stomach or thyroid.
3. Haemolytic anaemia—lymphoid malignancies, carcinomas of the ovary, stomach, colon, lung, cervix or breast.
4. Thrombocytosis and leucocytosis—bone marrow metastases.

Digestive disorders

1. Zollinger-Ellison syndrome—gastrinomas of the pancreas or duodenum, mucinous adenocarcinoma of the ovary.
2. Multiple endocrine neoplasia (MEN) syndromes.
3. Tumour-related diarrhoea—Zollinger-Ellison syndrome, carcinoid syndrome, vasoactive intestinal peptide-secreting tumours (VIPomas).

Renal dysfunction

1. Nephrotic syndrome—lymphoma, carcinomas of the lung, stomach, colon and ovary.
2. Tubular dysfunction—multiple myeloma.

Musculoskeletal disorders

1. Hypertrophic osteoarthropathy—see Section 1.24.
2. Dermatomyositis—carcinomas of the breast, lung, ovary or stomach, leukaemia, lymphoma and sarcomas.
3. Oncogenic osteomalacia—phosphaturic mesenchymal tumours.

Skin disorders

1. Acanthosis nigricans—gastric adenocarcinoma.
2. Pellagra-like lesions—carcinoid syndrome.
3. Porphyria cutanea tarda—hepatic adenoma or HCC.
4. Pemphigus vulgaris—pancreatic adenocarcinoma.

Neurological disorders

1. Progressive multifocal leukoencephalopathy—leukaemia, lymphoma, myeloma.
2. Cerebellar atrophy—carcinomas of the lung, breast, ovary and kidney; lymphomas.
3. Central pontine myelinolysis—leukaemia.
4. Myelopathy—visceral carcinomas.
5. Myasthenia gravis—thymoma, thymic hyperplasia.
6. Myasthenic syndrome—small cell carcinoma of the lung (Lambert-Eaton syndrome).
7. Opsomyoclonus (dancing eyes)—neuroblastoma (usually cervicothoracic).

Further reading

Rutherford, G.C., Dineen, R.A., O'Connor, A., 2007. Imaging in the investigation of paraneoplastic syndromes. Clin. Radiol. 62 (11), 1021–1035.

PHACE SYNDROME

Neurocutaneous disorder characterized by:

1. **P**osterior fossa malformations—e.g. Dandy-Walker, cerebellar hypoplasia.
2. **H**aemangioma (infantile)—on the face, orbit and scalp; present in all patients, usually large. Extracutaneous haemangiomas may also occur, e.g. intracranial or subglottic (risk of airway obstruction).
3. **A**rterial anomalies—of cerebral vessels: dysplasia, hypoplasia, aplasia, stenosis, occlusion and/or aneurysm, ± collaterals or persistent embryonic arteries.
4. **C**oarctation of aorta and cardiac anomalies (e.g. VSD).
5. **E**ye anomalies—e.g. choroidal haemangioma, coloboma, microphthalmos.
6. ± **S**ternal clefts and/or **S**upraumbilical raphe (PHACES syndrome)—other midline anomalies may also occur, e.g. of pituitary/thyroid.

Further reading

Rotter, A., Samorano, L.P., Rivitti-Machado, M.C., et al., 2018. PHACE syndrome: clinical manifestations, diagnostic criteria, and management. An. Bras. Dermatol. 93 (3), 405–411.

POLYARTERITIS NODOSA

Multisystem small–medium vessel vasculitis resulting in multiple microaneurysms, stenoses and occlusions. May be idiopathic or related to viral infection (e.g. hepatitis B). Usually presents in middle age. Clinical features include skin purpura or ulceration, mononeuritis multiplex, retinal vasculitis and constitutional symptoms. Imaging features include:

1. Multiple peripheral <1 cm aneurysms ± stenoses/occlusions of visceral arteries (renal > mesenteric > hepatic > splenic > pancreatic). Best seen on conventional angiography, though they may also be visible on CT angiography. CT may also show perivascular soft-tissue cuffing, visceral infarcts (especially renal and bowel) and/or haemorrhage from aneurysm rupture.
2. Coronary arteritis—with resultant aneurysms, stenoses, myocardial infarction or pericarditis.
3. Cerebral arteritis—with resultant aneurysms, stenoses and small peripheral cerebral infarcts.
4. Peripheral arteries in the arms or legs may also be involved.
5. Other rare sites of ischaemia—gallbladder, ureters, testes, ovaries, breasts.

Further reading

Jee, K.N., Ha, H.K., Lee, I.J., et al., 2000. Radiologic findings of abdominal polyarteritis nodosa. AJR Am. J. Roentgenol. 174, 1675–1679.

Stanson, A.W., Friese, J.L., Johnson, C.M., et al., 2001. Polyarteritis nodosa: spectrum of angiographic findings. Radiographics 21 (1), 151–159.

POLYCYSTIC KIDNEY DISEASE, AUTOSOMAL DOMINANT

Common hereditary multisystem disease that presents in the third/fourth decade. Commonest hereditary cause of end-stage renal failure. Can be diagnosed by screening family members or identified as an incidental finding.

Kidneys

1. Multiple renal cysts of varying sizes on imaging. Internal haemorrhage and wall calcification are common. Cyst infection or rupture can also occur. Diagnostic criteria for US screening of at-risk individuals include (NB: diagnosis is unreliable in children ≤14 years):
   (a) Age 15–39 years—≥3 renal cysts in total (uni- or bilateral).
   (b) Age 40–59 years—≥2 cysts in each kidney.
   (c) Age ≥60 years—≥4 cysts in each kidney.

2. Renal calculi—in 20%–35% of patients.
3. Increased incidence of RCC if on prolonged dialysis—may be multiple and bilateral.

Other organs

1. Polycystic liver disease—75% of patients will have hepatic cysts by age 60 years. >20 cysts = polycystic liver disease.
2. Cysts in other organs—seminal vesicles (very common), prostate, pancreas, spleen, testes, ovaries, thyroid, arachnoid cysts.
3. Intracranial berry aneurysms—important potential cause of mortality and morbidity. Diffuse dilatation (dolichoectasia) may also be seen.
4. Cardiovascular—bicuspid aortic valve, mitral valve prolapse, aortic aneurysm and dissection, atherosclerosis (related to renal failure).
5. Colonic diverticulosis.
6. Abdominal wall hernias.
7. Mild bronchiectasis—lower lobe predominance.

Further reading

Katabathina, V.S., Kota, G., Dasyam, A.K., et al., 2010. Adult renal cystic disease: a genetic, biological, and developmental primer. Radiographics 30 (6), 1509–1523.
Pei, Y., Obaji, J., Dupuis, A., et al., 2009. Unified criteria for ultrasonographic diagnosis of ADPKD. J. Am. Soc. Nephrol. 20 (1), 205–212.

POLYCYSTIC KIDNEY DISEASE, AUTOSOMAL RECESSIVE

Less common than autosomal dominant form. Main manifestations are renal and hepatic—the severity of these are inversely proportional and depend on the age of presentation:

1. Perinatal—severe renal disease (visible on prenatal US), minimal hepatic disease, oligohydramnios, pulmonary hypoplasia. Poor prognosis.
2. Neonatal—severe renal disease, minimal hepatic disease.
3. Infantile—moderate renal disease, moderate hepatic disease.
4. Juvenile—mild renal disease, severe hepatic disease. Some patients may present in adolescence or adulthood with cirrhosis and portal hypertension.

Renal disease

1. Bilateral smooth enlarged echogenic kidneys with loss of corticomedullary differentiation.
2. Cysts are usually too small to resolve individually (often seen as tiny echobright foci), though a few small (<1 cm) macrocysts may be seen. High-resolution US probes often show numerous small radially oriented dilated tubules.

3. Diffusely increased T2 signal in renal parenchyma on MRI, with multiple low signal fibrous septa.

Liver disease

1. Characterized by congenital hepatic fibrosis—heterogeneous liver echotexture on US ± periportal echogenicity. Poor visualization of peripheral portal veins.
2. Also associated with other ductal plate malformations—multiple biliary hamartomas, Caroli disease.
3. Signs of cirrhosis and portal hypertension—varices, splenomegaly, ascites.

Further reading

Avni, E., Guissard, G., Hall, M., et al., 2002. Hereditary polycystic kidney diseases in children: changing sonographic patterns through childhood. Pediatr. Radiol. 32, 169–174.

Dell, K., 2011. The spectrum of polycystic kidney disease in children. Adv. Chronic Kidney Dis. 18, 339–347.

Lonergan, G.J., Rice, R.R., Suarez, E.S., 2000. Autosomal recessive polycystic kidney disease: radiologic–pathologic correlation. Radiographics 20, 837–855.

POLYOSTOTIC BONE LESION SYNDROMES

Multiple bone cysts

1. Tuberous sclerosis—single or multiple bone cysts (especially in phalanges, metacarpals and metatarsals) and sclerotic lesions (especially in skull, spine, ribs and pelvis).
2. Cystic angiomatosis—multiple bone cysts (lymphovascular malformations) with thin sclerotic rims, most common in the axial skeleton, femora and humeri. Lymphangiomas may also be seen in other organs or tissues, most commonly in the spleen. Can present at any age, most often in adolescence; cysts may sclerose in older patients.
3. Nasu-Hakola disease—also known as polycystic lipomembranous osteodysplasia with sclerosing leukoencephalopathy (PLOSL). Polyostotic bone cysts (especially in carpals and tarsals) ± fractures. Early frontal lobe dementia.

Multiple nonossifying fibromas

1. NF1—with other features, e.g. tibial bowing and pseudarthrosis, multiple neurofibromas, etc.
2. Jaffe-Campanacci syndrome—with giant cell granulomas of the jaw and café-au-lait spots, ± other features, e.g. kyphoscoliosis, intellectual disability, precocious puberty, hypogonadism or cryptorchidism, and ocular or cardiovascular malformations. Now thought to be a manifestation of NF1.

3. Oculoectodermal syndrome—with giant cell tumours of the jaw, aortic coarctation, intracranial arachnoid cysts, seizures, epibulbar dermoids, aplasia cutis congenita and hyperpigmented naevi. Very rare.

Multiple enchondromas

Often have atypical appearances when multiple. Most common in hands and feet, may be unilateral or bilateral. Increased risk of malignant transformation to chondrosarcoma.

1. Ollier disease—also known as enchondromatosis. Increased risk of gliomas, acute myeloid leukaemia and juvenile granulosa cell tumours.
2. Maffucci syndrome—with soft-tissue haemangiomas (look for phleboliths). Increased risk of glial, pancreatic, haematologic, ovarian and breast tumours.
3. Metachondromatosis—with multiple osteochondromas.

Multiple osteochondromas

Increased risk of malignant transformation to chondrosarcoma.

1. Hereditary multiple exostoses—AD, presents in childhood.
2. Metachondromatosis—with multiple enchondromas.

Multiple bone islands

1. Osteopoikilosis—hereditary (AD). Most are located in the long bones, carpals/tarsals and pelvis, especially close to joints.
2. Mixed sclerosing bone dysplasia—osteopoikilosis + osteopathia striata + melorheostosis.
3. Dermatofibrosis lenticularis—osteopoikilosis + cutaneous connective tissue naevi.
4. Gunal-Seber-Basaran syndrome—osteopoikilosis + dacryocystitis.

Polyostotic fibrous dysplasia

Usually not syndromic. Rarely associated with:

1. McCune-Albright syndrome—with café-au-lait spots and precocious puberty ± other endocrine disturbances (hyper-thyroid/parathyroidism, Cushing's syndrome, acromegaly or hyperprolactinaemia).
2. Mazabraud syndrome—with multiple intramuscular myxomas.

Multifocal bone infarcts

See also Section 1.26. When multifocal, consider:

1. Sickle cell disease—usually with a shrunken calcified spleen.
2. Gaucher disease—with splenomegaly.

3. Corticosteroids—both exogenous and endogenous.
4. Drugs—including chemotherapy and chronic alcohol abuse.
5. Radiotherapy—limited to the radiation field, e.g. pelvis.
6. Thromboembolic—including vasculitis (e.g. SLE), antiphospholipid syndrome and dysbaric osteonecrosis.

Multifocal osteomyelitis

1. Multifocal bacterial, tuberculous or fungal osteomyelitis.
2. CRMO—noninfectious, typically in children. Most common in clavicles and metaphyses of long bones.
3. SAPHO syndrome—noninfectious, typically in adults. Most common in sternoclavicular region and spine.
4. Syphilis.

Others

1. Metastases—lytic or sclerotic.
2. Multiple myeloma.
3. Paget's disease.
4. Brown tumours—due to hyperparathyroidism.
5. Sarcoidosis.
6. Langerhans cell histiocytosis—usually in children.
7. Erdheim-Chester disease.
8. Gardner syndrome—multiple osteomas.
9. Epithelioid haemangioendothelioma—multifocal lytic lesions clustered in one area.
10. Amyloidosis.
11. Rosai-Dorfman disease.

Further reading

Northrup, B.E., Slat, D.F., Loomans, R.U., et al., 2014. The myriad of diseases that present with polyostotic bone lesions. Curr. Probl. Diagn. Radiol. 43 (4), 186–204.

POLYPOSIS SYNDROMES

A group of syndromes characterized by multiple polyps in the GI tract ± extraintestinal features. Polyps may cause bleeding, intussusception, obstruction and other symptoms. Polyps may be adenomatous, hamartomatous or hyperplastic. Inflammatory pseudopolyps occur in colitis (usually IBD) and are not true polyps.

Familial adenomatous polyposis (FAP)

Commonest polyposis syndrome, AD inheritance. Characterized by hundreds of adenomatous polyps carpeting the colon—nearly all patients will develop colorectal carcinoma by age 40 years unless total colectomy is performed. An 'attenuated' form can occur which presents with fewer polyps. FAP is also associated with an increased risk of other tumours:

1. Extracolonic polyps—stomach > duodenum (especially periampullary) > jejunum/ileum. These can also become malignant, especially periampullary adenomas.
2. Hepatoblastoma—in childhood.
3. Medulloblastoma—see Turcot syndrome (discussed later).

Gardner syndrome

A variant of FAP which has several additional extraintestinal features:

1. Multiple osteomas—especially of mandible and skull.
2. Epidermoid (sebaceous) cysts.
3. Desmoid tumours—of the mesentery, abdominal wall and soft tissues.
4. Dental anomalies—e.g. supernumerary teeth, dentigerous cysts, odontomas.
5. Papillary thyroid cancer.
6. Adrenal adenomas.
7. Subcutaneous lipomas and fibromas.
8. Nasopharyngeal angiofibroma.

Hereditary nonpolyposis colorectal cancer (HNPCC)

Also known as Lynch syndrome. Despite the name, adenomatous colonic polyps do occur, but diffuse polyposis is absent. Increased risk of various malignancies:

1. Colorectal carcinoma—develops in the majority, usually right-sided.
2. Endometrial carcinoma—common.
3. Small bowel adenocarcinoma—duodenum > jejunum > ileum.
4. Ureteric or renal pelvis transitional cell carcinoma.
5. Others—gastric cancer, ovarian tumours, CNS tumours (especially glioblastoma).

Turcot syndrome

Characterized by intestinal polyposis and brain tumours. Genetically associated with either FAP (brain tumours are usually medulloblastomas) or HNPCC (usually glioblastomas).

MYH-associated polyposis

AR. Numerous adenomatous colonic polyps, fewer than in FAP and usually presenting later in adulthood. High lifetime risk of developing colorectal carcinoma.

Hamartomatous polyposis syndromes

Most of these show AD inheritance, except Cronkhite-Canada syndrome which is an acquired disorder.

1. Juvenile polyposis syndrome—several or numerous hamartomatous polyps in the colon (especially rectum) ± stomach and small bowel. Polyps may degenerate into adenomas and carcinomas. Presents in childhood; may be associated with a range of congenital anomalies, e.g. malrotation, Meckel's diverticulum, mesenteric lymphangioma, cryptorchidism, hydrocephalus.
2. Peutz-Jeghers syndrome—solitary or numerous hamartomatous polyps in the small bowel (especially jejunum and ileum) ± colon and stomach. Mucocutaneous pigmentation on and around the lips is characteristic. Usually presents in childhood. Polyps may also be seen in the bronchi, urinary or biliary tract. Increased risk of GI tract carcinomas, sex cord tumours of the ovary, Sertoli cell tumours of the testis, and cancers of the pancreas, breast, uterus, cervix and lung.
3. PTEN hamartoma tumour syndromes—discussed separately. Can cause hamartomatous polyps in the stomach, small bowel and colon. Ganglioneuromas, adenomas, lipomas, hyperplastic and inflammatory polyps may also occur.
4. Cronkhite-Canada syndrome—numerous hamartomatous polyps in the colon and stomach ± small bowel (especially duodenum). Usually presents in middle age with watery diarrhoea, protein-losing enteropathy, skin hyperpigmentation, alopecia and nail dystrophy. Polyps may degenerate into adenomas and carcinomas (mostly left-sided in the colon).
5. Other syndromes associated with hamartomatous polyps—NF1, MEN 2B, Gorlin-Goltz, Birt-Hogg-Dubé.

Other polyposis syndromes

1. Serrated polyposis syndrome—multiple hyperplastic polyps and sessile serrated adenomas in the colon only. Increased risk of colon cancer (mostly right-sided). Usually presents in middle age.
2. Hereditary mixed polyposis syndrome—polyps occur in the colon only, and show mixed histological elements (hamartomatous, adenomatous and hyperplastic). Increased risk of colon cancer.

Further reading

Calva, D., Howe, J.R., 2008. Hamartomatous polyposis syndromes. Surg. Clin. North Am. 88 (4), 779.

Jelsig, A.M., Qvist, N., Brusgaard, K., et al., 2014. Hamartomatous polyposis syndromes: a review. Orphanet J. Rare Dis. 9, 101.

Groen, E.J., Roos, A., Muntinghe, F.L., et al., 2008. Extra-intestinal manifestations of familial adenomatous polyposis. Ann. Surg. Oncol. 15 (9), 2439–2450.

Shussman, N., Wexner, S.D., 2014. Colorectal polyps and polyposis syndromes. Gastroenterol. Rep. (Oxf) 2 (1), 1–15.

PSEUDOHYPOPARATHYROIDISM

End-organ unresponsiveness to parathormone. X-linked dominant inheritance.

1. Short stature, round face, thickset features, mental retardation and hypocalcaemia.
2. Short 4th and 5th metacarpals and metatarsals.
3. Basal ganglia calcification (50%).
4. Soft-tissue calcification.

PSEUDOPSEUDOHYPOPARATHYROIDISM

Similar clinical and radiological features to pseudohypoparathyroidism but with a normal plasma calcium.

PSORIATIC ARTHROPATHY

Usually preceded by skin and nail disease, but may precede these in 15%. Characterized by a proliferative erosive enthesopathy. Three clinical and radiological types:

1. Monoarthritis or asymmetric oligoarthritis with enthesitis.
2. Symmetric polyarthritis—resembling rheumatoid arthritis.
3. Axial disease—like ankylosing spondylitis but asymmetric.

Joint manifestations

1. Joints involved—DIP and PIP joints (hands > feet) > MCP/MTP joints, knees, ankles.
2. Proliferative bone erosions—erosions at joint margins and entheses with adjacent ill-defined bone proliferation and periostitis along diaphyses.
3. Acroosteolysis—associated with psoriatic nail changes.
4. Dactylitis (sausage digit)—digital oedema, arthritis of IP joints and tenosynovitis.
5. Ivory phalanx (diffuse sclerosis)—especially distal phalanx of hallux.
6. Ankylosis—common.
7. Pencil-in-cup and cup-and-saucer—due to severe erosive changes. Can give rise to 'arthritis mutilans'.
8. Preserved periarticular bone density (cf. rheumatoid arthritis)—though there is an increased risk of generalized osteoporosis.
9. Sacroiliitis—bilateral and asymmetrical. Large erosions with bone proliferation; ankylosis is rare.
10. Spondylitis—prominent asymmetrical 'comma' shaped paravertebral ossification.

Extraskeletal associations

1. Accelerated atherosclerosis.
2. Inflammatory bowel disease.
3. Autoimmune eye disease—uveitis, iritis.
4. Complications of therapy—e.g. methotrexate pneumonitis.

Further reading

Bennett, D.L., Ohashi, K., El Khoury, G.Y., 2004. Spondyloarthropathies: ankylosing spondylitis and psoriatic arthritis. Radiol. Clin. North Am. 42, 121–134.

Jacobson, J.A., Girish, G., Jiang, Y., Resnick, D., 2008. Radiographic evaluation of arthritis: inflammatory conditions. Radiology 248 (2), 378–389.

Jacobson, J.A., Girish, G., Jiang, Y., Sabb, B.J., 2008. Radiographic evaluation of arthritis: degenerative joint disease and variations. Radiology 248 (3), 737–747.

Klecker, R.J., Weissman, B.N., 2003. Imaging features of psoriatic arthritis and Reiter's syndrome. Semin. Musculoskelet. Radiol. 7 (2), 115–126.

PTEN HAMARTOMA TUMOUR SYNDROMES

A spectrum of inherited (AD) disorders including Cowden syndrome (CS), Bannayan-Riley-Ruvalcaba syndrome (BRRS) and Lhermitte-Duclos disease (LDD). These overlap significantly; LDD is now considered to be a manifestation of CS. Features common to both CS and BRRS include:

1. GI polyposis—in the stomach, small bowel and colon. Usually hamartomas, though ganglioneuromas, adenomas, lipomas, hyperplastic and inflammatory polyps can also occur.
2. Macrocephaly.
3. Increased risk of breast cancer, thyroid follicular carcinoma and benign thyroid nodules.

Features predominantly seen in CS include:

1. Clinical—trichilemmomas, acral keratoses, mucocutaneous papillomas and neuromas.
2. Glycogenic acanthosis—numerous small oesophageal nodules and plaques.
3. Testicular lipomatosis—multiple small echogenic lesions in both testes. Highly suggestive if present.
4. Dysplastic gangliocytoma of the cerebellum (LDD).
5. Increased risk of certain malignancies—colonic, endometrial, RCC.

Features predominantly seen in BRRS include:

1. Clinical—penile macules, mental retardation, joint hypermobility, hypotonia.
2. Soft-tissue lipomas and angiolipomas.

3. Vascular anomalies—including intracranial vascular anomalies.
4. Scoliosis and pectus excavatum.

Further reading

Pilarski, R., Burt, R., Kohlman, W., et al., 2013. Cowden syndrome and the PTEN hamartoma tumor syndrome: systematic review and revised diagnostic criteria. J. Natl. Cancer Inst. 105 (21), 1607–1616.

REACTIVE ARTHRITIS

Sterile inflammatory arthritis that follows infection at another site, especially urogenital or gut. Young adult males predominate.

1. Arthritis—similar features to psoriatic arthritis (bilateral asymmetric proliferative erosive enthesopathy + soft-tissue swelling), but tends to spare the upper limbs; see Section 3.2. The calcaneum is the commonest site involved. Can cause regional osteoporosis in acute disease but not in chronic or recurrent disease. Asymmetric sacroiliitis may also be seen.
2. Urethritis ± cystitis ± prostatitis/cervicitis ± circinate balanitis.
3. Conjunctivitis.
4. Keratoderma blenorrhagica—skin lesions on the palms and soles.
5. Aortitis and aortic regurgitation—rare, seen in chronic disease.

Further reading

Jacobson, J.A., Girish, G., Jiang, Y., Resnick, D., 2008. Radiographic evaluation of arthritis: inflammatory conditions. Radiology 248 (2), 378–389.

RENAL OSTEODYSTROPHY

Due to chronic renal failure. Consists of osteomalacia/rickets + secondary hyperparathyroidism + osteosclerosis.

Children

1. Changes most marked in the skull, pelvis, scapulae, vertebrae and metaphyses of tubular bones.
2. Vertebral sclerosis may be confined to the endplate regions ('rugger-jersey' spine).
3. Rickets—the epiphyseal plate is less wide and the metaphysis is less cupped than in vitamin D–dependent rickets.
4. Secondary hyperparathyroidism—subperiosteal erosions; 'rotting fence-post' appearance of the femoral necks ± SUFE.
5. Soft-tissue calcification—less common than in adults.
6. Delayed skeletal maturation.

Adults

1. Hyperparathyroidism—acroosteolysis, Brown tumours, etc.
2. Soft-tissue calcification is common, especially in arteries.
3. Osteosclerosis—including 'rugger-jersey' spine.
4. Osteomalacia—mainly evident as Looser's zones.

Further reading

Tigges, S., Nance, E.P., Carpenter, W.A., Erb, R., 1995. Renal osteodystrophy: imaging findings that mimic those of other diseases. AJR Am. J. Roentgenol. 165 (1), 143–148.

RHEUMATOID ARTHRITIS

Chronic multisystemic autoimmune disorder primarily causing an inflammatory arthropathy of synovial joints, with many other manifestations which are usually preceded by the arthropathy.

Joints

1. Symmetrical arthritis of synovial joints, especially the MCP/MTP and PIP joints of the hands and feet, wrists, knees, ankles, elbows, glenohumeral and acromioclavicular joints and hips. The synovial joints of the axial skeleton may also be affected, especially apophyseal and atlantoaxial joints of the cervical spine (± atlantoaxial subluxation). Less commonly the SIJs and TMJs are involved. The sequence of pathological/radiological changes at synovial joints is:
   (a) Synovial inflammation and effusion → soft-tissue swelling and joint space widening.
   (b) Hyperaemia and disuse → juxtaarticular osteoporosis; later generalized.
   (c) Destruction of cartilage by pannus → joint space narrowing.
   (d) Pannus destruction of unprotected bone at the joint capsule insertion → marginal erosions.
   (e) Pannus destruction of subchondral bone → widespread erosions and subchondral cysts.
   (f) Capsular and ligamentous laxity → subluxation, dislocation and deformity.
   (g) Fibrous and bony ankylosis.
   (h) Intraarticular loose bodies—rice bodies visible on MRI.
2. Cartilaginous joints, e.g. discovertebral junctions outside the cervical spine, symphysis pubis and manubriosternal joints, and entheses are less frequently and less severely involved (cf. seronegative spondyloarthropathies).
3. Periosteal reaction—uncommon.

4. Proliferative new bone formation does not occur—cf. seronegative arthropathies.
5. Secondary osteoarthritis in the major weight-bearing joints.
6. Pyogenic arthritis is a recognized complication.

Extraarticular musculoskeletal features

1. Subcutaneous rheumatoid nodules—over bony prominences; calcification rare.
2. Tendons—tenosynovitis, tendon rupture; especially extensor carpi ulnaris (± erosion of ulnar styloid), flexor carpi ulnaris and extensor carpi radialis.
3. Bursae—bursitis ± erosion of adjacent bone. Common sites: retrocalcaneal (± erosion of posterior calcaneal tubercle), olecranon and subacromial bursae.
4. Bones—osteopenia, avascular necrosis.
5. Carpal tunnel syndrome.

Systemic

1. Anaemia, lymphadenopathy, hepatosplenomegaly, leucocytosis and fever.
2. Felty syndrome—splenomegaly, leucopenia and rheumatoid arthritis.
3. Secondary amyloidosis.
4. Complications of therapy—e.g. methotrexate pneumonitis.

Pulmonary

1. Pleural thickening ± effusions—most common intrathoracic feature, often unilateral.
2. Interstitial pneumonitis and fibrosis—UIP or NSIP pattern.
3. Organizing pneumonia.
4. Rheumatoid lung nodules—single or multiple, usually peripheral, upper-mid zone predilection, may cavitate (± pneumothorax), may contain calcification.
5. Caplan syndrome—rheumatoid lung nodules + pneumoconiosis.
6. Airways—bronchiectasis, bronchiolitis obliterans (mosaic attenuation + air trapping), follicular bronchiolitis (centrilobular nodularity ± tree-in-bud).
7. Increased risk of lung infections, especially if on immunosuppressants.

Cardiac

1. Pericarditis ± effusion.
2. Myocarditis.
3. Pulmonary arterial hypertension.

Ocular

1. Secondary Sjögren's syndrome—dry eyes.
2. Episcleritis and scleritis.
3. Peripheral ulcerative keratitis (corneal ulcers).

Vascular

1. Accelerated atherosclerosis.
2. Vasculitis—small and medium vessels, resembling polyarteritis nodosa. Commonest manifestations: skin ulcers (especially in legs), digital ischaemia, mononeuritis multiplex (due to nerve ischaemia) and scleritis. Less commonly: stroke, myocardial infarction, bowel ischaemia, nephritis. Large vessels, e.g. aorta can rarely be involved.
3. Raynaud phenomenon.

Further reading

Jacobson, J.A., Girish, G., Jiang, Y., Resnick, D., 2008. Radiographic evaluation of arthritis: inflammatory conditions. Radiology 248 (2), 378–389.

Narvaez, J.A., Narváez, J., De Lama, E., De Albert, M., 2010. MR imaging of early rheumatoid arthritis. Radiographics 30 (1), 143–163.

Sommer, O.J., Kladosek, A., Weiler, V., 2005. Rheumatoid arthritis: a practical guide to state-of-the-art imaging, image interpretation and clinical implications. Radiographics 25, 381–398.

RICKETS

Increased noncalcified osteoid in the immature skeleton. Mainly a disorder of growth plates and equivalents (e.g. costochondral junction).

Causes of rickets

1. Vitamin D deficiency—due to poor dietary intake, lack of sunlight exposure or both. Occasionally from malabsorption (e.g. coeliac disease, IBD).
2. Dietary calcium deficiency—commoner than vitamin D deficiency in some developing countries, especially in dairy-free vegetarian diets.
3. Hypophosphataemic rickets—hereditary disorders of increased renal phosphate wasting.
4. Vitamin D–dependent rickets—hereditary disorders of vitamin D metabolism. Presents with severe rickets in infancy (but not at birth).
5. Oncogenic rickets—paraneoplastic phenomenon due to secretion of FGF23 by mesenchymal tumours such as nonossifying fibromas.
6. Other causes—e.g. prematurity, liver disease (e.g. biliary atresia), renal osteodystrophy.

Changes at the growth plate and cortex

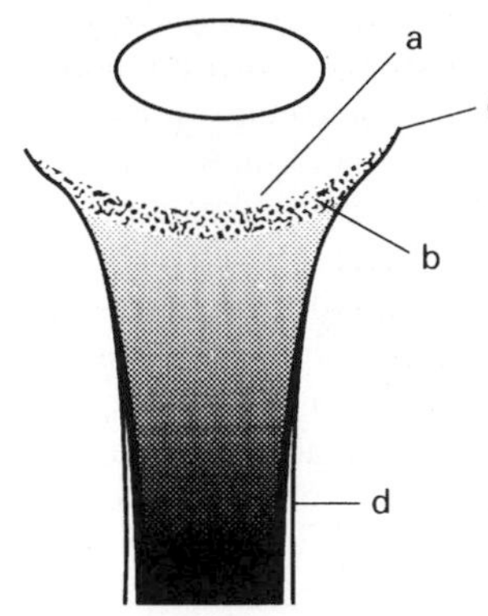

1. Widened growth plate (a).
2. Fraying, splaying and cupping of the metaphysis, which is of reduced density (b).
3. Thin bony spur extending from the metaphysis to surround the uncalcified growth plate (c).
4. Indistinct cortex because of uncalcified subperiosteal osteoid—mimics a periosteal reaction (d).
5. Rachitic rosary—cupping of the anterior ends of the ribs with abnormally large costochondral junctions.
6. Looser's zones—uncommon in children.

Changes due to bone softening (deformities)

1. Bowing of long bones.
2. Triradiate pelvis ± protrusio acetabuli.
3. Harrison's sulcus—indrawing of the lower chest wall due to soft ribs.
4. Spine—scoliosis, biconcave vertebral bodies.
5. Basilar invagination and platybasia.
6. Craniotabes—softening of the skull, resulting in flattening of the occiput and osteoid accumulation in the frontal and parietal regions.

General changes

1. Retarded bone maturation and growth.
2. Decreased bone density and increased fracture risk (if severe).

ROSAI-DORFMAN DISEASE

Also known as sinus histiocytosis with massive lymphadenopathy. Rare nonneoplastic non-Langerhans cell histiocytosis with multisystem manifestations. Most common in children and young adults. Can involve any organ or tissue, forming well-defined or infiltrative masses that tend to enhance homogeneously. Common sites include:

1. Lymphadenopathy—commonest manifestation, usually in the neck, large and bilateral. Axillary, inguinal, mediastinal or intraabdominal nodes can less commonly be involved. Involved nodes usually remain discrete and enhance homogeneously. Isolated nodal disease often resolves spontaneously.

2. Skin—often a sign of systemic disease. Well-defined or infiltrative subcutaneous masses which may infiltrate underlying muscle. Most common on trunk and proximal limbs. Homogeneous enhancement on MRI.
3. Head and neck—masses may arise within the sinonasal cavities (± bone destruction), orbits, tonsils, salivary or lacrimal glands, oropharynx or trachea.
4. Bone—usually occurs in the presence of nodal disease. Most common in metaphyses of long bones and skull; often multifocal. Typically lytic, though sclerotic and mixed lesions may be seen. Periosteal reaction and soft-tissue extension may also occur.
5. CNS—enhancing dural masses (intracranial > spinal) without underlying bony hyperostosis (cf. meningioma). The cavernous sinuses, pituitary, trigeminal nerves or ventricles may also be involved. Unlike other sites, CNS involvement usually occurs without nodal disease.
6. Respiratory tract—tracheobronchial masses/thickening, or less commonly lung nodules, masses or perilymphatic interstitial thickening. Mediastinal and hilar adenopathy is often also present. Pleural nodules and effusions can rarely occur.
7. Abdomen—visceral involvement often occurs in the presence of lymphadenopathy. The kidneys are the most common extranodal site, manifesting as infiltrative perihilar, intraparenchymal or perinephric masses. Other organs, e.g. liver (± biliary dilatation), pancreas (± peripancreatic extension), uterus or ovaries may rarely be involved. GI tract involvement is very rare and favours the colon/rectum, manifesting as masses, polyps or wall thickening. Infiltrative mesenteric, retroperitoneal or pelvic masses may also rarely occur.
8. Other rare sites—breasts (ill-defined hypoechoic mass lesions or architectural distortion), heart (intracardiac > pericardial, most commonly right atrium), thyroid (focal nodule or diffuse infiltration), testes, epididymides.

Further reading

Cheng, X., Cheng, J.L., Gao, A.K., 2018. A study on clinical characteristics and magnetic resonance imaging manifestations on systemic Rosai-Dorfman disease. Chin. Med. J. 131 (4), 440–447.

La Barge, D.V., III, Salzman, K.L., Harnsberger, H.R., et al., 2008. Sinus histiocytosis with massive lymphadenopathy (Rosai-Dorfman disease): imaging manifestations in the head and neck. AJR Am. J. Roentgenol. 191, W299–W306.

Mar, W.A., Yu, J.H., Knuttinen, M.G., et al., 2017. Rosai-Dorfman disease: manifestations outside of the head and neck. AJR Am. J. Roentgenol. 208, 721–732.

Raslan, O.A., Schellingerhout, D., Fuller, G.N., Ketonen, L.M., 2011. Rosai-Dorfman disease in neuroradiology: imaging findings in a series of 10 patients. AJR Am. J. Roentgenol. 196, W187–W193.

SAPHO SYNDROME

Acronym for **s**ynovitis, **a**cne, **p**ustulosis, **h**yperostosis, **o**steitis. A spectrum of conditions related to CRMO, but usually occurs in adults and more commonly involves sternoclavicular region and spine rather than long bones.

1. Anterior chest wall—bony sclerosis and hyperostosis around sternoclavicular joints ± involvement of costal cartilage of 1st and 2nd ribs. Erosions or ankylosis may be seen. 'Buffalo' sign on bone scan due to increased activity in the manubrium and sternum (head) and medial clavicles (horns).
2. Spine—bony sclerosis and hyperostosis of vertebral bodies and around costovertebral joints ± erosions or ankylosis ± paravertebral ossification causing bony bridging. Thoracic > lumbar or cervical.
3. Sacroiliitis—sclerosis and hyperostosis, frequently unilateral.
4. Flat bones—sclerosis and periostitis, e.g. ilium and mandible.
5. Long bones—sclerosis and periostitis, e.g. metadiaphyses of femur and tibia.
6. Skin—palmoplantar pustulosis and acne.

Further reading

Depasquale, R., Kumar, N., Lalam, R.K., et al., 2012. SAPHO: what radiologists should know. Clin. Radiol. 67 (3), 195–1206.

SARCOIDOSIS

A chronic multisystem disease of unknown aetiology characterized by noncaseating granulomas. Peaks in young adults, more common in Afro-Caribbean populations. Variable clinical presentation, with a huge variety of manifestations across all body systems.

Intrathoracic sarcoidosis

Thoracic disease occurs at some stage in >90% of patients. Nodal enlargement on CXR is most common manifestation and almost always occurs before lung infiltration. Stage I (adenopathy only), stage II (adenopathy + lung infiltrates), stage III (lung infiltrates only) and stage IV (lung fibrosis).

1. Lymphadenopathy—most commonly bilateral symmetrical hilar + right paratracheal adenopathy. Other mediastinal nodes may also be involved but not in isolation (think lymphoma or metastatic disease). Unilateral hilar adenopathy is uncommon. Punctate or 'egg-shell' calcification may occur in chronic disease.
2. Lung parenchymal disease manifests as:
   (a) Multiple bilateral 2–4 mm micronodules or reticulonodular opacities predominantly in the mid-upper zones. Perilymphatic

distribution is typical on CT: peribronchovascular ('beading'), along interlobular septa (± septal thickening) and subpleural/perifissural.

(b) Larger conglomerate nodules or masses (5–50 mm) may be seen ± nearby satellite micronodules ('galaxy' sign); may mimic progressive massive fibrosis. Cavitation is rare. May partially or completely regress.

(c) An 'alveolar' pattern (due to both air-space filling and interstitial thickening) may be seen as areas of consolidation or GGO ± air bronchograms.

(d) Mid-upper zone fibrosis occurs later in the disease, and tends to radiate from the hila to the periphery along bronchovascular bundles + traction bronchiectasis ± honeycombing or bullous change (risk of pneumothorax).

(e) Mosaic attenuation and air trapping (due to small airways involvement) can occur but is nonspecific.

3. Pleural involvement—rare. May cause effusion or thickening. Beware of confluent subpleural nodularity mimicking pleural thickening or plaques.
4. Tracheobronchial stenosis—rare; due to extrinsic compression or mural granulomas.

Skin

Second commonest site of disease involvement.

1. Erythema nodosum—almost always in association with bilateral hilar lymphadenopathy, ± fever and arthritis (Löfgren syndrome).
2. Lupus pernio, plaques and scar infiltration.
3. Discrete subcutaneous nodules or ill-defined fat stranding may be seen on imaging.

Head and neck

1. Cervical lymphadenopathy—posterior > anterior triangle.
2. Anterior uveitis.
3. Diffuse enlargement and inflammation of salivary and/or lacrimal glands—usually bilateral.
4. Uveoparotid fever (Heerfordt syndrome)—uveitis, parotitis, CN VII palsy + fever.

Cardiac

1. Most commonly causes arrhythmia ± sudden death.
2. Myocardial involvement is best seen on MRI, as focal areas of midwall or transmural LGE typically involving the basal septum and LV free wall. This is associated with T2 hyperintense oedema (acute phase) or myocardial thinning ± aneurysm (chronic phase).

Abdomen

1. Lymphadenopathy—periportal, paraaortic, left gastric, retrocrural. Usually in the presence of intrathoracic adenopathy. Mesenteric adenopathy (± fat stranding) can rarely occur.
2. Liver and spleen—numerous small hypovascular nodules, T2 hypointense on MRI. A granulomatous cholangitis can also rarely occur ± stricture formation.
3. Kidneys—nephrocalcinosis is the commonest manifestation, related to hypercalcaemia. Rarely, multifocal hypovascular lesions may be seen.
4. Testes—typically in Afro-Caribbean men; multiple bilateral hypoechoic lesions in the epididymides ± testes.
5. GI tract—rare. Most common in stomach, causing focal or diffuse thickening (especially in antrum). Can rarely cause small bowel or colonic strictures.
6. Other rare sites—pancreas (hypovascular masses or pancreatitis), ureters (filling defects), prostate (granulomatous prostatitis), peritoneal thickening.

Neurosarcoid

1. Strong predilection for the base of the brain, manifesting as:
   (a) Nodular thickening and enhancement of the basal leptomeninges—this can mimic TB or metastatic disease.
   (b) Cranial neuropathies—especially bilateral lower motor neuron CN VII palsies.
   (c) Thickening and enhancement of the optic nerves and/or chiasm.
   (d) Diabetes insipidus—due to involvement of posterior pituitary or hypothalamus.
2. Brain parenchyma—periventricular and deep white matter T2 hyperintensities. Single or multiple enhancing masses may also occur.
3. Spinal cord—intramedullary enhancing lesion + surrounding oedema.

Musculoskeletal

1. Bone involvement most often affects the hands and feet, causing multiple well-defined lytic lesions often with a characteristic 'lace-like' coarse trabecular pattern. Associated skin involvement is common; dactylitis and/or acroosteolysis may also be seen. In larger bones (e.g. spine, skull, ribs, long bones) the lesions are less specific, and may be lytic or sclerotic, mimicking bone metastases.
2. An acute transient symmetrical arthritis is common (e.g. as part of Löfgren syndrome), most often in the ankles, but this is occult on imaging. Chronic arthropathy is rare and may cause subluxations,

but erosions do not occur. Associated synovitis, tenosynovitis or bursitis may be seen.

3. Muscle involvement is rare, most often causing a chronic proximal myopathy (especially lower limbs) with marked fatty atrophy. Rarer manifestations include an acute myositis (diffuse nonspecific oedema and enhancement on MRI) or a nodular myositis (enhancing fusiform nodules oriented along muscle fibres; T2 hyperintense ± central hypointense fibrosis).

Further reading

Criado, E., Sánchez, M., Ramírez, J., et al., 2010. Pulmonary sarcoidosis: typical and atypical manifestations at high-resolution CT with pathologic correlation. Radiographics 30 (6), 1567–1586.

Koyama, T., Ueda, H., Togashi, K., et al., 2004. Radiologic manifestations of sarcoidosis in various organs. Radiographics 24 (1), 87–104.

SCHISTOSOMIASIS

Parasitic infection caused by various species of *Schistosoma*, most commonly:

1. *S. haematobium*—endemic in Africa and Middle East. Mainly infects GU tract.
2. *S. mansoni*—endemic in Africa, Middle East, Caribbean and northeastern parts of South America. Mainly infects colon and liver.
3. *S. japonicum*—endemic in southeast Asia. Mainly infects colon and liver.

Infection results in the deposition of parasite eggs in target organs, with a resultant granulomatous reaction which creates characteristic imaging appearances:

1. Urinary tract—acute infection typically involves bladder and distal ureters, causing diffuse nodular wall thickening which may appear polypoid or mass-like. Chronic disease typically results in diffuse bladder wall calcification and distal ureteric strictures (± calcification), though the upper tracts may also be involved. The prostate, seminal vesicles and vas deferens may also become calcified. Schistosomal granulomas may rarely be seen in the testes (heterogeneous on US + vascularity). Increased risk of bladder SCC.
2. Colon—typically involves rectosigmoid. Mural oedema and pseudopolyps may be seen in acute infection. Chronic infection can result in strictures and wall calcification, and an increased risk of colon cancer.
3. Liver—parasite eggs migrate to the liver via the portal veins, causing widening of hepatic fissures and periportal bands of fibrosis which are echogenic on US and enhance on CT/MRI. With

S. japonicum a network of septal and capsular calcification may also be seen on CT, giving a characteristic 'turtleback' appearance. Eventually results in cirrhosis and portal hypertension (especially *S. mansoni*) ± bile duct stenoses.

4. Lungs—during acute infection parasites migrate through the lung vasculature, which may cause a transient eosinophilic reaction manifesting as ill-defined nodules or GGO. Patients with chronic hepatic disease and associated portocaval shunting (especially with *S. mansoni*) may deposit parasite eggs in the lungs, leading to lung fibrosis and pulmonary hypertension.
5. CNS—rare. *S. japonicum* tends to affect the brain, causing enhancing nodular intracerebral lesions + surrounding vasogenic oedema, whereas *S. mansoni* and *S. haematobium* tend to affect the spinal cord, causing oedema and heterogeneous enhancement of the thoracic cord and conus.
6. Other rare sites—heart, skin, breast, female genitalia.

Further reading

Bilgin, S.S., Toprak, H., Seker, M., 2016. Imaging findings of hepatosplenic schistosomiasis: a case report. Radiol. Case Rep. 11 (3), 152–156.

Liu, H., Lim, C.C., Feng, X., et al., 2008. MRI in cerebral schistosomiasis: characteristic nodular enhancement in 33 patients. AJR Am. J. Roentgenol. 191, 582–588.

Niemann, T., Marti, H., Duhnsen, S.H., Bongartz, G., 2010. Pulmonary schistosomiasis—imaging features. J. Radiol. Case Rep. 4 (9), 37–43.

Sah, V.K., Wang, L., Min, X., et al., 2015. Human schistosomiasis: a diagnostic imaging focused review of a neglected disease. Radiol. Infect. Dis. 2 (3), 150–157.

Shebel, H.M., Elsayes, K.M., Abou El Atta, H.M., et al., 2012. Genitourinary schistosomiasis: life cycle and radiologic–pathologic findings. Radiographics 32 (4), 1031–1046.

SCLERODERMA (SYSTEMIC SCLEROSIS)

An autoimmune multisystem connective tissue disorder characterized by microvascular injury and deposition of collagen and extracellular matrix. Most commonly presents in middle-aged women. The most obvious clinical manifestation is skin induration and thickening, but involvement of other organ systems is very common.

Skin

1. Thickening, tightness and nonpitting induration—extent of skin disease defines two clinical subsets: limited cutaneous scleroderma (distal to elbows and knees ± face and neck; positive anticentromere antibodies) and diffuse scleroderma (diffuse skin involvement; positive anti-Scl70 antibodies).

2. Raynaud phenomenon—very common; may precede skin changes.
3. Soft-tissue atrophy in finger pads and digital pitting scars.
4. Subcutaneous calcinosis in the hands—punctate, globular or sheet-like.
5. Telangiectasia.
6. Hyperpigmentation, hypopigmentation or depigmentation.

Musculoskeletal

1. Acroosteolysis—associated with soft-tissue atrophy.
2. Joints—erosions and subluxation, especially at 1st CMC joint and IP joints.
3. Mandible—bone resorption (especially at angle), thickened periodontal ligament ± loss of lamina dura.
4. Ribs—symmetrical erosions on the superior surfaces of the posterior aspects of the 3rd to 6th ribs.
5. Osteopenia.
6. Soft tissues (on MRI)—fascial thickening, synovitis, tenosynovitis, myositis, enthesitis.

Cardiopulmonary

1. Lung disease is the commonest cause of death. Basal predominant fibrosis, NSIP > UIP pattern. Other patterns include organizing pneumonia and diffuse alveolar damage.
2. Aspiration pneumonia—secondary to gastrooesophageal reflux. Chronic aspiration can also cause basal fibrosis.
3. Pulmonary arterial hypertension—with or without coexistent lung disease.
4. Pericardial thickening ± effusion.
5. Restrictive cardiomyopathy—midwall LGE in the septum and RV insertion points on MRI.
6. Cardiac failure—due to any of the above.

Gastrointestinal system

1. Oesophagus—dilatation, dysmotility, gastrooesophageal reflux (with associated increased risk of Barrett's, stricture and adenocarcinoma). Commonest site of involvement in the GI tract. The presence of both oesophageal dilatation and bibasal lung fibrosis on CT should raise the suspicion of scleroderma.
2. Small bowel and colon—dilatation, atony, antimesenteric pseudosacculations, pseudoobstruction, pneumatosis cystoides intestinalis. In the small bowel, a 'hidebound' appearance due to dilatation and crowded mucosal folds is characteristic. Bacterial overgrowth may occur.
3. Stomach—gastroparesis, gastric antral vascular ectasia.
4. Anus—faecal incontinence due to internal anal sphincter atrophy.

Other features

1. Renal hypertensive crisis and renal failure.
2. Hypothyroidism—due to thyroid fibrosis.
3. Primary biliary cirrhosis.
4. Mixed connective tissue disease—overlapping features of scleroderma, SLE and polymyositis.

SCURVY

Due to vitamin C deficiency. Most common in young children, but not seen in infants <6 months of age due to prenatal stores. Rare in adults. Earliest signs are seen at the knees. Imaging features include:

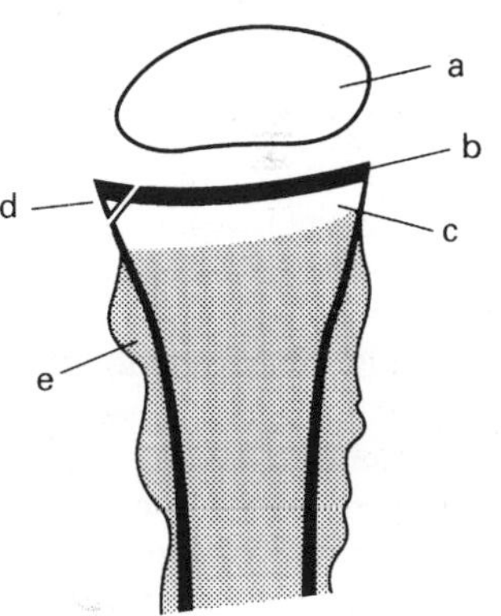

1. Osteoporosis—usually the only sign seen in adults.
2. Wimberger sign (a)—reduced epiphyseal density with a pencil-thin cortex.
3. Frankel line (b)—dense zone of provisional calcification in the metaphysis.
4. Trümmerfeld zone (c)—lucency under Frankel line.
5. Pelkan spurs (d)—represent healing metaphyseal corner fractures (caused by bone weakening), resulting in metaphyseal cupping.
6. Periosteal reaction (e)—due to subperiosteal haemorrhage.
7. Haemarthrosis.

Extraosseous features

1. Haemorrhage—subcutaneous, gingival, gastrointestinal, intramuscular, orbital, intracranial.
2. Impaired wound healing.
3. Poor dentition.
4. In adults, scurvy is usually seen with generalized malnutrition (e.g. alcoholism, anorexia, poverty) so other vitamin deficiencies may coexist.

SHOCK

Acute severe hypotension often results in a constellation of CT imaging findings termed the 'CT hypotension complex'. Causes include:

1. Hypovolaemic shock—due to significant blood loss, e.g. major trauma, postsurgical haemorrhage, large GI bleed, haemoperitoneum.
2. Neurogenic shock—severe head or spinal injury.
3. Cardiogenic shock—cardiac arrest.
4. Septic shock.
5. Distributive shock—e.g. anaphylaxis.
6. Bacterial endocarditis—combination of septic and cardiogenic shock.
7. Diabetic ketoacidosis.

CT features include, in decreasing order of frequency:

1. Collapsed IVC (AP diameter <9 mm)—most commonly seen in hypovolaemic shock. A fluid attenuation 'halo' is often also seen around the intrahepatic portion of the IVC. Other veins (e.g. renal, mesenteric) may also appear collapsed.
2. Shock bowel—diffuse submucosal oedema + intense mucosal enhancement throughout small bowel ± colonic involvement. Usually reversible.
3. Increased or persistent delayed renal cortex enhancement—contrast flow into the medulla is impaired due to tubular dysfunction; suggests a poorer prognosis. NB: absent renal enhancement may be seen in severe hypovolaemia in children (suggests an even worse prognosis).
4. Hyperenhancing adrenal glands—especially in children. Adrenal haemorrhage may also occur.
5. Small calibre aorta (<13 mm around level of renal arteries)—can be seen in severe hypovolaemia, but not a specific sign. Other arteries (e.g. SMA) may also appear narrowed.
6. Heterogeneously enhancing pancreas + peripancreatic fluid.
7. Hyperenhancing gallbladder wall.
8. Hypoenhancing spleen—in the absence of vascular pedicle injury/occlusion. Suggests a poorer prognosis.
9. Heterogeneously enhancing liver—in the absence of vascular occlusion.
10. Heterogeneously enhancing thyroid + surrounding fluid.

Further reading

Ames, J.T., Federle, M.P., 2009. CT hypotension complex (shock bowel) is not always due to traumatic hypovolemic shock. AJR Am. J. Roentgenol. 192 (5), W230–W235.

Higashi, H., Kanki, A., Watanabe, S., et al., 2014. Traumatic hypovolemic shock revisited: the spectrum of contrast-enhanced abdominal computed tomography findings and clinical implications for its management. Jpn. J. Radiol. 32 (10), 579–584.

Wang, J., Liang, T., Louis, L., et al., 2013. Hypovolemic shock complex in the trauma setting: a pictorial review. Can. Assoc. Radiol. J. 64 (2), 156–163.

SICKLE CELL DISEASE

Musculoskeletal

1. Marrow hyperplasia (red marrow persistence or reconversion) causes widening of medullary cavities, decreased bone density, coarsening of trabeculae, and cortical thinning and expansion. The changes are most marked in the axial skeleton.
   (a) Skull—coarse granular osteoporosis with widening of the diploë which spares the occiput below the internal occipital protuberance. 'Hair-on-end' appearance can rarely be seen.
   (b) Spine—osteoporosis, exaggerated vertical trabeculae and biconcave vertebral bodies (see also 2c, below).
2. Vascular occlusion results in osteonecrosis.
   (a) Sickle cell dactylitis (hand–foot syndrome)—in children aged 6 months to 2 years. Symmetrical soft-tissue swelling, patchy lucency and sclerosis of the shafts of metacarpals, metatarsals and phalanges, with periosteal reaction and bone shortening.
   (b) Long bones—diaphyseal or epiphyseal infarcts.
   (c) Spine—square-shaped compression infarcts of the vertebral endplates produce characteristic 'H-shaped' vertebrae.
3. Growth disturbances—retarded growth, delayed closure of epiphyses and tibiotalar slant.
4. Osteomyelitis and pyogenic arthritis—due to *Salmonella* in >50% of cases. NB: infarction is 50× more common than infection.
5. Subperiosteal haemorrhage.
6. Myonecrosis.
7. Extramedullary haematopoiesis—usually paraspinal or intrahepatic, but can occur anywhere. Less common than in thalassaemia.

Thorax

1. Acute chest syndrome—vasoocclusive crisis of lung vasculature, presenting with fever, leucocytosis, hypoxia and chest pain. Bilateral peripheral consolidation or atelectasis, usually in the lower lobes ± pleural effusions. Peak incidence at 2–4 years.
2. Pneumonia.
3. Chronic interstitial lung disease—peripheral fibrosis due to recurrent episodes of infection and acute chest syndrome.
4. Pulmonary embolism.
5. Cardiomegaly—due to chronic anaemia, microvascular ischaemia and restrictive cardiomyopathy.
6. Pulmonary hypertension—due to chronic haemolysis, hypoxia, microvascular occlusion, PE and LVF.

Spleen

1. Splenic sequestration—severe anaemia and hypovolaemia due to sudden accumulation of blood in the spleen, usually <6 years of age. Acute massive splenomegaly on imaging.

2. Autosplenectomy—shrunken calcified spleen, due to recurrent splenic infarction. Seen in nearly all patients by 8 years of age. Results in hyposplenism, increasing the risk of septicaemia.
3. Splenomegaly is rare in adults with sickle cell disease, but is common in other sickle variants, e.g. Hb SC and Hb S-beta thalassaemia.
4. Splenic abscess—rare, seen in those with splenomegaly or large infarcts.

Hepatobiliary

1. Gallstones—pigment type.
2. Hepatic crisis—acute vasoocclusive crisis; hepatomegaly on imaging ± infarcts. Acute hepatic sequestration is rare.
3. Secondary haemochromatosis—due to recurrent blood transfusions.
4. Cirrhosis—due to a combination of chronic microvascular occlusion, secondary haemochromatosis ± transfusion-related hepatitis B/C infection.
5. Portal hypertension—due to cirrhosis or NRH.
6. Ischaemic cholangiopathy.
7. Acute ischaemic pancreatitis—very rare.

Genitourinary tract

1. Large kidneys—in early disease.
2. Renovascular occlusion—papillary necrosis, renal infarcts, acute cortical necrosis and renal vein thrombosis. Results in renal scarring and atrophy over time.
3. Renal medullary carcinoma—mostly in patients with sickle cell trait.
4. Haemorrhagic cystitis.
5. Priapism.
6. Segmental testicular infarction.

GI tract

1. Peptic ulceration—due to chronic low-grade ischaemia.
2. Small or large bowel ischaemia—due to microvascular vasoocclusive crisis. Often resolves with conservative treatment, but can lead to necrosis and perforation.

CNS

1. Stroke—common cause of morbidity and death.
2. Chronic small vessel ischaemia and cerebral atrophy.
3. Intracranial arteries may be tortuous, aneurysmal, stenosed or occluded with secondary moyamoya syndrome.
4. Fat emboli—typically innumerable tiny foci of restricted diffusion ('starfield' pattern), due to bone marrow infarction.
5. Intraorbital haemorrhage.

Further reading

Ejindu, V.C., Hine, A.L., Mashayekhi, M., et al., 2007. Musculoskeletal manifestations of sickle cell disease. Radiographics 27 (4), 1005–1021.

Madani, G., Papadopoulou, A.M., Holloway, B., 2007. The radiological manifestations of sickle cell disease. Clin. Radiol. 62, 528–538.

SJÖGREN'S SYNDROME

Chronic autoimmune disorder mainly affecting salivary and lacrimal glands, typically presenting in middle-aged women with dry mouth and eyes. May be associated with other connective tissue diseases (RA > SLE > scleroderma) and PBC. On imaging:

1. Salivary glands (especially parotids)—diffusely enlarged and heterogeneous bilaterally in early disease, with areas of duct dilatation and stenosis ('beading') on sialography. In chronic disease, the glands undergo fatty atrophy and/or diffuse cystic change + calcifications. Solid hypoechoic nodules can also be seen, which may transform to lymphoma—look for cervical adenopathy.
2. Lacrimal glands—enlarged and heterogeneous in early disease. Fatty atrophy in chronic disease.
3. Lungs—manifestations are diverse:
   - (a) Interstitial lung disease—classically associated with LIP, but NSIP is actually the most common interstitial pattern. UIP and organizing pneumonia can also occur.
   - (b) Airways—involvement is common, resulting in bronchiectasis, bronchial wall thickening and/or bronchiolitis (follicular or obliterative).
   - (c) Benign lymphoproliferative lung disorders—including follicular bronchiolitis, LIP (mainly alveolar) and diffuse lymphoid hyperplasia (mainly perilymphatic, i.e. interlobular septal thickening). Can progress to MALT lymphoma, manifesting as masses or areas of nonresolving consolidation.
   - (d) Pulmonary amyloidosis—rare.
4. Mediastinum—lymphadenopathy, thymic hyperplasia and thymic cysts may be seen.
5. Chronic pancreatitis—can occur as part of the autoimmune exocrinopathy.
6. Synovitis—most common in the MCPJs, wrists and knees. Usually nonerosive.
7. CNS—can cause a cerebral vasculitis, leading to focal areas of infarction or nonspecific T2 hyperintensities.
8. Increased risk of lymphoma—especially MALT lymphoma arising in the lungs or salivary glands.

Further reading

Egashira, R., Kondo, T., Hirai, T., et al., 2013. CT findings of thoracic manifestations of primary Sjögren syndrome: radiologic-pathologic correlation. Radiographics 33 (7), 1933–1949.

STURGE-WEBER SYNDROME

Neurocutaneous disorder presenting clinically at birth with a unilateral facial port wine stain, usually involving the V1 territory of the trigeminal nerve. Seizures and hemiparesis then develop. Imaging manifestations are primarily in the CNS:

1. Leptomeningeal angioma—diffuse leptomeningeal enhancement, usually unilateral on the same side as the facial port wine stain.
2. Enlarged ipsilateral choroid plexus.
3. Choroidal angioma—ipsilateral choroidal enhancement in the globe.
4. Ipsilateral cerebral atrophy with characteristic cortical and subcortical 'tram-track' calcification—due to vascular steal phenomenon.
5. Ipsilateral skull thickening and sinus enlargement—secondary to cerebral volume loss.

SYPHILIS

Multisystem infection caused by *Treponema pallidum*. The primary and secondary stages of infection do not usually manifest on imaging, except for osteomyelitis (especially of skull) which can occur in secondary syphilis. Most imaging features are related to tertiary syphilis (in adults) or congenital syphilis (in children).

Tertiary syphilis

1. Musculoskeletal—many manifestations:
   (a) Chronic osteomyelitis.
   (b) Proliferative periostitis—most commonly involving tibia, ribs, skull and sternum. Often bilateral.
   (c) Gummatous bone lesions—mixed lytic and sclerotic + periostitis. Appearances are often variable and nonspecific.
   (d) Charcot arthropathy—due to neurosyphilis (tabes dorsalis).
2. Neurosyphilis—may be associated with concurrent HIV infection. Many manifestations:
   (a) Meningitis—leptomeningeal or pachymeningeal enhancement ± focal enhancing nodules.
   (b) Encephalitis—mimics herpes simplex encephalitis.
   (c) Myelitis—long-segment cord oedema ± nodular areas of enhancement.

(d) Meningovascular (arteritis)—leads to infarcts in the brain and/or spinal cord. Focal arterial stenoses or beading may be seen on angiograms.
(e) Gummas—focal enhancing granulomatous masses which may be intra- or extraaxial in the cranium (± vasogenic cerebral oedema), and intra- or extramedullary in the spine (± cord compression).
(f) Cerebral atrophy—late manifestation.
(g) Tabes dorsalis—a very late manifestation in the spinal cord, causing peripheral sensory neuropathy. Longitudinal T2 hyperintensity of the dorsal columns on MRI, representing demyelination.

3. Cardiovascular—classically causes aortitis, resulting in extensive 'tree-bark' calcification of the aortic wall ± saccular aneurysms especially involving the ascending aorta and/or coronary sinuses. Coronary ostial stenosis and aortic valve involvement (± regurgitation) may be seen.
4. Gummas—most common in skin, bone, brain, liver and testes, but can occur anywhere giving rise to granulomatous masses which usually have nonspecific appearances.

Congenital syphilis

Transmitted from an infected pregnant woman to her foetus, though most infants are asymptomatic at birth. On imaging:

Early onset (0–2 years)

1. Bones—most common, usually involving multiple sites (tibia > femur > humerus > other bones). Many features:
   (a) Periosteal reaction—commonest finding, usually bilateral and symmetrical.
   (b) Metaphyses—lucent bands ± irregularity or destructive lesions. Focal destruction of the medial proximal tibial metaphysis bilaterally is pathognomonic (Wimberger sign).
   (c) Diaphyses—cortical thickening ± destructive lesions. Anterior tibial cortical thickening and bowing ('sabre shin') may occur.
   (d) Pathological fractures—especially at metaphyses, often multiple.
   (e) Skull—lytic lesions.
2. Lungs—bilateral hazy consolidation. Complete lung opacification (pneumonia alba) is rare.
3. CNS—acute or chronic leptomeningitis.
4. Heart—myocarditis.
5. GI tract—enteritis, strictures ± obstruction.
6. Liver—hepatitis, which may lead to calcification.
7. Pancreas—pancreatitis and insufficiency.
8. Kidneys—glomerulonephritis.

Late onset (>2 years)

1. Bones—gummatous periostitis, sabre shin, frontal bossing, maxillary hypoplasia, saddle nose.
2. Synovitis—especially of knees, resulting in bilateral joint effusions.
3. Teeth—Hutchinson teeth (notched incisors), Mulberry molars (rudimentary enamel cusps on the permanent first molars).
4. Aseptic meningitis.

SYSTEMIC LUPUS ERYTHEMATOSUS

Multisystem autoimmune disorder with numerous manifestations, many of which are related to lupus vasculitis. Most commonly presents in young adult women. Most patients will have positive anti-dsDNA antibodies. Skin signs (e.g. malar rash, discoid rash and photosensitivity) are a common presenting feature.

Musculoskeletal

1. Polyarthritis—bilateral and symmetrical, involving the small joints of the hands, knees, wrists and shoulders. Soft-tissue swelling and periarticular osteopenia of the PIP and MCP joints. MCP subluxation, ulnar deviation, swan-neck and Boutonniere deformities and scapholunate dissociation can be seen due to ligamentous laxity (Jaccoud arthropathy)—this may mimic rheumatoid arthritis but erosions are typically absent.
2. Osteonecrosis—most frequently of the femoral head, especially if on steroids.
3. Terminal phalangeal sclerosis and resorption—due to lupus vasculitis.
4. Atlantoaxial subluxation.
5. Osteoporosis ± insufficiency fractures—especially if on steroids.
6. Tenosynovitis—due to steroids. Risk of tendon or ligament rupture.
7. Myositis—affects proximal limb muscles.
8. Increased risk of septic arthritis and osteomyelitis.
9. Subcutaneous calcification—may be linear or nodular.

Respiratory

1. Pleuritis and effusion—often recurrent and bilateral. May lead to pleural fibrosis.
2. Pneumonia—consider atypical organisms in patients on immunosuppressants.
3. Acute lupus pneumonitis—nonspecific consolidation or GGO, often bilateral and basal ± pleural effusions.
4. Diffuse pulmonary haemorrhage—due to pulmonary vasculitis, often with features of generalized vasculitis, e.g. rash, arthritis and renal failure.

5. Airways—bronchiectasis, bronchiolitis obliterans, tracheal thickening.
6. Chronic lung disease—variable patterns, e.g. NSIP, UIP, LIP, organizing pneumonia.
7. Pulmonary hypertension—either primary or secondary to chronic thromboembolic disease or lung fibrosis.
8. Shrinking lung syndrome—small lung volumes due to diaphragm dysfunction and elevation.

Cardiovascular

1. Pericarditis and effusion—may lead to calcification.
2. Nonbacterial thrombotic endocarditis (Libman-Sacks)—typically of mitral valve, resulting in regurgitation. Vegetations may embolize and cause infarcts (e.g. stroke, MI) or sepsis (e.g. brain abscesses).
3. Myocarditis—myocardial oedema and midwall LGE on MRI.
4. Accelerated atherosclerosis—especially if on steroids.

Abdominal

1. Peritonitis and ascites.
2. Oesophageal dysmotility ± reflux.
3. Small bowel dysmotility and dilatation ± pelviureteric dilatation ± biliary dilatation—termed 'generalized megaviscera of lupus' if all three are present.
4. Vasculitis—bowel ischaemia, acalculous cholecystitis, pancreatitis, splenic ± hepatic infarcts, gastric ulcers or antral vascular ectasia, visceral artery aneurysms ± haemorrhage.
5. Hepatosplenomegaly—may be due to hepatic vein thrombosis or venoocclusive disease, hepatitis, PBC or NRH.
6. Lupus nephritis—results in chronic renal atrophy. Kidneys may be enlarged and hyperechoic in the acute setting.
7. Adrenal haemorrhage or infarction.
8. Lupus cystitis—diffuse bladder wall thickening ± bilateral VUJ obstruction.

Neurological

1. Vasculitis—ischaemic stroke, small vessel disease, arterial stenoses.
2. Subarachnoid and intracerebral haemorrhage.
3. Myelopathy—transverse myelitis, optic neuritis or both (NMO).
4. Lupus psychosis and delirium.
5. Septic or aseptic meningoencephalitis.
6. PRES—rare, associated with renal involvement.

Malignancy

Increased risk of lymphoma (especially NHL), hepatobiliary, lung and thyroid cancers.

Antiphospholipid syndrome (APS)

Seen in 27%–42% of SLE patients; positive lupus anticoagulant and/or anticardiolipin antibodies. Can present with:

1. Recurrent miscarriages.
2. Recurrent venous/arterial thromboses—dural venous sinus thrombosis, stroke, moyamoya syndrome, DVT and PE, MI, Budd-Chiari syndrome, portal vein thrombosis, ischaemic bowel, renal vein/artery thrombosis.
3. Thrombotic microangiopathy—haemolytic anaemia, thrombocytopenia and organ damage (especially renal failure).
4. Catastrophic APS—simultaneous thrombosis in ≥3 organs or tissues. High mortality.

Further reading

Goh, Y.P., Naidoo, P., Ngian, G.S., 2013. Imaging of systemic lupus erythematosus. Part I: CNS, cardiovascular, and thoracic manifestations. Clin. Radiol. 68 (2), 181–191.

Goh, Y.P., Naidoo, P., Ngian, G.S., 2013. Imaging of systemic lupus erythematosus. Part II: gastrointestinal, renal, and musculoskeletal manifestations. Clin. Radiol. 68 (2), 192–202.

Kirby, J.M., Jhaveri, K.S., Maizlin, Z.V., et al., 2009. Abdominal manifestations of systemic lupus erythematosus: spectrum of imaging findings. Can. Assoc. Radiol. J. 60 (3), 121–132.

Lalani, T.A., Kanne, J.P., Hatfield, G.A., Chen, P., 2004. Imaging findings in systemic lupus erythematosus. Radiographics 24, 1069–1086.

THALASSAEMIA

Imaging features are more severe in thalassaemia major than minor.

Skeletal

1. Marrow hyperplasia causes widening of medullary cavities, decreased bone density, coarsening of trabeculae ('cobwebbing'), and cortical thinning and expansion. These features are more pronounced than in sickle cell disease. Initially both axial and appendicular skeleton are affected (e.g. ribs, clavicles and tubular bones of hands and feet) but as marrow regresses from the appendicular skeleton at puberty the changes in the latter diminish.
   (a) Skull—granular osteoporosis, widening of the diploë, thinning of the outer table and 'hair-on-end' appearance. Involvement of the facial bones produces obliteration of the paranasal sinuses, hypertelorism and malocclusion of the teeth. These changes are rare in other haemoglobinopathies so are important differentiating signs.

   (b) Spine—osteoporosis, exaggerated vertical trabeculae and fish-shaped vertebrae.
2. Growth disturbances, including those due to desferroxamine treatment—dysplasias, irregular physeal–metaphyseal junction, e.g. distal ulna.
3. Fractures.

Extraskeletal

1. Extramedullary haematopoiesis—typically paravertebral or in the liver or spleen, but can occur anywhere.
2. Iron overload—in the liver, spleen, bone marrow, pancreas and heart. Due to recurrent blood transfusions. Reduced T2 signal on MRI with signal loss on opposed-phase T1 sequences.
3. Cardiomyopathy—due to iron overload. May be dilated or restrictive.
4. Gallstones—pigment type.

Further reading

Tunaci, M., Tunaci, A., Engin, G., et al., 1999. Imaging features of thalassaemia. Eur. Radiol. 9, 1804–1809.

Tyler, P.A., Madani, G., Chaudhuri, R., et al., 2006. The radiological appearances of thalassaemia. Clin. Radiol. 61 (1), 40–52.

TUBERCULOSIS

Granulomatous infection caused by *Mycobacterium tuberculosis*. Primary infection typically occurs in the lungs, and patients with extrapulmonary TB will often have evidence of previous lung infection. Huge variety of manifestations; can involve nearly any part of the body.

Lungs

1. Primary TB most commonly occurs in childhood and typically presents as an area of consolidation + ipsilateral hilar or mediastinal adenopathy. Involved nodes are typically necrotic centrally and may occur without lung involvement. During resolution, calcification often develops in the lung (Ghon focus) and/or nodes. Less common manifestations include unilateral pleural effusion (may result in pleural thickening and calcification) or miliary TB (usually in the elderly, infants or immunocompromised; manifests as numerous randomly distributed micronodules throughout both lungs).
2. Postprimary TB represents reactivation of infection, usually occurring several years later during a period of reduced immunity. Typically manifests as tree-in-bud opacities and/or cavitating consolidation, usually in the upper zones. Adenopathy is less common than in primary TB. Pleural involvement results in an

effusion/empyema + pleural thickening ± calcification. Less common manifestations include miliary TB or tuberculoma formation (well-defined mass ± cavitation ± satellite nodules).

3. Complications of pulmonary TB include:
   (a) Secondary fungal infection of lung cavities (e.g. aspergilloma).
   (b) Bronchial stenosis and bronchiectasis.
   (c) Erosion of a calcified focus into a bronchus (broncholith) ± obstruction.
   (d) Bronchopleural fistula.
   (e) Extension of empyema into chest wall (empyema necessitans) ± pleurocutaneous fistula.
   (f) Bronchial/pulmonary artery pseudoaneurysm.
   (g) Cardiac involvement—usually manifests as tuberculous pericarditis, causing irregular pericardial thickening (>3 mm) and a small effusion, often with mediastinal adenopathy ± signs of constrictive pericarditis. Myocardial tuberculomas are rare.

Abdomen

1. Lymphadenopathy—typically involving mesenteric, periportal, peripancreatic and/or paraaortic nodes, usually with central necrosis. Nodes often calcify with healing.
2. GU tract—commonest extrapulmonary extranodal site of infection. Can involve any part:
   (a) Kidneys—usually unilateral. Causes papillary necrosis and infundibular stenosis resulting in dilated moth-eaten or clubbed calyces, which can be large and mimic cysts. Abscesses can also form if the caseating papillary necrosis does not rupture into the collecting system. Atrophy and calcification occur in the chronic phase, leading to a 'putty kidney'.
   (b) Ureters—nodular wall thickening and strictures ± 'beaded' appearance; most common in distal ureter. Usually secondary to renal TB.
   (c) Bladder—diffuse wall thickening ± irregular mucosal masses in the acute phase. Contracted thick-walled bladder ± calcification in the chronic phase. Nearly always secondary to renal involvement, so the presence of normal kidneys practically excludes TB.
   (d) Female genital tract—typically causes bilateral fallopian tube strictures and occlusions ± tuboovarian abscesses ± tuberculous peritonitis. Endometrial involvement results in adhesions and distortion of the cavity.
   (e) Prostate—causes granulomatous prostatitis ± abscess; may lead to volume loss and calcification.
   (f) Seminal vesicles and vas deferens—may be thickened and dilated (due to strictures) ± calcification.

(g) Scrotum—may cause diffuse epididymoorchitis or a focal abscess/mass ± sinus tract to the scrotal skin. Usually occurs in the presence of GU tract involvement elsewhere.

(h) Urethra—rare; can cause strictures of the anterior urethra ± multiple perineal and scrotal fistulas ('watering can' perineum).

3. Peritonitis—classically three types have been described (wet, dry and fibrotic), but there is significant overlap between them. Generally manifests as diffuse smooth or nodular peritoneal thickening ± adhesions matting bowel loops together ± omental stranding, nodularity or caking ± adenopathy. Ascites may be present (wet type) or absent (dry type); when present, the fluid is often of high attenuation (20–45 HU) due to protein content and cellularity.
4. Liver and spleen—most commonly manifests as numerous tiny (miliary) hypovascular nodules, usually associated with miliary lung disease. Macronodular involvement is less common, manifesting as larger hypovascular nodules or masses. Involvement of the biliary tree (strictures) or gallbladder (mural thickening) is rare.
5. Adrenals—typically bilateral due to haematogenous spread. Enlarged adrenals, usually with central necrosis. May cause an Addisonian crisis. In the chronic phase the adrenals are atrophic and calcified.
6. GI tract—typically involves the ileocaecal region, causing mural thickening, stricturing and caecal contraction ('conical' caecum) ± fistulae ± necrotic ileocolic nodes. Other sites can rarely be involved, e.g. stomach (especially antrum, causing ulceration ± stricturing), rest of small and large bowel (causing mural thickening and stricturing) or oesophagus (usually from adjacent mediastinal adenopathy).
7. Pancreas—rare; may cause discrete masses, collections or diffuse infiltration.

Head and neck

1. Most commonly manifests as cervical lymphadenopathy (scrofula), usually with central necrosis ± cutaneous fistula. Calcification can occur in chronic cases. Extranodal TB in the neck is rare.
2. Larynx—infiltrative soft-tissue thickening of the paraglottic and pre-epiglottic spaces.
3. Otomastoiditis—soft-tissue thickening ± bony/ossicular erosion ± pachymeningeal thickening and enhancement ± dural venous sinus thrombosis. Cervical adenopathy is often also present.
4. Pharynx and sinonasal cavity—nonspecific soft-tissue thickening ± masses ± bone erosion.
5. Eyes—usually manifests as a unilateral choroidal mass.
6. Thyroid—very rare. May manifest as a necrotic mass, abscess, miliary involvement or chronic diffuse fibrosis.

CNS

Most commonly seen in immunocompromised patients.

1. Meningitis—leptomeningeal enhancement usually involving the basal meninges ± communicating hydrocephalus ± cranial nerve involvement ± vascular involvement causing cerebral infarcts. Pachymeningitis is rare.
2. Cerebral tuberculoma—round/lobulated nodule with solid or ring enhancement + surrounding vasogenic oedema ± calcification. Internal T2 hypointensity and lack of restricted diffusion can aid differentiation from pyogenic abscesses.
3. Less common intracranial manifestations include tuberculous abscess (indistinguishable from pyogenic abscesses), miliary TB (numerous enhancing micronodules) and cerebritis.
4. Spinal meningitis—manifests as arachnoiditis, resulting in thick linear enhancing adhesions distorting the lumbar nerve roots. May be complicated by a syrinx.

Musculoskeletal

1. Spine—commonest site. Typically causes destruction of the anterior vertebral body and endplate, often spreading in a subligamentous fashion to other vertebrae, with minimal reactive sclerosis and relative sparing of the disc (cf. pyogenic infection). Rim-enhancing paraspinal collections are very common and often large ± calcification. Eventually leads to vertebral collapse ± acute kyphosis (gibbus deformity).
2. Arthritis—typically a monoarthritis of large weight-bearing joints. Causes synovitis, marginal erosions and periarticular osteopenia ± joint space narrowing in later stages. Sinus tracts and soft-tissue collections may be seen.
3. Osteomyelitis—usually occurs in the presence of tuberculous arthritis. Isolated bone involvement most commonly involves the femur, tibia or short tubular bones of the hands and feet (dactylitis). Typically causes ill-defined metaphyseal lysis with minimal sclerosis or periosteal reaction. A less common pattern is multiple well-defined metaphyseal cystic lucencies.
4. Dactylitis—fusiform soft-tissue swelling (finger > toe) ± bony expansion, cortical thickening and trabecular coarsening. Acroosteolysis and sinus tracts may also be seen. Bony sclerosis occurs after healing.
5. Soft tissues—tenosynovitis, bursitis or myositis. Rare.

Breasts

Tuberculous mastitis is very rare. May manifest as an ill-defined mass (± calcification), abscess, or diffuse soft-tissue thickening/fibrosis ± reduction in breast size. Overlying skin thickening and sinus tracts may be seen and are suggestive. Axillary adenopathy is common and may be calcified.

Further reading

Burrill, J., Williams, C.J., Bain, G., et al., 2007. Tuberculosis: a radiologic review. Radiographics 27 (5), 1255–1273.

Da Rocha, E.L., Pedrassa, B.C., Bormann, R.L., et al., 2015. Abdominal tuberculosis: a radiological review with emphasis on computed tomography and magnetic resonance imaging findings. Radiol. Bras. 48 (3), 181–191.

Jung, Y.Y., Kim, J.K., Cho, K.S., 2005. Genitourinary tuberculosis: comprehensive cross-sectional imaging. AJR Am. J. Roentgenol. 184, 143–150.

TUBEROUS SCLEROSIS (TS)

A hamartomatous neurocutaneous syndrome with AD inheritance. Clinical features include seizures, mental retardation and skin lesions.

Central nervous system

1. Cortical tubers—benign hamartomas located at or just beneath the cortex; present in nearly all patients. T2 hyperintense, usually nonenhancing. May calcify.
2. Subependymal hamartomas—usually calcified on CT, with variable enhancement. Typically <1 cm. Seen in nearly all patients.
3. Radial migration lines—T2 hyperintense bands of neuroglial heterotopia extending from the periventricular region to the subcortical white matter. Cystic white matter lesions may also be seen.
4. Subependymal giant cell astrocytoma—benign slow-growing tumour (usually >1 cm) arising from subependymal nodules, typically located at the foramen of Monro ± hydrocephalus. Often enhance avidly.
5. Retinal astrocytic hamartomas—can calcify, appearing as 'giant drusen' on CT.
6. Other rare manifestations—cerebral atrophy, arterial occlusion or aneurysm, corpus callosum dysgenesis, Chiari malformation, arachnoid cyst, chordoma.

Thoracic

1. Cardiac rhabdomyomas—commonest cardiac tumour in children; occurs in most children with TS (usually <1 year, or detected prenatally). Most regress spontaneously.
2. Lymphangioleiomyomatosis (LAM)—numerous thin-walled cysts throughout both lungs, ± pneumothorax ± chylous pleural effusions. Rarely, mediastinal nodes may also be involved.

3. Multifocal micronodular pneumocyte hyperplasia—multiple benign subcentimetre lung nodules in a random distribution.
4. Aortic or pulmonary artery aneurysms—rare.

Kidneys

1. Angiomyolipomas—seen in most patients, usually multiple and bilateral. Risk of haemorrhage increases with size.
2. Cysts—often multiple and bilateral.
3. RCC—no increased risk overall, but has a younger age of onset and slower growth.

Other abdominal manifestations

1. Retroperitoneal LAM—thin or thick-walled lymphatic cysts ± chylous ascites.
2. Hepatic AML—much less common than renal AML. Other hepatic lesions (lipoma, hamartoma, fibroma) have rarely been described.
3. GI tract polyps—benign; often multiple, can occur anywhere. Other GI tract lesions (adenocarcinoma, leiomyoma, fibrous tumour, vascular malformation) have rarely been described.
4. Other rare lesions—e.g. splenic hamartoma, pancreatic NET or hamartoma.

Skeletal

1. Discrete sclerotic lesions in the skull, spine, ribs and pelvis. Hyperostosis of the skull can also be seen.
2. Hypertrophic osteoarthropathy—especially in the hands and feet.
3. Cyst-like lesions in phalanges, metacarpals and metatarsals.
4. Distal phalangeal erosion by subungual fibroma.
5. Scoliosis.

Further reading

Manoukian, S.B., Kowal, D.J., 2015. Comprehensive imaging manifestations of tuberous sclerosis. AJR Am. J. Roentgenol. 204 (5), 933–943.

Umeoka, S., Koyama, T., Miki, Y., et al., 2008. Pictorial review of tuberous sclerosis in various organs. Radiographics 28 (7), e32.

Von Ranke, F.M., Faria, I.M., Zanetti, G., et al., 2017. Imaging of tuberous sclerosis complex: a pictorial review. Radiol. Bras. 50 (1), 48–54.

TURNER SYNDROME

Females with 45XO chromosome pattern. Presents with short stature and primary amenorrhoea.

Skeletal

1. Delayed bone maturation.
2. Osteoporosis.

3. Arms—cubitus valgus, Madelung deformity, short metacarpals (especially 4th).
4. Knees—overgrown medial femoral condyle, undergrown medial tibial plateau ± metaphyseal beaking.
5. Feet—short metatarsals (especially 4th), pes cavus, congenital lymphoedema.
6. Spine—kyphoscoliosis, hypoplasia of C-spine.
7. Skull—short and flat skull base, small maxilla and mandible.
8. Chest—thin ribs and clavicles, mild pectus excavatum, broad chest, congenital diaphragmatic hernia.

Extraskeletal

1. Cardiovascular—aortic coarctation, bicuspid aortic valve.
2. Renal anomalies—horseshoe, duplex or pelvic kidney.
3. Ovarian dysgenesis—small 'streaky' uterus and ovaries.
4. GI tract—omphalocoele, pyloric stenosis, telangiectasia, IBD.
5. Cystic hygroma (lymphangioma).
6. Pituitary hyperplasia or adenoma.
7. Hashimoto's thyroiditis.
8. Diabetes (type 2).

VACTERL ASSOCIATION

A sporadic constellation of congenital anomalies which tend to occur together without a recognized genetic cause. ≥3 of the following are required for the diagnosis.

1. **V**ertebral anomalies—e.g. block, butterfly or hemivertebrae, caudal regression, dysraphism. Rib anomalies may also be seen.
2. **A**norectal malformations—anal atresia ± fistula.
3. **C**ardiac anomalies (VSD, ASD, PDA, tetralogy of Fallot), cleft lip and/or choanal atresia.
4. **T**racheo-**E**sophageal fistula ± atresia. Other GI tract anomalies may also be seen, e.g. microgastria, duodenal atresia, malrotation, Meckel's diverticulum.
5. **R**enal anomalies (agenesis, cystic dysplasia, ectopia, horseshoe) and radial ray anomalies (dysplastic or absent radius, thumb hypoplasia, absent scaphoid).
6. **L**imb anomalies—poly/syn/oligodactyly.

VON HIPPEL-LINDAU DISEASE

Hereditary (AD) disorder associated with multisystem manifestations and neoplasms.

1. Haemangioblastoma—cerebellar > retinal > spinal cord > brainstem. Often multifocal; >1 haemangioblastoma is diagnostic.

A single haemangioblastoma + a related visceral tumour or family history is also diagnostic. In the CNS these typically present as a cystic mass with an avidly enhancing mural nodule, though the cystic component may occasionally be absent. In the spine there may be associated flow voids and/or a syrinx. In the retina these may be seen as a tiny enhancing nodule or may present with haemorrhagic retinal detachment.

2. Renal lesions—present in most patients.
   (a) Cysts—usually multiple and bilateral. May be simple or complex, representing early RCC.
   (b) Clear cell RCC—often multiple, bilateral and slow-growing. Tend to be followed up until >3 cm, at which point they are resected via nephron-sparing surgery.
   (c) AML.
3. Pancreatic lesions—common.
   (a) Cysts—usually multiple. Unlike most other pancreatic cystic lesions, these are true benign epithelial cysts.
   (b) NET—usually nonfunctional and low-grade, often multiple. Hypervascular mass.
   (c) Serous cystadenoma—single or multiple. Microcystic lesion ± central scar.
4. Phaeochromocytoma—common. Adrenal > extraadrenal (paraganglioma; may occur in the abdomen, chest, or head and neck).
5. Papillary cystadenomas of the epididymis (men) or rarely the broad ligament (women)—these are benign tumours that are mixed solid-cystic on US with internal vascularity on Doppler. If bilateral, very suspicious for vHL.
6. Endolymphatic sac tumour (cystadenoma)—infiltrative lytic mass in the petrous temporal bone centered on the vestibular aqueduct ± calcific spicules. T2 hyperintense on MRI with enhancement. If bilateral, almost pathognomonic for vHL.

Further reading

Ganeshan, D., Menias, C.O., Pickhardt, P.J., et al., 2018. Tumors in von Hippel-Lindau syndrome: from head to toe – comprehensive state-of-the-art review. Radiographics 38 (3), 849–866.

WEGENER'S GRANULOMATOSIS

Now known as granulomatosis with polyangiitis, though Wegener's is still in common use amongst radiologists. Necrotizing small–medium vessel granulomatous c-ANCA positive vasculitis with multisystem manifestations, typically involving the respiratory tract and kidneys ± other sites. Most commonly presents in middle age.

1. Lungs—classically causes multiple lung nodules/masses ± cavitation ± radiating linear scars. Patchy peripheral consolidation, diffuse pulmonary haemorrhage, pleural effusions, interstitial fibrosis and mediastinal adenopathy may also be seen.
2. Sinonasal cavities—typically causes mucosal thickening and soft-tissue nodules with bony destruction (especially nasal septum, turbinates and lateral nasal wall) ± hyperostosis.
3. Airways—usually with concurrent lung involvement. Typically causes focal circumferential subglottic stenosis, though focal/ diffuse circumferential thickening and stenosis may occur elsewhere in the trachea or bronchi, ± bronchiectasis.
4. Kidneys—necrotizing glomerulonephritis; kidneys may appear enlarged and echogenic in early disease, and atrophic in chronic disease. Rarely, a renal pseudotumour may be seen.
5. Joints—common; causes a nonerosive migratory polyarthropathy, most commonly involving the wrists, fingers, knees and ankles.
6. Orbits—most commonly causes a granulomatous orbital pseudotumour (usually unilateral, either extraconal or trans-spatial) which often extends from the paranasal sinuses via erosion of the lamina papyracea. The mass may involve the orbital apex and cavernous sinus and cause optic nerve atrophy. The vasculitis may cause ischaemic optic neuropathy, scleritis, episcleritis, uveitis or conjunctivitis.
7. Temporal bones—sinonasal disease may occlude the eustachian tubes, causing a serous otitis media. Granulomatous inflammation may also occur, causing bone destruction.
8. CNS—several possible manifestations:
   (a) Vasculitis—can cause cerebral infarcts and/or haemorrhage.
   (b) Granulomatous meningitis—mainly involves the dura, causing either diffuse pachymeningeal thickening and enhancement, or focal thickening due to direct intracranial extension from a sinonasal granuloma through the skull base (± cranial nerve involvement, especially CN I and II).
   (c) Pituitary—gland enlargement ± loss of the posterior pituitary T1 bright spot ± heterogeneous enhancement ± cystic change ± stalk thickening and enhancement.
9. Heart—most commonly causes pericarditis. Other manifestations include coronary arteritis (± myocardial ischaemia), valve thickening and dysfunction, myocarditis, cardiomyopathy and heart failure.
10. Spleen—focal or diffuse infarction may rarely occur.
11. GI tract—rare; may cause inflammation, ischaemia and/or perforation.
12. Other rare sites—large vessels (e.g. aortitis, pulmonary arteritis), salivary glands (heterogeneous enlargement), pancreas (granulomatous masses), breasts (irregular masses), adrenals

(infarction), ureters (stricture), prostatitis, epididymoorchitis, periostitis (tibial or fibular), myositis.

Further reading

Allen, S.D., Harvey, C.J., 2007. Imaging of Wegener's granulomatosis. Br. J. Radiol. 80, 757–765.

Martinez, F., Chung, J.H., Digumarthy, S.R., et al., 2012. Common and uncommon manifestations of Wegener granulomatosis at chest CT: radiologic-pathologic correlation. Radiographics 32 (1), 51–69.

Pakalniskis, M.G., Berg, A.D., Policeni, B.A., et al., 2015. The many faces of granulomatosis with polyangiitis: a review of the head and neck imaging manifestations. AJR Am. J. Roentgenol. 205, W619–W629.

Index

Page numbers followed by "*f*" indicate figures and "*t*" indicate tables.

B

E

F

H

J

K

L

M

N

O

P

R

S

W

X

Y

Z